Tobacco or Health:

Status in the Américas

A report of the Pan American Health Organization

Scientific Publication No. 536

PAN AMERICAN HEALTH ORGANIZATION
Pan American Sanitary Bureau, Regional Office of the
WORLD HEALTH ORGANIZATION

525 Twenty-third Street, NW
Washington, DC 20037, USA

Published also in Spanish (1992) with the title:
Tabaco o salud: situación en las Américas.
Un informe de la Organización Panamericana de la Salud
Publicación Científica   No. 536
ISBN 92 75 31536 1

PAHO Library Cataloguing in Publication Data

Pan American Health Organization
  Tobacco or health : status in the Americas :
a report of the Pan American Health Organization
/ Pan American Health Organization
  Washington, D.C. : PAHO, 1992. — 401 p.
  (Scientific Publication ; 536)

ISBN 92 75 11536 2

I.   Title   II. (Series)
1.   SMOKING—prevision
2.   TOBACCO USE DISORDER   3. AMERICA
NLM   QV137

> Given the need to set a closing date in order to send this book to press, we were unable to incorporate some valuable comments that unfortunately arrived after that date.

ISBN 92 75 11536 2

Contents

Preface
from the Director,
Pan American Health Organization

Each year, health problems linked to tobacco consumption lead to more than one-half million premature deaths in the Region of the Americas. Moreover, their cost in terms of disease, disability, loss of productivity, and use of health services is beyond measure.

Unfortunately, there is good reason to fear that this situation may worsen. The huge transnational corporations that control the tobacco industry in Latin America and the Caribbean have flooded the Hemisphere with advertising, expanding their markets and imposing the consumption of ''blond'' tobacco in every corner.

Furthermore, to varying degrees throughout the Region, the population is aging and migrating to urban areas, women are increasingly becoming part of the work force, and lifestyles are changing. Within this context, tobacco consumption is growing, particularly among urban women and young people. The long-term toll of this trend in terms of disease, disability, and deaths may become apparent in the next few decades.

And yet, there is room for optimism. There are countries in the Hemisphere that have decreased tobacco consumption and have managed to maintain those lower levels over time, demonstrating that the prevention and control of smoking is an attainable goal. Not only is there greater awareness of the problem, but governments also have gathered an increased political will, public opinion is better informed, and broad intersectoral and multidisciplinary programs for the control of smoking have been set in motion. The countries of the Americas and the Pan American Health Organization are fully engaged in this struggle, joining forces so that future generations may be tobacco-free.

This report caps the hard work of many persons and agencies, whose invaluable contributions we gratefully acknowledge. This publication not only offers descriptive information; perhaps more importantly, it represents a landmark for measuring progress attained and an incentive for pursuing additional Regionwide joint efforts. The reduction and, in time, the eradication of smoking will contribute significantly toward achieving the goal of health for all by the year 2000.

Carlyle Guerra de Macedo
Director

Preface

from the Surgeon General,
United States Department of Health and Human Services

"Smoking is hazardous to your health." That warning, though now common-place, is still invisible to many. There remains a gap between what we know and what we need to accomplish.

We need no longer be mired in demonstrating the harmful effects of smoking. We have informed the public of these effects, and ongoing surveys demonstrate that many have acquired the knowledge. We must now provoke action based on that knowledge: abandonment of smoking by those who do; prevention of initiation by those who contemplate smoking; and regulation of the environment for everyone.

This report, a country-by-country analysis of the status of smoking and the programs to prevent it in the Americas, is a milestone for such action. Compiled over several years with the collaboration of all the Pan American Health Organization member countries, the report documents the current status of smoking prevention and control, and—as it should—points to both triumphs and gaps. It represents the starting point for a concerted, coherent, and coordinated effort to eliminate smoking where it has taken hold, and prevent its appearance where it has not.

The issuance of this report coincides with the publication of the 1992 Report of the Surgeon General on Smoking and Health in the Americas, which provides an overview of smoking in the Western Hemisphere. These companion reports were the result of sustained collaboration between PAHO and the U.S. Department of Health and Human Services, a collaboration in which I have been honored to be a part. It is with the greatest enthusiasm and anticipation that I look forward to the dissemination of these reports, and to the action which our collaboration will generate.

Dr. Antonia C. Novello
Surgeon General

Acknowledgments

This report was prepared by the Pan American Health Organization (PAHO), under the general direction of:

Carlyle Guerra de Macedo, M.D., M.P.H., Director of PAHO

Francisco López-Antuñano, M.D., Area Director of Health Programs, PAHO

Helena E. Restrepo, M.D., M.P.H., Coordinator, Health Promotion Program, PAHO

Eric S. Nicholls, M.D., M.P.H., Regional Advisor in Non-Communicable Diseases, Health Promotion Program, PAHO

Thomas E. Novotny, M.D., M.P.H, Senior Editor, U.S. Centers for Disease Control and Consultant to PAHO

The subregional editors were as follows:

Aloyzio Achutti, M.D., University of Rio Grande do Sul, *Southern Cone and Brazil*

Neil Collishaw, M.A. Department of National Health and Welfare, Canada, *Canada and the Caribbean*

Sylvia Robles, M.D., M.Sc., University of Costa Rica, *Central America, Latin Caribbean and Mexico*

Margarita Ronderos Torres, M.D., M.Sc., National Cancer Institute, Colombia, *Andean Subregion*

Bernadette Theodor-Gandhi, M.D., Caribbean Epidemiology Center, PAHO, *Caribbean Subregion*

Country collaborators are listed below:

Argentina
Carlos Alvarez Herrera, M.D.
Public Health Foundation
Buenos Aires, Argentina

Marcela Porcellana
Public Health Foundation
Buenos Aires, Argentina

Bahamas
Hanna Gray
Ministry of Health
Nassau, Bahamas

Barbados
Bernadette Theodor-Gandhi, M.D.
Caribbean Epidemiology Center
Port-of-Spain, Trinidad and Tobago

Belize
Claudia Cayetano
Belize City Hospital
Belize City, Belize

Bolivia
Jaime L. Ríos-Dalenz, M.D.
Chief, Department of Pathology
La Paz, Bolivia

Brazil
Vera Luiza da Costa e Silva, M.D.
Ministry of Health
Rio de Janeiro, Brazil

British Territories
Cecilia Staut
Pebbles Hospital
Roadtown, British Virgin Islands

Alla Kumar, M.D.
Ministry of Health
Cayman Islands

Vernice E. Hendrickson
Department of Health
Basseterre, St. Kitts and Nevis

Stephenson Rogers
Ministry of Health
Anguilla

John Cann, M.D.
Ministry of Health
Paget, Bermuda

Canada
Thomas Stephens, Ph.D.
Consultant
Ontario, Canada

Chile
María Cecilia Sepúlveda, M.D.
Ministry of Health
Santiago, Chile

Colombia
Margarita Ronderos Torres, M.D.
National Cancer Institute
Bogotá, Colombia

Costa Rica
Gonzalo Vargas Chacón, M.D.
National Cancer Council
San José, Costa Rica

Cuba
Patricia Varona Pérez, M.D.
National Health and Epidemiology Institute
Havana, Cuba

Dominican Republic
Tabaré de los Santos, M.D.
Secretariat of Public Health and Social Welfare
Santo Domingo, Dominican Republic

Ecuador
Nelson Edwin Samaniego S., M.D.
Ministry of Public Health
Quito, Ecuador

El Salvador
Ernesto A. Urquilla Milián, M.D.
Ministry of Public Health and Social Welfare
San Salvador, El Salvador

French Overseas Departments and Territories
Jocelynne Amourgon
Health Programs Service
Basse-Terre, Guadeloupe

Lowell Lewis, M.D.
Ministry of Health
Montserrat

Jacques de Thoré
Regional University Hospital Center
Fort-de-France, Martinique

Guatemala
Romeo Lucas Medina, M.D.
Ministry of Health
Guatemala City, Guatemala

Guyana
Kenforth Danns
Georgetown, Guyana

Haiti
Pierre Denicé
APAAC
Port-au-Prince, Haiti

Honduras
Carlos Alberto Fortín Metzger, M.D.
Honduran Institute for Alcoholism, Drug
   Addiction and Drug Dependency
Tegucigalpa, D.C., Honduras

Jamaica
Loraine Barnaby, M.D.
Ministry of Health
Kingston, Jamaica

Mexico
Magdalena Labrandero, M.D.
Institute for Respiratory Diseases
Mexico, D.F., Mexico

Organization of Eastern Caribbean States
Sheila Piggott
Ministry of Health
Antigua and Barbuda

Roderick Fortune
Ministry of Health
Goodwill, Dominica

Carl F. Brown, M.P.H.
Ministry of Health and Environment
Kingstown, St. Vincent and the Grenadines

Debra Louisy-Charles, M.D.
Ministry of Health
Castries, Saint Lucia

Angela Gittens
Ministry of Health
St. George's, Grenada

Panama
Nilda Chong, M.D., M.P.H.
Ministry of Health
Panama City, Panama

Paraguay
Gilberto Chaparro Abente, M.D.
Paraguayan Anti-Smoking League
Asunción, Paraguay

Peru
Edgar Amorín Kajatt, M.D.
National Institute of Neoplastic Diseases
Lima, Peru

Puerto Rico
Anabel Santiago, M.P.H.
Department of Public Health
San Juan, Puerto Rico

Suriname, Aruba, and Netherlands Antilles
Wim Bakker, M.D.
Bureau of Public Health
Paramaribo, Suriname

Ferdinand A. Vorst, M.D.
Ministry of Public Health
Oranjestad, Aruba

Trinidad and Tobago
Gloria Beckles, M.D.
Caribbean Epidemiology Center
Port-of-Spain, Trinidad and Tobago

Uruguay
Roberto Silva Sosa, M.D.
Ministry of Health
Montevideo, Uruguay

U.S. Virgin Islands
Ann Hatcher, M.P.H.
Department of Health
St. Croix, U.S. Virgin Islands

Venezuela
Manuel Adrianza, M.D.
Ministry of Health and Social Welfare
Caracas, Venezuela

Natasha A. de Herrera
Medical Training Center La Trinidad
Caracas, Venezuela

Reviewers and other contributors included those listed below:

Argentina
Enrique Nájera, M.D.
PAHO/WHO Country Representative
Buenos Aires, Argentina

Emma Balossi, M.D.
National Institute for Social Services for Retired
   Persons and Pensioners
Buenos Aires, Argentina

Bahamas
Barry Whalley, M.D.
PAHO/WHO Country Representative
Nassau, Bahamas

Belize
César Hermida, M.D.
PAHO/WHO Country Representative
Belize City, Belize

Bolivia
Germán Perdomo, M.D.
PAHO/WHO Country Representative
La Paz, Bolivia

Brazil
Cesar Gomes Victora, Ph.D.
Universidade Federal de Pelotas
Pelotas, Brazil

Rodolfo Rodríguez, M.D.
PAHO/WHO Country Representative
Brasília, Brazil

Jose Rosenberg, M.D.
Universidade Católica de Sorocaba
São Paulo, Brazil

British Virgin Islands
Cora Christian, M.D., M.P.A.
Department of Health
St. Croix, U.S. Virgin Islands

Canada
Murray J. Kaiserman, Ph.D.
Health and Welfare Canada
Ottawa, Canada

Wayne Millar
Canadian Center for Health Information
Ottawa, Canada

Fernand Turcotte, M.D., M.P.H., FRCPC
Department of Social and Preventive Medicine
Laval University
Quebec, Canada

Chile
Sergio Bello, M.D.
Coordinator of the Smoking Control Commission
Chilean Society for Respiratory Diseases
Santiago, Chile

Ernesto Medina, M.D.
School of Public Health
University of Chile
Santiago, Chile

Gustavo Mora, M.D.
PAHO/WHO Country Representative
Santiago, Chile

Colombia
Antero Coelho Neto, M.D.
PAHO/WHO Country Representative
Bogotá, Colombia

Mauricio Restrepo, M.D.
National Institute of Health
Bogotá, Colombia

Juan Manuel Zea, M.D., F.A.C.S.
National Cancer Institute
Bogotá, Colombia

Costa Rica
Guido Miranda, M.D.
Public Health Department
University of Costa Rica
San José, Costa Rica

Raul Penna Melo, M.D.
PAHO/WHO Country Representative
San José, Costa Rica

Cuba
Miguel Angel Márquez, M.D.
PAHO/WHO Country Representative
Havana, Cuba

Nery Suárez-Lugo, Ph.D.
Cuban Institute of Research and Public
   Demand Orientation
Havana, Cuba

Dominican Republic
Hugo R. Mendoza, M.D.
Director, CENISMI
Santo Domingo, Dominican Republic

Mirta Roses, M.D.
PAHO/WHO Country Representative
Santo Domingo, Dominican Republic

Ecuador
Italo Barragán, M.D.
PAHO/WHO Country Representative
Quito, Ecuador

Carlos Salvador García, M.D.
President of the CILA
Quito, Ecuador

Juan Carlos Zevallos, M.D.
Quito, Ecuador

French Overseas Departments and Territories
Monique Karan, M.D.
Regional Observatory of the Health of French
 Guiana
Cayenne, French Guiana

J. L. Grangeon
Regional Medical Health Inspector
Fort-de-France, Martinique

Guatemala
Juan Antonio Casas, M.D.
PAHO/WHO Country Representative
Guatemala, Guatemala

Carlos Tejada, M.D.
University of the Valle
Guatemala, Guatemala

Guyana
Peter R. Carr
PAHO/WHO Country Representative
Georgetown, Guyana

Haiti
Xavier Leus, M.D.
PAHO/WHO Country Representative
Port-au-Prince, Haiti

Honduras
Juan Almendares Bonilla, M.D.
National Committee for the Control of Smoking
Tegucigalpa, D.C., Honduras

Luis Antonio Loyola, M.D.
PAHO/WHO Country Representative
Tegucigalpa, D.C., Honduras

Jamaica
Samuel Aymer
PAHO/WHO Country Representative
Kingston, Jamaica

Carol Gayle
Ministry of Health
Kingston, Jamaica

Mexico
Julio Frenk, M.D.
National Institute of Public Health
Mexico City, Mexico

Jaime Sepúlveda, M.D.
Director General of Epidemiology
Mexico City, Mexico

Juan Manuel Sotelo, M.D.
PAHO/WHO Country Representative
Mexico City, Mexico

Nicaragua
Carlos Linger, M.D.
PAHO/WHO Country Representative
Managua, Nicaragua

Organization of Eastern Caribbean States
Stella Horsford
Permanent Secretary
Ministry of Social Services
The Valley, Anguilla

Panama
Vicente Bayard, M.D.
Ministry of Health
Panama City, Panama

Oscar Fallas, M.D.
PAHO/WHO Country Representative
Panama City, Panama

Paraguay
Armando López-Scavino, M.D.
PAHO/WHO Country Representative
Asunción, Paraguay

Claudio Prieto, M.D.
Paraguayan Physicians' Group
Asunción, Paraguay

Peru
Julio Burbano
PAHO/WHO Country Representative a.i.
Lima, Peru

Elmer Huerta, M.D.
Fellow, Division of Cancer Prevention and Control
National Cancer Institute
Bethesda, Maryland (USA)

Luis Pinillos Ashton, M.D.
Chairman, Latin American Coordinating
 Committee on Smoking Control
Lima, Peru

Puerto Rico
Evelyn Santos de Rodríguez
Puerto Rican Lung Association
Hayo Rey, Puerto Rico

John Rullan, M.D., M.P.H.
Territorial Epidemiologist
San Juan, Puerto Rico

Miguel Angel Sisamone Rodríguez
American Cancer Society
San Juan, Puerto Rico

List of countries and other political entities included in the report

Latin America
Andean Subregion
Bolivia
Colombia
Ecuador
Peru
Venezuela
Southern Cone Subregion
Argentina
Chile
Paraguay
Uruguay
Brazil
Central America
Belize
Costa Rica
El Salvador
Guatemala
Honduras
Nicaragua
Panama
Mexico
Latin Caribbean
Cuba
Dominican Republic
Haiti
Puerto Rico

Caribbean
Anguilla
Antigua and Barbuda
Aruba
Bahamas
Barbados
Bermuda
British Virgin Islands
Cayman Islands
Dominica
French Guiana
Grenada
Guadeloupe
Guyana
Jamaica
Martinique
Netherlands Antilles
St. Kitts and Nevis
St. Vincent and the Grenadines
Saint Lucia
Suriname
Trinidad and Tobago
Turks and Caicos Islands
U.S. Virgin Islands

North America*
Canada
Saint Pierre and Miquelon

The designations employed and the presentation of the material in this publication do not imply the expression of any opinion whatsoever on the part of the Secretariat of the Pan American Health Organization or the U.S. Department of Health and Human Services concerning the legal status of any country, territory, city, or area of its authorities, or concerning the delimitation of its frontiers or boundaries.

*Because so much material is available on smoking and health in the United States (more than 60,000 articles and 22 previous Reports of the U.S. Surgeon General on tobacco and health), this Report focuses on Canada, Latin America, and the Caribbean. Most of the information contained in this publication cannot be found in any other single source.

Overview

Introduction

Rationale for the Report

Background of the Report

Methodology
    Roles of various contributors
    Country collaborator reports
    Central data sources and their limitations
    Chapter outline

General Results
    Progress against tobacco use in the United States and Canada
    Sociodemographic changes
    The tobacco industry
    Tobacco use
    Smoking and health
    Tobacco use prevention and control activities

Summary and Recommendations

References

Introduction

This document is comprised of individual reports on smoking and health for nations, territories, and other political entities in the Region of the Americas. The purpose of this Report was to compile available information on tobacco use, tobacco-related disease, and tobacco-use prevention and control efforts for each of these political entities as of late 1990. It is intended to accompany the 1992 Report of the U. S. Surgeon General, entitled *Smoking and Health in the Americas*, that was prepared by the U.S. Department of Health and Human Services (USDHHS) in collaboration with the Pan American Health Organization (PAHO). Because so much material is available on smoking and health in the United States (more than 60,000 articles and 22 previous Reports of the U.S. Surgeon General on tobacco and health), this Report focuses on Canada, Latin America, and the Caribbean. Most of the information contained in this publication cannot be found in any other single source.

Rationale for the Report

Lifestyle and personal behaviors are primary determinants of morbidity and mortality for chronic diseases such as cardiovascular disease and neoplasms (Mosley 1990). Many of the noncommunicable disease risk factors, such as tobacco use, become more prevalent with increasing urbanization and changing lifestyles. However, most primary disease prevention activities in developing countries are still directed toward acute and infectious diseases or maternal and child health problems. As these health problems come under control, longevity increases and the population ages. These changes in health and disease patterns interact with changes in economic and sociologic determinants to constitute what has come to be known as the "epidemiologic transition." This transition, in which chronic noncommunicable diseases displace infectious diseases as the primary causes of morbidity and mortality, is evident in developed countries and is evolving in developing countries (Omran 1971).

On the basis of changes in age structure of the Latin American population, chronic disease occurrence among adults relative to acute diseases among infants and children is expected to more than double (Mosley 1990). The rapidly emerging epidemic of smoking-related diseases, particularly lung cancer, that nations of the Americas likely will face in the next few decades will be superimposed on health systems designed to control infectious diseases and maternal and child health problems (Lopez 1990). Thus, it is increasingly important that the nations of the Americas understand the historical, economic, political, and public health aspects of tobacco use and tobacco production. This understanding will facilitate planning for control measures needed to alleviate the impending burden of smoking-related diseases.

In response to declining tobacco sales in the developed world, the transnational tobacco corporations have opened foreign markets. The history of this market penetration into Latin America is well documented in the 1992 Report of the U.S. Surgeon General. What is less evident is the disease impact of tobacco use in these nations. To a large extent, the disease burden related to long-term exposure to tobacco is yet to come in most countries of the Americas. However, the implication is obvious for increased burdens of chronic disease morbidity due to smoking on health care systems. What also should be obvious is the potential to prevent much of this burden through concerted public health efforts against tobacco use and other risk factors. These efforts often are given little significance in the face of perceived economic benefits associated with growing and producing tobacco in less developed countries (Barry 1990).

Information, knowledge, and skills that target tobacco as a public health problem are essential elements of the primary prevention effort against tobacco-related diseases. These elements include understanding the current sociodemographic environment, data collection on tobacco use and its determinants, analysis of disease outcomes associated with tobacco use, regulation and legislation, cigarette taxes, and direct investments in Government tobacco control programs. The chapters in this publication summarize the current state of tobacco control efforts in Canada, Latin America, and the Caribbean.

Background of the Report

Although PAHO has been concerned with tobacco and health since the early 1970s, specific program activities began in the mid-1980s. In 1984, PAHO held a meeting in Punta del Este, Uruguay, on programs for control of noncommunicable diseases. This effort was followed by an advisory group recommendation to hold subregional workshops on tobacco control in member countries.

Workshops were subsequently held for the Southern Cone and Brazil in 1985, the Andean subregion in 1986, the English-speaking Caribbean in 1987, and Central America in 1988. In 1988, during its 33rd Meeting, the Directing Council of PAHO approved a Resolution entitled "The Fight Against Tobacco" that was endorsed by the Ministers of Health of the Americas. In 1989, a Regional Plan of Action for the Prevention and Control of the Use of Tobacco (Resolution CD 34/12) was approved by the Directing Council of PAHO at its 34th Annual Meeting in Washington, D.C. (see *Smoking and Health in the Americas*, Chapter 6 [USDHHS 1992]). This plan calls for public health actions at the Regional and national levels to prevent and control the use of tobacco as well as to protect the health of nonsmokers. The plan includes the development of national policies, plans, and programs; mobilization of resources; management and dissemination of information; training; research; and development of technical advisory services.

As a result of PAHO's Health Promotion Program efforts to support the Regional plan and the international interests of the Centers for Disease Control's (CDC) Office of Smoking and Health (OSH), detailed reports on smoking and health in the Americas were developed. This Status Report is part of a larger project initiated in 1988 by former U.S. Surgeon General C. Everett Koop, M.D., Sc.D., and the Director of PAHO, Carlyle Guerra de Macedo, M.D., M.P.H. Staffing and support for the project were provided by OSH, National Center for Chronic Disease Prevention and Health Promotion, CDC, Public Health Service, and the Health Promotion Program, PAHO (Regional Office for the Americas of the World Health Organization).

The 1992 U.S. Surgeon General's Report is published by the USDHHS in collaboration with PAHO. It contains a broad overview of historical, social, economic, and regulatory aspects of smoking in the Americas, and it defines current tobacco control activities in countries of the Americas. This Regional Status Report is published solely by PAHO.

Methodology

Roles of Various Contributors

Numerous contributors have participated in the preparation of this Report. Overall responsibility for the production of the Report has been with the PAHO Health Promotion Program and its component Tobacco or Health Program. Primary contributors were individuals identified in each country or political entity who had specific knowledge of tobacco-related issues and programs. These "country collaborators" were usually public health workers or epidemiologists. In all cases, PAHO solicited the cooperation of each Ministry of Health in support of these persons. In the case of Caribbean territories and dependencies, the Caribbean Epidemiology Center (CAREC), a PAHO Center in Port-of-Spain, Trinidad and Tobago, helped select collaborators. For the U.S. Territories (U.S. Virgin Islands and Puerto Rico), the territorial health departments were contacted to supply the names of collaborators. The collaborators' primary responsibility was to complete a detailed survey form that contained questions on various aspects of tobacco use.

Because of the sheer size of the Region, subregional editors were selected to oversee the data collection and to produce initial drafts of specific country chapters. After collecting preliminary data, the collaborators met with PAHO staff, OSH staff, subregional editors, and other support staff in February and March of 1990. After review of the initial data, collaborators completed their data collection and submitted final reports to the subregional editors. Central data sources, described below, were used to supplement the collaborators' reports. The editors then completed initial draft chapters which were translated into English by PAHO when necessary. The editorial staff revised these chapters, and chapters on Spanish-speaking countries were translated into Spanish for the review process. Each was then reviewed by the country collaborator, the PAHO representative in each member country (who solicited comments from the Ministry of Health), one or more experts on tobacco in each country or political entity, and a panel of reviewers at PAHO Headquarters. Review comments were incorporated by the editorial staff. See the acknowledgments section for a complete list of editors, collaborators, reviewers, and other contributors.

Country Collaborator Reports

PAHO and OSH staff developed a detailed questionnaire that outlined data to be supplied by the individual country collaborators. This questionnaire was reviewed by a panel of international experts and translated into Spanish by PAHO and into French by Health and Welfare Canada. Specific items on the questionnaire included: adult and adolescent tobacco use surveillance; data on the public's tobacco-related attitudes and knowledge; data on other forms of tobacco use; and data on smoking-related mortality and hospital discharges. In addition, per capita cigarette consumption, cigarette tax data, and other information on the tobacco industry were reported. Summaries of legislation to control tobacco use, limit tobacco product advertising, restrict access to tobacco by young people, report tar and nicotine content of commercial cigarettes, and mandate product labelling were submitted. Finally, Government and nongovernmental tobacco prevention and control activities were described.

In most cases, collaborators were not asked to provide information that was available from central data sources (see section below on data sources), but in some cases, such as tobacco production and cigarette manufacturing data, collaborators reported locally obtained data to validate those obtained from central sources. Collaborators were asked to provide copies of reports, surveys, legislation, and publications used for their reports.

Central Data Sources and Their Limitations

Several data sources were explored for the production of this Report. Literature searches in both the English- and Spanish-language medical literature were performed by the OSH Technical Information Center and PAHO; articles obtained through these searches were forwarded to subregional editors for use in their reports. Information on general health and economic indicators for each country was obtained from documents published by the World Bank (1989, 1990), the Centro Latinoamericano de Demografía (CELADE) (1990), and PAHO (1986, 1990). Country-specific mortality data were obtained from the PAHO data bank for use in the analysis of smoking-related mortality. As a general rule, only data for the 10 years prior to the report (usually from 1978 or 1979) were included in the country chapters.

Data on tobacco production, importation, exportation, manufacturing, and consumption were obtained from the U.S. Department of Agriculture's (USDA) computerized data base (USDA 1990). These data are collected by USDA Overseas Emissaries attached to U.S. Embassies in various countries. In addition, data on the tobacco industry in each country were obtained from reports of the Tobacco Merchants' Association (1989), the Maxwell Consumer Report (1989), the Euromonitor

Consultancy (1990), Agro-economics and Tabacosmos, Ltd. (1987), and the United Nations Food and Agriculture Organization (1990). These data were compared whenever possible to data collected by the country collaborators.

Finally, newspaper reports, tobacco industry publications (such as *Tobacco Journal International*), USDA reports (*World Tobacco*), and unpublished reports of surveys on tobacco use were included as references.

In many cases, the methodology for the surveys reported by country collaborators was unstandardized and undocumented; therefore, it was impossible to validate the reported results of many surveys. In some cases, the face validity of consumption and production data was in question. For example, in many smaller countries, USDA data on production are exactly the same for several years in a row; large jumps in consumption or production are reported in some cases, and these may be simply reporting artifacts that make specific year-to-year analysis difficult.

Many countries in the Americas experience problems in national representation of mortality data. These problems result from underregistration of deaths, lack of physician ascertainment of cause of death, and deficiencies in coding. These issues have been examined in some detail in past PAHO reports (e.g., *Health Conditions in the Americas* [PAHO 1990]), and they are important in understanding the true disease impact of tobacco use. In particular, mortality data for older persons and for those living in rural areas suffer from underregistration and poor cause-of-death ascertainment. Because tobacco-related mortality primarily affects older persons, it is difficult to estimate accurately the disease impact of tobacco based on reported mortality. Some countries, and specific areas within countries, have excellent mortality data; therefore, trend analyses of tobacco-related mortality were presented for these countries.

Chapter Outline

Because of the difficulties mentioned above, country chapters may not contain uniform data or content coverage. In addition, many small countries and territories in the Caribbean subregion were combined for the sake of convenience. These combined chapters include those on the Organization of Eastern Caribbean States (Antigua and Barbuda, Dominica, Grenada, St. Kitts and Nevis, Saint Lucia, and St. Vincent and the Grenadines);

the French overseas departments and territories (Guadeloupe, Martinique, French Guiana, and St. Pierre and Miquelon in North America); Suriname, Aruba, and the Netherlands Antilles; and the British territories (Anguilla, Bermuda, the British Virgin Islands, the Cayman Islands, and the Turks and Caicos Islands). The U.S. Territories (U.S. Virgin Islands and Puerto Rico) were presented in separate chapters because of the greater quantity of information available.

Each chapter has the following basic outline:

General Characteristics: This section contains geographic, demographic, general health, and economic information from central data sources. Table 1 typically provides a summary of these data for each country. In some cases, population pyramids appear as Figure 1.

The Tobacco Industry: This section contains information on tobacco agriculture and production, employment in the tobacco industry, manufacturing and trade, advertising/marketing, and taxation.

Tobacco Use: This section contains information on per capita (usually age 15 and older) consumption, adult prevalence, adolescent prevalence, and public attitudes and beliefs.

Smoking and Health: This section reports data on mortality trends, proportionate mortality, and smoking-attributable mortality for tobacco-related diseases. When available, analyses are reported of hospital discharge data and economic costs related to chronic diseases caused by smoking.

Tobacco Use Prevention and Control Activities: Information on the executive structure of Government tobacco control programs is reported in this section. Activities of nongovernmental organizations (NGOs) and voluntary agencies are also reported, including school- and media-based educational programs, cessation programs, and policies. Legislation to regulate tobacco use, access to tobacco by minors, tobacco product advertising, and labeling is reported in this section and, in some cases, the *Tobacco Industry* section as well.

Summary and Conclusions: A brief summary of the chapter is presented with three or more conclusions for each country. Many countries share similar conclusions.

References: All chapters are referenced with respect to the author and date for each statement of fact. Many references derive from unofficial publications and unpublished data. These references were usually supplied by the country collaborators and are not yet available in the medical literature. Copies of collaborators' reports and most of these unpublished reports have been retained in the PAHO Health Promotion Program's data base.

General Results

The Region of the Americas is heterogeneous with respect to tobacco use, tobacco economics, tobacco-related disease impact, and tobacco control measures. However, several common themes emerge from the individual country reports. Although these common themes are covered in more detail in the 1992 Report of the U.S. Surgeon General, some of them are summarized below.

Progress against Tobacco Use in the United States and Canada

In the United States and Canada, the epidemic of tobacco use and its related diseases has been recognized and confronted in various degrees. The results of public health efforts to prevent and control tobacco use are increasingly visible in these nations, and much has been written concerning this epidemic, particularly in the United States.

The 1989 Report of the U.S. Surgeon General emphasized the progress made against smoking in the United States in the 25 years since the publication of the first report of the Surgeon General of the Public Health Service in 1964 (U.S. Department of Health and Human Services [USDHHS] 1989). Annual adult (18 years of age and older) per capita cigarette consumption decreased 26 percent, from 4,345 cigarettes in 1963 to 3,196 in 1987 (Figure 1). The prevalence of cigarette smoking declined substantially among men and slightly among women, but hardly at all among those with low levels of education. By 1987, nearly half of all persons who ever smoked cigarettes had quit. Unfortunately, because of differential rates of quitting and initiation, it is predicted that by the mid-1990s, the prevalence of smoking among women will be higher than that among men in the United States (Pierce 1989).

In addition to, or possibly as a result of, changes in tobacco-use behavior, widespread changes in public knowledge of the health consequences of smoking have occurred since 1964. At present, the vast majority of U.S. residents believes that smoking is both harmful to health and a cause of serious illness. A majority favors policies restricting smoking in public places and worksites, prohib-

Figure 1. Adult per capita cigarette consumption (in thousands of cigarettes per year) and major events, United States, 1900 to 1990

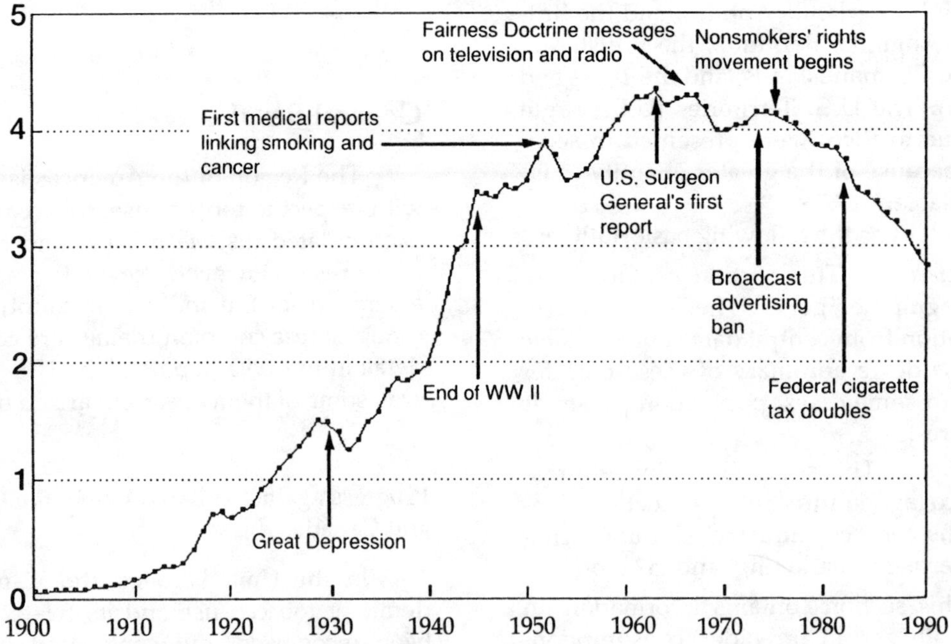

Source: U.S. Department of Agriculture, 1990.

iting the sale of cigarettes to minors, and increasing the cigarette tax to support medical care. About half the public supports a ban on cigarette advertising. These policy activities have increased substantially in recent decades, but enactment and enforcement of effective laws to limit access to tobacco by young persons remain particularly limited (Choi 1992).

Smoking accounts for 87 percent of lung cancer deaths, 82 percent of chronic obstructive pulmonary deaths, 21 percent of coronary heart disease deaths, and 18 percent of stroke deaths in the United States. In 1988, smoking was responsible for 434,000 premature deaths, or nearly one-fifth of all U.S. mortality (CDC 1991). However, because of widespread lifestyle changes and improvement in medical treatments, the mortality rate for ischemic heart disease has declined since the 1960s, and lung cancer mortality rates among men have declined since 1985 (Rothenberg 1990). Because of the reduction in tobacco use in the United States, an estimated 789,000 deaths were avoided or delayed during the period from 1964 to 1985 (USDHHS 1989). Because of long lag times between population exposure to tobacco and beneficial changes in smoking-attributable mortality, smoking will remain for

decades the single most important preventable cause of death in the United States.

Despite advances in tobacco control policies and wider application of cessation programs, school-based health education, and public information campaigns, the United States lacks a coordinated Government approach to preventing tobacco use and its subsequent health impact. Recently, the State-oriented nature of the public health delivery system in the United States has fostered extensive tobacco-use prevention and control efforts by individual States (Novotny 1992). The public health practice of tobacco control increasingly will be located at the State level.

The most important antitobacco public health effort ever undertaken by the U.S. Government commenced in 1991. This effort, the American Stop Smoking Intervention Trial, is a $US117 million project funded by the U.S. National Cancer Institute to support 17 of the 50 States in developing intensive community-based interventions (McKenna 1989). In addition, the State of California initiated a massive intervention effort in 1989 through a $US0.25 per pack increase in the cigarette tax that was earmarked partially for education against tobacco use. The State budget for the first year of this effort was $US155 million. Preliminary results indicate that there already may be 750,000 fewer smokers in California since introduction of the tax and education campaign in 1989. The prevalence of smoking declined to 21.2 percent in 1990 from a 1987 baseline of 26.3 percent (University of California, San Diego 1990).

A comprehensive intersectoral effort to control tobacco use began in Canada in the late 1960s. The national strategy included incentives to farmers to cease cultivation, heavy tobacco-product taxation, extensive restrictions on smoking in public places and worksites, health education and health promotion directed toward high-risk groups, development of communication and information resources, and vigorous Government support for a social milieu that discourages smoking.

The Canadian Government support of non-smoking is evident in recent legislative efforts. The 1989 Tobacco Products Control Act and the Non-smokers' Health Act included significant increases in Federal tobacco taxes, designated as both revenue-raising and public health measures (Rogers 1991). In addition, stiff new advertising restrictions and labeling regulations may have had an impact on smoking. These restrictions have been challenged in the Canadian courts by multinational tobacco companies, but the unfavorable ruling is under appeal by the Government.

After a steady decline from 50 percent in 1965 to 34 percent in 1985, the proportion of smokers in the Canadian population changed little from 1985 to 1989. However, the amount of tobacco consumed daily has declined over this period (Taylor 1991). Rates of smoking-related mortality are beginning to decline for men but are still rising for women. In 1989, more than 38,000 deaths were attributable to smoking in Canada (Collishaw 1991).

Canada has demonstrated bold leadership as one of the few countries in the world with a Government-supported crop substitution program to lessen the economic dependence of farmers on tobacco (Rogers 1991). Because of the importance and innovation of the Canadian tobacco control program, considerable space in this Report has been devoted to descriptive and analytical information on Canada.

Sociodemographic Changes

Several important sociodemographic changes are noted in each country, especially for the more developed ones. These include decreases in all-cause mortality rates, infant mortality rates, and fertility rates, as well as increases in life expectancy at birth and aging of the population. These changes result from general improvement of health conditions, control of infectious diseases, and progress against maternal and child health problems. They facilitate the emergence of chronic diseases as the dominant cause of disease, disability, and death in most countries of the Americas. In addition, urbanization, increased literacy, and the entry of women into the work force have facilitated the adoption of consumer patterns more akin to those in developed countries; these patterns include among others increased tobacco use. However, most countries, especially those in Central and South America, report severe economic crises in the late 1980s that may be associated with decreases in per capita consumption of manufactured cigarettes. It is clear that higher prices have reduced demand among smokers in South America and the Caribbean. In fact, the effects of increased prices on decreased consumption have been cited as the basis for including increased tobacco taxes as health policy in the Third World (Warner 1990).

The Tobacco Industry

It is clear that the multinational tobacco companies have established market dominance in most countries of the Americas and that recent sociodemographic changes in these countries have facilitated the expansion of markets for manufactured cigarettes. Prior to the widespread diffusion and adoption of manufactured cigarettes made with blond tobacco (i. e., Virginia blend, bright tobacco, light tobacco, tabaco rubio), the consumption of dark tobacco (i.e., black tobacco, tabaco negro) was dominant in the Americas. In most countries, particularly in South America, dark tobacco consumption is decreasing and that of blond tobacco is increasing. Cigarettes containing blond tobacco now dominate most markets in the Americas, and the marketing and advertising of manufactured cigarettes made with blond tobacco proliferated in the 1970s and 1980s.

Today, multinational tobacco companies saturate environments throughout the hemisphere with tobacco product advertising. In addition, tobacco companies use cultural and sports events, and even health care, to promote good will and product identification. Recently, some nations have moved to limit tobacco product advertising. Canada has banned all forms of advertising, but this ban is being challenged in the courts. Venezuela banned television advertising of tobacco products, but found it necessary to shut down television stations when indirect advertising (logo presentation without mentioning tobacco) was used by tobacco companies to subvert the intent of the regulation.

The economic impact of the tobacco industry in various countries ranges from negative, due to a negative balance of trade for tobacco products and goods used in tobacco production and manufacture, to substantial, for countries such as Brazil with major tobacco manufacturing and exporting industries. Most countries report minimal percentages of the agricultural and industrial work forces being involved in tobacco production and manufacturing. It is impossible to conduct cost-benefit analyses of tobacco use in countries of the Americas because the costs, in terms of health care for tobacco-related diseases, disability, premature mortality, lost productivity, and diversion of expenditures from other products, have not been examined fully.

Tobacco Use

Although PAHO sponsored a standardized survey of tobacco use and its determinants in eight cities of Latin America in 1971 (Joly 1977), few standardized surveys of adult and adolescent tobacco use are reported for the Americas outside of Canada and the United States. Most surveys cover individual cities, urban populations, or specific subgroups such as health department employees. Thus, few reported data are nationally representative or comparable. However, several general statements can be made regarding smoking in countries other than the United States and Canada. Smoking is more prevalent in urban as opposed to rural areas, is more common among groups with higher income than among those with the least education and economic capability, and is decreasing somewhat among men but increasing substantially among women. In general, smokers in Latin America and the Caribbean smoke fewer cigarettes per day than do smokers in the United States and Canada. Cigarette consumption data reported by the USDA and other sources probably substantially underestimate true consumption because of unreported sales, illegal trade in cigarettes, and substantial duty-free sales (particularly in the Caribbean).

Few countries report nationally representative data on tobacco use among adolescents, and most surveys have been performed on school popula-

tions only. Tobacco use by adolescents is included on several drug use surveys by countries in Latin America and the Caribbean. In general, adolescents report low percentages of daily cigarette use. However, initiation and experimentation with cigarettes appear to be most common in the middle and late teenage years, just as in the United States and Canada.

In general, the few surveys that covered attitudes, beliefs, and knowledge about tobacco and its health effects in countries in the Americas other than Canada and the United States reported widespread knowledge of the health effects of smoking. However, a tolerance of smoking and a lack of concern for personal risk were also evident. For most countries of the Americas, smoking still appears to be socially acceptable.

Smoking and Health

Because of limitations in the quality of mortality data for many countries in Latin America and the Caribbean, trend analyses, proportionate mortality analyses, and smoking-attributable mortality calculations are difficult to interpret. When mortality data were adequate, estimates of smoking-attributable mortality, that is, the proportion of deaths preventable in the absence of smoking in a population, were found to be similar to those in the United States (where 20 percent of all deaths are attributable to smoking). Using cancer registry data, some countries or areas were able to demonstrate mortality rates increasing over time for lung and other cancers related to smoking. These patterns are typical of populations heavily exposed to tobacco during the previous 20 to 30 years.

Several countries reported lung cancer mortality rates for men and women aged 45 to 54 and 55 to 64. In these age groups, it is unlikely that anything but smoking caused lung cancer deaths. Thus, these data may help demonstrate the impact of smoking in populations where mortality reporting is incomplete or inaccurate. Most countries reporting such data show increasing lung cancer mortality rates for men but not for women.

Cardiovascular disease appears to be one of the most common causes of death in countries of the Americas. Much of this mortality is due to lifestyle factors such as smoking, but it is impossible to separate the effects of the various risk factors and improvements in medical management without longitudinal studies in defined populations. Nonetheless, past increases in cigarette use in the Americas contributed to the expression of these diseases in the 1980s, but to a lesser extent than to lung and other cancers. Mortality rates for cardiovascular disease are beginning to decrease in some Latin American countries and the Caribbean, as they have in the United States and Canada. The decline in cardiovascular disease mortality in the United States and Canada has been attributed to declines in smoking as well as to changes in other lifestyle-related risk factors and to improvements in medical management (Rothenberg 1990).

Tobacco Use Prevention and Control Activities

For most countries of the Americas, tobacco use has not been assigned the same status as a public health problem as has the control of infectious diseases or maternal and child health problems. A few countries have established Government structures for the control of tobacco use, but in general, these efforts have been poorly funded and staffed. In some cases, cigarette tax revenues have been used to fund research on or interventions against smoking. In many countries, Non Governmental Organizations [NGOs] such as medical associations, anticancer associations, and churches have provided leadership in policy, school-based education, and public information on tobacco-related issues. Specific evaluations of the effects of these programs have been rare, owing in part to the lack of data on tobacco use in targeted populations.

In general, most countries have in place a basic structure to assume a public health approach to tobacco prevention and control. Many have enacted laws designed to limit smoking in public places, tobacco product advertising, and access to tobacco by young persons. However, in general, compliance with these laws is unsubstantiated. The very presence of these efforts to control tobacco use, whether educational or legislative, indicates a favorable environment for changing the current social norms that support smoking. Additional financial and personnel resources as well as improved data collection are essential to strengthen these efforts.

Summary and Recommendations

This Status Report has collected information from hundreds of individuals and documents that has never appeared before in a single publication.

The process of data collection and collaboration by so many diverse agencies, Governments, and individuals has in itself served to increase the awareness that tobacco is one of the most important health issues in the Americas for the 1990s. In recent decades, the public health community has focused most of its attention on communicable diseases and infant mortality but it is clear from this Report that chronic noncommunicable diseases, especially those caused by smoking, will need to be addressed more aggressively by Governments and international health agencies.

This Report will serve as a baseline data source, particularly for Latin American and Caribbean nations as they address the complex issues involved in preventing and controlling tobacco use. Certainly the epidemic of lung cancer and other diseases caused by tobacco use that has been painfully evident in the United States and Canada does not need to be repeated throughout the hemisphere before prevention is enacted. Countries of the Americas can learn from each other, and they can join in combatting an industry that thrives on complacency and economic dependence.

Impressive progress against public health problems caused by infectious diseases and maternal and child health problems has been made in recent years in the Americas. However, these public health problems were never a source of profit for multinational corporations and governments, nor were they supported by extensive advertising expenditures and the promotion of social activities such as sports and cultural programs. It was relatively easy to identify these problems as harmful to national progress, personal well-being, and productivity. It is more difficult to identify tobacco use as a public health problem when positive images associated with smoking are common in television and radio advertising and on billboards, street signs, and kiosks throughout the hemisphere. Many governments, farmers, and retailers depend on taxes and profits from tobacco.

In several countries, individuals with the most education and income (including physicians), who are presumably the change agents for healthy lifestyles, smoke at higher rates than those in lower socioeconomic strata. The health consequences of smoking may not be as apparent in Latin America and the Caribbean because insufficient data are available to demonstrate the effects of smoking on the population's health. In addition, insufficient data are available to demonstrate changes in behaviors and attitudes necessary to diminish tobacco use. Finally, resources and personnel assigned are not proportionate to the magnitude of the issue of tobacco and health, even when health indicators increasingly show the potential for substantial disease effects.

The Region of the Americas can use the information presented in this Status Report and the 1992 Report of the U.S. Surgeon General to build an international coalition against what may be the most important public health issue of the 1990s. Based on information in this Report, recommendations for action are as follows:

1. Data collection on behavior, attitudes, knowledge, and beliefs associated with tobacco use should be improved and standardized. These data should be published regularly and used to help support changes in public opinion and political action against tobacco use.
2. Data on mortality and morbidity should be improved, collected, and analyzed systematically in nations of the Americas to understand and communicate fully the current and future burden of smoking-related diseases. Without such data, policy makers and the public will not appreciate the public health burden of tobacco use.
3. Efforts to divert economic and human resources away from dependence on tobacco production and manufacture should be supported, even though short-term costs for this diversion may be appreciable.
4. Policies and legislation that prohibit smoking in public places, advertising and promotion of tobacco products, and access to tobacco by young persons should be strengthened and enforced. These actions serve to decrease the social acceptability of smoking and are essential to changing individual behavior.
5. Ad valorem taxes on cigarettes should be increased substantially and periodically as a means of decreasing consumption.
6. Public health agencies should mobilize monetary and personnel resources dedicated to the prevention and control of tobacco use. Increasing the stature of tobacco control efforts is essential to changing individual behavior and preventing chronic diseases associated with tobacco use.
7. Comprehensive, intersectoral and multidisciplinary tobacco prevention and control programs should be established, including innovative tobacco control activities in schools.

References

AGRO-ECONOMICS SERVICES, LTD. *The Employment, Tax Revenue, and Wealth that the Tobacco Industry Creates.* Agro-Economics Services, Ltd., September 1987.

BARRY, M. The influence of the U.S. tobacco industry on the health, economy, and environment of developing countries. *New England Journal of Medicine* 324(13):917–920, 1990.

CENTERS FOR DISEASE CONTROL. Smoking-attributable mortality and YPLL—United States, 1988. *Morbidity and Mortality Weekly Report* 40:60–71, 1991.

CENTRO LATINOAMERICANO DE DEMOGRAFIA. *Boletín Demográfico.* No. 45. Santiago, Chile, January 1990.

CHOI, W.S., NOVOTNY, T.E., THIMIS, A.T. Restricting minors' access to tobacco: a review of state legislation, 1991. *American Journal of Preventive Medicine* 8(1):19–21, 1992.

COLLISHAW, N.E., LEAHY, K. Mortality attributable to tobacco use in Canada, 1989. *Chronic Diseases in Canada* 12(4):46–49, 1991.

EUROMONITOR CONSULTANCY. *The World Market for Tobacco: Strategy 2000.* Volumes I–II. August 1989.

FOOD AND AGRICULTURE ORGANIZATION OF THE UNITED NATIONS. *Tobacco Supply, Demand, and Trade Projections, 1995 and 2000.* FAO Economic and Social Development Paper 86. Rome: Food and Agriculture Organization of the United Nations, 1990.

JOLY, D.J. *Encuesta sobre las características del hábito de fumar en América Latina.* Washington, D.C.: Pan American Health Organization. Scientific Publication No. 337, 1977.

LOPEZ, A.D. Causes of death in the industrialized and the developing countries: Estimates for 1985. *Health Sector Priorities Review* HSPR-20. Washington, D.C.: Population, Health and Nutrition Division, Population and Human Resources Department, The World Bank, November 1990.

MAXWELL, J.C. *The Maxwell Consumer Report. International Tobacco 1989.* Wheat First Securities, Butcher and Singer, 1990.

MCKENNA, J., CARBONE, E. Huge tobacco control project begun by NCI, ACC. *Journal of the National Cancer Institute* 81:93–94, 1989.

MOSLEY, W.H., JAMISON, D.T., HENDERSON, D.A. The health sector in developing countries: problems for the 1990s and beyond. *Annual Review of Public Health* 11:335–358, 1990.

NOVOTNY, T.E., ROMANO, R.A., DAVIS, R.M., MILLS, S.E. The public health practice of tobacco control: lessons learned and directions for the States in the 1990s. In press, *Annual Review of Public Health*, 13:287–318, 1992.

OMRAN, A.R. The epidemiological transition: a theory of the epidemiology of population change. *Milbank Memorial Fund Quarterly* 49:509–538, 1971.

PAN AMERICAN HEALTH ORGANIZATION. *Health Conditions in the Americas—1981–1984*. Washington, D.C.: Pan American Health Organization. Scientific Publication No. 500, 1986.

PAN AMERICAN HEALTH ORGANIZATION. *Health Conditions in the Americas—1990 Edition*. Washington, D.C.: Pan American Health Organization. Scientific Publication No. 524, 1990.

PIERCE, J.P., FIORE, M.C., NOVOTNY, T.E., HATZIANDREU, E.J., DAVIS, R.M. Trends in cigarette smoking in the United States: projections to the year 2000. *Journal of the American Medical Association* 261:61–65, 1989.

ROGERS, B. Public health gains against smoking and the economic health of the Canadian tobacco industry. *Chronic Diseases in Canada* 12(4):53–55, 1991.

ROTHENBERG, R.B., KOPLAN, J.P. Chronic disease in the 1990s. *Annual Review of Public Health* 11:267–296, 1990.

TAYLOR, L., STEPHENS, T. Smoking in Canada—1989: down but not out. *Chronic Diseases in Canada* 12(4):63–64, 1991.

TOBACCO MERCHANTS ASSOCIATION OF THE U.S., INC. *Special Report—Production and Consumption of Tobacco Products for Selected Countries 1979–1988*. Special Report 89-3. Princeton, New Jersey: Tobacco Merchants' Association of the U.S., September 28, 1989.

U.S. DEPARTMENT OF AGRICULTURE (Unpublished data). Washington, D.C.: Tobacco, Cotton, and Seeds Division, Foreign Agricultural Service, U.S. Department of Agriculture, April 1990.

U.S. DEPARTMENT OF HEALTH AND HUMAN SERVICES. *Reducing the Health Consequences of Smoking—25 Years of Progress. A Report of the Surgeon General 1989*. Rockville, Maryland: U.S. Department of Health and Human Services, Public Health Service, Centers for Disease Control, Center for Chronic Disease Prevention and Health Promotion, Office on Smoking and Health; DHHS Publication No. (CDC) 89-8411, 1989.

U.S. DEPARTMENT OF HEALTH AND HUMAN SERVICES. *Smoking and Health in the Americas—A Report of the Surgeon General*. Atlanta, Georgia: U.S. Department of Health and Human Services, Public Health Service, Centers for Disease Control, National Center for Chronic Disease Prevention and Health Promotion, Office on Smoking and Health, 1992; DHHS Publication No. (CDC) 92-8419.

UNIVERSITY OF CALIFORNIA, SAN DIEGO. *Tobacco Use in California—1990*. Sacramento: California Department of Health Services, 1990.

WARNER, K.E. Tobacco taxation as health policy in the Third World. *American Journal of Public Health* 80(5):529–530, 1990.

WORLD BANK. *World Development Report 1989*. New York: Oxford University Press, 1989.

WORLD BANK. *World Development Report 1990—Poverty*. New York: Oxford University Press, 1990.

Argentina

General Characteristics

Argentina is a federal republic located on the Atlantic coast of South America. The estimated 1991 mid-year population was 32,370,298 (unpublished data, Instituto Nacional de Estadísticas y Censos 1991). The population is increasingly urban, with 83 percent of the 1980 population living in communities larger than 2,000, and 88 percent projected to live in such communities by the year 2000. Most residents live in the capital city, Buenos Aires. The age structure of the population is similar to that of most industrialized countries: 69.9 percent are older than 15 years, and the age groups that show the greatest growth per year are those 65 years and older (27.6 percent) and those 5 to 14 years old (23 percent) (Pan American Health Organization [PAHO] 1990).

The per capita gross domestic product (GDP) ($US2,640 in 1989) ranks in the upper middle level of the world economic community (World Bank 1990); even so, the foreign debt ($US56,813 million in 1987) is proportionately very high (68 percent of the gross national product). Inflation was severe during the 1980s, ranging from 82 percent in 1986 to 372 percent in 1988. The average annual rate of inflation for the period 1980 to 1987 was 298.7 per-

cent, three times the average rate of all other countries in the comparable economic subgroup. In the Americas, this rate was exceeded only by Bolivia during the same period (PAHO 1990). The per capita GDP decreased by 15.2 percent between 1981 and 1988 (PAHO 1990).

Despite these severe economic conditions, the social and health indicators for Argentina have been maintained at relatively high levels (Table 1). For example, literacy among persons 15 years and older is 94.9 percent; overall life expectancy at birth increased from 65.5 years in 1960 to 71.4 years in 1990 (68.1 for males and 74.8 for females); and infant mortality fell from 59.7 per 1,000 live births in 1960 to 28.8 in 1990 (CELADE 1990). The availability of medical care is quite high: the ratio of population to hospital beds is 186:1, and the ratio of persons to physicians 370:1 (Encyclopedia Britannica 1989).

In 1983, after a long period of military rule and socioeconomic instability, Argentina adopted a directly elected form of civilian Government. Privatization and a more open economy now characterize this political system (PAHO 1990). Since 1982, exports have outpaced imports, leading to a favorable balance of trade ($US3.3 billion in 1988).

The Tobacco Industry

Agriculture

Argentina is one of the major tobacco-producing countries in the hemisphere (Maxwell 1990). Both production and exportation of raw tobacco grew consistently over the last decade, accompanied by a drop in imports and domestic consumption (Table 2). In 1946, almost 60 percent of the tobacco consumed domestically was imported. In 1955, however, imports began to be replaced by domestic production. Today, almost half the tobacco produced is exported, mainly to the United States and England (Misdorp 1990b). The value of exported tobacco in 1989 was $US54 million.

In 1988, 110,000 farmers were involved in tobacco growing in some way. This figure represented 43,900 full-time equivalent farmers (1.2 percent of the agricultural workforce) working on 52,267 ha (0.14 percent of the arable land surface) (Alvarez-Herrera 1990). Production occurs almost entirely in the northern subtropical portion of the country. Three provinces (Jujuy, Salta, and Corrientes) account for nearly 75 percent of production (Misdorp 1990a). Tobacco sales account for 7.4 percent of Argentina's GDP and 4.5 percent of its industrial production (Banco Velox 1988).

Table 1. Health and economic indicators, Argentina, 1980s

Indicator	Year	Value
Population	1991	32,370,298
Percentage < 15 years old	1988	30.1
Percentage urban	1988	86.0
Percent literate (≥ 15 years)	1988	94.9
Total fertility rate	1988	2.9
Crude mortality rate per 1000 persons	1988	9.0
Infant mortality rate per 1000 live births	1989	28.8
Life expectancy from birth		
Men	1990	68.1
Women	1990	74.8
Gross national product ($US millions) per	1988	83.0
capita ($US)	1989	2,640
Annual rate of inflation	1980–1987	298.7
Persons/physician	1985	370:1
Persons per hospital bed	1980	186:1

Sources: Instituto Nacional de Estadísticas y Censos, 1991; World Bank, 1990; Encyclopedia Britannica, 1989.

Table 2. Leaf tobacco production, exports, imports, and domestic consumption, in metric tons, Argentina, 1979–1989

Year	Production	Exports	Imports	Consumption
1979	68,558	21,635	266	40,600
1980	61,839	17,402	1,094	40,400
1981	50,680	16,938	1,322	35,064
1982	65,667	26,281	205	35,506
1983	70,717	29,156	515	37,385
1984	77,925	24,963	487	37,468
1985	60,453	28,531	315	37,790
1986	60,361	22,363	154	33,883
1987	70,231	23,487	27	36,874
1988	72,235	27,292	103	33,559
1989	80,455	30,927	1	33,915

Source: U.S. Department of Agriculture, 1990.

In response to domestic and external market trends, including the increasing numbers of women who smoke, the percentage of dark tobacco grown has declined. In the mid-1970s, 40 percent of tobacco grown was dark tobacco; in the 1980s, this percentage fell to one-half that level (Tobacco Merchants Association [TMA] 1989). In the same period, the percentage of dark tobacco consumed declined from almost 25 percent in 1975 to 14 percent in 1989 (Maxwell 1990).

Leaf tobacco is purchased by provincial farming cooperatives for export or by two multinational cigarette companies for domestic production. The cooperatives provide technical assistance to farmers. They also assist in establishing supplementary nontobacco winter crops such as tomatoes, cucumbers, and melons. Thus, agricultural technical assistance by the tobacco industry is not limited to tobacco (Bickers 1990). There are no Government programs to substitute other crops for tobacco. In fact, the President of the Republic recently emphasized the socioeconomic importance of expanding tobacco production (Misdorp 1990c).

Manufacturing, Production, and Trade

Argentina provides a good example of the oligopolistic annexationist model of the tobacco industry (United Nations Conference on Trade and Development [UNCTAD] 1978. In the 1920s, the Argentine tobacco industry comprised approximately 30 locally owned companies and 1 British company. By the 1960s, the smaller companies had gradually merged to form five large companies. In the 1980s, they consolidated even further into two

multinational companies (PAHO 1986). These companies share the market almost equally: Nobleza-Picardo, associated with British-American Tobacco Co., has 54.8 percent of the domestic market, and Messalin-Particulares, associated with Philip Morris Co., has 45.2 percent of the domestic market.

In 1985, 127 factories manufactured tobacco products in Argentina (Alvarez-Herrera 1990). According to a tobacco industry analysis, 2.6 percent of the nonagricultural labor force is involved with tobacco manufacture in some way (Agro-Economics 1987).

Between 1979 and 1988, mean cigarette production declined 0.9 percent per year. However, in just one year, (the 1987–1988 season), production fell by almost 3.5 billion units, a decline of nearly 9.1 percent (TMA 1989; U.S. Department of Agriculture [USDA] 1990) (Table 3).

The Government has no official tobacco development program. Since 1972, however, the Tobacco Industry Council, a National Advisory Committee of manufacturers, producers, and Government officials, has defined pricing policies for tobacco (U.N. Food and Agriculture Organization [FAO] 1990).

Despite the cessation of imports in 1985, an extensive illegal trade in cigarettes exists in Argentina (Alvarez-Herrera 1990). According to the Cámara de la Industria del Tabaco (CIT), Argentina is part of an extensive black market circuit involving Panama, Cuba, Chile, Colombia, Brazil, Paraguay, and Antigua (Washington Times 1990; CIT 1991). The illegal market comprises 12 percent of cigarette sales in Argentina (CIT 1991).

Advertising and Marketing

All types of advertising and promotional activities are permitted in Argentina. However, tobacco advertisements on television and radio are not permitted between 8:00 A.M. and 10:00 P.M. in an attempt to avoid viewing times used most often by children and youth (Chapman 1990). In 1988, the Philip Morris Co. spent $US25 million and BAT Industries $US16 million on advertising; these expenditures placed them first and third, respectively, on the list of top ten advertisers in Argentina.

Taxes

In December 1989, 75 percent of the average retail price of a package of cigarettes was federal

Table 3. Manufactured cigarettes, production, exports, imports, total consumption in millions of units, and per capita consumption, Argentina, 1979–1989

Year	Production	Exports	Imports	Consumption	Per capita consumption
1979	38,168	34	114	38,248	2,000
1980	37,972	200	400	38,172	2,000
1981	35,204	10	416	35,610	1,800
1982	32,455	0	32	32,487	1,600
1983	34,576	26	0	34,550	1,700
1984	38,926	31	3	38,898	1,900
1985	39,105	28	0	39,077	1,900
1986	40,108	30	0	40,078	1,900
1987	37,694	7	0	37,687	1,800
1988	34,267	5	6	34,268	1,600
1989	32,618	6	168	32,780	1,500

Sources: U.S.Department of Agriculture, 1990; Maxwell, 1990.

tax. No state or local taxes are levied. According to a tobacco industry correspondent (Misdorp 1990c), tax revenue from tobacco represents 15 percent of total Government revenue (approximately $US1 billion), an increase from the 10 percent reported for 1986 (PAHO 1986). This increased proportion may be explained both by an absolute increase in tobacco excise taxes between 1986 and 1990, and also by a decline in other sources of tax revenue. Rapid inflation may also affect the estimates of the proportions. Since 1967, approximately seven percent of tobacco tax revenues have been dedicated to a Special Tobacco Fund, the purpose of which is to support growers' prices.

Tobacco Use

Consumption Data

In 1989, at 1,500, the yearly per capita cigarette consumption among persons aged 15 years and older in Argentina was higher than in all other Latin American countries except Uruguay (1,800) and Cuba (approximately 3,500), and was about one-half the U.S. per capita consumption (2,800). Per capita consumption increased three percent between 1970 and 1985 (Chapman 1990) but declined substantially between 1975 and 1989 (from 2,100 to 1,500). This rate of decline (two percentage points per year) was equal to the average yearly rate of decline observed in the United States for the same period (Maxwell 1990; Table 3). Global per capita cigarette consumption fell 4.1 percentage points per year between 1974 and 1976 and 1984 to 1986 (FAO 1990). The trend in consumption in the early 1980s (five years of marked decline followed by a

period of recovery) bears strong resemblance to the trend observed in Brazil and other tobacco-exporting countries. This suggests that such trends are driven by a common mechanism independent of domestic changes in the socioeconomic environment. It is likely that these trends also reflect shared economic conditions in several countries of the Americas.

Almost all cigarettes consumed in Argentina are filter-tipped (97 percent). The tar content of the leading cigarette brand in Argentina (Jockey Club; market share of 33 percent) is 18.1 mg. Interestingly, the tar content of the second leading cigarette brand (Marlboro; market share of 10.2 percent) is reported as 25.5 mg (Hauger-Klevene 1989). In the United States, where Marlboro is the leading cigarette brand, the U.S. Federal Trade Commission (FTC) reports the tar level to be 16 to 17 mg (FTC 1988). Thus, Argentines may have altered their consumption patterns in response to several factors: economic, advertising, and cultural. Curiously, tar levels are markedly higher for cigarette brands marketed in Argentina than for identical brands marketed in the United States; the implication of this finding is unclear.

An estimated seven percent of all tobacco consumed is in the form of loose-cut tobacco used for hand-rolled cigarettes; pipes and cigars each account for an additional one percent of total tobacco consumption. Approximately 90 percent of tobacco consumed in Argentina is manufactured cigarettes (Alvarez-Herrera 1990).

Behavioral Surveys

Several sources of data on the prevalence of smoking are available for Argentina (Table 4). Each

Table 4. Behavioral surveys on tobacco use, Argentina, 1971–1990

Year	Author (Sponsor)	Sample area	N	Age group	Prevalence (%) Smokers	Prevalence (%) Ex-smokers
1971	Joly	La Plata	1,540	15–74	36.2	8.7
1980	Hauger-Klevene	La Plata	217	12–17	13.9	
1981	Hauger-Klevene	La Plata (males)	455	12–15	12.6	
1981	Alvarez-Herrera	Buenos Aires	306	15+	32.6	
1981	LALCEC	Buenos Aires Schools	NA	15–21	13.5	
1982	Balossi	Zárate city	899	15–80	34.8	
1986	Boddewyn	Children	1,008	7–15	1	
1987	Hayes	District 9 de Julio (women)	94	20–59	8.5	
1988	Gallup	Buenos Aires	826	15+	35.0	17.0
1988	Costa de Robert	Zárate blue-collar workers	873	20–64	43.0	
1988		Pediatric Hospital staff	128	20–55	48	
80–90	Maxwell	NA	NA	NA	37.0–32.0	
1990*	Misdorp	NA	23,634	NA	58	
1991	Catterberg and Assoc.	Buenos Aires	800	18–80	34	
1991	LALCEC (INZA)	Azul city	2,490	Secondary students	14.5	

* Year reported; actual year of survey unknown.
NA = Not available.

of these surveys is limited to a city or to a small sample of the population. Because little information is available on sampling methodology for most of the surveys, generalizations to the national level are not possible, and comparisons between surveys are difficult to substantiate.

Prevalence of smoking among adults

The Joly (1977) study was a population-based survey of the city of La Plata. Because of consistencies of methodology and sampling, comparisons among the eight Latin American cities surveyed by Joly at the same time (1971) are possible. The La Plata study sample included 1,540 men and women 15 to 74 years old.

The overall prevalence of current smokers was 54.4 percent among men and 20.0 percent among women, and the prevalence of ex-smokers was 15.3 percent and 2.8 percent, respectively, for men and women. Current smoking prevalence ranged from a low of 56.8 percent among men and 31.1 percent among women in the 15 to 24 year age group to a peak of 68.8 percent among men and 31.1 percent among women in the 25 to 39 year age group. Prevalence was lower among persons in older age groups (Table 5). Of all eight cities in the Joly survey, La Plata had the highest prevalence of smoking among men and the third highest prevalence of smoking among women.

The number of cigarettes smoked per day by male smokers was higher in La Plata compared with the other cities surveyed in the Region: 38.2 percent of smokers smoked 20 or more cigarettes per day. Only smokers in São Paulo and Caracas had a higher proportion of heavy smokers (51.5 and 50.9 percent, respectively). Among women, most smokers smoked fewer than 20 cigarettes per day; only 17.5 percent of female smokers smoked

Table 5. Prevalence of current and former smoking (percent) by age group and sex, La Plata, Argentina, 1971

Category	Age group	Current smokers	Former smokers
Men		54.4	15.3
	15–24	56.8	5.3
	25–39	68.8	9.5
	40–54	52.9	17.8
	55–74	39.4	27.5
Women		20.0	2.8
	15–24	31.1	2.1
	25–39	31.2	6.1
	40–54	14.3	1.5
	55–74	6.1	1.6
Both	15–74	36.2	8.7

Source: Joly, 1977.

Table 6. Prevalence (percent) of current smoking by sex and age group, Buenos Aires, Argentina, 1981

Age group	Both sexes	Men	Women
15–74	32.6	39.1	27.2
15–19	23.7	31.0	16.7
20–24	54.3	56.5	32.2
25–34	55.0	57.1	53.1
35–44	45.5	62.9	34.0
45–54	27.5	32.7	22.6
55–64	22.1	25.7	19.0
65–74	11.7	16.1	8.7

Source: Alvarez-Herrera, 1981.

20 or more cigarettes per day. Almost all smokers (92.2 percent) smoked filter cigarettes (Joly 1977).

The second study was a telephone survey of 306 Buenos Aires adults aged 15 to 74 years (Alvarez-Herrera 1981). The prevalence of current smoking among men (39.1 percent) was less than that reported by Joly 10 years earlier but was higher among women (27.2 percent) (Table 6). The prevalences again were highest among the young-adult age group: 57.1 percent among men and 53.1 percent among women aged 25 to 34.

A third study of 899 persons in the Province of Buenos Aires (Zárate city) was reported by Balossi for 1982 (Balossi 1987). Of this urban sample, 46.8

percent of men and 22.9 percent of women were smokers of at least three cigarettes per day. By age, the highest prevalence of smoking reported was among men 31 to 35 years old (69.2 percent) and among women 26 to 30 years old (53.1 percent).

The fourth available data source is the 1988 Gallup survey commissioned by the American Cancer Society (Gallup 1988). This survey targeted Buenos Aires adults aged 18 to 50 years and older. The prevalence of current smoking among men (45.5 percent) was similar to that reported in Zárate in 1982 (Balossi 1987) and 1987 (Hauger-Klevene 1987) (Table 4) and much higher than reported by Joly in 1971. Among women, the prevalence of current smoking (30.5 percent) was four percentage points higher than in the 1981 Alvarez survey (Tables 6, 7) and the 1982 Balossi survey. The lack of available methodological information for the Gallup survey does not permit conclusions as to whether these differences are real or simply a sampling artifact. It seems likely, however, that the increase in the prevalence of smoking among women over the last two decades is a real observation, similar to that seen in other countries of South America such as Chile and Uruguay.

Of particular interest is the higher prevalence of current smoking (54 percent) seen among men 18 to 24 years old, compared with older men in the Gallup survey: 48 percent among 25 to 49 year-olds, and 32 percent among men 50 years and

Table 7. Prevalence (percent) of current and former smoking, by sex, age group, educational attainment, and socioeconomic level, Buenos Aires, 1988

Category	Age group	Current smoking	Ex-smoking	N
Total	18–50+	35	17	826
Men	18–50+	45.3		403
Women	18–50+	30.5	9	423
Men	18–24	54	4	59
	25–34	48	25	86
	35–49	48	19	106
	50+	32	38	152
Women	18–24	31	10	49
	25–34	47	7	71
	35–49	29	15	137
	50+	15	5	166
Primary education		32	16	534
Secondary education		40	18	245
Tertiary education		32	21	47
High socioeconomic level		38	17	86
Low socioeconomic level		30	20	169

Source: Gallup, 1988.

older. In 1971, the highest current smoking prevalence occurred among men aged 25 to 39 (68.8 percent); in 1981, the highest current smoking prevalence among men was also in the 25 to 34 year age group (57.1 percent). The higher prevalence among young men in 1988 suggests that younger men initiated smoking at higher rates in 1988 than in the past. Among women in the Gallup survey, the highest prevalence of current smoking was observed among members of the group aged 25 to 34 years (47 percent), a rate similar to that among men (48 percent) in the same age group. Among persons less than 25 years of age in 1981, the prevalence of current smoking was markedly higher among men than among women; the prevalence of current smoking was similar for men and women in the age group 25 years and older. The Gallup survey also reported that the prevalence of former smoking among men was higher than that among women, a pattern similar to that seen in the 1971 Joly survey.

By education and "social class" (definition not provided), the prevalence of current smoking among persons with higher educational attainment and high social class was higher than among those with less educational attainment and lower social class on the Gallup survey (40 percent among persons with secondary education vs. 32 percent among persons with primary education; 38 percent among members of "high social class" vs. 30 percent among members of "low social class"). These data differ from those reported for 1971. At that time, the prevalence of smoking among men was inversely related to education (39.2 percent among men with primary education, 33.3 percent among men with secondary education, and 26.4 percent among men with tertiary education). Among women, the highest prevalence was observed for those with secondary education (42.5 percent) compared to those with primary education (29.1 percent) or tertiary education (26.3 percent). This suggested change in the demographics of smoking may in fact be linked to recent socioeconomic changes in Argentina; persons in lower socioeconomic strata in 1988 may not be as able to purchase consumer items such as tobacco as were persons in 1971.

Staff members (N=128) of the Buenos Aires Pediatrics Hospital aged 20 years and older were surveyed via personal interview in 1988 (Hospital de Pediatría 1988). By sex, the prevalence of current smoking was similar for men and women: 48 percent and 49 percent, respectively (Table 8). Administrators and physicians had higher reported rates of current smoking (68 percent and 46 percent) than

Table 8. Prevalence (percent) of current smoking among staff of the Hospital de Pediatría, by sex and job category, Buenos Aires, 1988

Category	Current smoking prevalence	N
Men	48.0	52
Women	49.0	76
Physicians	45.7	
Technicians	31.0	
Nurses	40.0	
Administrative	68.0	

Source: Hospital de Pediatría, 1988.

did nurses and technicians (40 percent and 31 percent). These data support the notion that smoking is more common among persons with the highest socioeconomic status in Argentina. Almost all respondents to this survey smoked fewer than 20 cigarettes per day.

In 1990, a tobacco industry analyst reported a series of prevalence data without supporting methodologic documentation (Maxwell 1990). The data suggest a downward trend between 1980 and 1988 in prevalence of current smoking among men and a relatively stable level of current smoking among women (Table 9). The prevalences reported by Maxwell were higher for both sexes (48 percent among men and 28 percent among women) than those reported in the Alvarez-Herrera study and lower than those in the 1988 Gallup survey (38 percent among men and 25 percent among women). It is difficult to evaluate the quality of these data without additional methodologic documentation. Another tobacco industry source (Misdorp 1990c) reportedly obtained data from a sample of 23,634

Table 9. Prevalence (percent) of current smoking, by sex, Argentina, 1980–1988

Year	Both sexes	Men	Women
1980	37.0	46.0	28.0
1981	38.0	48.0	29.0
1982	37.0	49.0	27.0
1983	34.0	47.0	23.0
1984	36.0	47.0	25.0
1985	NA		
1986	35.0	43.0	29.0
1987	NA		
1988	32.0	38.0	25.0

Source: Maxwell, 1990.

Argentineans, but again the methodology and sample frame are unknown. The prevalences of smoking among men (58 percent) and women (42 percent) based on this survey are much higher than those based on the previously cited studies.

Two studies related to cardiovascular risk factors included smoking prevalence data in their reports (Hayes 1990; Costa de Robert 1990). In a small sample of women in District 9 de Julio, Hayes reported that only 8.5 percent of the sample were smokers in 1987; cardiovascular mortality is relatively low in this district, and the prevalence of smoking as well as that of other risk factors were found to be comparatively low as well (Hayes 1990). In contrast, Costa de Robert reported that among blue-collar paper industry workers in Zárate, 43 percent were smokers in 1988, and that the mean daily number of cigarettes smoked increased with age (from 15.3 cigarettes per day among persons 20–29 years old to 24.1 cigarettes per day among persons 60–64 years old) (Costa de Robert 1990).

Finally, Catterberg (1991) conducted a survey of 800 randomly selected Buenos Aires adults (aged 18–80 years). This survey also collected important information on knowledge and attitude toward smoking and tobacco-use controls such as advertising restrictions. The proportion of current smokers was 34 percent overall, 40 percent among men and 28 percent among women (Table 10). These levels are almost identical to those of the 1988 Gallup survey. The highest prevalence of current smoking

was reported for persons age 25–34 years (48 percent).

Prevalence of smoking among adolescents

Several sources of data are available on tobacco use among adolescents in Argentina (Table 4). Two specific studies have been performed by the Liga Argentina de Lucha Contra el Cancer (LALCEC). In 1981, a survey was performed in a sample of students aged 15 to 21 years from the third, fourth, and fifth grades in one Buenos Aires secondary school. The overall prevalence of current smoking among the responding students was 13.5 percent; data from the survey also suggested a positive correlation between smoking among adolescents and parents who smoke (LALCEC 1981). In 1991, LALCEC surveyed 2,490 secondary school students in Azul city in the province of Buenos Aires. The overall prevalence of ever smoking was similar (14.5 percent) (Inza 1991).

Hauger-Klevene reported on the prevalence of cardiovascular risk factors among students in Mar del Plata in 1980 and 1981 (Table 4). In 1980, the prevalence of smoking among both male and female students aged 12 to 17 years was only 12.6 percent (Hauger-Klevene 1984). In 1981, the same investigator reported that the prevalence of smoking among male students from blue-collar families age 12 to 15 was similar (12.6 percent) (Hauger-Klevene 1985).

Another tobacco-industry-sponsored survey sought to explain "why adolescents smoke." Largely a justification for tobacco advertising, this 1986 survey was performed by the International Advertising Association using a sample of 1,008 youths aged seven to 15 years (Boddewyn 1987). According to this study, only one percent of respondents were smokers of at least one cigarette per week, a rate similar to youth in Hong Kong and lower than that reported by seven other countries. The 1971 survey (Joly 1977) reported that 36.6 percent of smokers initiated smoking before age 16, and that another 37.6 percent began smoking between age 16 and 20 years. Based on this reliable data source, it seems unlikely that the prevalence of smoking one cigarette per week was only one percent in urban areas of Argentina in 1987.

Attitudes and beliefs about smoking

In the Joly study, several questions were asked of respondents regarding attitudes and beliefs about smoking. The main reason for initiating smoking reported by male smokers was peer group

Table 10. Prevalence (percent) of current smoking, by sex, age group, and educational attainment, Buenos Aires, 1991

Category	Current smoking prevalence
Total	34
Men	40
Women	28
Age group	
18–24	31
24–34	48
35–54	39
55–80	15
Educational level	
Low	27
Middle	42
High	32

Source: Catterberg y Asociados, 1991.

pressure (75.4 percent); this reason was only reported by 56.2 percent of women. Of smokers, 47.2 percent of men and 35.6 percent of women intended to quit smoking. This level of intention was intermediate with respect to smokers in the other eight cities in the study. With regard to the hazardous effects of smoking, 53.7 percent of male smokers and 58.4 percent of female smokers responded that smoking "was not hazardous." This proportion increased to 75 percent among men and 86 percent among women with less than high school education (Joly 1977).

Catterberg (1991) reported that 98 percent of Buenos Aires respondents knew that smoking is dangerous to health. In addition, 88 percent (including 85 percent of current smokers) believed that cigarette advertising must include health warnings, but only 48 percent felt that tobacco product advertising should be banned.

Smoking and Health

Data on mortality for Argentina apparently are a reliable health indicator for the population in recent years. In 1982, approximately three percent of deaths were due to signs, symptoms, and ill-defined conditions (ICD 780–799); in 1986, this figure was two percent. This proportion, which reflects the general quality of mortality data, compares favorably with the most developed countries of the hemisphere. Proportionally, the most common causes of death in Argentina are those that may have links to smoking: heart disease (ICD 390–429, 32.6 percent), malignant neoplasms (ICD 140–208, 18.1 percent), and cerebrovascular disease (ICD 430–438, 10.4 percent) (PAHO 1990). In 1991 Balossi reported that cardiovascular diseases were the principal cause of death in Argentina, with 36.1 percent of all deaths (Balossi 1991). In addition, she noted that the mortality rates for infectious disease and accidents, violence, and poisoning decreased significantly (52.4 percent and 55.0 percent, respectively) while the mortality rates for cardiovascular disease decreased somewhat in men (9.4 percent) and increased slightly in women (1.3 percent). This mortality pattern suggests that Argentina has undergone the epidemiologic transition from a country in which mortality is dominated by infectious diseases to one in which chronic diseases linked to behavioral risk factors are the dominant causes of death.

Lung cancer mortality (ICD 162) is a specific indicator of the impact of smoking in a population. In 1986, 7,193 deaths due to lung cancer were recorded in Argentina, accounting for three percent of all deaths. The age-adjusted rate for this cause of death (12.3 per 100,000 persons) was among the highest of all countries in the Americas, surpassed only by the United States (21.2 per 100,000), Canada (21.1 per 100,000), Cuba (16.2 per 100,000), and Uruguay (16.0 per 100,000). Thus, Argentina, with a long tradition of tobacco use by its population, demonstrates the mortality effects of this exposure, just as other countries with high prevalence of smoking, high per capita cigarette consumption, strong tobacco economic interests, and advanced socioeconomic conditions have demonstrated these effects.

Trends in age-adjusted mortality rates for cardiovascular disease in Argentina suggest that Argentines may have decreased several risk factors for death due to this cause over the last two decades. Balossi reported in 1987 that the age-adjusted coronary heart disease mortality rate increased by 36.1 percent among men and by 33.4 percent among women aged 35 to 64 years in 1962 to 1978. This increase was in part due to increasing cigarette consumption during this period. However, in 1990, Hauger-Klevene reported that the age-adjusted mortality rate for coronary heart disease in Argentina decreased by 5.1 percent between 1977 and 1985, and she attributed the change to decreases in dietary and other risk factors, including smoking (Hauger-Klevene 1990).

Because of the similarities between the tobacco exposure history of Argentines and residents of the United States, an attributable risk calculation using U.S.-based attributable risk percentages from studies performed in the 1950s and 1960s was reported in 1986 (PAHO 1986). This report, based on 1981 Argentine mortality, estimated that 49,128 of 242,000 deaths (20.3 percent) were attributable to smoking. By comparison, a study using similar risks for 1984 U.S. mortality data estimated that 15.6 percent of all deaths were attributable to smoking (CDC 1987). The Argentine study may have overestimated the total by including certain causes of death due to gastrointestinal disease (smoking-attributable deaths = 3,781), but the smoking-attributable fractions due to cancer, respiratory disease, cardiovascular disease, and perinatal conditions may provide a reasonable estimate of the number of deaths that could be postponed or prevented if smoking were eliminated in Argentina (PAHO 1986). The total number of smoking-attributable deaths for these conditions was 43,648, or 18 percent of all deaths in 1981. Because Argentina may demonstrate a "mature" exposure to tobacco, it is not unreasonable to expect a high proportion of adult deaths to be caused by tobacco, the leading preventable cause of death in the United States and Canada.

A follow-up study of smoking-attributable mortality performed on 1988 mortality data using updated relative risk data from the United States (U.S. Department of Health and Human Services [USDHHS] 1989) reported that 38,375 deaths were attributable to smoking (Fundación Salud Pública 1991). Thus, calculations using different methodology and prevalence data show that the mortality burden caused by smoking among Argentines is substantial.

A study on smoking and pregnancy among 545 pregnant women in Argentina found an inverse correlation between number of cigarettes smoked per day and birth weight. Most important, the relative rate of infant mortality was 9.1 for children born to smokers of 20 or more cigarettes per day compared with nonsmokers (Aguirre 1984).

No other longitudinal or case-control studies on smoking and mortality have been reported for Argentina, but additional analyses of Argentine mortality data may be found in the companion document, *Smoking and Health in the Americas. 1992 Report of the Surgeon General*, Chapter 3.

Tobacco Use Prevention and Control Activities

Argentina has one of the most developed tobacco prevention and control movements in the Americas. Most activities and antismoking campaigns originate through nongovernmental organizations (NGOs). These include LALCEC, the Public Health Foundation, and the Argentine Antitobacco Union, which includes 40 representatives of social organizations such as medical associations, the Rotary Club, the Mainetti Foundation, and the Favaloro Foundation as well as 40 health professionals (Alvarez-Herrera 1990). The effect of these organizations can be seen in Federal legislation that prohibits advertising of tobacco products on television and radio before 10:00 P.M. and that mandates warnings on cigarettes manufactured in Argentina (Consumidores y Desarrollo 1991). In addition, several provinces and cities have passed legislation restricting smoking in public places (Table 11).

Government Action and Legislation

Argentina does not have an official, financed office dedicated to tobacco prevention and control. However, legislative activities on tobacco have been particularly noteworthy in Argentina. In 1970, Law No. 18.604 was passed in the National Congress banning all cigarette advertising for a period of one year. It was not renewed because of lack of public concern for the problem and because of strong lobbying activities by the tobacco industry.

In 1972, Law No. 19.800 was passed to regulate the production and marketing of tobacco in Argentina. This law was designed to protect producer

Table 11. Listing of provincial and city legislation restricting smoking in public places, Argentina

Locale	Law number	Date
Buenos Aires City	(Several)	Since 1984
Jujuy Province	4.292	June 1987
Buenos Aires Province	10.600 (transport)	November 1987
Balcarce City	222/87	December 1987
Córdoba City	8425	October 1988
San Isidro-Valle Viejo City	366	October 1988
San Luis City	2057	October 1988
Mendoza Province	5.374	December 1988
San Fernando del Valle City	1912	August 1989
Cordoba Province	7827	September 1989
Chaco Province	3.515	November 1989
Bahía Blanca City	1119	November 1989
Posadas City	44	May 1990
Pinamar City	803	August 1990

Source: Alvarez-Herrera, 1990.

and manufacturer interests. It created the Permanent National Assessing Commission on Tobacco, consisting of representatives of workers and traders. This commission regulates prices paid to growers, and it may draw on a Special Tobacco Fund (financed by a seven percent tax on tobacco) to support prices to growers. Law No. 3.764 regulates cigarette excise taxes; these are set at 66.5 percent of the retail price for either locally produced or imported cigarettes.

Argentina, along with Peru, has one of the few dedicated taxes on cigarettes in the Americas. In 1984, Law No. 23.102 created the National Fund for Medicines, which is supported in part by a 2-percent surtax on cigarettes (PAHO 1986).

In 1986, Law No. 23.344 of July 31, made it mandatory to include health warnings on cigarette packs (República Argentina 1986). The warning "Smoking is Harmful to your Health" appears only on cigarette packs; billboards, posters, and other forms of advertising are exempt from this requirement.

Numerous activities against environmental tobacco smoke arose in Argentina during the 1980s. The Argentine Academy of Environmental Sciences proposed national legislation for the protection of the nonsmoker, citing the negative health consequences of environmental tobacco smoke components. This law would have prohibited smoking in theaters, restaurants, schools, health care facilities, and other public places. The municipality of Buenos Aires passed legislation restricting smoking by students in schools, in taxis and on public transportation, while transporting flammable substances, in sports arenas, in theaters, in food processing centers, and factories. This legislation is particularly important given that most of the country's population lives in the capital city. Other provincial Governments and municipal Governments have also placed restrictions on smoking in health facilities, schools, on public transportation, and in enclosed public areas (Table 11).

In 1990, the Argentine Anti-Tobacco Union proposed comprehensive legislation that would regulate smoking in public places, tobacco sales to minors, and all advertising and promotion of tobacco products. The legislation also called for a public education program and guaranteed the right of nonsmokers to breathe smoke-free air. The law passed through the House of Representatives and was being considered by the Argentine Senate as of late 1991 (Consumidores y Desarrollo 1991).

Educational Activities

In 1981, the Ministry of Justice, the Ministry of Health and Social Action, and LALCEC joined in an antismoking educational program. Under the supervision of a coordinating committee, 561 educational institutions (93 percent were secondary schools) were enrolled, and an instructor was designated to coordinate activities in each institution. The committee provided for training and distribution of instructional and scientific material through these on-site coordinators (PAHO 1986). Thirty percent of institutions participated in the program; more than half of these were in the capital city. Most institutions included the materials in curricular activities, and most reported that the materials were helpful in prevention education against tobacco use. Additional surveys of students and staff were performed in conjunction with the educational program.

In 1978 and 1983, a national antismoking campaign supported by LALCEC targeted youth, using the slogan "For a new generation of non-smoking Argentines." In conjunction with this campaign, LALCEC developed several mass-media and school-based activities, including an organization named "chao pucho" ("bye-bye smoking"). This campaign was partially funded by the Ministry of Health in 1979, 1980, and 1982. Since 1990, the Secretary of Prevention and Help for Drug Addiction incorporated tobacco-related material into the primary school curriculum. This move demonstrated a significant advance in the recognition of tobacco as an addictive drug.

The Public Health Foundation developed and produced several 40-second television and radio spots. In addition, several institutions have provided press releases concerning tobacco's harmful consequences on health.

Cessation Services

Smoking cessation programs have been provided by the Public Health Foundation, the Argentine Anti-Smoking Union, and LALCEC. The Seventh Day Adventist Church provides its 5-day smoking cessation course as it does in many countries of the Americas.

An evaluation of 383 smoking cessation classes directed by LALCEC from 1978 to 1983 showed a 40-percent rate of success and a 40-percent relapse rate after 6 months. In 701 smoking-cessation classes sponsored by the Adventist Church between 1978 and 1985, a short-term success rate of 85 percent was reported among 70,759 participants (Alvarez-Herrera 1990).

Summary and Conclusions

Argentina demonstrates a major commitment to growing and exporting tobacco and a major, primarily nongovernmental movement to educate Argentines about the health consequences of smoking. Surveys have shown that almost all residents of Buenos Aires at least recognize the health consequences of smoking. Still, more than one-third of urban Argentines are current smokers. The mortality patterns for lung cancer and other smoking-related diseases indicate that the disease impact of smoking on the population is substantial. Increased prevalence of smoking among women and somewhat decreased smoking prevalence among men between 1971 and 1991 suggest that the disease burden among women has not yet peaked. Among men, the burden will persist for decades because the prevalence of smoking among younger men is still very high.

Substantial gains in the control of advertising and smoking in public places are reported, and comprehensive national anti-tobacco legislation is pending.

Based on the data reported in this chapter, the following conclusions can be drawn:

1. Argentina demonstrates a high level of health despite serious economic problems due to inflation and foreign debt.
2. Argentina is one of the main producers and exporters of tobacco in the Americas, but domestic tobacco consumption declined in the 1980s. The prevalence of smoking is higher among younger men and women and higher among those with higher educational attainment and higher socioeconomic status than among those with less education and lower socioeconomic status. The prevalence of smoking among women increased between 1971–1991.
3. The mortality pattern for diseases associated with smoking in Argentina is similar to that for nations with sustained high population exposure to tobacco. Yearly smoking-attributable mortality has been estimated at approximately 38,000 to 49,000. As many as 20 percent of all deaths may be caused by smoking in Argentina. The relative rate of infant mortality for children born to smoking mothers in Argentina is nine times that for children born to nonsmoking mothers.
4. Argentina has one of the most developed tobacco-use prevention and control movements in the Americas. Most activities are initiated by nongovernmental organizations such as the Argentine Union Against Smoking and the Liga Argentina de Lucha Contra el Cancer.
5. Legislative restrictions on television advertising prohibit ads before 10:00 P.M. Numerous provincial and local legislative actions restrict smoking in many public places. Comprehensive legislation with restrictions on advertising, tobacco sales to minors, and smoking in public places is under consideration at the national level.

References

AGRO-ECONOMICS SERVICES, LTD. *The Employment, Tax Revenue, and Wealth that the Tobacco Industry Creates.* Agro-Economics Services, Ltd. September 1987.

AGUIRRE, E.B. *Tabaco y embarazo.* Doctoral Thesis in Medicine. Faculty of Medicine. University of Buenos Aires. Buenos Aires, 1984.

ALVAREZ-HERRERA, C. Country Collaborator Report, Argentina, unpublished data, Pan American Health Organization, 1990.

ALVAREZ-HERRERA, C. Prevalencia del hábito de fumar en la Republica Argentina. Estimación a principios de 1981. Unpublished manuscript, Buenos Aires, 1981.

BALOSSI, E.C., HAUGER-KLEVENE, J.H. Mortalidad por enfermedad isquémica coronaria en la República Argentina (1962–1978): su relacion con los factores de riesgo cardiovascular. *Revista Argentina Cardiología,* 55(4): 196–200, 1987.

BALOSSI, E.C., HAUGER-KLEVENE, J.H. Tendencias de la mortalidad por grandes grupos de causas. Argentina. (1977–1985). *La Semana Médica* 175(4):67–73, 5 de abril de 1991.

BANCO VELOX. La industria del tabaco. *Reseña* Año IV-No. 48. Mayo 1988.

BICKERS, C. Argentine growers reap cash rewards. *World Tobacco,* March 1990, p. 55.

BODDEWYN. *Why Adolescents Smoke.* International Advertising Association, 1987.

CAMARA DE LA INDUSTRIA DEL TABACO. *Revista Noticias.* Junio 1991.

CATTERBERG Y ASOCIADOS. Unpublished report, Survey of 800 Buenos Aires Residents. May 1991.

CELADE. *Boletín Demográfico.* No. 45. Santiago, Chile, January 1990.

CENTERS FOR DISEASE CONTROL. Smoking-attributable mortality and years of potential life lost. United States—1984. *Morbidity and Mortality Weekly Report* 36(42): 693–697, October 30, 1987.

CHAPMAN, S., WONG, W.L. *Tobacco Control in the Third World—A Resource Atlas.* Penang: International Organization of Consumers Unions, 1990.

CONSUMIDORES Y DESARROLLO. Estrategias legislativas para controlar la epidemia mundial del tabaquismo. ¿Por qué legislar? *Consumidores y Desarrollo* (5): 1–6, Junio-Julio, 1991.

COSTA DE ROBERT, S., GENTILLINI, N., VEROQUI, L., BARROS, C. Cardiovascular risk factors among workers of the paper industry of Zarate, Argentina (1988). *CVD Newsletter* 46:115, 1990.

ENCYCLOPEDIA BRITANNICA. *Year Book—1989.*

FUNDACION SALUD PUBLICA. Mortalidad por causa, sexo y edad. Unpublished data, 1991.

GALLUP ORGANIZATION, INC. *The Incidence of Smoking in Central and Latin America.* Princeton, New Jersey, 1988.

HAUGER-KLEVENE, J.H., BALOSSI, E.C. Descenso de la tasa de mortalidad por enfermedad coronaria. Argentina, 1977–1985: posibles explicaciones. *Revista Argentina de Cardiología,* Julio-Agosto, 58(4):170–176, 1990.

HAUGER-KLEVENE, J.H., BALOSSI, E.C. La adolescente fumadora: estudio Mar del Plata, 1980. *Boletín Epidemiológico Nacional* 1:3–6, 1984.

HAUGER-KLEVENE, J.H., BALOSSI, E.C. Prevalence of cardiovascular risk factors: The Mar del Plata Study, 1981. *CVD Epidemiology Newsletter* 38:165, 1985.

HAUGER-KLEVENE, J.H., BALOSSI, E.C. Prevalence of the smoking habit in an urban community of Argentina. *CVD Epidemiology Newsletter* 42(55), 1987.

HAUGER-KLEVENE, J.H., BALOSSI, E.C. Tobacco in Argentina. Unpublished manuscript, 1989.

HAYES, M., MELI, S., HAUGER-KLEVENE, J.H. Trends in cardiovascular mortality and prevalence of coronary risk factors in women of District 9 de Julio, Argentina (1987). *CVD Epidemiology Newsletter* 46:115, 1990.

HOSPITAL DE PEDIATRIA. Encuesta sobre el tabaquismo en el Hospital de Pediatria (unpublished document). Buenos Aires, 1988.

INZA, F.A., LANDENA, J., PAGLIER R. Encuesta de tabaquismo en los colegios secundarios de la ciudad de Azul. *Boletín LALCEC,* pp. 13–14, 1991.

JOLY, D.J. *Encuesta sobre las características del hábito de fumar en América Latina.* Scientific Publication No. 337, PAHO/WHO, Washington, D.C., 1977.

LALCEC. Observaciones sobre un estudio en escuela secundaria sobre el hábito de fumar en estudiantes y sus familias. Unpublished document. Buenos Aires, 1981.

MAXWELL, J.C. *The Maxwell Consumer Report. International Tobacco 1989 Part One.* Wheat First Securities, Butcher and Singer, May 18, 1990.

MISDORP, S. Jujuy has the right stuff to produce quality tobaccos. *Tobacco International,* June 1, pp. 38–41, 1990a.

MISDORP, S. Record production and exports continue to be set off by inflation. *Tobacco International,* June 1, pp. 42–45, 1990b.

MISDORP, S. Tobacco contributes heavily to revenue in Argentina. *Philip Morris Magazine,* May 1, p. 64, 1990c.

PAN AMERICAN HEALTH ORGANIZATION. *Control del Hábito de Fumar. Taller sub-regional para el Cono Sur y Brasil, November 18–22, 1985.* Technical Paper No. 2, PAHO/WHO, Washington, D.C., 1986.

PAN AMERICAN HEALTH ORGANIZATION. *Health Conditions in the Americas—1990 Edition.* Scientific Publication No. 524. PAHO, Washington, D.C., 1990.

REPUBLICA ARGENTINA. Ley No. 23.344. *Boletín Oficial de la República Argentina de 29 de agosto de 1986.*

TOBACCO MERCHANTS ASSOCIATION OF THE U.S., INC. *Production and Consumption of Tobacco Products for Selected Countries 1979–1988.* Special Report 89–3, September 28, 1989.

U.N. CONFERENCE ON TRADE AND DEVELOPMENT. *Marketing and Distribution of Tobacco.* Geneva, Switzerland: United Nations, June 16, 1978.

U.N. FOOD AND AGRICULTURE ORGANIZATION. *Tobacco: Supply, Demand and Trade Projections, 1995 and 2000.* FAO Economic and Social Development Paper 86. FAO, Rome, 1990.

U.S. DEPARTMENT OF AGRICULTURE. Tobacco production, imports, exports, and total domestic consumption. U.S. Department of Agriculture, Foreign Agricultural Service, Tobacco, Cotton, and Seeds Division, unpublished tabulations. April 1990.

U.S. DEPARTMENT OF HEALTH AND HUMAN SERVICES. *Reducing the Health Consequences of Smoking—25 Years of Progress. A Report of the Surgeon General.* U.S. Department of Health and Human Services, Public Health Service, Centers for Disease Control, Center for Chronic Disease Prevention and Health Promotion, Office on Smoking and Health. DHHS publication no. (CDC) 89–8411. January 1989.

U.S. FEDERAL TRADE COMMISSION. *Federal Trade Commission Report. "Tar," Nicotine, and Carbon Monoxide of the Smoke of 272 Varieties of Domestic Cigarettes.* December 1988.

WASHINGTON TIMES. *Trail of phony Winstons leads to Noriega, Cuba.* July 5, p. A3, 1990.

WORLD BANK. *World Development Report 1990—Poverty.* Oxford University Press, New York, 1990.

Bahamas

General Characteristics

The Commonwealth of the Bahamas is an archipelago of approximately 700 islands and cays located south of the Florida keys. Of these islands, 29 are inhabited; the capital, Nassau, is located on the most densely populated island, New Providence. The estimated 1987 midyear population was 240,000 (Table 1). Only 4.5 percent of Bahamians are aged 65 years and older, and in general, the population is quite young: 38 percent are younger than age 15 years. Although most of the Bahamas is rural, 82 percent of the total population resides in the urban areas of New Providence and Grand Bahama. Life expectancy increased overall from 65 years in 1970 to 70 years in 1988, while total fertility declined during the same period. Thus, the Bahamian population is aging rapidly (Ministry of Health 1986).

In 1987, the crude birth rate was 25.7/1,000 population. In that same year, the infant mortality rate was 29.3/1,000 live births. The crude death rate was 5.7/1,000 persons (Department of Statistics, Ministry of Finance 1990). However, because of under-registration of both births and deaths in the outlying cays and islands, vital statistics data may not be accurate for the nation as a whole. Because the Bahamas is an independent member of the British Commonwealth, the Ministry of Health is responsible for implementing national health policies and providing health care.

The Bahamas' extremely open economy is related to its dependence on tourism and offshore banking and commerce. Of the total 1988 gross domestic product (GDP) of US$2,863.2 million, tourism accounted for 75 percent of economic activity (Gray and Fountain 1990).

The Tobacco Industry

Tobacco is neither grown nor manufactured in the Bahamas. Cigarettes are imported for local consumption and for extensive duty-free sales to tourists. The major brands imported are Rothman's, Salem, Kool, Marlboro, Winston, Benson and Hedges, and DuMaurier. The illegal trade in cigarettes reported by several other Caribbean countries apparently is negligible in the Bahamas (Gray and Fountain 1990).

Duty-free cigarettes are purchased frequently by the 3 million tourists who visit the islands each year. However, cigarettes sold for domestic consumption are heavily taxed. In 1988, tax accounted for 47.5 percent of the average retail price of $US2.65 per pack of 20. Most of the tobacco consumed in the Bahamas is in the form of cigarettes. However, cigars and cheroots accounted for 10 percent (in dollar value) of all tobacco sold in the Bahamas in 1988, pipe and smokeless tobacco accounted for 1.1 percent, and fine-cut tobacco for roll-your-own cigarettes was 0.2 percent of the total (Gray and Fountain 1990).

No laws restrict tobacco product advertising in the Bahamas and tobacco companies commonly support sporting events (Gray and Fountain 1990). By law, tobacco product advertising in printed or electronic media must include a health warning that reads,

**"Warning—Tobacco smoking may
cause heart disease or lung cancer
among other diseases."**

Cigarette packages imported for sale in the Bahamas must also include this warning (Ministry of Health 1976). It is not clear whether duty-free

Table 1. Health and economic indicators, Bahamas, 1980s

Indicator	Year	Value
Population	1987	240,000
% < 15 years	1980	38
% ≥ 65 years	1980	4.5
% Urban	1990	82
Crude mortality rate per 1,000 persons	1987	5.7
Crude birth rate per 1,000 persons	1987	25.7
Infant mortality rate per 1,000 live births	1987	29.3
Life expectancy at birth	1988	70 years
Gross domestic product (GDP) million	1988	$US2,863.2
Per capita GDP	1986	$US9,378

Sources: Gray and Fountain 1990; PAHO 1990; Department of Statistics, Ministry of Finance 1990.

Figure 1. Adult* per capita cigarette consumption, Bahamas, 1979–1988

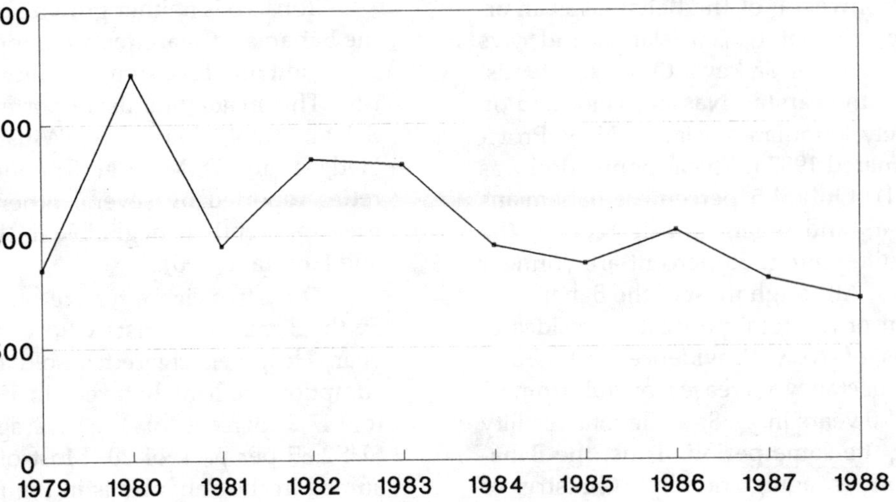

Source: Gray and Fountain, 1990.
*Age 15 and older.

cigarettes must display this warning, or whether the law is enforced. The enforcement of the law depends on a $100 fine applicable to persons who fail to comply.

Tobacco Use

Consumption Data

Data on per capita cigarette consumption among persons aged 15 and older suggest that Bahamians consumed 700 to 1,000 cigarettes per adult in 1979 to 1988, with no evident change or trend (Figure 1). Anomalous high rates of per capita consumption for 1980, 1982, and 1983 may result from tourists having purchased greater quantities of taxable cigarettes in those years. However, the data collection system for reporting of excise taxes may lack precision (Gray and Fountain 1990).

Behavioral Surveys

Prevalence of smoking among adults

Two carefully performed surveys of tobacco use are available for the Bahamas. The first, the 1988 National Health and Nutrition Survey of adults aged 15 and older, was conducted by the national Health Information Coordinating Services Unit (Ministry of Health 1988). Among the 1,894 respondents, 11.4 percent were current regular smokers (19.9 percent of men and 4.6 percent of women) (Table 2). The prevalence of smoking was slightly higher on the urbanized island of New Providence (11.4 percent), compared with the Family Islands (10.9 percent) and Grand Bahama (10.8 percent). The prevalence of smoking among Bahamian blacks was less than one-half that of Bahamian whites and non-Bahamian residents (9.8 percent vs. 23.5 percent vs. 24.3 percent, respectively). Most respondents (53.4 percent) began smoking between 15 and 19 years of age, and the mean ages of initiation were 20.4 for women and 18.7 for men. Only 3 percent of smokers smoked cigars and 0.5 percent smoked pipes (Gray and Fountain 1990).

In 1989, a survey on drug use that included tobacco was conducted by the Ministry of Health (1989) among 1,000 persons aged 16 to 59 years. The data on tobacco use from this survey may be compared to those of the 1988 survey even though the precise definitions used for classifying smokers (current, former, occasional, never, etc.) were somewhat different. Of all respondents, 60.4 percent reported never having smoked (Table 3). The prevalence of smoking among men was more than four times that among women (19.3 vs. 3.8 percent), similar to levels reported for 1988. The percentage of current regular smokers was greater among those aged 35 to 54 compared with those

Table 2. Prevalence (%) of current and former smoking, by sex, age, ethnicity, and educational attainment among adults, aged 15 years and older, Bahamas, 1988

Category	Current smoking prevalence (%)	Former smoking prevalence (%)	N
All adults	11.4	15.2	875
Men	19.9	24.7	392
Women	4.6	7.5	483
Women aged 15–44	4.8	6.4	374
Age groups			
Men 15–24	8.4	13.4	119
25–44	23.9	27.8	65
45–64	28.8	31.5	73
≥65	12.5	50.0	16
Women 15–24	1.3	5.2	154
25–44	7.3	7.3	220
45–64	3.8	10.0	80
≥65	3.7	14.8	27
Ethnicity			
Bahamian blacks	9.2	14.3	725
Bahamian whites	23.5	29.4	51
Non-Bahamians	24.3	20.0	70
Educational attainment			
Primary or less	8.2	20.4	98
Secondary	11.7	13.6	566
>Secondary	12.6	18.1	199

Source: Ministry of Health 1988.

aged 20 or younger (14 vs. 9 percent). The prevalence of current regular smoking by occupation was highest among those employed in "blue-collar" jobs compared with those in professional jobs (22.8 vs. 9.9 percent). The frequency of quitting (as measured by the prevalence of former smoking) was positively related to age and highest among persons aged 55 to 59 years. The mean number of cigarettes smoked per day was similar for men and women (14 vs. 12 per day). The mean age of initiation of smoking on this survey was also 18 years (Gray and Fountain 1990).

Based on these two surveys, performed a year apart, the overall prevalence of current regular smoking appears to be approximately 10 percent among adults in the Bahamas. Prevalence is higher among those employed in blue-collar jobs, and is also much higher among whites and non-native Bahamians.

Prevalence of smoking among adolescents

A 1987 anonymous self-administered survey of 4,800 schoolchildren aged 10 to 19 years was performed by the Ministry of Health's Department of Psychiatric Social Services (Bahamas National Drug Abuse Council 1987). The sample comprised 25.3 percent of the school-attending population in this age group. The use of tobacco ever in the lifetime, in the past year, and in the past month was ascertained (Table 4). Overall, 14.5 percent of adolescents had ever used tobacco (20.4 percent of boys and 9.7 percent of girls). Only 0.7 percent were current regular smokers.

Of those aged 10 to 14 years, twice as many boys as girls reported ever having used cigarettes (17 vs. 8 percent). Prevalence of ever smoking increased by 50 percent for the age group 15 to 19 years, indicating that experimentation and the onset of regular use by smokers occur at this age. The prevalence of ever smoking was higher in urban than in rural areas (16 vs. 11 percent).

A small sample of 74 delinquents aged 10 to 16 years who resided at an industrial school was surveyed in 1988 by the same agency (Bahamas National Drug Abuse Council 1988). In this "high risk" population, the overall prevalence of ever smoking was 32.4 percent, and the prevalence of

Table 3. Prevalence (%) of current, former, and occasional smoking by sex, age, income, educational attainment, and occupational status among adults, aged 16–59 years, Bahamas, 1989

Category	Current smoking (%)	Former smoking (%)	Occasional smoking (%)	N
All adults	10.0	6.3	2.7	1,000
Men	19.3	10.5	4.0	400
Women	3.8	3.5	1.8	600
Women aged 15–44	3.7	2.0	2.3	484
Age groups				
Men 16–24	3.3	2.2	3.3	90
25–44	23.1	10.0	4.8	229
45–59	26.4	23.6	2.8	72
Women 16–24	0.7	—	2.7	148
25–44	5.1	3.0	2.1	336
45–59	3.9	10.8	—	102
Income				
<National average	8.2	5.1	1.7	293
>National average	11.1	6.9	3.3	606
Educational attainment				
Primary or less	14.7	6.3	3.7	190
Secondary	7.5	5.4	2.0	597
>Secondary	12.6	8.6	3.5	198
Occupational status				
Professional/mgr.	9.9	8.0	2.4	212
Clerical/sales	6.0	4.8	1.6	249
Service	6.5	5.0	2.7	260
Blue-collar/agr.	22.8	9.2	4.4	206
Housewife/unemp.		1.4	1.4	68

Source: Ministry of Health 1989.

Table 4. Prevalence (%) of ever smoking, smoking in the last year, smoking in the last month, and current regular smoking among adolescents aged 14–19 years, by sex, age group, and island of residence, Bahamas, 1987

Category	Ever used (%)	Last year (%)	Last month (%)	Current regular smoking (%)	N
All respondents	14.5	5.0	3.0	0.7	4,767
Boys	20.4	7.6	4.7	0.8	2,102
Girls	9.7	2.9	1.7	0.4	2,665
Age 10–14 years					
Boys	16.8	6.5	3.7	0.5	
Girls	8.3	2.0	1.1	0.2	
Age 15–19					
Boys	24.5	8.8	5.7	1.7	
Girls	11.5	4.0	2.5	0.6	
Residence					
Family Islands	10.7	4.0	2.7	0.5	
New Providence/Grand Bahama	15.9	5.4	3.2	0.8	

Source: Bahamas National Drug Council (Alcohol, Smoking, and Drug Use Among Students) 1987.

smoking within the year prior to admission was 28.8 percent. Because of the small sample size, additional stratification of the results is not possible.

Knowledge and Attitudes towards Smoking

The 1989 National Adult Drug Use Survey described above (Ministry of Health 1989) asked about perceived risk and addictiveness associated with cigarettes. Preliminary results from this survey suggest that most Bahamians (82.1 percent) agree that a person who smokes one or more packs of cigarettes per day is at "moderate" or "great" risk. In addition, 80.9 percent of respondents thought that cigarettes are addictive.

Smoking and Health

Mortality Data

In 1987, of a total of 1,411 reported deaths, only 2.5 percent were classified as symptoms, signs and ill-defined conditions (ICD 780–799). Thus, mortality data for the Bahamas may be quite reliable. The mortality structure for this population reflects both the high degree of development and the high prevalence of chronic diseases that may be caused by lifestyle-related risk factors (Table 5). Of the total number of deaths, one-fifth were due to malignant neoplasms; of these 277 deaths, lung cancer accounted for 34 (12.3 percent). The age-specific lung cancer mortality rate has been consistently higher for men than for women, in accordance with the much higher reported preva-

Table 5. Leading causes of death, Bahamas, 1987

Cause (ICD-9 Code)	Number of deaths	Percentage of total
All causes	1,411	100
Ill-defined conditions (780–799)	35	2.5
Malignant neoplasms (140–208)	277	20.1
Heart disease (398–429)	250	18.2
Accidents (E800–949, E980–989)	155	11.3
Cerebrovascular disease (430–499)	115	8.4
Respiratory disease	94	6.8

Source: World Health Organization 1991.

Table 6. Age-specific mortality rates (per 100,000 persons) for lung cancer and heart disease by sex, Bahamas, 1984 and 1987

Disease rate	Age group	1984 mortality rate	1987 mortality rate
Men			
Lung cancer	45–54	78.7	21.1
	55–64	50.8	174.6
	65–74	200	179.5
Heart disease	45–54	146	253.4
	55–64	525.2	364.5
	65–74	1,000	1,105.4
Women			
Lung cancer	45–54	10.5	39.6
	55–64	29	68.9
	65–74	46.5	41.3
Heart disease	45–54	94.8	89.2
	55–64	188.5	289.3
	65–74	767.5	661.2

Source: World Health Organization 1991.

lence of smoking by men compared with women (Table 6). Malignant neoplasms have been the leading cause of death since 1982, when these causes of death surpassed heart disease (Ministry of Health 1986). The age-adjusted mortality rate for neoplasms increased from 83/100,000 persons in 1982 to 115/100,000 persons during 1987 (Pan American Health Organization [PAHO] 1990). The average Bahamian at birth has approximately a 20–percent chance of dying from malignant neoplasms (World Health Organization [WHO] 1991).

Heart diseases (ICD 398–429) were the second leading cause of death, with a proportionate mortality of 18.2 percent. Heart disease mortality rates overall were essentially unchanged between 1984 and 1987. However, the age-specific mortality rate among persons aged 55 years and older increased during this short time period (Table 6).

Morbidity

Aside from childbirth, neoplasms and heart disease are the main causes cited on hospital admission records in the Bahamas. Of the 6,076 admissions to the main hospital, 63 were diagnosed as coronary heart disease, 52 were chronic obstructive lung disease (including asthma), and 8 were lung cancer. These diseases all may have at least some relationship to smoking; most admissions for these chronic diseases were among adults aged 45 years and older.

Tobacco Use Prevention and Control Activities

Government Structure and Policy

No official policy on tobacco use has been published by the Government of the Bahamas, and no specific office is dedicated to the prevention and control of tobacco use. Administratively, the Ministry of Health devotes resources to tobacco issues from within the Health Information Coordinating Unit and the Social Services department. As in several other Caribbean nations, drug-use prevention and tobacco-use prevention and control are closely linked, especially for the adolescent population; however, the National Drug Abuse Council deals mainly with illegal drug use.

Legislation

Although no specific legislation has been enacted to restrict smoking in public places or to restrict retail cigarette sales to minors, voluntary restrictions on smoking have been reported for health-care facilities, educational facilities, cinemas, some public transport vehicles, and some restaurants (Gray and Fountain 1990). In 1987, the Ministry of Transport enacted an ''Administrative Directive'' prohibiting smoking during domestic inter-island flights of the national airline (Bahamas Air) (PAHO 1988).

The Health Services (Amendment) Act of 1976 is one of the most forceful legislative interventions passed to warn consumers of the harmfulness of cigarettes (see tobacco advertising section above). This law mandates a fairly clear warning for cigarette packages and tobacco product advertising (Ministry of Health 1976). However, the warning is not likely to be visible during the promotion of sports events that receive wide media coverage and that generally attract young people in the Bahamas.

Economic Disincentives

The average price of a pack of 20 cigarettes is $US2.65, of which $US1.26 is national tax (47.5 percent of import cost). In 1988, retail cigarette sales generated $US4.7 million in revenue compared with $1.8 million in 1979 and $6 million in 1982. From 1979 to 1982, tax revenues varied from $3.9 million to $5.3 million. Retail cigarette sales prices are among the highest in the Caribbean, but the average worker's wage in the Bahamas is likely among the highest also. Because tobacco is not a commercial agriculture or manufacturing product for the Bahamas, substantial savings in foreign exchange could be anticipated with lower consumption of tobacco. In 1986, it was estimated that almost $US3 million in foreign exchange currency might be saved if all imports of tobacco were discontinued (PAHO 1988).

Insurance companies provide discounts on premiums to nonsmokers of 15 to 35 percent in the Bahamas. Smokers are not considered eligible for rate differentials until they have quit smoking for at least 12 months (PAHO 1988).

Educational Activities

Health education on tobacco use is not required in the school system. As increasing numbers of the very young population of the Bahamas reach the documented age of experimentation with tobacco use (15 to 19 years), the low prevalences of adult smoking reported in this chapter may change dramatically. Children are told in schools that they should not smoke, but they are not taught specific antismoking skills.

Public education on the health consequences of tobacco use has been supported by the Bahamas Cancer Society through brochures, posters, t-shirts, and the World Health Organization's ''World No Tobacco Day'' on May 31. During the entire month of May, the Society also sponsors seminars and telethons during which local and international speakers promote nonsmoking. The Bahamas Heart Association sponsors television-based public service announcements dealing with smoking and other risk factors. The Seventh Day Adventist Church sponsors 5-day smoking cessation classes in the Bahamas just as it does throughout the Caribbean region (PAHO 1988).

Summary and Conclusions

The prevalence of current regular smoking among adult and adolescent native Bahamians is very low. However, the high prevalence among white Bahamians and non-native Bahamians serves as an extremely dangerous example for the rest of the population. Surveys conducted in 1988 and 1989 indicate that the prevalence of smoking among professional adults is quite low, and that as in other developed nations, the prevalence is higher among blue-collar employed persons.

The lung cancer mortality rate among middle-aged and older persons, as a marker for long-term population exposure to tobacco, is still quite low in the Bahamas, but chronic diseases, including those caused by lifestyle-associated risk factors, are increasing in importance. Thus, if consumption data indicate a continued level of moderate exposure in the Bahamas, it can be expected that lung cancer mortality and mortality due to other smoking-associated risk factors will increase.

Aside from a moderately strong requirement for a health warning, little Government action against tobacco use has been reported in the Bahamas. Voluntary efforts by groups traditionally interested in cancer and heart disease prevention have been reported, but the effect of specific programs is unknown.

Based on the data presented above, the following conclusions can be drawn:
1. The prevalence of tobacco use among adults is approximately 10 percent in the Bahamas. The prevalence among men is four times that among women. The prevalence of current regular smoking is much higher among white Bahamians and non-native residents than among black Bahamians.
2. Chronic diseases, led by neoplasms and heart disease, are the most important causes of death in the Bahamas. Many of these diseases may be attributable to smoking and the mortality rate for these diseases can be expected to increase as the Bahamian population ages.
3. No legislative or policy-based controls on smoking in public places, minors' access to tobacco, health education against tobacco use, or advertising are reported for the Bahamas. A moderately strong requirement for a health warning on cigarette packages and in tobacco product advertisements has existed since 1976.

References

BAHAMAS NATIONAL DRUG ABUSE COUNCIL. Alcohol, Smoking and Drug Use among Delinquent Students at an Industrial School, unpublished. 1988.

BAHAMAS NATIONAL DRUG COUNCIL. Alcohol, Smoking and Drug Use among Students, 1987. Unpublished.

DEPARTMENT OF STATISTICS, MINISTRY OF FINANCE, unpublished data. 1990.

GRAY, H., FOUNTAIN, T. Country Collaborator's Report—Bahamas. Unpublished data, Pan American Health Organization, 1990.

MINISTRY OF HEALTH. *Basic Health Information, Commonwealth of the Bahamas*, Ministry of Health. 1986.

MINISTRY OF HEALTH. National Drug Use Survey, Health Information Coordinating Services Unit, Ministry of Health, unpublished. 1989.

MINISTRY OF HEALTH. National Health and Nutrition Survey, Health Information Coordinating Services Unit, Ministry of Health, unpublished. 1988.

MINISTRY OF HEALTH. *The Health Services (Amendment) Act, 1976 (No. 15 of 1976)*. Official Gazette. S.I. No. 130 of 1976.

PAN AMERICAN HEALTH ORGANIZATION. *Health Conditions in the Americas, 1990 Edition*. Washington, D.C., Pan American Health Organization. Scientific Publication No. 524, 1990.

PAN AMERICAN HEALTH ORGANIZATION. *Smoking Control—Third Subregional Workshop, Caribbean Area*. Kingston, Jamaica, 8–11 December 1987. Tech. Paper No. 20. Washington, D.C.: Pan American Health Organization, 1988, pp. 15–19.

WORLD HEALTH ORGANIZATION. *1990 World Health Statistics Annual*. Geneva, Switzerland: World Health Organization, 1991.

Barbados

General Characteristics

Barbados is the easternmost Caribbean island, occupying 430 km² due east of St. Vincent in the Lesser Antilles. The Government is a parliamentary democracy within the Commonwealth of Nations (MacMillan 1988). The per capita gross national product (GNP) reached US$6,110 in 1988 after an annual growth of 2.3 percent between 1965 and 1988 (World Bank 1990). The economy is based on tourism, services, light manufacturing, and agriculture. Tourism grew steadily from $US93 million in 1983 to US$169 million in 1990 (United Nations Economic Commission on Latin America and the Caribbean [UNECLAC] 1990). Sugar cane has been the main crop grown in Barbados for some 300 years. Crop diversification programs now include sea island cotton, tropical flowers, vegetables, and livestock farming. The fishing industry is also expanding. Light manufacturing of furniture, garments, packaging supplies, and data processing and electronic equipment help reduce unemployment. Nonetheless, unemployment increased from 13.7 percent in 1989 to 14.7 percent in 1990 (UNECLAC 1990).

With 590 persons per km², Barbados is one of the most densely populated islands in the Caribbean. In 1988, the estimated mid-year population was 255,000; the annual growth rate averaged 0.3 percent between 1980 and 1988 (World Bank 1989). Recent population changes have been marginal, with a 0.001-percent decrease between 1987 and 1988. Of the total 1988 population, 11.3 percent is aged 65 and older, and 24.6 percent is less than 15 years old (Table 1). The proportion of the Barbadian population aged 65 years and older has increased from 6.4 percent in 1960 to 11.3 percent in 1988 (UNECLAC 1990). Thus, Barbados has a very high proportion of elderly people compared with its Caribbean neighbors (see Table 1 in chapter on the Organization of Eastern Caribbean States in this report).

General health indicators for the Barbadian population suggest an advanced state of health conditions in Barbados. Between 1983 and 1987, the birth rate declined steadily from 18 to 15 per 1,000 population, and the fertility rate declined from 77 to 59 per 1,000 women aged 15 to 44 years. This change was probably due to an ongoing family planning and family life education program (Pan American Health Organization [PAHO] 1990). The 1987 infant mortality rate was 21.6 per 1,000 live births, and the 1988 crude death rate was 8.8 per

Table 1. Health and economic indicators, Barbados, 1980s

Indicator	Year	Level
Population	1988	255,000
% < age 15	1988	24.6
% ≥ age 65	1988	11.3
Crude birth rate per 1,000 persons	1987	15
Fertility rate per 1,000 women aged 15–44 years	1987	59
Infant mortality rate per 1,000 live births	1987	21.6
Crude death rate per 1,000 persons	1988	8.8
Life expectancy at birth		
Men	1988	73
Women	1988	77
Per capita GNP US$	1988	6,110

Source: UNECLAC, 1990.

1,000 population (PAHO 1990). Life expectancy at birth was 73 years for men and 77 years for women (World Bank 1990) (Table 1).

The growing elderly population coupled with life expectancies comparable to those of industrialized countries suggests that Barbados will suffer an increasing burden of morbidity and mortality from chronic diseases, particularly cardiovascular diseases, respiratory diseases, and cancer. These diseases, many of which are caused by smoking, impose a significant financial burden on health care facilities as well as on individuals and families. However, Barbados is well prepared to implement effective health promotion activities because of the high adult literacy rate (98 percent) (World Bank 1990). The success of family planning and family life education in Barbados might suggest that other health education activities also could be successful.

The Tobacco Industry

No tobacco is grown in Barbados. The British-American Tobacco Company, Ltd. (BAT) found the soil unsuitable for tobacco agriculture. The privately owned BAT (Barbados), Ltd., a subsidiary of BAT in the United Kingdom, is the only tobacco company operating in Barbados. The company employs 70 persons in management, production, sales, and advertising; this total does not include retail outlet employees (Theodore-Gandhi 1991).

In 1990, 116,365 kg of raw tobacco was imported from the United Kingdom, Canada, the

Table 2. Imports, production, exports, and domestic consumption of cigarettes, Barbados, 1980–1990

Year	Imports	Production	Exports	Total domestic consumption
1980	27,599	224,000	96,029	155,570
1981	27,864	260,000	134,899	153,005
1982	17,394	271,000	117,248	171,146
1983	23,385	241,000	93,559	170,826
1984	125,845	238,000	219,376	144,469
1985	13,345	143,000	79,575	76,770
1986	9,677	172,000	73,225	108,452
1987	10,054	163,000	38,158	134,896
1988	11,554	149,000	78,638	81,916
1989	17,904	143,000	120,398	40,506
1990	59,793	135,000	43,591	151,202

Source: Barbados Central Statistical Office, 1990.

United States, Brazil, Netherlands, Cuba, and Greece. Most of this was used in the production of tobacco products for the local market, but 200 kg was re-exported (Barbados Central Statistical Office 1990). Small quantities of cigars, cheroots, cigarillos, and snuff are also imported.

According to Barbadian sources, domestic cigarette production steadily decreased during 1981 to 1990 from 260 million to 135 million units (Barbados Central Statistical Office 1990). However, this decline is not corroborated by U.S. Department of Agriculture (USDA) data (1990). The USDA reported that production of cigarettes increased from 240 million in 1981 to 260 million in 1989. Both sources indicated that imports of manufactured cigarettes (15 million per year) did not change significantly during the 1980s (Table 2). The visible trade balance from cigarettes declined during the decade 1980 to 1990 (Figure 1). (Imports are valued at the market value of goods at the time of importation

Figure 1. Visible trade balance for cigarettes, Barbados, 1980–1990, in Barbados dollars (thousands)

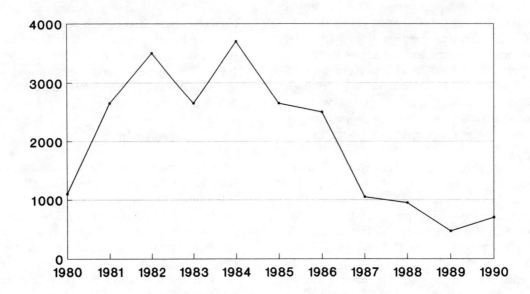

Source: Theodore-Gandhi, 1991.
*B$2.00 = US$1.00

plus cost of insurance and freight (CIF). Exports are valued at the cost of goods to the purchaser abroad, including all charges up to the point where the goods are put on board (FOB). The visible trade balance is the difference between the Value of Exports (FOB) and the Value of Imports (CIF).) The foreign exchange needed for the imported inputs into production of cigarettes, such as raw tobacco leaf, machinery, paper, and boxes, is not included in this calculation. The input costs of these items comprise a significant component of production costs and hence reduce the overall value of the exported product (Theodore-Gandhi 1991).

BAT (Barbados) produces four brands of cigarettes: Benson and Hedges, 555's, Embassy, and Mayfair. Cigarettes are sold in packs of 10 and 20; packs of 10 are the most popular. Distribution is limited to Barbados and other Caribbean islands. It has been reported to be difficult for the locally produced cigarettes to compete in European and North American markets. Cigarettes are imported from the United Kingdom, the United States, Canada, Trinidad, Jamaica, and Guyana. There is no evidence of an illegal trade in cigarettes in Barbados (Theodore-Gandhi 1991).

Consumption tax on cigarettes is BD$15 per kg, with stamp duty at 15 percent of the total cost.

Therefore, a pack of cigarettes costs approximately BD$4.90 (US$2.50), and 41.2 percent of the package price is tax (PAHO 1988). No data are available on the proportion of total Government revenue that is contributed by cigarette taxes.

There are no restrictions on tobacco advertising, but the local tobacco company voluntarily does not advertise on television or in cinemas. However, tobacco advertising on the radio is common. In addition, BAT (Barbados) sponsors the National Cultural Society and various sports such as horseracing, football, and cricket. While the local company does not sponsor local teams, the transnational parent company sponsors major sports events (Theodore-Gandhi 1991). Many homes in Barbados now receive cable television directly from the United States; thus, viewers also have access to anti-tobacco media messages.

Tobacco Use

The apparent per capita cigarette consumption among persons aged 15 years and older decreased from 1,218 in 1980 to 285.9 in 1989 and increased to 1,051 in 1990 (Figure 2). These figures were based on the assumption that the amount of cigarettes available for local consumption is equal

Figure 2. Adult* per capita cigarette consumption, Barbados, 1980–90

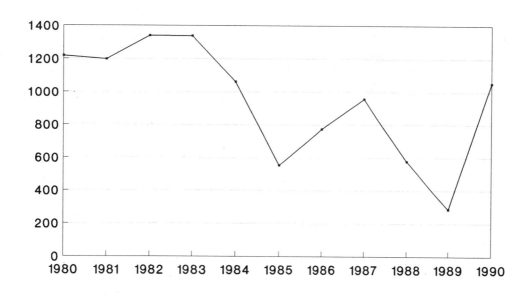

Source: USDA 1990.
*Age 15 and older

to the total imports plus local production less domestic exports and re-exports. This estimated per capita consumption does not account for increased domestic availability of duty-free cigarettes purchased outside Barbados by tourists and returning residents. Similarly, the denominator does not include tourists to Barbados. Fluctuations in duty-free purchases could account for the wide variation in apparent per capita consumption of duty-paid cigarettes. However, the data suggest that the per capita consumption of cigarettes in Barbados is falling over the long term. This notion is further supported by the decline in local cigarette production and the reduction in cigarette imports.

There have been no surveys on tobacco use among either adolescents or adults in Barbados. An undocumented estimate of the prevalence of smoking (9 percent of the population) was reported in 1988 (PAHO 1988). To substantiate this estimate, per capita cigarette consumption was calculated for Barbadian smokers aged 15 and older. If 9 percent of the population aged 15 and older (17,300 persons) smoked an average of 10 cigarettes per day, then 63 million cigarettes would have been smoked in Barbados in 1988. The total 1988 domestic consumption was 82 million, according to the conservative estimates by the Barbados Statistical Services. Using this estimate, the 9 percent adult prevalence is probably reasonable. However, the USDA estimate of yearly consumption (265 million) is more than three times as high (USDA 1990), suggesting a threefold higher prevalence of smoking as well. If it were possible to deduct tourist purchases of cigarettes, the yearly consumption by Barbados residents would be substantially less. Thus, the true estimate of current smoking prevalence probably lies somewhere between 9 and 27 percent. A survey of schoolchildren aged 11 to 18 years was planned for 1991.

Smoking and Health

Mortality

Heart disease (ICD 393–398, 410–429) is the leading cause of death in Barbados, accounting for 20.3 percent of total mortality in 1985 to 1989. Malignant neoplasms (ICD 140–208) ranks second and accounts for 18.6 percent of all deaths. Cerebrovascular disease (ICD 430–438), diabetes mellitus (ICD 250) and "other" diseases of the circulatory system (ICD 440–459) were the third, fourth, and fifth causes of death during the same period, accounting for 8.9 percent, 5.1 percent, and 4.8 percent of mortality, respectively (Theodore-Gandhi 1991).

Among smoking-related cancers in men aged 35 or older during 1985 to 1989, stomach cancer was the leading cause of death (2.9 percent of total mortality); lung cancer and esophageal cancer were the second and third leading causes of cancer death (1.8 and 1.5 percent of total mortality, respectively). Among women aged 35 and older, cervical cancer was the leading cause of cancer death, accounting for 2.3 percent of total mortality. Stomach cancer and lung cancer were the second and third principal causes of cancer death, accounting for 2 percent and 0.6 percent of all deaths, respectively (Theodore-Gandhi 1991) (Table 3).

Too few mortality events occur in Barbados to permit meaningful trend analyses of smoking-related diseases. There may be substantial under-reporting of these causes of death due to lack of diagnostic or pathology services. However, almost 100 percent of deaths are registered in Barbados (Massiah 1985). The accuracy of cause-of-death assignation is unknown, but the percentage of deaths attributed to "signs, symptoms, and ill-defined causes" is small (3.8 percent).

Morbidity

The Queen Elizabeth Hospital is the main acute care hospital in Barbados. During 1987 to 1989, 12 smoking-related disease categories (U.S. Department of Health and Human Services [USDHHS] 1989) accounted for approximately 10 percent of total admissions to this hospital (Table 4). However, total admissions included obstetric care and admissions for social reasons. It is difficult to estimate the smoking-attributable percentage of these admissions (i.e., those that would be prevented in the absence of smoking), but it is certain that a substantial proportion of the disease burden is directly related to smoking. The prevalence of smoking among the admitted patients is unknown. In addition, hospital admissions do not reflect smoking-attributable morbidity in the entire community because many patients who have these diseases will not be hospitalized. Admissions depend on the referral policy of general practitioners and on the admitting policy of hospital clinicians. The same individual may have repeated admissions in the year for the same diagnosis. These data therefore provide only a minimal estimate of the tobacco-attributable disease burden on acute hospital services.

The smoking-attributable cost to the commu-

Table 3. Number of deaths and proportionate mortality from smoking-related diseases in Barbados 1985–1989 in persons 35 years and over

Cause	Male No.	Male (%)	Female No.	Female (%)	Total No.	Total (%)
Total deaths from all causes	4,704		5,299		10,003	
Coronary heart disease (ICD 410–414)	566	(12)	527	(10)	1,093	(10.9)
Other heart disease (ICD 390–398, 401–405, 415–417, 421–429)	600	(12)	775	(14.6)	1,375	(13.7)
Cerebrovascular disease (ICD 430–438)	584	(12)	808	(15.2)	1,392	(13.9)
Other circulatory disease (ICD 440–448)	190	(4)	348	(6.6)	538	(5.4)
Chronic obstructive disease (ICD 490–492)	51	(1)	38	(0.7)	149	(1.5)
Other respiratory disease (ICD 010–012, 480–487, 493)	133	(2.8)	103	(1.9)	236	(2.4)
Malignant neoplasms Lip, oral cavity, pharynx (ICD 140–149)	40	(.85)	21	(0.4)	61	(0.6)
Esophagus (ICD 150)	72	(1.5)	14	(0.3)	86	(0.9)
Stomach (ICD 151)	152	(3.2)	104	(1.9)	256	(2.6)
Lung (ICD 162)	85	(1.8)	35	(0.7)	120	(1.2)
Cervix (ICD 180)	N/A		118			
Other cancers (ICD 157, 161, 188, 189)	56	(1.2)	71	(1.3)	127	(1.3)
Symptoms, signs, or ill-defined disease	178	(3.8)	204	(3.8)	382	(3.8)

Sources: PAHO, 1990; Theodore-Gandhi, 1991.

Table 4. Admissions to the Queen Elizabeth Hospital in Barbados 1987–1989 for smoking-related diseases 15 years and over

Cause	No.	Percentage of total admissions
Total admissions all causes	68,828	
Coronary heart disease (ICD 410–414)	1,056	1.5
Other heart disease (ICD 390–398, 401–405, 415–417, 421–429)	3,017	4.4
Cerebrovascular disease (ICD 430–438)	859	1.2
Other circulatory disease (ICD 440–448)	318	0.46
Chronic obstructive disease (ICD 490–492, 496)	512	0.74
Other respiratory disease (ICD 010–012, 480–487, 493)	409	0.59
Malignant neoplasms. Lip, oral cavity, pharynx (ICD 140–149)	84	0.12
Esophagus (ICD 150)	78	0.11
Stomach (ICD 151)	143	0.21
Lung (ICD 162)	109	0.15
Cervix (ICD 180)	230	N/A
Other cancers (ICD 157, 161, 188, 189)	153	0.22
Total (smoking-related diseases)	6,968	9.7

Source: Theodore-Gandhi, 1990.

nity and to the individual and family is difficult to measure. However, the information on admissions provides a minimum estimate of the smoking-attributable economic burden for hospital costs in Barbados. The daily hospitalization cost per patient in Barbados was approximately BD$200 in 1988. This estimate does not include laboratory, x-rays, and treatment. Annual admissions averaged 2,322 for adult smoking-related diseases at the Queen Elizabeth Hospital from 1987 to 1989. The average length of stay for patients is approximately 12 to 14 days (Chief Medical Officer 1986). Using a conservative length-of-stay of 10 days, the estimated cost for all smoking-related admissions in 1987 to 1989 is approximately BD$4,644,000. In the United States, it has been estimated that 60 percent of all hospital costs for cardiovascular disease, malignancies, and respiratory disease are attributable to smoking (Hodgson 1992). Thus, the smoking-attributable hospital cost in Barbados may be as high as BD$2.7 million. This cost does not include outpatient medical treatment, lost workdays, nursing home costs, or other social and economic costs to individuals. In view of the demographic changes in Barbados over the decade 1980 to 1990 that forecast an increasing proportion of elderly persons, it is likely that the economic burden of tobacco use will increase substantially.

Tobacco Use Prevention and Control Activities

The Government has no specific policy or program to prevent and control tobacco use. A Health Services Regulation on Smoking and Tobacco has been drafted but not yet enacted. This legislation will prohibit smoking in public places and require a health warning on all cigarette packages. BAT (Barbados) preempted enactment of the proposed legislation by voluntarily introducing warning labels on the cigarette packages. The warning reads: ''The Chief Medical Officer has determined that tobacco smoking is injurious to health'' (Theodore-Gandhi 1991).

While there are no restrictions on smoking in public places, the Health Services (Food Hygiene) Regulations prohibit any person from using tobacco, including snuff, while handling food or while in a room where uncovered food is present. Smoking is restricted through policies in certain industries which use or store flammable material and in private offices of health organizations such as those of the Barbados Cancer Society. There are no

specific laws regulating nicotine and tar levels in cigarettes, but BAT (Barbados) produces cigarettes according to the standards of the parent company in the United Kingdom.

Efforts are made by both Government Ministries and nongovernmental organizations to implement specific educational programs when funds are available. The World Health Organization's No-Tobacco Day (May 31) is a regular focus for these activities. ''No Smoking'' posters and signs prepared by the Ministry of Health have been distributed to hospitals, post offices, supermarkets, stores, and public transportation facilities (Theodore-Gandhi 1991). The Barbados Cancer Society sponsors antismoking television messages (PAHO 1988).

The National Drug Abuse Council of Barbados addresses drug abuse on the island. Its jurisdiction includes tobacco and alcohol as well as illegal drugs and prescription drugs. The Council was established in response to the CARICOM Secretariat's Initiative for a Regional Program on Drug Abuse Abatement and Control. The Council plans to collect data on the prevalence of drug use and abuse in the future (Theodore-Gandhi 1991).

The Barbados Cancer Society conducts 5-week smoking cessation clinics based on the American Cancer Society model. Clients are recruited through advertisements and health care providers. In addition, the Society also gives lectures about the dangers of smoking, provides antismoking leaflets and posters, and distributes ''nosmoking'' signs to various public places and agencies.

At the 1990 Annual Meeting of the Barbados Association of Medical Practitioners, members decided to lobby for nonsmoking flights on British West-Indian Airways and Leeward Islands Airline Travel. In addition, the Association plans to advocate smoke-free public places. These initiatives are in the planning stages, and activities were intended to be launched during 1991 (Theodore-Gandhi 1991).

Summary and Conclusions

No data are available on knowledge, attitudes, and behavior concerning tobacco use for either adolescents or adults in Barbados. However, the per capita consumption of cigarettes of persons 15 years and older in Barbados indicates that consumption of cigarettes decreased during 1980 to 1990. Estimates based on per capita consumption data suggest that the adult prevalence of smoking is between 9 and 27 percent.

Barbados had a positive but declining balance of trade for tobacco during the 1980s. The foreign exchange needed for imported production inputs is not included in this calculation, and deduction for these goods will reduce the overall value of tobacco exports substantially. The total Government revenue generated from excise duties and taxes on tobacco is unknown.

Chronic noncommunicable diseases (i.e., cardiovascular disease and malignancies) are the leading causes of death in Barbados. A conservative estimate of annual hospital expenditures for the care of selected smoking-related chronic diseases is BD$2.7 million. This estimate does not include the costs of outpatient primary health and social services, lost working days, or social and economic costs to the individual and family. Barbados has an increasing elderly population. This demographic shift is likely to increase the financial burden of smoking-related diseases in the future.

Few regulatory activities have been implemented in Barbados, although health legislation to mandate package warnings and clean indoor air regulations has been drafted. No current or proposed legislation bans tobacco sales to children or restricts advertising of tobacco products. However, the domestic tobacco company in consultation with the Ministry of Health voluntarily agreed to place warnings on cigarette packs manufactured in Barbados.

As yet, there are no sustained education and prevention programs in Barbados, but Government and nongovernmental organizations have taken individual actions. World No-Tobacco Day is a focus for communications on tobacco and health. The Barbados Cancer Society provides smoking cessation clinics. The Barbados Association of Medical Practitioners has plans for advocacy activities in clean indoor air and smokefree air travel.

Barbados is well situated to prevent additional chronic diseases caused by tobacco through coordinated educational, regulatory, advocacy, and research programs. The small size of the country, the high literacy rate, and the relative affluence of the population provide an encouraging setting in which to prevent diseases associated with tobacco. Hypertension and diabetes, conditions worsened with tobacco use, are particularly notable health problems in Barbados. As childhood and infectious diseases are controlled in this relatively healthy nation, chronic diseases will require more attention. Smoking is the chief preventable cause of these chronic diseases, and this risk has already affected the health of Barbadians.

Based on the data presented above, the following conclusions can be drawn:

1. Few data are available on tobacco use, knowledge, attitudes, and beliefs for Barbados. Per capita consumption of cigarettes in Barbados has decreased from 1981 to 1989. Based on cigarette consumption data, the estimated adult prevalence of smoking is between 9 and 27 percent.
2. Because the per capita consumption of cigarettes is low compared with that of developed countries, Barbados is well situated to reduce the future impact of tobacco-related diseases through multisector prevention approaches.
3. Chronic noncommunicable diseases are the leading causes of death in Barbados. Health and demographic data indicate that the impact of these diseases will grow over the next few decades.
4. Effective clean indoor air legislation and policies are lacking in Barbados, and there are no restrictions on the purchase of tobacco by minors. A voluntary health warning is placed on packages of cigarettes manufactured in Barbados.
5. Nongovernmental organizations have been active in providing political leadership and smoking cessation classes in Barbados.

References

BARBADOS CENTRAL STATISTICAL OFFICE. Trade Statistics, unpublished data. 1980–1990.

CHIEF MEDICAL OFFICER. *Annual Report for the Year 1986.* Ministry of Health, Barbados, 1988.

HODGSON, T.A. Cigarette smoking and lifetime medical expenditures. *Milbank Memorial Quarterly*, 1992.

MACMILLAN. *Caribbean Certificate Atlas.* Macmillan Publishers Ltd., London, 1988.

MASSIAH, J. *Recent Trends in Mortality in Barbados, 1970–1984: A Report to PAHO.* Institute of Social and Economic Research (Eastern Caribbean) University of the West Indies, Cave Hill Barbados. December 1985.

PAN AMERICAN HEALTH ORGANIZATION. *Health Conditions in the Americas, 1990 Edition.* Pan American Health Organization, Washington, D.C., Scientific Publication No. 524, 1990.

PAN AMERICAN HEALTH ORGANIZATION. *Smoking Control—Third Subregional Workshop, Caribbean Area.* Kingston, Jamaica, December 8–11, 1987. Technical Paper No. 20. Pan American Health Organization, Washington, D.C., 1988.

THEODORE-GANDHI, B. Country Collaborator's Report, Barbados. Unpublished data, Pan American Health Organization, 1991.

UNITED NATIONS ECONOMIC COMMISSION ON LATIN AMERICA AND THE CARIBBEAN. *Selected Statistical Indicators of Caribbean Countries.* Vol. II, 1990. Subregional Headquarters for the Caribbean. Caribbean Development Co-operation Committee (CDCC), Port-of-Spain, Trinidad. Publication No. LC/CAR/G.293, March 19, 1990.

U.S. DEPARTMENT OF AGRICULTURE. Foreign Agricultural Service; Tobacco, Cotton, and Seeds Division. Unpublished tabulations, 1990.

U.S. DEPARTMENT OF HEALTH AND HUMAN SERVICES. *Reducing the Health Consequences of Smoking: 25 Years of Progress. A Report of the Surgeon General.* U.S. Department of Health and Human Services, Public Health Service, Centers for Disease Control, Center for Chronic Disease Prevention and Health Promotion, Office on Smoking and Health. DHHS Publication No. (CDC)89–8411, 1989.

WORLD BANK. *The World Bank Atlas—1989.* The World Bank, Washington, D.C., November 1989.

WORLD BANK. *World Development Report 1990—Poverty.* Oxford University Press. New York, 1990.

Belize

General Characteristics

The Tobacco Industry
    Agriculture
    Manufacturing and marketing
    Advertising and promotion
    Sales and taxes

Tobacco Use
    Total consumption data
    Behavioral surveys

Smoking and Health

Tobacco Use Prevention and Control Activities
    Public education and cessation programs
    Education in schools

Summary and Conclusions

References

General Characteristics

Belize is situated south of Mexico's Yucatan Peninsula on the Caribbean coast of Central America, and is bordered on the north by Mexico, on the west by Guatemala, and on the south and east by the Caribbean Sea. Belize gained its independence from the United Kingdom in 1981 and is now a sovereign and democratic state ruled by a parliamentary system with a Prime Minister as Head of Government. It is the only English-speaking country in Central America. Belize has an area of 23,003 km² with 280 km of coastline. The estimated 1990 population was 180,793 with an annual average growth of 2.4 percent per year over the previous decade. Thus, Belize is one of the least densely populated countries in the world, with 8 persons/ km². Forty-eight percent of the population lives in eight urban centers and 25 percent lives in Belize City. There are eight ethnic groups in the country, including Creoles (40 percent), Mestizos (33 percent), Garinagu (8 percent), Maya Mopan (7 percent), Maya Ketchi (3 percent), and smaller groups of Chinese, East Indians, and whites (Pan American Health Organization [PAHO] 1990).

In 1988, 44.5 percent of the population was under age 15, 49.8 percent was 15 to 64 years old, and 5.7 percent was 65 years and older. The large proportion of the population that is of working age (15 to 64 years) suggests that the dependency ratio will decline significantly in future decades, from 981/1,000 persons of working age in 1980 to 408 to 427 by 2015 (United Nations Economic Commission for Latin America and the Caribbean [UNECLAC] 1990b). The infant mortality rate for Belize was 19.4/1,000 live births in 1989. Overall life expectancy at birth was 70.8 in 1990 (69.9 for men and 71.8 for women) (Ministry of Health 1991), and the crude mortality rate was 4.2 in 1988 (PAHO 1990) (Table 1).

The principal economic activities in Belize are agriculture and manufacturing. The main agricultural products are sugar, citrus fruits, and bananas. Garment exports have increased in recent years. Tourism has become a major source of income, especially on the offshore islands (Keys), where exists the second largest barrier reef in the world. The per capita gross domestic product was $US1,132 in 1987, up from $US1,082 in 1982 (PAHO 1990).

The Tobacco Industry

Agriculture

There are no commercial tobacco farms in Belize. However, tobacco has been grown for many years on a small scale by Indians in the Northern and Toledo Districts. Most of this tobacco is grown for personal or local consumption, but the extent of this activity is unknown. Likewise, tobacco is not cured in Belize for commercial purposes (Cayetano 1990).

Manufacturing and Marketing

Prior to independence from the United Kingdom, tobacco was produced as part of Government-sponsored experimental agricultural programs and small commercial enterprises. These small-scale attempts sought to develop various indigenous tobaccos for blending with other tobacco types (Secretariat for British Honduras 1955). These efforts all failed.

Until recently, there was only one tobacco company in Belize, the Caribbean Tobacco Company Ltd. (CTC), which has no relationship to multinational tobacco companies. There is no Government program to support sales of tobacco. However, CTC, as well as other companies, have access to foreign exchange. In 1989, for example, the company used an estimated $US1.89 million to purchase imported goods and services related to cigarette sales and manufacturing. Most of this hard currency was spent on tobacco. At the end of

Table 1. Health and economic indicators, Belize, 1980s

Indicator	Year	Level
Population	1990	180,793
% < age 15	1988	44.5
% ≥ age 65	1988	5.7
% Urban	1990	48.0
Crude birth rate per 1,000 persons	1988	38.5
Crude mortality rate per 1,000 persons	1988	4.2
Infant mortality rate per 1,000 live births	1989	19.4
Life expectancy at birth	1990	70.8
Men		69.9
Women		71.8
Per capita gross domestic product	1987	$US1,132

Sources: PAHO, 1990; Ministry of Health, 1991; Cayetano, 1990; UNECLAC, 1990a.

1990, a new tobacco company, the National Tobacco Company, Ltd., began operations with headquarters in Belmopan (Cayetano 1990).

Information is available from the Central Statistical Office on the value of unmanufactured tobacco imports as well as cigarettes over the last 6 years (Table 2). A small amount of cigarettes is reexported to Mexico each year (4,900 kg in 1989). The most popular brands of manufactured cigarettes sold in Belize are in order Independence, Winston, Millport, Benson & Hedges, and Colonial. In addition, National Tobacco now produces two brands—National and Coral. Winston and Benson & Hedges are imported from the United States and United Kingdom, respectively; the other brands are manufactured by the CTC. Data on relative market share are not available (Cayetano 1990).

The vast majority of tobacco consumed in Belize is in the form of manufactured cigarettes. Less than 1 percent is snuff, chewing tobacco, or pipe tobacco. The only fine-cut tobacco for "roll-your-own" cigarettes in Belize is brought in by British soldiers for their own consumption.

Advertising and Promotion

Tobacco advertising is not permitted on radio but is permitted and used on television, in magazines and newspapers, on billboards and posters, and preceding movies. Most advertising is for foreign brands, with local television channels advertising foreign cigarettes at night only. The local tobacco company supports sports and cultural events, donating approximately B$3,000 per year to the Sports Council, and makes other political and corporate donations (Cayetano 1990). Distribution of free samples is also used to promote cigarettes. The distributors of Winston spend approximately B$15,000 per year on promotions and advertising. The distributors of Benson & Hedges spend B$10,000 per year on advertising. Their promotion policy is dictated by the regional office in Barbados (Cayetano 1990).

Sales and Taxes

The price of the most popular locally produced brand of cigarettes, Independence, ranges from B$1.75 to $2.00 for a pack of 20 cigarettes, compared to a price of B$2.00 for a pack of 10 imported cigarettes and B$4.00 for a pack of 20 cigarettes. Cigarettes are also sold singly by street vendors, and there are no vending machines. An illegal trade in cigarettes is active in Belize, and this trade is facilitated by the small size of the country with easy access across its international borders. The extent of this trade is difficult to determine (Cayetano 1990).

In 1987, 28 percent of the retail price of cigarettes was tax, and tobacco provided 2 percent of all national tax revenue. However, national tax revenues provided by cigarettes over the last few years declined from B$1.2 million in 1984 to B$689,000 in 1988. Because the tax per package of cigarettes (B$0.50) has not changed since 1984, a decline in the number of cigarettes sold or in the number of

Table 2. Domestic production, imports, exports, and total consumption of manufactured cigarettes (in metric tons) 1979–1988, and hard currency spent on imports of tobacco (in $US), Belize, 1984–1989

Year	Domestic production	Imports	Exports	Total consumption	Hard currency spent on imports
1979	90	20	5	170	
1980	90	20	5	170	
1981	90	20	5	170	
1982	90	20	5	170	
1983	90	20	5	170	
1984	90	20	5	170	$648,000
1985	100	20	5	175	702,000
1986	100	20	5	175	651,000
1987	100	20	5	175	770,000
1988	100	21	5	175	568,000
1989	116	49		191	637,000

Sources: Cayetano, 1990; USDA, 1990.

cigarettes taxed has occurred in Belize (Cayetano 1990).

The average industrial wage in Belize is B$3.00/hr. Salaried Government employees work 39.5 hr/week, whereas other employees work 40 hr. Wage labor is 45 to 48 hr/week. Thus, an average worker who smoked one pack of locally made cigarettes per day in Belize would spend approximately 40 minutes each day working to support his addiction to tobacco (Cayetano 1990).

Tobacco Use

Total Consumption Data

Varying estimates of population sizes aged 15 years and older preclude accurate estimates of yearly adult per capita cigarette consumption in Belize. However, according to U.S. Department of Agriculture data (U.S. Department of Agriculture 1990), total domestic cigarette consumption increased from 170 MT in 1979 to 175 MT in 1988. Of this total, 100 MT are domestically produced cigarettes. Based on these data, the adult (aged 15 years or older) per capita cigarette consumption in Belize was 1,744 in 1988.

Behavioral Surveys

Data on tobacco use are available for school-aged children from surveys conducted in 1986 and 1989 (Adams 1986; Comstock 1989). The surveys were sponsored by the Parents Resource Institute for Drug Education (PRIDE/Belize) which is funded by the U.S. Agency for International Development. The surveys sampled students in Standards 4 through 6 (aged 10 to 13 years), Forms 1 through 4 (13 to 17 years) and Forms 5 and 6 (16 to 19 years). The PRIDE/Belize questionnaire was based on a similar PRIDE questionnaire used in the United States, but included modifications to reflect specific conditions in Belize. The 1986 survey used a simple random sample of all schools in the country. Approximately 85 percent of the target population (13,000) was surveyed. Of these, 12,500 (96 percent) of the questionnaires were usable. The final sample included 5,800 males and 6,300 females aged 10 to 19 years. Information on tobacco use as well as use of alcohol, cocaine, marijuana, and other drugs was ascertained.

In 1989, 17.9 percent of students overall used tobacco at least occasionally. Most were "light" smokers (1 to 6 times per year) (Table 3). A comparison of results on tobacco use from the 1986 PRIDE survey with the 1989 PRIDE survey suggests that an increasing number of students experimented with cigarettes between 1986 and 1989. Some of the differences between the class groups seen during the period 1986 to 1989 may be attributable to a cohort effect.

Table 3. Prevalence (%) of cigarette smoking by grade level and frequency of smoking, Belize, 1986 and 1989

Year and grade level	Reported cigarette smoking				
	No use	Total use	Light	Moderate	Heavy
Standard 4–6					
1986	90.8	9.2	6.6	1.3	1.3
1989	87.1	12.9	9.3	1.6	2.0
Form 1–4					
1986	76.2	23.8	14.1	4.5	5.2
1989	75.2	24.8	15.2	4.1	5.5
Form 5–6					
1986	62.7	37.3	12.1	6.0	19.2
1989	74.6	25.4	17.0	1.8	6.6
Total					
1986	88.7	11.8	7.5	2.6	1.7
1989	82.1	17.9	11.8	2.6	3.5

Sources: Adams, 1986; Comstock, 1990.
Light = 1–6 times per year.
Moderate = 1–2 times a month.
Heavy = 1–3 times a week or daily.

Smoking and Health

The quality of mortality data in Belize is reasonably good, with 85 to 90 percent of all deaths registered and 98 percent of these certified by a physician. Only 5.9 percent of all deaths in Belize were classified as due to "symptoms and ill-defined causes" (ICD 780–799) in 1988. However, the percentage of deaths from ill-defined causes among persons aged 35 years and older is twice as high at 12 percent, suggesting that the quality of mortality data is not as good as for persons dying at older ages.

Data are insufficient to analyze trends over time in the evolution of smoking-related morbidity and mortality. However, in 1987, there were seven deaths from lung cancer (six men and one woman). Coronary heart disease and respiratory diseases, which may be smoking-related conditions, ranked among the five leading causes of death in Belize for the years 1985 to 1987. Heart and lung disease also ranked fifth in 1987 as a cause of admission to hospital and seventh in 1988 (PAHO 1990; Cayetano 1990).

Tobacco Use Prevention and Control Activities

The National Drug Abuse Advisory Council was commissioned in 1988. The Council is currently assigned to the portfolio of the Ministry of Home Affairs with participation of many other branches of the Government as well as other private sector and nongovernmental agencies. The Council's broad objectives are to educate the public about the dangers of drug abuse and to prevent the indiscriminate use of drugs. The main focus of the Council's activities is related to illicit drugs, but the reduction of tobacco use is also addressed as part of its wider mandate. Otherwise, no officially sanctioned antitobacco activities are sustained in Belize (Cayetano 1990).

Belize has no laws pertaining to tobacco control and none are proposed. Neither is there an active lobby to promote laws or policy regarding tobacco use or tobacco trade. In practice, however, there are many restrictions on cigarette smoking. All health care institutions have unwritten restrictions on smoking within their buildings. Smoking is prohibited in cinemas and confined to the front area of buses. Many buses display "No Smoking" signs. Some private worksites have "No Smoking" signs, but the enforcement of these restrictions is unknown. Smoking is not allowed in classrooms. No restrictions on smoking are reported for restaurants, and only voluntary restrictions are operative in Government buildings (Cayetano 1990).

Health warnings are placed on locally manufactured cigarettes and read "Cigarette smoking may be harmful to your health." Apparently, this warning is not mandated by law, but is applied independently by the local tobacco company (Cayetano 1990).

Public Education and Cessation Programs

There are no smoking cessation programs available in Belize, but a variety of educational programming exists against tobacco use on television and radio. Antismoking messages are shown on cable television broadcasts originating in the United States. Antismoking messages are broadcast on local radio and television on an irregular basis (Cayetano 1990).

The Belize Drug Abuse Advisory Council and PRIDE/Belize recently have developed antidrug pamphlets as well as antitobacco pamphlets. The Medical and Dental Association has begun campaigning against smoking and in 1989 spearheaded an antismoking campaign that included panel discussions on local television and the distribution of antismoking bumper stickers (Cayetano 1990).

Education in Schools

PRIDE/Belize and the Curriculum Development Unit of the Ministry of Education have developed a School Health Education Program during which children are taught the dangers of tobacco, alcohol, and drug use. The curriculum is aimed at developing values and skills that will help children avoid substance abuse (Cayetano 1990). Three levels of materials have been developed: for young children, juniors, and seniors.

Summary and Conclusions

Tobacco prevention and control activities in Belize are limited, although there is spillover from the United States through messages on cable television. The National Drug Abuse Advisory Council has as part of its wider mission the prevention of tobacco use, but this organization has concentrated more heavily on illicit drugs than on tobacco. The School Health Education Program, which has had input from the United Nations (UNICEF), may provide most antitobacco efforts among young persons in the future.

Data are quite limited on tobacco use and per capita consumption in Belize, as are mortality and morbidity data on tobacco-related diseases. However, the 1988 adult per capita cigarette consumption level in Belize is similar to that of most other countries in Central America. Total cigarette consumption has not declined in recent years, and the reported illegal trade in cigarettes may in fact mean that consumption has increased. Behavioral surveys of adults would help clarify current tobacco use patterns in Belize.

Based on the data presented above, the following conclusions can be made:

1. Continuing health promotion activities targeted at children and young adults in Belize encompass education on tobacco use as part of broad drug abuse prevention programs.
2. Surveillance to monitor the prevalence of tobacco use in Belize will be necessary to evaluate the impact of education programs.
3. An active multidisciplinary, multiministerial approach is needed at the national level to address legislative and policy issues related to tobacco in Belize.

References

ADAMS, R. Report on PRIDE/Belize Survey 1986, unpublished manuscript. 1986.

CAYETANO, M. Country Collaborator's Report, Belize. Unpublished data, Pan American Health Organization. 1990.

COMSTOCK, M. *Drug Awareness Household Survey Final Report.* Drug Awareness Education Project, PRIDE/Belize, 1989.

MINISTRY OF HEALTH. *Health Activities in Belize.* MOH-PAHO-WHO Newsletter No. 6, May 1991.

PAN AMERICAN HEALTH ORGANIZATION. *Health Conditions in the Americas, 1990 Edition.* Scientific Publication No. 524. Pan American Health Organization, Washington, D.C. 1990.

SECRETARIAT FOR BRITISH HONDURAS. *Tobacco Production in British Honduras.* Commodity Series Paper No. 8, File No. 118, August 1955.

UNITED NATIONS ECONOMIC COMMISSION FOR LATIN AMERICA AND THE CARIBBEAN. *Selected Statistical Indicators of Caribbean Countries.* LC/CAR/G.293, Vol. 11, 1990a.

UNITED NATIONS ECONOMIC COMMISSION FOR LATIN AMERICA AND THE CARIBBEAN. *Population Projections for Eight Caribbean Countries 1980–2015.* LC/CAR/G.311, 1990b.

U.S. DEPARTMENT OF AGRICULTURE. Tobacco, Cotton, and Seeds Division. Foreign Agricultural Service (unpublished tabulations), April 1990.

Bolivia

General Characteristics

The Tobacco Industry
    Agriculture
    Manufacturing
    Marketing

Tobacco Use
    Consumption
    Behavioral surveys
    Prevalence of smoking among adults
    Prevalence of smoking among adolescents
    Smoking among physicians
    Other uses of tobacco
    Attitudes, knowledge, and opinions about smoking

Smoking and Health
    Mortality
    Morbidity

Tobacco Use Prevention and Control Activities
    Government actions
        Policies and executive structure
        Legislation
        School-based antismoking education
        Public information campaigns
        Taxes
    Nongovernmental activities

Conclusions

References

General Characteristics

Bolivia is one of the poorest countries in Latin America. Since 1981, negative growth in the gross domestic product (GDP) has been reported, while the external debt increased between 1985 and 1987 by $US643 million to total $US3.93 billion (PAHO 1990). The population density is only 5.1 inhabitants per km². Of the estimated 1988 population (6.9 million), 48.9 percent are rural and largely indigenous or mestizo. The social and economic development differences between rural and urban areas are enormous, with 50 percent of the population receiving only 17 percent of total national income. This poverty is reflected in a life expectancy at birth of 53 years, an infant mortality rate of 108/1,000 live births, a literacy rate for the population of 46.0 percent, and a legal minimum wage in 1987 of $US24 a month. In 1988, the per capita gross national product (GNP) was only $US570 (Table 1). There has been a gradual trend toward urbanization, and it is estimated that by the year 2000, 56 percent of the population will live in cities.

Bolivia's principal sources of foreign exchange are oil and coal, followed by minerals such as copper. As in Peru and Colombia, coca production, spurred by a growing international drug trade, has led to an increase in black market foreign exchange. A democratic form of Government was established after several violent political takeovers. In 1985, highly unpopular anti-inflationary measures threatened major social disruption. Health expenditures declined from 9.7 percent of total public spending in 1984 to 5.2 percent in 1986. In 1984, 92.2 percent of health funding came from the national treasury, but by 1988 only 50.1 percent was from that source. A substantial proportion (27.8 percent) derived from foreign aid.

Tobacco use prevention and control activities have been remarkably visible in the face of these difficult conditions. Individual and organizational strength in the public health sector have enabled these activities.

Tobacco Industry

Agriculture

The total land area planted in tobacco in Bolivia has declined sharply to 24,000 ha in 1988, representing less than one percent of the country's total arable land (2,335,000 ha) (Chapman and Leng 1990). The principal tobacco-growing areas are in eastern Bolivia, and their dwindling size can be largely explained by two phenomena. First, increased planting of highly profitable coca was reported during the 1980s (Ríos-Dalenz 1989); in fact, coca leaf was the fastest growing agricultural product of the decade (Ministry of Social Services and Public Health 1989). Second, there has been an increase in imports of contraband cigarettes since 1979; this illegal trade reduced national cigarette production and subsequently reduced demand for locally grown leaf tobacco (El Diario 1986; Misdorp 1990).

The principal tobacco-producing department, Santa Cruz, accounts for 65 to 75 percent of total production. The Corporación Cruceña de Desarrollo (Santa Cruz Development Corporation—CORDECRUZ) is a semipublic entity that acts as the purchasing and sales agent for the tobacco growers and the manufacturing industry. CORDECRUZ supports agricultural research in *tabaco rubio*, although at present, most tobacco grown is *tabaco negro*.

Despite the fact that Bolivia is a predominantly rural country, the economic importance of minerals has shifted employment to mining. Even so, in 1985, 500,000 persons were engaged in agriculture; approximately 600 (0.1 percent) of these grew tobacco (Instituto Nacional de Estadísticas 1985). In addition, corn is planted during the 6 months needed to recover from tobacco. In this

Table 1. Health and economic indicators, Bolivia, 1980s

Indicator	Year	Value
Population	1988	6,900,000
Percent urban	1988	51.1
Percent < 15 years	1988	43.9
Percent ≥ 65 years	1988	3.2
Adult literacy rate (%)	1985	46
Life expectancy at birth	1988	53
Infant mortality rate per 1000 live births	1988	108
Crude mortality rate per 1000 persons	1988	14
Total fertility rate (per 1000 women)	1988	6.0
Per capita gross national product ($US)	1988	570

Source: World Bank, 1990.

way tobacco farmers diversify their activity and their land use.

According to the Ministry of Agriculture and Livestock, tobacco production has declined since 1980 (Table 2). However, data from the U.S. Department of Agriculture (USDA) indicate that production has been stable since 1979. It is likely that raw tobacco production decreased because of the previously mentioned economic decline, the decline in the cigarette market, and the reduction in land planted with tobacco. Tobacco exports were not important in the Bolivian tobacco sector (Table 2).

According to tobacco industry sources Bolivia imports approximately 800 MT of tobacco annually, mainly from the United States and Brazil (Chapman and Leng 1990). The tax on imported leaf tobacco is 17 percent, excepting tobacco from Brazil, which is subject only to an 8 percent ad valorem tax. The data on imports reported by the USDA (Table 2) are lower than those provided by the tobacco industry for the last few years. Moreover, the USDA reports that the ad valorem tax is only 10 percent on imports (USDA 1989). It is possible that the USDA information covers only trade with the United States.

Table 2. Domestic production (in metric tons), imports, exports, and total domestic consumption of leaf tobacco, Bolivia, 1960–1989

Year	Raw tobacco 1	Raw tobacco 2	Imports 1	Exports 1	Exports 2	Total domestic consumption 1
1960	800		322	0		900
1961	800		355	0		942
1962	875		363	0		912
1963	896		379	0		992
1964	900		359	0		1,084
1965	836		400	0		1,164
1966	1,144		421	0		1,200
1967	1,398		458	0		1,632
1968	1,608		533	0		1,884
1969	2,011		415	0		2,099
1970	2,146		539	0		2,337
1971	2,280		494	0		2,423
1972	2,350		617	0		2,524
1973	2,392		600	0		2,625
1974	2,970		700	0		2,730
1975	2,569		800	0		2,840
1976	2,230		800	0		2,955
1977	2,270		1,000	0		2,900
1978	1,700		1,000	0		2,400
1979	1,600		1,000	0		2,400
1980	1,800	1,825	1,000	0		2,400
1981	1,800	1,395	1,000	0	45	2,500
1982	2,000	1,105	1,000	0		2,300
1983	1,250	1,179	557	0	4	1,660
1984	1,250	1,126	107	0		1,316
1985	1,250	975	205	0		1,405
1986	1,250	840	157	0		1,357
1987	1,250	890	227	0		1,327
1988	1,250	950	250	0		1,350
1989	1,250		250	0		1,350

Sources: 1. USDA, 1990.
2. Ministry of Agriculture, Department of Statistics, 1990.

Manufacturing

The Compañía Industrial de Tabacos (CIT), a private monopoly, has been in operation since 1934. Other companies operating as licensees of British-American Tobacco (BAT) and Liggett and Myers have tried to enter the Bolivian market, but these efforts have been short-lived because of "expulsions for political or economic reasons" (Misdorp 1990). CIT is a concessionaire of Philip Morris International and Massalin Particulares (Philip Morris Argentina). Its main cigarette factory is in La Paz, with a second in Santa Cruz. The company also produces filtered cigarettes for export. In 1983, cigarettes represented only 2.6 percent of all manufacturing output (Instituto Nacional de Estadísticas 1985).

Cigarette production data reported by USDA (Table 3) show a progressive increase in production through 1976, followed by a gradual decline that levels off in the 1980s. This report differs from all others available since 1973 (El Diario 1986; Maxwell 1989; Instituto Nacional de Estadísticas 1985) that indicate that cigarette production held steady at around 1 billion units a year until 1981, when it began a steep 3–year descent to 368 million units. There appears to have been a gradual recovery in production beginning in 1985. This agrees with the situation described above for agricultural production: during the 1980s production was undermined by a massive influx of contraband cigarettes at prices lower than those produced locally. In addition, Bolivia's weak economy from 1982 to 1986 caused a lack of foreign currency necessary for the importation of the *tabaco rubio* needed for modern cigarette production.

These discrepancies in reported production and consumption are important to consider in attempting to ascertain the population's exposure to tobacco. Consumption levels are quite different depending on which set of production data is used and whether or not contraband cigarettes are included in the calculations.

The Bolivian tobacco industry produces about 20 brands of cigarettes; while some are national brands, most are produced under license to transnational corporations. Bolivia has never exported cigarettes, and since 1969 there has been no record of legal cigarette imports (Table 2). However, since 1978 contraband cigarettes have been imported mainly from neighboring countries, principally Argentina, Brazil, and Chile. At the same time that national production declined, imports of contraband cigarettes increased from 180 million units in 1978 to 1.72 billion in 1984, the year of lowest national production in recent history (El Diario 1986). In 1990, contraband cigarettes accounted for 40 to 50 percent of the total Bolivian cigarette market. However, in 1985 contraband cigarettes represented 75 percent of the domestic market. Information about contraband cigarettes is available only from an unsubstantiated report in a daily newspaper (El Diario 1986). The local industry, whose interests are threatened by contraband cigarettes, may tend to exaggerate the problem to invoke Government action. A thriving black market in cigarettes raises the specter of losses of foreign currency and tax revenues as well as jobs.

Marketing

Cigarette advertising has been prohibited since September 1988 in "audiovisual media" airing before 9:00 p.m. However, it is not clear whether this prohibition includes radio or is limited only to television advertising. Cigarette advertising in all mass media is also regulated so that it does not encourage smoking or show people in the act of smoking. It seems that advertising of cigarettes in a monopolistic market is moot in terms of the well-stated intent of tobacco companies to use advertising to encourage consumers only to switch brands. However, the illegal trade in cigarettes as well as the need to recruit new young smokers apparently encourages advertising of cigarettes in Bolivia. Cigarette trademarks are commonly evident at sports events such as soccer matches.

Tobacco Use

Consumption

According to an 1982 International Agency for Research on Cancer (IARC) report on smoking and cancer in 110 countries, Bolivia ranked 96th in the per capita consumption of cigarettes (206 per person aged 15 and older) among cited countries of the Americas (World Health Organization 1986). This figure differs from those derived from USDA data and CELADE population estimates in Table 3. If estimated contraband cigarettes are included in the consumption totals, per capita consumption rises to 550 cigarettes in 1982; using USDA data alone (excluding contraband estimates), per capita cigarette consumption was 348.

Including contraband consumption estimates, the data suggest that there has been a steady and alarming rise in per capita cigarette consumption since 1968: between 1973 and 1985, per capita consumption increased 73 percent. However, using USDA data alone, per capita consumption decreased 23 percent between 1970 and 1988; this decline in consumption may be accounted for by the economic recession of the 1980s. It is much more likely that per capita cigarette consumption in-

creased with increased purchases of cheap contraband cigarettes during times of economic recession. It is clear that the illegal cigarette trade poses a major health hazard to Bolivians through easier access to cigarettes.

Consumption preferences have shifted from *tabaco negro* to filtered *tabaco rubio* cigarettes, al-

Table 3. Production, imports, contraband, total domestic consumption[1], and per capita consumption[2] of manufactured cigarettes, Bolivia, 1960 to 1989

Year	USDA*				Other sources**			
	Production[3]	Imports[3]	Total domestic consumption[3]	Per capita consumption[4]	Production[3]	Contraband[3]	Total domestic consumption[3]	Per capita consumption[4]
1960	449	50	499	255				
1961	471	60	531	265				
1962	456	53	509	248				
1963	496	67	563	268				
1964	542	73	615	286				
1965	582	50	632	288				
1966	600	37	637	283				
1967	612	20	632	275				
1968	710	10	720	306				
1969	805	3	808	335				
1970	900	0	900	365				
1971	1,000	0	1,000	396				
1972	1,125	0	1,125	435				
1973	1,250	0	1,250	471	900	0	900	339
1974	1,375	0	1,375	506	1,000	0	1,000	368
1975	1,500	0	1,500	539	1,120	0	1,120	402
1976	1,650	0	1,650	578	1,150	0	1,150	403
1977	1,336	0	1,336	457	1,320	0	1,320	451
1978	1,400	0	1,400	467	1,300	180	1,480	494
1979	1,260	15	1,275	415	1,281	340	1,621	527
1980	1,265	0	1,265	402	1,263	520	1,783	566
1981	1,155	0	1,155	357	1,162	700	1,862	576
1982	1,555	0	1,155	348	624	1,200	1,824	550
1983	1,200	0	1,200	353	628	1,380	2,008	590
1984	1,200	0	1,200	344	368	1,720	2,088	598
1985	1,200	0	1,200	335	520	1,580	2,100	586
1986	1,200	0	1,200	326	800	554	1,354	368
1987	1,200	0	1,200	317	900	623	1,523	403
1988	1,200	0	1,200	309	1,000	692	1,692	453

Sources: * United States Department of Agriculture.

**Production 1973 to 1978, and contraband, 1973 to 1985 from El Diario 1986; production 1979 to 1985 from Instituto Nacional de Estadística de Bolivia; production 1986 to 1988 from Maxwell 1989; estimated contraband, 1986 to 1988 based on the assumption that 45 percent of cigarettes consumed in Bolivia are illegal.

[1]There are no exports of manufactured cigarettes.
[2]Age ≥ 15 years (population figures from CELADE 1990).
[3]Metric tons.
[4]Cigarette/person/year.

though 16.6 percent of the domestic cigarettes were unfiltered and 35 percent were made with *tabaco negro* (Maxwell 1989). It appears that all contraband cigarettes are filtered and made with *tabaco rubio*. Cigarettes are sold only in packs of 20, and there are no vending machines in Bolivia.

From 1981 to 1983 the World Health Organization and the Addiction Research Center of Canada analyzed the nicotine, tar, and carbon monoxide yields for 50 brands of cigarettes smoked in developing countries. The study included eight brands from Bolivia, five imported and three domestic. The nicotine yield of the well-known international brands ranged from 0.9 to 1.1 mg, while the most widely sold domestic brand yielded 0.9 mg. However, the tar yield of the international brands, which held only a small proportion of the Bolivian market, was between 11.1 and 16.6 mg, and the yield in the domestic brand was 18.1 mg. Carbon monoxide ranged from 11.1 to 17.5 mg in the international brands but was 20 mg in the domestic brand.

The average cost of a pack of cigarettes in 1990 was $US0.32. Thus, a person who smoked one pack a day would have spent $US10 per month on cigarettes, or 30 percent of the minimum wage ($US30 in 1990).

Behavioral Surveys

In 1983, the Fundación Boliviana de Lucha Contra el Cáncer (FBLC) (Bolivian Anti-Cancer Foundation) selected a sample of 2,263 persons in the following social strata: 802 business employees, 1,074 high school students, 160 university students, and 227 housewives. A final sample of 963 adults in La Paz were surveyed, although it is not clear how this group was selected. As may be inferred from the demographic distribution of the survey population, this study is not representative of the entire population of La Paz. This survey also does not represent the 20 percent unemployed and informally employed persons in La Paz, but simply reports tobacco use among a subgroup of largely male middle- to upper-middle-class young adults (De Osorovic and Pereira 1983).

In 1986 the Department of Mental Health in the Bolivian Ministry of Social Welfare and Public Health conducted a survey of 1,058 adults in the urban area of La Paz, 1,060 in the rural areas surrounding La Paz, and 1,745 in the city of Sucre (De la Quintana 1987; PAHO 1987). Although the methodology used for sample selection is unclear, the results of this survey for La Paz may be comparable to those of the 1983 FBLC study. The 1986 survey suffers from some of the same problems of representation as does the 1983 survey in La Paz.

Both the 1983 FBLC survey and the 1986 Ministry of Social Welfare and Public Health survey included students aged 13 to 18 years who were enrolled in private and public secondary schools in La Paz. In 1983, 754 adolescents and young people were surveyed with a response rate of 93.8 percent. In 1986, 1,359 adolescents and young people were surveyed. The 1989 National Education and Housing Survey estimated the rate of school nonattendance among the 5- to 19-year age group at 38.5 percent in the urban area. Thus, these surveys cover only the population of young people and adolescents who attend school and are still enrolled after they complete elementary school.

In 1983, the Liga Tarijeña de Lucha Contra el Cancer (Tarija Anti-Cancer League) conducted several surveys on smoking behavior among 120 students in four educational institutions (average age, 18 years) in the city of Tarija.

In 1987, De Osorovic and Ríos-Dalenz conducted a survey among hospital physicians in La Paz to determine the prevalence of smoking as a function of their knowledge and attitudes about smoking. The total sample was 154 physicians, but the response rate for this survey was only 47 percent.

Between 1979 and 1980, the Consejo de Lucha Contra el Narcotráfico (Council Against Drug Traffic) conducted a survey on the prevalence of drug use among young persons receiving institutional education; the results of this survey have not been published. A total of 18,956 young persons between the ages of 14 and 22 were surveyed. Tobacco use per se was not investigated, but the survey did find tobacco being used in combination with coca paste (cocaine sulfate).

Prevalence of Smoking among Adults

In the 1983 FBLC survey, 70.7 percent of the 945 persons who responded to the question, "Have you smoked in the last six months?" answered in the affirmative; of these, 40.8 percent of the men and 31.7 percent of women smoked daily; 36.7 percent of men and 32.9 of women said they smoked occasionally. The ratio of male to female smokers was 1:4. The FBLC did not publish data on persons who had "smoked at some time" (ever smoking).

Persons with higher levels of education had higher prevalences of smoking than did persons with lower educational attainment (Table 4). How-

Table 4. Prevalence (percent) of daily smoking in the last six months by level of schooling, La Paz, 1983

Years of schooling	Daily smokers		Total
	n	Prevalence	n
Up to 5 years	11	20.0	55
6 to 11 years	26	25.5	102
12 or more years	310	38.4	806
Total	347	36.0	963

Source: Fundación Boliviana de Lucha Contra el Cancer, 1983.

ever, the survey sample is biased toward more persons with higher educational levels, as evidenced by the size of the samples for each educational level. It can be assumed that the variation in actual prevalence in the sample at lower levels of schooling is greater than at the higher levels. Of daily smokers, 59 percent smoked fewer than 10 cigarettes a day, 29 percent smoked 10 to 20 cigarettes per day, and 12 percent smoked more than 20 cigarettes per day.

The 1986 Ministry of Social Forecasting and Public Health survey conducted in urban La Paz, with results comparable to those of the 1983 FBLC survey, found that 38.3 percent of respondents smoked daily (46 percent among men and 28.6 percent among women). An additional 35.7 percent smoked occasionally (37.8 percent among men and 33 percent among women). The prevalence of daily smoking was slightly higher on the 1986 survey than on the 1983 survey, more so among men, but the percentage of daily smokers apparently declined somewhat among women.

Of the 1,060 persons surveyed in the rural area around La Paz in 1986, only 5.6 percent smoked daily (6.4 percent among men and 3.3 percent among women), while 47.7 percent smoked occasionally. With regard to occasional smoking, the author noted that this generally involves traditional forms of tobacco used in indigenous ceremonies and thus does not constitute addictive use. Of particular note is the large difference observed between the urban and rural areas, which reflects the enormous differences between these two cultures in Bolivia. These differences also suggest that the 1983 and 1986 surveys overestimated the prevalence of smoking in urban La Paz because the population surveyed is biased toward higher social

strata. The smoking prevalence among the marginal and informal sectors probably falls between the rates for urban La Paz and the rural area.

In Sucre, a city of approximately 85,000 inhabitants in southeast Bolivia where 1,723 persons were surveyed, the prevalence of daily smoking was found to be 28.4 percent (34.5 percent among men and 18.2 percent among women) and of occasional smoking, 41 percent. This survey reported a higher prevalence of occasional smokers and a lower prevalence of daily smokers than in urban La Paz both among men and women. In addition, smoking prevalence by occupation was ascertained on this survey (Table 5). Although sample sizes were small, the prevalence of daily smoking over the 6 months prior to the survey was generally in the mid-30–percent range for most employees.

Prevalence of Smoking among Adolescents

The 1983 FBLC survey found that 8.7 percent of 707 respondents were daily smokers at the time of the survey (10.5 percent of males and 7.5 percent of females) and that 35 percent smoked occasionally (41 percent of males and 25.9 percent of females). The absolute difference between adolescent males and females who were daily smokers was 34 percentage points, while in occasional smokers that difference was 15.1 percentage points. Among the adults in this same survey, the greatest differences between the sexes were in daily smoking. It appears as though more males than

Table 5. Prevalence (percent) of daily smoking in the last six months, by occupation, Sucre-Chiquisaca, 1986

Occupation	Daily smokers		Total
	n	%	n
Retail	13	48.0	27
Professional	63	36.4	173
Administrator/ managers	6	36.3	22
Craftsmen	36	36.0	100
Office workers	132	35.6	370
Transport workers	16	32.0	50
Workmen and laborers	14	31.0	45
Personal services	14	22.0	63
Not specified	46	26.9	178
Total	340	33.0	1,028

Source: PAHO, 1987.

females progress from occasional smoking (adolescent experimentation) to daily smoking. As expected, the prevalence of daily smoking increases with age, from 1 percent among those less than age 13, to 7 percent among 15-year-olds, 16 percent among 16-year-olds, and 21 percent among 18-year-olds. The same phenomenon occurs with occasional smokers: 17 percent of those less than age 13, 37 percent of 15-year-olds, and 54 percent of 18-year-olds.

Of the adolescents surveyed, 401 attended private schools and 306 attended public schools. Of those enrolled in private schools, 14.5 percent were daily smokers compared with only 2.6 percent of public school students. Among occasional smokers, however, there was little difference: 34.7 percent of the private school students vs. 35.6 percent of public school students. Eighty-nine percent of the young daily smokers smoked fewer than 10 cigarettes a day.

In the 1986 survey of adolescents and young people in La Paz, the only reported results are for those who had "smoked at some time" (72 males and 61 females). Four percent of those under the age of 14 had smoked, while 56 percent of 15- to 17-year-olds and 40 percent of 18- to 20-year-olds had ever smoked. It is likely that the 15- to 17-year age group represents the peak ages for experimentation with cigarettes. The 1983 survey in Tarija reported that 8.3 percent of 120 respondents smoked daily, while 55.1 percent were occasional smokers; only one smoker smoked more than 10 cigarettes a day.

Smoking among Physicians

Although the sample of physicians in the study by De Osorovic and Ríos-Dalenz (1987) was not representative, the responses do suggest a major problem among physicians in La Paz. Of the 72 respondents, 34.7 percent smoked daily and 16.7 percent smoked occasionally. Overall, 93 percent of the physicians surveyed had "smoked at some time." It is difficult to draw any conclusions from this survey because of the low response rate (47 percent), however.

Other Uses of Tobacco

In the 1979–1980 survey of drug use among persons aged 14 to 22 years in nine Bolivian cities, 3.1 percent of respondents had smoked a mixture of tobacco and coca paste called "pitillo." It is important to note that the tobacco smoking is still strongly linked to Bolivia's indigenous traditions.

A large percentage of the population smokes during traditional celebrations, which explains the high rates of occasional smoking observed, especially among men. To bring good luck, cigarettes are lighted and placed in the mouth of an "ekeko"—a symbolic figure that protects the family. This statue has a tube in its mouth and "smokes" when a lighted cigarette is placed at the end of it. This ritual is performed at the beginning of each year so that throughout that year the family will enjoy good luck.

Attitudes, Knowledge, and Opinions about Smoking

The 1983 FBLC survey asked about knowledge of the health effects of cigarettes only among the 344 daily smokers. Of these, 67 percent considered smoking to be "hazardous," 16 percent thought that cigarettes were "very hazardous," 13 percent thought cigarettes were "harmless," and 3 percent considered cigarettes to be "beneficial." These results were similar among both men and women. Nearly half the daily smokers (46 percent) had tried to stop smoking, which corresponds closely to the proportion believing that it is dangerous for their health. This group was also asked if, given the choice to be smokers or nonsmokers at this point in their lives, they would take up smoking. Of these, 58 percent responded that they would have preferred not to get started. When they were asked whether or not they would smoke in the future, 7 percent responded that they would not, 35 percent said that they would be cutting back, 28 percent answered that they would probably stop smoking, and only 28 percent said that they would continue to smoke.

In the physicians' survey of 1987, almost all the respondents (88 percent) agreed that smoking is bad for one's health, but only half of them routinely questioned their patients about their smoking. Only pregnant women and patients with clinical respiratory or cardiovascular disease or peptic ulcer were warned to give up smoking.

In the 1983 Tarija survey, 43.3 percent of respondents said that smoking is "very dangerous," 52.6 said it was "harmful," and 4.1 percent said it was "harmless"; none of the respondents said that cigarettes were "beneficial." While 65 percent of the daily or occasional smokers considered cigarettes to be "harmful," 65 percent of the nonsmokers felt that they were "very hazardous," and none of this group rated cigarettes as "harmless." When asked if they thought that they would continue smoking in the future, 20 percent of the daily smokers, 57 percent of the occasional smokers, and 78 percent of the nonsmokers answered "no" or "probably not."

In the 1983 FBLC survey in La Paz, when young adult and adolescent daily or occasional smokers were asked if they thought they would still be smoking at age 21, 78 percent of the daily smokers and 39 percent of the occasional smokers answered "yes" or "probably."

Results from these two surveys suggest that there is more awareness of the harmful effects of cigarettes on health among adolescents than among adults. Although many of the adolescent occasional smokers, particularly males, will become daily smokers, it is clear that not all are aware of the addictive nature of cigarettes.

Smoking and Health

Mortality

The most recent data available on overall mortality by cause of death are for 1980 and 1981; only proportional mortality by cause was published for those years (PAHO 1990) (Table 6). Given that 70 percent of deaths are unreported, it is likely that the apparent mortality structure during 1980 and 1981 is biased toward the urban population and that a large number of deaths that were not certified by a physician were registered as "heart dis-

Table 6. Proportionate mortality for defined causes (registered deaths), Bolivia, 1980–1981

Cause and ICD code	Proportion (percent)
All infections (001–139, 464–487, 320–322)	36.4
Cardiovascular disease (390–459)	19.5
Accidents and adverse effects of violence (E800–E999)	9.8
Conditions originating in the perinatal period (760–779)	7.4
Malignant tumors (140–239)	4.0
Other causes	22.9

Source: PAHO, 1990.

eases." Even so, infectious diseases rank high, while the proportion of neoplasms is low; the most common neoplasms are those of the female genital system. No data are available that permit trend analyses or the assessment of changes in mortality structure due to urbanization.

Bolivia has 11,077 hospital beds, with 70 percent of these located in the country's four most developed departments. Hospital mortality statistics available for 1970, 1979, 1982, and 1987 shed some light on possible changes in the structure of Bolivian mortality (Table 7). Deaths due to respiratory disease and tuberculosis are remarkable for 1987, and there was an increase in intestinal infections throughout the period. In addition, trauma has become more important as a cause of hospital death. The total absence of malignant neoplasms during 1970 to 1987 suggests that these causes of death still are not common, whereas diseases of the circulatory system are. According to data from the La Paz cancer registry, the incidence of malignant neoplasms is low in this population; among men it is the lowest of all cities that have cancer registries in the Americas. The impact of high rates of smoking on cancer incidence in Bolivia has not yet become evident.

Morbidity

The principal source of information on the incidence of cancer in Bolivia is the cancer registry in La Paz. This registry was established in 1978 and is considered to have acceptable coverage, especially in the population under age 64. Cancer incidence was reported to be one of the lowest in the world among men, but was quite high among women due to the high rates of cervical cancer (PAHO 1990). For cancer of the trachea, bronchi, and lung, the rate was 2.32/100,000 men and 1.25/100,000 women between 1978 and 1982; 10 years later, in 1988 and 1989, these rates were 2.35 in men and 1.0 in women. This is noteworthy in view of the increase in the rate for all cancer sites in this registry (from 42.3/100,000 to 46.6/100,000 in men, and from 86.3/100,000 to 92.8/100,000 in women) during these same periods. However, the per capita cigarette consumption among adults doubled between 1960 and 1975 in Bolivia, and a significant portion of this increase must have been concentrated in the city of La Paz. Thus, the under-reporting or misdiagnosis of lung cancer must be extensive; it is likely that the high incidence of pulmonary tuberculosis confounds the diagnosis of lung cancer. Still, there may be other confounders observed in

Table 7. Hospital mortality rates per 1,000 discharges, by 10 leading causes, Bolivia, 1970, 1979, 1982, 1987

Causes	1970		1979		1982		1987	
	Deaths	Rate	Deaths	Rate	Deaths	Rate	Deaths	Rate
Tuberculosis	224	4.8	250	2.4	132	1.2	297	3.8
Other pneumonias	154	3.3	254	2.4	156	1.4		
Circulatory disease and other heart disease	114	2.5	261	2.5	120	1.1	1,249	16.2
Vitamin deficiency and other nutritional disorders	89	1.9	119	1.1	131	1.2		
Intestinal infections	80	1.7	301	2.8	379	3.4	381	4.9
Other digestive tract diseases	78	1.7	104	1.0	238	2.2		
Intestinal obstruction and hernia	53	1.1						
Head injury	49	1.0	144	1.3	260	2.4	246	3.2
Meningitis	42	0.9	99	0.9				
Cirrhosis of the liver	42	0.9	92	0.9				
Other bacterial diseases			174	1.6				
Septicemia					191	1.7		
Chronic respiratory disease							452	5.8
Other diseases of the respiratory tract					107	1.0	413	5.3
Other cardiovascular diseases					96	0.9	217	2.8
Perinatal conditions							361	4.7
Endocrine diseases, metabolic diseases, and immunologic diseases							106	1.4
Other lesions and complications due to trauma							104	1.3
Total	1,774	38.3	3,336	31.5	3,494	31.7	7,586	98.2

Source: Division Nacional de Bioestadística, Ministerio de Previsión Social y Salud Pública de Bolivia.

some studies, such as high altitude in La Paz, that may affect the usually observed association between population exposure to tobacco and lung cancer in Bolivia.

In 1981, Ríos-Dalenz compared the incidence of smoking-related cancers in three Latin American cities (La Paz, São Paulo, and Cali). In general, the incidence rate for these diseases was lowest in La Paz (Table 8).

In 1986 the Instituto Boliviano de Biología de Altura (Bolivian Institute of High-Altitude Biology) in La Paz (Speilgovel et al. 1990) compared 33 resident smokers (25 men and 8 women) with a nonsmoking population at sea level for lung function, electrocardiographic alterations, hemoglobin and hematocrit, carbon dioxide and oxygen levels, cholesterol, triglycerides, carboxyhemoglobin, and blood pressure. The preliminary conclusions were that smoking at high altitudes appears to have a greater effect on the respiratory than on the circula-

Table 8. Incidence rates* for smoking-related malignant neoplasms among the populations aged 35–64 years in three Latin American cities, by sex, 1980

Site	Men			Women		
	La Paz	Cali	São Paulo	La Paz	Cali	São Paulo
Lung	13.7	24.4	41.1	3.2		
Larynx	1.9	9.6	28.7	0.6		
Mouth	2.2	3.7	14.6	4.2	2.2	2.0
Esophagus	4.7	3.9	22	0.8	1.6	3.0
Bladder	2.6	8.2	15.8	0.8	3.5	1.9

Source: Ríos-Dalenz, 1981.
* Standardized to the world population.

tory system and that women may be more sensitive than men to physiologic changes produced by smoking.

Tobacco Use Prevention and Control Activities

Government Actions

Policies and executive structure

The 1978 Health Code of the Republic of Bolivia explicitly recognizes that tobacco is harmful to health (República de Bolivia 1978). In 1983 the Comisión Nacional de Lucha Antitabáquica (CONLAT) (National Anti-Smoking Commission) was created on the basis of a recommendation by the Jornadas Nacionales "Cigarrillos y Cancer" in September 1983. This meeting was promoted by the International Union Against Cancer (UICC) and sponsored by the FBLC. CONLAT was created by the Ministry of Social Welfare and Public Health and the Ministry of Education and Culture, and included representatives from the professional, civil, legislative, and private sectors. Its stated objectives were to support antismoking legislation, to protect the rights of nonsmokers, to reduce cigarette advertising until it is prohibited, to report on the health hazards of smoking, to conduct population studies on the prevalence of smoking, and to coordinate with other national and international organizations interested in preventing and controlling smoking (Ríos-Dalenz 1987). In 1986, the Ministry of Social Welfare and Public Health officially designated CONLAT as coordinator of health sector activities against smoking. CONLAT was also preparing an official plan for smoking control. In addition, the resolution assigned CONLAT the duty of coordinating its activities with the Bureau of Health, the Ministry of Education and Culture, and the National Board of Solidarity and Social Development.

CONLAT has branches in La Paz, Oruro, Sucre, Potosí, Cochabamba, and Santa Cruz—six of the capital cities of Bolivia's nine departments. CONLAT prepared the tobacco control plan mentioned above and has experienced important gains in the areas of legislation, information, education, and data collection.

Legislation

The Regulations on the Use of Tobacco contained in the Health Code (Decree-Law 15,629) of July 1978 entrust health authorities, through the Division of Health Education, to establish national mass education programs about the harmful effects of tobacco use, to prevent indiscriminate promotion of smoking, and to require that advertising not show smoking. This regulation also prohibits smoking in schools and health facilities, in enclosed public places, and on mass transit. All cigarette packs must clearly and visibly display the warning "This product is hazardous to your health." The regulation provides for sanctions ranging from warnings to fines. It appears, however, that with the exception of the warning printed on cigarette packs, there is little or no compliance with the regulations.

In October 1984, Ministerial Resolution No. 883 of the Ministry of Education and Culture was issued, prohibiting smoking in both public and private educational establishments throughout Bolivia. In November 1987, Ministerial Resolution No. 1095 of the Ministry of Social Forecast and Public Health was passed prohibiting smoking in public and private hospital centers. Earlier, in July 1987, Ministerial Resolution No. 2049 of the Ministry of Education and Culture prohibited smoking in all of Bolivia's educational establishments as well as the offices of the Ministry. This was the third time that legislation was passed prohibiting smoking in educational centers, which may indicate the difficulty of putting such legislation into practice.

Ministerial Resolution No. 0894 of the Ministry of Social Welfare and Public Health, passed in September 1988, limits tobacco-related advertising on audiovisual media to after 9:00 p.m.

Several local jurisdictions have regulated smoking in public places. Municipal Ordinance No. 015 of La Paz in October 1988 prohibited smoking in enclosed public places and on mass transit. This ordinance also made it mandatory to display visible signs to this effect. Violation of these provisions may be penalized at the discretion of the local authority. In March 1990 the municipal government of Oruro issued Municipal Ordinance No. 26 under which smoking is prohibited in enclosed public spaces and on mass transit. Penalties are imposed at the discretion of local authorities depending on the severity of the violation. The municipality of Cochabamba also issued an ordinance in May 1990 (Ordinance No. 792) which prohibited advertising on any of the mass media in the city and set up "Departmental Mass Education Programs" to discourage tobacco use.

The evolution of legislation aimed at controlling the smoking problem shows that there is growing interest among authorities in using this tool in Bolivia. However, as is true in almost every country, there are difficulties in terms of surveillance and compliance. Successful implementation of antismoking legislation depends to a great extent on citizens' awareness of the benefits to be gained from such legislation and of how important it is to get involved in antismoking activities at the local level.

School-based antismoking education

The National Curriculum Department in the Ministry of Education and Culture developed teaching materials on tobacco and its harmful effects on health for use in the natural science curricula in the third and fifth years of primary school. CONLAT offers informative lectures on a regular basis in primary and secondary schools in La Paz, Cochabamba, Sucre, Santa Cruz, and Oruro.

Public information campaigns

Since the first campaign on Cigarettes and Cancer in September 1983, CONLAT has promoted national "Tobacco or Health" Days on a biennial basis. At these events, health personnel meet to discuss new knowledge about smoking and health, as well as any achievements in the fight against tobacco. At the same time, news about the activities associated with these meetings is disseminated through the mass media (El Diario 1990; La Patria 1990).

In addition, since 1983 a "Smokeout," or "Pure Air Day," has been held on the third Thursday of November. Since 1989, May 31 has been celebrated as "World No-Tobacco Day." These events help stimulate national interest. Two children's antismoking poster contests have been sponsored in conjunction with these events in La Paz and Sucre.

Taxes

Tax accounts for 61 percent of the final retail cigarette pack price. There is also a 17–percent surtax on imported tobacco (Ministry of Finance 1990). Tobacco and cigarette taxes declined as a percentage of the country's internal revenue between 1984 and 1987, from 7.8 percent to 1.4 percent.

Nongovernmental Activities

Although CONLAT is the Bolivian Government's authorized agency for tobacco control, nongovernmental organizations (NGOs) working in conjunction with the Ministry of Social Forecast and Public Health have acted as prime movers of tobacco control and have been instrumental in its management. One of the most important of these organizations is the FBLC.

The other NGO that has made important contributions to the antismoking campaign is the Adventist Mission of Bolivia, an arm of the Seventh Day Adventist Church. This group supports a temperance program designed to eliminate alcohol, tobacco, and drug use in the community. Numerous initiatives have been conducted in coordination with CONLAT, most notably their standard 5–day smoking cessation program.

Conclusions

1. Bolivia has one of the lowest levels of per capita cigarette consumption in the world. Nevertheless, after the 1960s, per capita consumption increased sharply, doubling by the mid-1970s. The use of tobacco continued to rise steadily in the late 1980s.
2. Bolivia is predominantly rural, with sporadic tobacco use associated with popular traditions.

However, a substantial proportion of the urban population, particularly persons of high socioeconomic status, has acquired western smoking patterns, similar to those in developed countries.

3. Inadequate health-related data preclude detailed analyses of the epidemiologic transition in Bolivia. At present, the negative impact of smoking on the Bolivian population is minimal.

4. Bolivia has engaged in extensive antitobacco activity since the 1980s. The country has an efficient national organization with community involvement. Major efforts have been made in legislation. The tolerant attitudes of the population toward smoking and the lack of political initiative to control smoking are still major obstacles to overcoming the increasing problem of tobacco use in Bolivia.

References

CENTRO LATINOAMERICANO DEMOGRAFICO. *Boletín Demográfico*. Año XXII, No. 45. Santiago de Chile, January 1990.

CHANDLER, W.U. Banishing tobacco. *World Watch Paper*, 68, January 1986.

CHAPMAN, S., WONG, W.L. *Tobacco Control in the Third World—A Resource Atlas*. Penang, Malaysia: International Organization of Consumers Unions, 1990.

DE LA QUINTANA, M. Incidencia y prevalencia de tabaco en ciudades y area rural. *Boletín Epidemiológico del Ministerio de Previsión Social y Salud Pública*. 138, 1987.

DE OSOROVIC, G., PEREIRA, R. *Incidencia del consumo de tabaco en la población adulta de la ciudad de La Paz*. Report of the National Meeting on Cigarettes and Cancer, La Paz, Bolivia, September 26–27, 1983; organized by the Fundación Boliviana contra el Cáncer and the International Union against Cancer, 1983.

DE OSOROVIC, G., RIOS-DALENZ, J. *El hábito de fumar en médicos*. Unpublished manuscript, 1987.

EL DIARIO. *El contrabando: un mal evitable?* May 4, 1986.

EL DIARIO. *Inauguración jornadas nacionales de tabaco o salud en Oruro*. March 25, 1990.

FRECKER, R.C., PISCHKIT, H. *Constituents of Cigarettes from Developing Countries: Nicotine, Tar, and Carbon Monoxide Values for 50 Brands Selected by the World Health Organization*. WHO/SMO/84.4, 1984.

INSTITUTO NACIONAL DE ESTADISTICAS. *Bolivia en cifras: 1985*. Cuadro No. 83: Bolivia: Producción anual de bienes seleccionados del sector manufacturero, 1985.

INSTITUTO NACIONAL DE ESTADISTICAS. *Bolivia: indicadores demográficos por área de residencia*. Departamento de Estadísticas Sociales, p. 43, 1991.

LA PATRIA. *Inaguraron IV jornada de lucha antitabáquica*. March 25, 1990.

MAXWELL, J.C. *The Maxwell Consumer Report—International Tobacco Part One*. Wheat First Securities/Butcher and Singer. WFS-2557, March 30, 1989.

MINISTRY OF FINANCE. Unpublished Data, Department of Direct Collections of Internal Revenue, January 1990.

MINISTERIO DE PREVISION SOCIAL Y SALUD PUBLICA. *Informe sobre consumo de sustancias psicoactivas*, 1988.

MINISTERIO DE PREVISION SOCIAL Y SALUD PUBLICA. *Bolivia: situación de salud y sus tendencias*. Working Paper. La Paz: Representación de la Organización Panamericana de la Salud y Organización Mundial de la Salud en Bolivia. Imprenta Offset Prisa Publicidad, 1989.

MISDORP, S. Bolivia report. Bolivian inflation rate is down. Tobacco industry stabilizes. *Tobacco International*, March 15, 1990, pp. 24–30.

PAN AMERICAN HEALTH ORGANIZATION. *Control del hábito de fumar. Informe de Bolivia*. Segundo Taller Subregional del Area Andina. Washington, D.C.: Pan American Health Organization. Cuaderno Técnico No. 9, 1987.

PAN AMERICAN HEALTH ORGANIZATION. *Health Conditions in the Americas—1990 Edition*. Washington, D.C.: Pan American Heatlh Organization. Scientific Publication No. 524, 1990.

REPUBLICA DE BOLIVIA. *Decree-Law 15629*, July 18, 1978.

RIOS-DALENZ, J. Actividades de la Comisión Nacional de Lucha Antitabáquica (CONLAT). *Revista Médica El Sajama*, 1987, pp. 2–4.

RIOS-DALENZ, J. El tabaquismo y sus características en Bolivia. In: *Historia y perspectivas de la salud pública en Bolivia*. La Paz, Bolivia: Sociedad Boliviana de Salud Pública, PAHO/WHO, UNICEF, CIMA, 1989.

RIOS-DALENZ, J., CORREA, P., HAENSZEL, W. Morbidity from cancer in La Paz, Bolivia. *International Journal of Cancer* 28:307–314, 1981.

ROBERTSON, T.J. *Encuesta de cigarrillos y cancer*. Mimeo, Tarija: September 1, 1983.

SPEILGOVEL, H., APARICIO, O., BELLIDO, D., GALARA, M., NALLAR, N., QUINTELA, A., PEÑALOZA, R., TÉLLEZ, A., VARGAS, E., VILLENA, M., RÍOS-DALENZ, J. *The Effects of Smoking on a High Altitude Popu-*

lation (*La Paz, Bolivia, 3600 m or 12,200 ft*). Presented at the Seventh World Conference on Tobacco or Health. Perth, Australia, April 1990.

U.S. DEPARTMENT OF AGRICULTURE. *Tariffs and Other Import Duties on Tobacco Leaf and Cigarettes, 1988.* FAS-5–89, 1989.

WORLD BANK. *World Development Report 1990—Poverty.* New York: Oxford University Press, 1990.

WORLD HEALTH ORGANIZATION. Tobacco smoking. *IARC Monographs on the Evaluation of the Carcinogenic Risk of Chemicals to Humans* 38:70. Lyon, France: International Agency for Research on Cancer, 1986.

Brazil

General Characteristics

The Tobacco Industry
    Agriculture
    Manufacturing and trade
    Advertising and marketing
    Taxation of tobacco products

Tobacco Use
    Consumption
    Surveys of adults
    Prevalence of smoking among adolescents
    Beliefs, attitudes, and opinions toward smoking

Smoking and Health

Tobacco Use Prevention and Control Activities
    Government executive structure and policies
    Antitobacco legislation and executive actions
    Educational activities
    Nongovernmental action against tobacco

Summary and Conclusions

References

General Characteristics

Brazil is a federal republic of 8,512,000 km² on the Atlantic coast of South America, extending from approximately 5 degrees north of the equator to the temperate regions of the Southern Hemisphere. It ranks third in land surface and second in population among countries of the Americas. Brazil is the world's third largest producer of tobacco, and, as of 1989, the second largest exporter of tobacco. The cultural and economic importance of tobacco in Brazil is reflected in the presence of a sheaf of tobacco (along with a coffee branch) on the official Seal of the Republic. Of Brazil's massive territory, 66.6 percent is forested, 19.6 percent is pasture and range lands, and 9 percent is used for agriculture.

Brazil's estimated 1990 mid-year population of 150,368,000 is ethnically and sociologically diverse. Within the forested regions near the Amazon River reside the remnants of aboriginal peoples. Many of these people retain shamanistic practices involving tobacco use dating to pre-Columbian times (U.S. Department of Health and Human Services [USDHHS] 1992). Most of the population (75 percent) is urban, however, and very poor families account for the majority of the country's population (Table 1).

Table 1. **Demographic and economic indicators, Brazil, 1980s**

Indicator	Year	Value
Population	1990	150,368,000
Percentage < 15 years old	1988	35.2
Percentage ≥ 65 years old	1988	4.5
Percentage urban	1988	75.0
Infant mortality rate per 1,000 live births	1988	61.0
Crude birth rate per 1,000 persons	1988	28
Total fertility rate	1988	3.4
Crude mortality rate per 1,000 persons	1988	8.0
Life expectancy at birth per 1,000 live births	1988	65.0
Percent literate (age > 15)	1985	79.3
Gross national product		
$US millions	1988	328,860
Per capita ($US)	1988	2,280
Mean annual inflation rate (%)	1980–88	188.7

Source: World Bank, 1990.

Since World War II, Brazil has undergone a major social transformation from a largely rural society (50 percent in 1965) to one of the most industrialized, urban societies in Latin America (World Bank 1990). Brazil is one of the top 10 economies in the Western Hemisphere (Pan American Health Organization [PAHO] 1990) and the per capita gross national product ($US2,280 in 1988) is the fifth highest among Latin American countries (World Bank 1990). Included in Brazil's social transformation has been the development of an extensive, modern system of mass communication that has fostered cultural homogenization. The transformation has also produced significant socioeconomic instability; a burgeoning foreign debt ($US124 million in 1987); massive inflation (mean annual inflation rate of 188.7 percent from 1980 to 1988); and significant fluctuations in wages, cost of living, and purchasing power of the residents (World Bank 1989, 1990). This instability is reflected in a very apparent socioeconomic imbalance in Brazil. The richest 10 percent of the population receives 53.2 percent of all income, while the poorest 10 percent receives only 0.6 percent of all income (Instituto Brasileiro de Geografia e Estatistica [IBGE] 1990). In 1985, it was estimated that 53 million Brazilians (40.1 percent) lived in poverty (PAHO 1990).

In 1985, Brazil returned to a democratically elected form of Government. This change was accompanied by a restructuring of Government health programs in 1986. Following prolonged debate, a new national constitution was approved in 1988 that contained restrictions on advertising of tobacco and other potentially harmful consumer products (Constitution of Brazil 1988). However, because of marked economic deterioration in 1988 and 1989, the new Government of 1990 sought drastic cutbacks in federal expenditures. The National Program Against Tobacco, which was organized in 1986 (Costa e Silva 1988), was reduced in scope in 1990.

Young adults predominate in the population of Brazil, with almost 65 percent aged 15 years or older and only 4.5 percent aged 65 or older. The declining total fertility rate (3.4 in 1988) has helped slow the annual population growth from 2.4 percent in 1965 to 1980 to a projected 1.8 percent in 1988 to 2000. The shift from rural to urban population growth (almost 4.5 percent annually) has encouraged the emergence of huge cities, primarily in the south, such as São Paulo and Rio de Janeiro. These cities are now burdened by extensive slums with deteriorating health conditions (PAHO 1990).

The Tobacco Industry

Agriculture

Brazil has been a producer and exporter of tobacco since its colonization in the 1500s. Until 1987 Brazil was the fourth largest producer of tobacco; as of 1990, it is the third largest producer, surpassed only by the United States and China. Approximately 160,000 farms (2.6 percent of the national total) were involved in growing tobacco in the late 1980s. These farms occupied 296,678 ha (0.57 percent of arable land) and employed full- or part-time approximately 600,000 farmers, or 4.2 percent of the rural work force (Associaçao Brasileira das Indústrias do Fumo [ABIFUMO] 1990; IBGE 1989). Tobacco production has grown from 135,700 MT in 1966 to 450,000 MT in 1990, accounting for 6.3 percent of world production (U.S. Department of Agriculture [USDA] 1990; IBGE 1990; ABIFUMO 1990). Approximately half of this tobacco was consumed domestically (Table 2). Tobacco is Brazil's third leading export product, behind coffee and soybeans. Most tobacco production (80 percent) occurs in the southern states of Rio Grande do Sul, Santa Catarina, and Paraná. Light tobacco for manufacturing cigarettes is the predominant type grown in these states. The northeastern states of Alagoas and Bahia annually produce approximately 43,000 MT of dark tobacco, which is used in Brazil for cigars and pipes.

The Government itself has not sponsored crop substitution programs for tobacco, but tobacco manufacturing companies have explored alternatives on their own. A recent study on farm economics (Konzen 1987) concluded that the only viable substitute crop that would not produce economic loss would be the white (Irish) potato. Switching to this crop would use only about 30 percent of the labor used in tobacco growing.

Light tobacco is flue cured using wood fuel. This practice has a detrimental impact on the country's already threatened forests as well as on the efforts to replenish them. The tobacco industry has implemented some programs to support reforestation (Crescenti 1990a), but these have been limited in scope. Although almost two-thirds of the country is covered by forests, tobacco-growing states are already greatly deforested (Jungbluth 1988; Chapman 1990). More than 93,000 ovens are used for tobacco curing in Brazil (Chapman 1990). Approximately 25 kg of wood are needed to cure each kg of tobacco; thus, the ecologic impact of curing a light tobacco harvest of over 400,000 MT per year is substantial (Bianco 1982).

Manufacturing and Trade

Four companies, three of which are linked to multinational firms, controlled cigarette production in Brazil during the 1970s and 1980s (Table 3). Consequently, they have also influenced tobacco agriculture and industry through their control of the market and through organized promotion and support actions for farmers (Chapman 1990). The British-American Tobacco Company (BAT) subsidiary, Souza Cruz, S.A., has the largest domestic market share (79.4 percent in 1988). In fact, Souza Cruz Trading is the largest individual tobacco exporter in the world. The other two multinational companies were the Philip Morris Company, with 8 percent of the domestic market, and R.J. Reynolds, with 9.5 percent. R.J. Reynolds recently sold out to Philip Morris Company (Zimmerman 1990). The only private domestic company (Sudan) held 2.8 percent of the market in 1988 (Costa e Silva 1990). In 1988, 219 factories were involved in tobacco processing, including 99 for leaf tobacco, 107 for twist (or pigtail) tobacco, and 13 for cigar and cigarette manufacturing. Approximately 16,000 persons, or 0.4 percent of the total industrial work force, were employed in tobacco manufacturing activities (IBGE 1988). However, including persons involved in tobacco agriculture, persons indirectly involved in tobacco trade activities such as in transportation, and persons employed by the 350,000 establishments selling tobacco, an estimated 2.5 million persons may be di-

Table 2. Unmanufactured tobacco, production, exports, imports, and total domestic consumption (MT), Brazil, 1979 to 1989

Year	Production	Exports	Imports	Total domestic consumption
1979	422,891	140,188	338	283,041
1980	405,537	143,555	352	262,334
1981	362,250	148,609	251	213,892
1982	421,532	165,718	379	256,193
1983	395,485	176,827	649	219,307
1984	414,808	187,438	33	227,403
1985	410,918	198,662	58	212,256
1986	386,827	175,658	70	211,099
1987	397,845	173,684	180	224,341
1988	429,955	199,436	302	230,217
1989	446,266	207,000	302	238,964

Source: IBGE, 1991.

Table 3. Tobacco companies, market shares, and relationship to multinational companies, Brazil, 1988

Company	Type	Market share	Relationship to multinationals
Souza Cruz	Multinational	79.4	British-American Tobacco, Ltd., Subsidiary
Philip Morris	Multinational	8.0	Philip Morris Co. Subsidiary
R.J. Reynolds	Multinational	9.5	R.J. Reynolds Subsidiary
Sudan	Private national	2.8	None

Source: Costa y Silva, 1990.

rectly or indirectly involved in the tobacco industry (ABIFUMO 1990).

With 20.3 percent of world exports, Brazil is the world's second largest exporter of tobacco, surpassed only by the United States with 23.9 percent. In 1989, tobacco exports yielded approximately $US570 million (1.66 percent of total exports) (ABIFUMO 1990). The Government does not subsidize tobacco production or exports. Because of low production costs, Brazilian tobacco prices are very competitive on the international market, at one-half the cost of U.S. tobacco (Food and Agriculture Organization of the United Nations [FAO] 1990). The low price helps explain the success of Brazilian tobacco exports. The United States and countries of the European Economic Community have been the major recipients of Brazil's tobacco exports.

The Government has no formal program to develop further tobacco manufacturing. Prices paid for cigarettes are regulated, however, by the central Government via the Government Price Control Agency negotiations with ABIFUMO. The average price of a pack of the most popular brand of cigarettes was $US0.34 in 1989 (Costa e Silva 1990). In 1991, the Government increased cigarette prices 776 percent, or three times the rate of inflation in 1990.

Advertising and Marketing

The 1988 constitutional provision restricting the advertising of potentially harmful products has not been implemented yet. However, the Ministry of Health issued an executive order that limits times when tobacco commercials may be broadcast; the order also makes mandatory health warnings on all types of tobacco-product advertising and bans the sale of tobacco to minors (Regulation No. 731 of May 31, 1990). The actual package and advertisement warnings are quite small and often difficult to read. Prior to this order, all types of advertising and promotional activities were permitted and used. Radio commercials are the only format that is not used, having been canceled in response to the Ministry of Health executive order demanding a spoken health warning as part of the commercial (Crescenti 1990b). In addition to television advertising, the tobacco companies use other promotional activities, including several that serve to divert attention away from the health consequences of tobacco use and away from public support of Government tobacco control activities. For example, Souza Cruz (BAT) sponsored polio vaccination campaigns in northern states (except Bahia and Paraíba), using their support staff and vehicles that displayed the Hollywood cigarette logo. The campaign served as a grassroots advertising campaign for tobacco in the guise of a humanitarian effort. In addition, Souza Cruz utilized a religious event, the Passion Play in Pernambuco State in the Northeast, to promote tobacco. Other events promoting specific cigarette brands include the Hollywood Motocross and Rock Festival; the Free Jazz Festival; the Carlton Dance Festival; the Camel Motor Rally Trophy; Oktoberfest in Santa Catarina state; sponsorship of Formula 1 race car drivers; and the distribution of free samples at trade fairs, conventions, and universities.

Although the tobacco industry ignores no segment of Brazilian society in its advertising, tobacco was only the eleventh leading advertiser in Brazil in 1987 (Hijjar 1991). This low rank may result from the industry's independent decision to suspend all types of advertising between mid-1986 and the end of 1987. This decision reportedly was taken because of decreased profits resulting from the Government's centrally regulated pricing policy. The advertising budget increased dramatically (685 percent) from $US8,686,000 in 1987 to $US68,197,200 in 1988. The tobacco industry now ranks firmly among the top 10 advertisers in Brazil, and the per capita expenditure for tobacco advertising may be higher than in any other developing country in the Americas (Chapman 1990).

Table 4. Manufactured cigarettes, production, exports, total domestic consumption (millions), and per capita consumption, Brazil, 1979 to 1989

Year	Production	Exports	Total domestic consumption	Per capita consumption (15 years and older)
1979	139,500	518	139,500	1890
1980	142,700	462	142,700	1890
1981	134,900	613	134,900	1740
1982	132,300	615	132,300	1660
1983	129,200	708	129,200	1580
1984	127,800	1,058	127,800	1520
1985	146,300	1,252	146,300	1690
1986	168,900	1,601	168,900	1920
1987	161,400	2,807	161,400	1780
1988	157,900		157,900	1700
1989	162,300		162,300	1690
1990	164,600		162,300	

Source: Costa e Silva, 1990a; USDA, 1990; ABIFUMO, 1990.

Taxation of Tobacco Products

Accounting for 73 to 76 percent of the selling price of cigarettes in Brazil, the cigarette tax comprises the following components: 53.4 percent is the federal tax on manufactured goods (IPI), 2.4 percent is the federal tax FIMSOCIAL, and 17.0 percent is state excise tax (ICM). At the federal level, cigarette taxes account for 5 to 7 percent of overall tax revenues (Costa e Silva 1990a).

Tobacco Use

Consumption

Between 1935 and 1985, the per capita consumption of tobacco tripled for persons aged 15 and older in Brazil (Chapman 1990). Between 1970 and 1986, the population grew 49 percent, and total cigarette consumption increased 132 percent (Costa e Silva 1988). In 1989, adult per capita cigarette consumption was estimated at 1,690 per year, representing a decrease from the 1979 level of 1,890. Annual variations of up to 32.1 percent occurred in 1979 to 1989 (Table 4). These variations may be attributed to fluctuations in the purchasing power of currency and wages. As observed in other countries, variations occurred not only in the volume of cigarettes consumed but also in preferences.

Lower-cost cigarettes became more popular as buying power and subsequent per capita cigarette consumption declined (Crescenti 1990b); higher-cost cigarettes were popular prior to 1986 (Hijjar 1991).

In 1988, an estimated 11.6 percent of consumption was loose-cut tobacco used in pipes and roll-your-own cigarettes; consumption of twist (or pigtail) tobacco was approximately 50 tons (Costa e Silva 1990a).

Surveys of Adults

Brazil's sheer geographic size and huge population, combined with its sociocultural heterogeneity, create difficulties in collecting population-based data with adequate national representation. Preliminary national data on tobacco use for 65,000 persons aged 5 years and older are available from the Pesquisa Nacional sobre a Saúde e Nutrição sponsored by Instituto Brasileiro de Geografia e Estatística (IBGE 1991). Several other studies that have examined tobacco use behavior (Table 5) have been limited to specific population groups or geographical areas.

São Paulo was included as one of the eight surveyed cities in the 1971 survey of adults aged 15 to 74 that was sponsored by PAHO (Joly 1977) (Table 6).

São Paulo adults aged 15 to 59 were also surveyed as part of a 1987 assessment of noncommunicable chronic diseases in several Latin American cities (Ramos 1988) (Table 7).

One of the most representative Brazilian studies surveyed the adult populations aged 18 to 55 years in 12 state capitals for smoking and other lifestyle variables (Ministry of Health 1988); these data can be compared to the 1971 survey of the São Paulo urban population (Table 8).

One investigator collected data on a rural population in Rio Grande do Sul State in 1978 (Table 9) (Achutti 1978) and on the urban population of that state in 1987 (Achutti 1988) (Table 10).

The Gallup Organization surveyed 1,297 adults aged 18 and older in Rio de Janeiro and São Paulo in 1988, but little information was provided on the methodology used for the survey (Gallup 1988) (Table 11).

Finally, the nationally representative 1989 IBGE survey included data on smoking by children and adults (Table 12). For all respondents (age 5 years and older), the prevalence of smoking was higher in rural areas than in urban areas (26.5 percent vs. 23.2 percent). The prevalence of smoking among adults age 15 and older (39.9 percent among

Table 5. Prevalence of current smoking among adults reported by surveys from 1971 to 1989, Brazil

Sponsor/author	Year	Age group	Sample area	N	Men	Women	Both
PAHO/Joly	1971	15–74	São Paulo	1450	53.8	20.2	36.0
Achutti	1978	15–74	Rio Grande do Sul (Urban and Rural)	4557	61.4	27.1	38.5
Rosemberg*	1979		Sorocaba Catholic University M.D.s		28	33	
Saltz*	1981		Porto Alegre M.D.s		26	40	
Rosemberg*	1982		Brazilian Medical Association		32	27	
DeLucia**	1983	18–60	Workers in Cubatao Employees, Families, Retirees				51.2
Brazilian Air Force**	1986	18–63	Active Duty and Reserves		32.1		
Achutti	1987	20–64	Porto Alegre	1041	51.7	34.4	40.8
Rodrigues	1987	15–59	São Paulo	1471	45.0	31.0	38.0
Bank of Brazil Feitosa**	1988	Adults					29.7
Gallup/ACS	1988	18–50+	São Paulo and Rio de Janeiro	1297	40	36	38
Health Ministry	1988	18–55	Twelve State Capitals	2003	45	33	38.7
Pohlmann	1988	15–64	Porto Alegre	407			41.7
Ribeiro**	1989		Employees, Construction workers of Sergen SA, Office Workers			47.2	30.6
Campos et al.*	1989		Lung Institute M.D.s U. of Rio de Janeiro		11	17	
Campos et al.*	1989		Cascavel, Parana M.D.s		34	23	
Campos et al.*	1989		Sobradinho, Brasilia M.D.s		25	20	
Campos*	1989		Rio de Janeiro State M.D.s		28	23	
IBGE	1989	15+	National	65,000	39.9	25.4	32.6

*Physician surveys. Source: Rosemberg, 1990.
**Worker surveys. Source: Hijjar, 1991.

Table 6. Prevalence (%) of never, current, and ex-smoking, by sex and age group, São Paulo, 1971

Category		Never smokers	Current smokers	Ex-smokers
Men	15–74		53.8	9.6
	15–24	44.7	53.6	1.7
	25–39	33.5	58.9	7.6
	40–54	34.1	49.2	16.7
	55–74	31.9	48.3	19.8
Women	15–74	20.2	4.0	
	15–24	76	20.3	3.7
	25–39	72.5	23.9	3.6
	40–54	78.8	17.3	3.9
	55–74	79.8	14.5	5.7
Both	15–74		36.0	6.6

Source: Joly, 1977.

Table 7. Prevalence (%) of current smoking by age group, sex, and educational attainment, São Paulo, 1987

Age group	Men	Women	Both
15–59	45.0	31.0	38.0
15–24	34.3	31.0	
25–34	54.7	41.7	
35–44	47.8	17.9	
45–49	43.9		
Education			
Primary			35.7
Secondary			63.5
Tertiary			68.2

Source: Ramos, 1988.

Table 8. Prevalence of never smoking, current smoking, and former smoking (%) among adults age 18 to 55 in 12 state capitals, by age group, education, social class, occupation, and region, Brazil, 1988

Category	Never smokers	Current smokers	Former smokers	N
Men	35.6	45	19.5	999
Women	52.0	33	15.3	1,004
Both (age 18–55)	43.7	38.7	17.4	2,003
Age groups				
18–24	58.5	29.7	11.8	458
25–34	34.2	45.4	20.9	617
35–44	39.2	42.9	17.8	510
45–55	47.6	33.7	18.7	418
Educational attainment				
Primary	43.1	40.7	16.2	636
Secondary	48.0	35.1	16.9	490
Tertiary	39.5	37.8	22.7	172
Social class				
(low)	42.8	37.4	19.8	495
(high)	43.0	40.5	16.5	805
Occupation				
Unskilled	31.6	48.1	20.3	79
Retired	38.8	45.0	16.3	129
Commercial	43.5	40.4	16.1	230
Laborer and military	44.3	38.3	17.4	149
Housekeeper	52.5	30.9	16.7	606
Region				
North	42	40	18	137
Northeast	50	33	18	387
South	43	42	15	98
Southeast	43	40	17	1,335
East Central	30	39	30	45

Source: Ministry of Health, 1988.

men and 25.4 percent among women) was similar to that reported for most of the other surveys.

Because health care providers should reflect the leading edge in changes in smoking behavior, seven surveys of physicians were performed between 1979 and 1989 in Brazil (Rosemberg 1990) (Table 5). Methodological differences make it impossible to compare results internationally, but the data in general suggest that the prevalence of smoking among Brazilian physicians is slightly lower than that of the general Brazilian population; the prevalence is intermediate between countries with high prevalence levels among physicians (such as Poland at 70 percent) and low levels (such as the United States at 8 percent).

Despite differences in methodology and limitations on the comparability of the various studies, several consistent findings can be observed regarding the adult prevalence of smoking in Brazil. The prevalence of current smoking among men is higher than that among women; the prevalence of former smoking also appears to be higher among men. The prevalence of current smoking consistently appears to be higher among young adults (25 to 34 years, 25 to 39 years, etc.); older age groups have lower prevalences of smoking. The prevalence of current smoking is related inversely to level of education and social class. Unskilled workers and construction workers demonstrate a higher prevalence of current smoking than do physicians, office workers, housewives, and military employees and their families. The 1988 survey of lifestyle and health risk behavior in 12 state capitals reported that the prevalence rate is higher (42.0

Table 9. Prevalence (%) of never smoking, current smoking, and former smoking, by sex, age group, educational attainment, area of residence, and occupation, Rio Grande do Sul State, Brazil, 1978

Category		Never smokers	Current smokers	Former smokers
Men	20–74	23.8	61.4	14.8
	20–34	30.9	61.3	7.8
	35–54	18.8	62.8	18.3
	55–74	14.3	58.5	27.2
Women	20–74	66.1	27.1	6.8
	20–34	60.2	33.0	6.7
	35–54	68.7	24.4	6.9
	55–74	77.3	15.7	6.9
Both	20–74	53.3	38.5	10.9
Education				
Primary		47.8	38.6	9.7
Secondary		40.6	44.9	12.3
Tertiary		49.2	34.4	12.7
Rural		55.6	36.0	9.3
Urban		44.4	38.6	12.3
Occupation				
Unskilled		24.0	60.4	13.7
Dependent		70.8	20.1	5.4
Agriculture		47.3	38.8	10.2
Service		44.9	39.9	11.2
Public administration		30.1	45.5	19.9
Transport and communication		26.9	49.3	19.4

Source: Achutti, 1978.

Table 10. Prevalence (%) of never, current, and former smoking, Porto Alegre City, by sex and age group, Brazil, 1987

Sex	Age group	Never smokers	Current smokers	Former smokers
Men	20–64	33.1	51.7	15.2
	15–19	55.3	39.5	5.3
	20–34	42.3	47.8	9.9
	35–54	26.1	59.6	14.3
	55–64	20.4	38.6	40.9
Women	20–64	57.9	34.4	7.6
	15–19	61.9	20.6	17.5
	20–34	52.5	40.1	7.2
	35–54	68.1	31.9	7.5
	55–64	69.8	30.9	9.3
Both	20–64	48.7	40.8	10.4

Source: Achutti, 1988.

percent) in the more developed (and tobacco-growing) southern region where consumer purchasing power is greatest; the proportion of heavy smokers is also highest in this region. Overall, 20 percent of men and 10 percent of women smoke more than 20 cigarettes a day. In the northeast, the current smoking prevalence among adults is 33 percent.

The 1988 Ministry of Health survey provided additional detailed data on the initiation of tobacco use among Brazilians. When asked about the age of initiation, 82 percent of men and 69.4 percent of women reported having begun smoking before the age of 19. Smoking appears to be positively associated with higher consumption of alcohol and a sedentary lifestyle.

Based on the older study that obtained data from rural as well as urban areas in Rio Grande do Sul (Achutti 1978), the prevalence of current smoking was slightly lower among rural populations than urban populations (36.0 vs. 38.6 percent). The generalizability of this survey is uncertain, and the urban-rural difference was reversed in the data reported for the 1989 nationally representative IBGE survey.

Smoking has adverse effects on reproductive outcomes, and 10 surveys of reproductive-age women (15 to 44 years) who were pregnant, non-pregnant, or using oral contraceptives were performed in 1970 to 1990 (Table 13). Prevalence of

Table 11. Prevalence (%) of current and former smoking among adults by sex, age group, educational attainment, social class, and place of residence in Rio de Janeiro and São Paulo, Brazil, 1988

Category	Current smokers	Former smokers	N
Men	40	18	643
Women	36	6	654
Both	38	12	1,297
Age group			
18–29	38	8	511
30–49	45	11	512
50+	25	22	274
Education			
Primary	37	15	499
Secondary	39	9	598
Tertiary	39	13	200
Social class			
Low	38	12	508
High	33	15	109
São Paulo	39	11	673
Rio de Janeiro	37	13	624

Source: Gallup, 1988.

Table 12. Prevalence (%) of current smoking by age group and sex, Brazil, 1989

| Age group | Prevalence of current smoking | | |
	Men	Women	Both
15–19	18.0	13.9	16.3
20–29	40.9	27.3	34.7
30–49	48.0	30.9	39.7
50+	41.9	21.8	30.1
15+	39.9	25.4	32.6

Source: IBGE, 1991.

smoking among pregnant women was less than among the general female population. Younger pregnant women appeared to smoke at higher rates than did older women (Gross 1983). The 1970 study of smoking by pregnant women in the city of Pelotas, Rio Grande do Sul (Procianoy 1970), showed that 19.4 percent of women patients in a maternity ward smoked, and that there was a correlation between smoking and both low birth weight and smaller head circumference of their babies.

Another population-based study from the city of Pelotas carried out in 1982 showed that 35.6 percent of approximately 6,000 women giving birth in

that year had smoked during pregnancy. The prevalence of smoking decreased with increasing family income, from 43.7 percent among the poorest to 22.4 percent among women in the highest income group. Low birth weight (under 2,500 grams) ranged from 7.5 percent among nonsmokers to 16.3 percent among women smoking 15 or more cigarettes per day during the entire pregnancy. This difference remained after adjustment for socioeconomic factors (Victoria 1988).

Follow-up surveys of reproductive-aged women were performed on a national sample and on residents of São Paulo, Southern Brazil, and Northern Brazil through the U.S. Centers for Disease Control (CDC) sponsorship in the late 1980s. In general, these surveys show that the prevalence of smoking among women 15 to 44 years increased from that reported in the early 1980s.

Several general conclusions about the trends in current smoking prevalence for men and women in urban areas are suggested by the data in Tables 7 to 12. Like the United States and Canada, the use of tobacco in Brazil appears to be more common among less educated persons and among those employed in blue-collar jobs. The prevalence of smoking may be lower among those with the lowest disposable incomes, especially in rural areas, but data on tobacco use behavior among these groups are insufficient to characterize fully their behavior. It seems, however, that the current smoking prevalence among men remained stable between 1971 and the late 1980s. The prevalence of smoking among women appears to have increased substantially. Smoking cessation (i.e., the prevalence of former smoking) appears to be more common among men and among those with the highest educational attainment. The prevalence of smoking among physicians is lower than that in the general population (Table 5).

Prevalence of Smoking among Adolescents

Because of the increasing trend in current smoking prevalence among women and the sustained high levels of smoking among men in Brazil, it is important to consider adolescent smoking patterns in some detail. In 1987 and 1989, primary and secondary school students aged 10 to 18 years and older in 10 state capitals were surveyed about their use of drugs, including tobacco. Data were collected by a multistaged random sample technique, and grouped data for the 1987 study were analyzed using multivariate logistic regression for determinants of tobacco use among adolescents (Barbosa

Table 13. Prevalence of smoking among reproductive-aged women, Brazil, 1970–1990

Sponsor/author	Year	Sample area	N	Pregnant	Non-pregnant	Using OCs	Total
					Current smoking prevalence		
Procianoy	1970	Pelotas maternity hospital Rio Grande do Sul	838	19.4			
Candelas	1979	São Paulo maternity hospital	404	27.9			
Simoes	1979	Ribeirao Preto	6,203		29.0		
Gross et al.	1981	Ribeirao Preto	516		37.0		
Centers for Disease Control	1981	Southern Brazil	4,047	20.8	24.9	27.7	24.7
Centers for Disease Control	1982	Piaui State	3,293	27.1	26.6	25.5	26.7
Centers for Disease Control	1982	Amazonas State	2,099	18.8	22.6	26.4	22.3
Segre et al.	1986	São Paulo State	9,348	43.3			
CLAP*	1987**	National	3,786	36			
Viggiano et al.	1990	Goias State	155	33.5			

*(Centro Latinoamericano de Perinatologia y Desarrollo Humano, PAHO, Montevideo, Uruguay).
**Date reported; actual survey year unknown.

1989). Overall, 19.5 percent of students reported smoking at some time in the past; 15.9 percent had smoked in the last year; 10.5 percent had smoked in the last month; and 9.8 percent were regular smokers. Bivariate analysis revealed positive associations between the use of tobacco and the student's employment, night school attendance, poor school performance, and parental smoking. Multivariate analysis included poor school performance and parental smoking in the final model.

Unpublished data for each city sample show that the prevalence of current smoking (i.e., smoked within the last year) varied from 16.2 percent among young men in Salvador to 27.5 percent in Fortaleza. Among young women, the prevalence varied from 16.3 percent in Curitiba to 24.7 percent in São Paulo. The prevalence of current smoking increased dramatically with age, from 3.8 percent among 10- to 12–year-olds in Salvador to 54.3 percent among 18–year-olds in Belo Horizonte (Table 14) (Barbosa et al. 1989).

The 1989 survey of 10 state capitals showed

Table 14. Current smoking prevalence (%) among students in 10 state capitals, by age group, Brazil, 1987

Capital	10–12	13–15	16–18	18+	N
		Current smoking prevalence			
Belem	5.6	15.3	34.2	41.2	1,356
Belo Horizonte	9.8	21.2	33.2	54.3	1,613
Brasilia	4.7	21.8	32.8	45.0	1,566
Curitiba	5.6	15.3	34.2	41.2	1,825
Fortaleza	4.0	13.9	29.2	38.4	1,688
Porto Alegre	8.9	22.8	38.2	39.1	1,146
Recife	5.4	11.5	27.5	47.6	1,750
Rio de Janeiro	7.3	18.4	33.0	38.4	1,775
Salvador	3.8	14.2	22.0	31.4	1,271
São Paulo	5.9	25.2	39.7	53.8	2,159

Source: Barbosa et al., 1989.

that the prevalence of regular smoking (i.e., at least six times in the last month) varied between 2.2 percent in Curitiba and 7.5 percent in São Paulo (Hijjar 1991). Current smoking (i.e., at least once within the last year) varied between 16.7 percent in Curitiba and 32.9 percent in São Paulo. Sex-specific data are not available, but the prevalence of smoking within the last year appears to have increased among students in the 10 survey cities during the interval between 1987 and 1989. "Street boys" in the three cities of Porto Alegre, São Paulo, and Salvador were surveyed by Carlini-Cotrim in 1989 as an extension of the 10-city study of school youth. The prevalence of smoking at least once in the last month among this small sample of high-risk youth was 72 percent in Porto Alegre, 86 percent in São Paulo, and 36 percent in Salvador.

Achutti surveyed students aged 11 to 20 in Porto Alegre for 5 consecutive years for smoking behavior and knowledge of the health consequences of smoking (Achutti 1986) (Table 15). Data from this study indicate that the prevalence of current smoking among youth of both sexes increased with age beginning at age 13, and the age of initiation was earlier among girls than among boys. The prevalence of current smoking in 1984 was significantly lower for both sexes and for all ages when compared with the initial survey done in 1980. During 1984, there was a concomitant general decline in per capita cigarette consumption throughout the country. In 1988, Rosito used the same survey methodology and extended the sample to the rest of the state. The prevalence of smoking in Rio Grande do Sul in 1988 apparently was similar to the level in 1984, despite the fact that national per capita cigarette consumption had reached record levels

in 1986 (Table 4). The percentage of students who recognized that smoking was hazardous to health was relatively high (more than 50 percent). Knowledge of the health consequences of smoking appeared to increase among Porto Alegre students over the 5 years of observation. There was no difference in level of knowledge between smokers and nonsmokers (Achutti 1986).

Additional data have been collected on the prevalence of regular and occasional smoking (combined) among male and female medical students between 1979 and 1989 (Table 16). In each survey, the prevalence of smoking generally increased between the first and sixth years of medical school. However, the prevalence of regular and occasional smoking appeared to be lower in the late 1980s than in the period from 1979 to 1983 (Rosemberg 1990).

The 1989 IBGE survey collected data on children aged 5 to 10 years and adolescents aged 10 to 14 years. The prevalence of smoking among children was 0.2 percent, while the prevalence of smoking among adolescents was 2.2 percent (IBGE 1991).

Finally, the U.S. CDC sponsored six Young Adult Reproductive Health Surveys of youth aged 15 to 24 in the late 1980s (U.S. Department of Health and Human Services [USDHHS] 1992). Prevalence among men ranged from 22.5 percent in Rio de Janeiro to 33.7 percent in São Paulo. The prevalence of smoking among young women was, for the most part, similar to that among men (Table 17).

As part of an antitobacco poster contest sponsored by the Ministry of Health, data were collected on the prevalence of smoking among parents of

Table 15. Prevalence (%) of daily smoking among students, by age, Porto Alegre, 1980 to 1984

Age	1980*	1980	1981	1982	1983	1984
11	0.8	2.40	0	0	0	
12	2.7	2.8	0	3.1	2.4	4.5
13	4.6	4.8	3.4	2.5	5.5	2.7
14	9.5	9.3	7.4	8.5	6.3	7.7
15	16.7	16.8	10.8	8.5	9.8	14.7
16	18.7	20.9	18.6	17.4	17.1	15.5
17	29.7	27.7	22.1	17.4	20.3	23.5
18	34.3	39.0	22.7	26.9	21.9	17.3
19	36.5	37.9	35.5	37.5	25.0	14.8
20	45.5	50.0	20.0	28.6	13.3	22.7

Source: Achutti, 1986.
*Pre-test.

Table 16. Prevalence (%) of current smoking among medical students in year 1 and year 6 of studies, Brazil, 1979 to 1989

Location	Year	Men Year 1	Men Year 6	Women Year 1	Women Year 6	Both Year 1	Both Year 6
Sorocaba	1979	33.9	50.9	29.5	58.8	31.2	54.8
Ribeirao Preto	1980	15.7	18.9	25.7	0	20.7	9.4
São Paulo	1983					17.8	38.8
Ribeirao Preto	1986	3.4	31.0	4.2	10.7	4.0	21.1
Ribeirao Preto	1988	6.3	12.9	0	14.3	3.1	13.6
Sorocaba	1989	14.0	30.0	8.3	32.3	11.1	31.1
Porto Alegre	1989					14.0	20.2
Fortaleza	1989					9.4	22.2

Source: Rosemberg, 1990.

Table 17. Prevalence (%) of smoking among men and women 15 to 24 years of age, Brazil, 1986 to 1989

Area	Year	Men Sample size	Men Prevalence	Women Sample size	Women Prevalence
Brazil	1986	—	—	2,479	27.3
Salvador	1987	871	13.9	956	14.1
São Paulo	1988	750	33.7	804	26.2
Curitiba	1989	950	24.4	913	22.0
Rio de Janeiro	1989	848	22.5	831	22.0
Recife	1989	1,154	23.9	989	12.0

Source: U.S. Department of Health and Human Services, 1992.

71,941 school-aged entrants. Approximately half of the children reported at least one smoker per household. The average number of smokers per household was 1.7, with no differences between rural and urban families (Costa e Silva 1990a).

Beliefs, Attitudes, and Opinions toward Smoking

Few data are available concerning the beliefs, attitudes, and opinions on tobacco for Brazilians. Several unpublished reports suggest that Brazilians generally believe that smoking is harmful to health. According to an unpublished 1988 study of 407 randomly selected adults aged 15 to 64 years from Porto Alegre (Pohlmann 1988), almost 100 percent of the population agreed that environmental tobacco smoke is hazardous to children. Of respondents, 78 percent believed that smoking reduces physical performance; 83 percent believed that smoking is a cause of chronic cough; 88 percent believed that smoking is hazardous to the fetus; and 79 percent believed that smoking increases the risk of adverse reproductive outcomes. Surprisingly, only 48 percent believed that the life ex-

pectancy of smokers is less than that of non-smokers. Finally, the majority of women either disagreed with (17.1 percent) or did not know (48.6 percent) about the negative interaction of oral contraceptives and smoking.

In a survey of 1,156 adults in Porto Alegre on the prevention of noncommunicable diseases (Bordin 1990), almost all respondents agreed that smoking should be banned in enclosed areas. Fewer respondents believed that warnings should be more pervasive, that tobacco advertising should be banned, and that cigarettes should be subjected to higher prices. Approximately 50 percent suggested banning the sale of cigarettes. These data were obtained from the survey on risk factors for adult population sponsored by PAHO (1987).

Smoking and Health

Mortality registers in Brazil are subject to region-specific limitations in quality and percent registration. Vital statistics data collection is more developed in the relatively affluent regions of the

Figure 1. Proportionate mortality for registered deaths among men, 35 years and older, Brazil, 1986

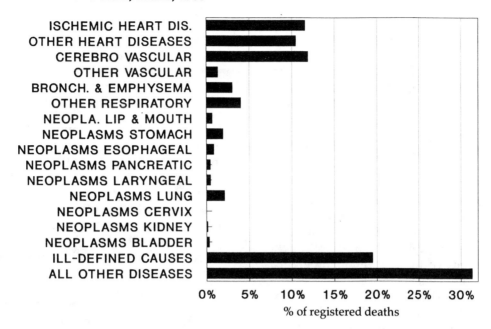

south and southeast. Although the number of registered deaths is high (approximately 800,000 nationally per year), underreporting is still estimated at 20 percent overall. "Signs, symptoms, and ill-defined causes of death" account for 20.3 percent of all causes. Thus, it is difficult to achieve national representation using these data.

Despite limitations in the quality of cause-of-death data, the mortality profile for Brazil suggests the relative importance of cardiovascular diseases and neoplasms that are at least partially related to smoking (Figure 1). Proportionately, circulatory diseases account for one-third of all Brazilian deaths, malignant neoplasms account for 11.4 percent, and diseases of the respiratory system account for 10.3 percent (PAHO 1990). Mortality registers from areas with adequate data show a proportionate mortality profile similar to that of developed countries. In 1985, the World Health Organization reported that Brazil had become the first developing country to have tobacco-caused diseases surpass other causes of death in total mortality (New Scientist 1985).

The age-adjusted mortality rates for lung cancer for men and women have increased over time, and these patterns may suggest a temporal link with historically increasing rates of cigarette consumption in Brazil. The increase in age-adjusted lung cancer mortality among men is more dramatic

than among women. Men have had historically higher rates of smoking prevalence than have women; therefore, this sex difference in lung cancer mortality rates is expected. The sex-specific trends roughly have followed the growth curve of per capita cigarette consumption from 1935 to 1970 by a lag of approximately 20 to 30 years. Although mortality rates are still lower than those found in countries where cigarette consumption was higher for a longer period of time, given the apparent upward trend, the mortality rates for lung cancer among either men or women likely have not yet peaked. (US Department of Health and Human Services [USDHHS] 1992).

Based on a report by Rosemberg in 1979 (Hijjar 1991), an estimated 100,000 deaths, or 7 percent of total deaths, are attributed annually to smoking in Brazil. More recent adjusted estimates of smoking-attributable mortality yield an estimated 32,400 smoking related deaths in Brazil (USDHHS 1992). Brazilians, like residents of the United States, have a long history of exposure to tobacco. Using U.S. attributable risk fractions, an estimated 66,000 deaths from 10 main causes of death may be attributed to smoking.

On a related topic, Brazil uses 80,000 to 100,000 tons of toxic agricultural products each year (PAHO 1990). A study of pesticide use by tobacco farmers in the Itajaí Valley, Santa Catarina, reported that 79.3 percent of the 563 farmers interviewed had suffered intoxication by chemical agents used for tobacco farming (APREMAVI 1988).

Tobacco Use Prevention and Control Activities

Government Executive Structure and Policies

In 1985, the Ministry of Health established the Advisory Group on the Control of Smoking, a multidisciplinary group with interinstitutional representation (from the Senate and the Chamber of Deputies, the Press Association, the Bar Association, the National Conference of Bishops, the Evangelical Movement, the Medical Association, the Consumer Defense Council, and six academic experts). The goals of the Advisory Group were to propose standards and legislation to control smoking, to provide advice for prevention programs, and to assess the implementation of a National Program to Control Smoking. The program had an executive secretariat and was linked directly to the Ministry of Health. Institutional reforms in the country's health system caused the National Program to be subsumed under the National Division of Chronic-Degenerative Diseases of the Ministry of Health in 1990.

In April 1989, the USDA reported that "The Brazilian Ministry of Health had just begun an antismoking campaign through the local radio, television, and printed press. This campaign was not very strong and had not had a significant effect on reducing the number of Brazilian cigarette smokers. . ." (Burr 1989). Even so, this program is one of the most advanced in the Americas. It has distributed five million copies of an antismoking comic book for children and has sponsored courses for health workers in all state capitals. The Ministry of Health has published for health professionals "Tabagismo e Saúde," a booklet of information on smoking (Rosemberg 1987). Grants, educational materials, and communications campaigns have also been sponsored by the National Program (Chapman 1990). On National Anti-Smoking Day, the National Program and local committees sponsor a foot race with the slogan "Run Away from Smoking." In 1990, more than 400 cities across the country participated in the event. For the last 3 years the National Program has published a newsletter that provides information and a means of communication between local groups. A nationwide antitobacco poster contest is held each year through schools.

In 1991, the Ministry of Health's Advisory Group succeeded in persuading the National Mail Service of Brazil to issue antismoking postage stamps. This issue was commemorated in a ceremony on April 9, 1991 (Alvarez-Herrera 1991).

Antitobacco Legislation and Executive Actions

Between 1952 and 1988, the National Congress considered 194 bills aimed at restricting tobacco use; only one was approved: Federal Law No. 7488 (1986) proclaiming National Anti-Smoking Day. In the country's new constitution, ratified in October 1988, Article 220 refers specifically to the commercial advertising of tobacco and other potentially harmful products, stipulating that restrictions will be made by the Ministry of Health and that a warning must always appear on tobacco advertisements stating the harmful effects arising from tobacco use. In 1988, the Ministry of Health issued an order (No. 490 of August 25, 1988) requiring cigarette packs and advertisements to display a warning and limiting the time when commercials may be broadcast on television and radio (only after 9:00 p.m.) (Chapman 1990).

The Ministry of Health has further restricted tobacco use through executive order, banning smoking in specific environments (e.g., libraries, classrooms, health centers, on public transportation, and on domestic flights lasting less than 2 hours), and also banning the sale of cigarettes to minors and the distribution of free samples. The extent to which these prohibitions have been enforced in the absence of legal penalties is not known.

Between 1980 and 1991, 10 states and 48 cities have passed various laws restricting cigarette smoking in specific environments such as Health Department premises, public transportation, shops, schools, cinemas, theaters, and elevators. For example, the city of São Paulo has recently made it mandatory for restaurants larger than 100 m² to provide a separate, no-smoking area (Costa e Silva 1990a).

Educational Activities

The introduction of antitobacco material into the school curriculum has been irregular and has occurred only through the initiative of individual states or schools. National policies or legislation do not mandate antitobacco school education. States and schools have, in general, responded to guidance from parent and teacher groups on this issue. The availability of educational material from the Ministry of Health has helped promote antitobacco education in many schools. No data are available on the evaluation or implementation of these programs.

Nongovernmental Action against Tobacco

In 1985, the Comite Coordenador do Controle do Tabagismo no Brasil (Brazilian Coordinating Committee on Smoking Control) was created: activities of this national organization include public information campaigns, scientific research, and collaboration with the Latin American Coordinating Committee on Smoking Control (Rosemberg 1990). In addition, the Associação de Mulheres da America Latina para o Controle do Tabagismo (AMALTA) (Latin American Women's Association on Smoking Control) has recently been organized in several Brazilian cities (Hijjar 1991).

The Brazilian Medical Association (AMB) has organized a Commission for the Fight against Smoking, and activities of the Association have increased in recent years. These include workshops and symposia in several states; two national professional conferences on smoking and health; and numerous articles on tobacco and health in the Jornal Brasileiro de Medicina (JBM) (Costa e Silva 1990b). However, in the 1988 Porto Alegre survey by Pohlmann (Pohlmann 1988), more than three-quarters of respondents who were smokers had not received any advice from physicians on the health consequences of smoking before they began to smoke. Approximately half remembered receiving some warning after beginning to smoke, but almost one-third of smokers were never advised by their physicians to stop smoking. In the survey of employees of SERGEN SA, 29 percent of respondents had received advice from physicians on smoking and health (Ribeiro 1989).

Several private companies have offered seminars and sponsored smoking cessation programs for their employees in recent years. In some cases, these activities have been designed to prevent work-related accidents such as fires. However, others are integrated into broader health promotion programs. For example, in 1988 the Banco do Brazil launched an antismoking educational campaign at all its offices throughout the country. This program followed the 1988 prevalence survey cited above. Follow-up data are not yet available regarding the possible effect of this educational program.

Summary and Conclusions

Brazil is one of the world's leading growers and exporters of tobacco. Its struggle for economic recovery prolongs its substantial dependence on tobacco exports. Domestic consumption virtually exploded in the post World War II decades, but during the 1980s, economic forces created a decreased demand for tobacco. Unfortunately, the mortality effects of the population's exposure to smoking are already evident, especially with respect to increasing rates of lung cancer among both men and women.

Numerous legislative attempts to influence tobacco use have faltered in Brazil, but a rather open-ended mandate to control the advertising of harmful products was included in the 1988 Constitution. This article permitted health authorities to regulate some of the advertising of tobacco over the electronic media; one success of this regulation has been the abandonment of tobacco advertisements on radio. However, tobacco advertising in Brazil appears to be a prolific enterprise, and promotions include otherwise beneficial health activities by both Government and nongovernmental agencies.

Because of decentralized state governments, other actions have been taken on a state or local level to regulate smoking in public places and to control access to tobacco by minors, but the degree of implementation and compliance with these regulations is unknown. The health care community has assumed important leadership activities in tobacco control, but, unfortunately, physicians appear to be lagging behind in both cessation of smoking and the application of preventive clinical activities.

Brazil has produced numerous studies on tobacco and health, on the health consequences of environmental tobacco smoke, and on the prevalence of tobacco use, and has also demonstrated both a Government and a scientific commitment to understanding and controlling the use of tobacco by its citizens. The National Anti-tobacco Program, though reduced in size, maintains a highly visible presence both in Brazil and in the world anti-tobacco community.

Based on the data presented in this report, the following can be concluded about tobacco and health in Brazil:

1. The impact of prolonged exposure to tobacco is evident in the mortality patterns of the Brazilian population. At least 32,400 deaths annually are attributable to smoking in Brazil.
2. Tobacco agriculture and export are important in the economy of Brazil. Crop substitution programs may be feasible, but these programs have not been supported thus far. Domestic consumption has declined in the 1980s due both to

economic pressures and to a growing domestic tobacco prevention and control effort.

3. The environmental impact of deforestation and agricultural chemical use in tobacco agriculture is substantial in Brazil. Efforts to reforest by tobacco growers have been ineffective.

4. The prevalence of smoking among men has been nearly 50 percent for almost 20 years. The prevalence of smoking among women has increased substantially over the last 20 years until the current rate among urban women is similar to that among urban men. Recent national data report the smoking prevalence among men as 39.9 percent and among women as 25.4 percent.

5. The proportion of reproductive-aged women who smoke is approximately one-third. The reproductive outcome of this exposure is documented by two studies that show increased rates of low birth weight as a complication of maternal smoking.

6. National and local efforts to control tobacco exist and have succeeded in disseminating widely public information, school programs, and communications efforts in Brazil. The effects of these programs are not yet evident.

References

ABIFUMO. *O Perfil da Cultura do Fumo no Brasil*, 1988.

ABIFUMO. *O Perfil da Indústria do Fumo no Brasil*, 1990.

ACHUTTI, A. *Fatores de Risco em Porto Alegre—1987*. Informe Preliminar, Washington, D.C.: Organização Panamericana da Saúde, 1988.

ACHUTTI, A., MEDEIROS, A.M.B., AZAMBUJA, M.I.R., COSTA, E. A., KLEIN, C. H. *A Hipertensão Arterial e outros Fatores de Risco no Estado do Rio Grande do Sul*. B. SAUDE, Porto Alegre 12(1):6–54, 1985.

ACHUTTI, A., et al. Smoking habit in schoolchildren of Porto Alegre. A five year project evaluation, 1980–1984. In: *Control del Hábito de Fumar, Taller Subregional para el Cono Sur Brazil*. Organization Panamerica de Salud. Cuaderno Técnico No. 2, 1986.

ANDERSON, J.E. Smoking during pregnancy and while using oral contraceptives. Data from seven surveys in Western Hemisphere populations. Presented at the International Conference on Smoking and Reproductive Health. San Francisco, CA, October 15–17, 1985. Atlanta, Georgia: Centers for Disease Control, 1985.

APREMAVI. *Newsletter No. 3*. June 5, 1988, Ibirama, 1988.

BARBOSA, M.T.S., CARLINI-COTRIM, B., SILVA-FILHO, A.R. O uso de tabaco por estudantes de primeiro e segundo graus em dez capitais brasileiras: possiveis contribuições da estatística multivariada para a compreensão do fenômeno. *Rev Saúde Publica S. Paulo* 23:401–409, 1989.

BIANCO, A.P., DE COSTA, E.C. *Goodness of Thermal Efficiency of Tobacco Curing Barns*. Santa Cruz: AP Santa Cruz do Sul SAFRA, 1982.

BORDIN, R., CORTILLETI, S. Prevençao e Control o doenças não transmissiveis. Porto Alegre. *Jornal Brasileiro Medicina* 61(2):90–97, 1991.

BURR, P.W. *Special Report: The Brazilian Tobacco Industry*. World Tobacco Situation Circular Series, FT 4–89, U.S. Department of Agriculture, April 1989.

CANDELAS, N.M.F. Fumo durante a gestação: Aspectos educativos de um problema comportamental. *Rev Saúde Publica* 13:244–253, 1979.

CHAPMAN, S., WONG, W.L. *Tobacco Control in the Third World—A Resource Atlas*. Penang, Malaysia: International Organization of Consumers Unions, 1990.

CONSTITUTION OF BRAZIL. Brasília: Republic of Brazil, 1988.

COSTA E SILVA, V.L. Country Collaborator's Report. Unpublished data, Washington, D.C.: Pan American Health Organization, 1990a.

COSTA E SILVA, V.L. Tabagismo—um problema de saúde pública no Brasil. *Jornal Brasileiro Medicina* 59(2):14–24, August, 1990b.

COSTA E SILVA, V.L., ALMEIDA, S.M. Tabagismo nos domicílios de crianças em idade escolar. 8th World Conference on Tobacco and Health, Poster, Buenos Aires, 1992.

COSTA E SILVA, V.L., CAMPOS, G.P., ROMERO, L.C., GERHARDT, F.G. Smoking modification behavior—an approach to teenagers in the Brazilian antismoking program. In: Aoki, M., Hisamichi, S., Tominaga, S. (eds.) *Smoking and Health 1987*. Amsterdam: Elsevier Science Publishers B.V., 1988.

CRESCENTI, R. Farmers in Brazil set example in ecology. *Tobacco International*. February 1990a, p. 20.

CRESCENTI, R. Brazilian smokers favour cheaper brands. *Tobacco International*. February 1990b, p. 56.

DELUCIA, R., SILVA PLANETA, C., ALMEIDA, N.S. Consumo de medicamentos, bebidas alcohólicas e cigarros por operários de Cubatão. *Revista Asociação de Medicina do Brasil* 33(11–12):215–218, 1987.

FEITOSA, T.M. Pesquisa sobre o hábito de fumar. Respostas as preguntas sobre conhecimento e medidas de controle do tabagismo em relação ao local de trabalho. Unpublished data. Agosto de 1988.

FOOD AND AGRICULTURE ORGANIZATION. *Tobacco: Supply, Demand and Trade Projections, 1995 and 2000.* FAO Economic and Social Development Paper 86. Rome: Food and Agriculture Organization of the United Nations, 1990.

GALLUP ORGANIZATION. *The Incidence of Smoking in Central and Latin America.* Conducted for: American Cancer Society. GO 87333. Princeton, New Jersey: The Gallup Organization, Inc., April 1988.

GROSS, R., FILHO, F.M., NETTO, A.R., SOBRINHO, F.M., FERREIRA, D.L.B., GORSON, M., MARTINEZ, A.R. Tabagismo e Gravidez—I. Prevalência do hábito de fumar entre gestantes. *Revista Asociación de Medicina do Brasil* 29(1–2):4–6, Jan–Feb 1983.

ALVAREZ-HERRERA, C. Brazil: Mail service issues antismoking stamps. *Globalink News Bulletin,* July 9, 1991.

HIJJAR, M.A., COSTA E SILVA, V.L. Tobacco epidemiology in Brazil. *Jornal Brasileiro de Medicina* 60(1–2):50–71, Jan–Feb 1991.

INSTITUTO BRASILEIRO DE GEOGRAFIA E ESTATISTICA (IBGE). *Anuario Estatístico.* Rio de Janeiro: IBGE, 1989.

INSTITUTO BRASILEIRO DE GEOGRAFIA E ESTATISTICA (IBGE). *Censo Agropecuario.* Rio de Janeiro: IBGE, 1989.

INSTITUTO BRASILEIRO DE GEOGRAFIA E ESTATISTICA (IBGE). *Pesquisa Nacional Sobre a Saúde e Nutrição 1989.* Rio de Janeiro: IBGE, 1991.

JOLY, D.J. *Encuesta sobre las características del hábito de fumar en América Latina.* Washington, D.C.: Pan American Health Organization. Scientific Publication 337, 1977.

JUNGBLUTH, G.A. Southern Brazil: A survey of devastation and conservation. *Tobacco International,* June 24 1988, p. 15.

KINZEN, O.G., ROHR, E.J. Produção de Fumo em Folha no Brasil e Substituição Potencial do Fumo por Outras Culturas. Anais Do Congreso da Sociedade Brasileira de Economia e Sociología Rural, Brasília, 1988.

LATIN AMERICAN CENTER FOR PERINATOLOGY AND HUMAN DEVELOPMENT (CLAP). Tabaquismo y embarazo: hay que ayudar a parar. *Salud Perinatal* 2(7):65–77, 1987.

MINISTERIO DA AERONAUTICA. Uma pesquisa de opinião. Ordem Interna de Serviço No. 001/DSA/84. Curitiba, September 14, 1984.

MINISTRY OF HEALTH. Projeto Saúde. Estudo sobre estilos de vida. Divisão Nacional de Doenças Crônico-degenerativas. LPM-61.88-2909. Brasília: November 28, 1988.

MINISTRY OF JUSTICE, MINISTRY OF HEALTH. Consumo de drogas psicotrópicas no Brasil, em 1987. Brasília: Centro de Documentação de Ministério da Saúde, 1989.

NEW SCIENTIST. Brazil tops Third World league for deaths from smoking. *New Scientist* 14, Feb 1985.

PAN AMERICAN HEALTH ORGANIZATION. *Health Conditions in the Americas.* Volume I and Volume II. Washington, D.C.: Pan American Health Organization, Scientific Publication 524, 1990.

POHLMANN, P., LOSS, S.F., FLORES, C., BOLZONI, DUNCAN, B. Tabagismo em Porto Alegre: Prevalência e o papel dos profissionais da saúde na prevenção. *Rev. Ass. Med. Brasil* 37(1), 1991.

PROCIANOY, G., MAULAZ, P.B., SCHLEE, J.C. Influência do fumo durante a gestação sobre o recem-nascido. *Jornal Brasileiro de Medicina* Maio, 88–105, 1970.

RAMOS, L. *Fatores de Risco em São Paulo—1987.* Informe preliminar. Washington, D.C.: Organização Panamericana da Saúde, 1988.

RIBEIRO, L.F. Typescript Report of survey of SERGEN S/A. Rio de Janeiro: Programa Nacional de Combate ao Fumo, Ministério da Saúde, November 1989.

ROSEMBERG, J. *Tabagismo e Saúde. Informação para Profissionais de Saúde.* Ministério da Saúde, Grupo Assessor Para O Controle Do Tabagismo No Brasil, Secretaria Nacional de Programas Especiais de Saúde. Brasília: Centro de Documentação do Ministério da Saúde, 1987.

ROSEMBERG, J. *Tabagismo, Sério Problema de Saúde Publica* (pamphlet). São Paulo: Ministério da Saúde, 1987.

ROSEMBERG, J., PERON, S.O. Tabagismo entre estudantes da Faculdade de Ciências Médicas de Sorocaba. Tabagismo nos Académicos de Medicina e nos Médicos. *Jornal da Pneumologia,* 1990.

SEGRE, C.A.M., et al. *Revista Paulista Pediatria* 4:1075, 1986.

SIMOES, M.J.S. Estudo da frequencia do hábito de fumar durante a gestação. Ribeirão Preto-SP. *Rev Cienc Biomed* 6:61–69, 1985.

STEWIEN, G.T.M. *O Adolescente e o Fumo.* Masters in Public Health Thesis. São Paulo: São Paulo University, Faculty of Public Health, 1977.

TOBACCO MERCHANTS ASSOCIATION OF THE U.S. 1979. *Production and Consumption of Tobacco Products for Selected Countries, 1979–1988.* Special Report 89-3. Princeton, New Jersey: Tobacco Merchants Association of the U.S. Inc., September 28, 1989.

U.S. DEPARTMENT OF HEALTH AND HUMAN SERVICES. *Smoking and Health in the Americas. A Report of the*

Surgeon General. Atlanta, Georgia: U.S. Department of Health and Human Services, Public Health Service, Centers for Disease Control, National Center for Chronic Disease Prevention and Health Promotion, Office on Smoking and Health, 1992, DHHS Publication No. (CDC) 92-8419.

VICTORIA, C.G., BARROS, F.C., VAUGHAN, J.P. Epidemiologia da Desiqualdade: Um Estudo Longitudinal de 6,000 Crianças Brasileiras. São Paulo: Cebeas-Hucitec, 1988.

VIGGIANO, M.G.C., et al. *Jornal Brasileiro Ginecologia* 100:147, 1990.

WORLD BANK. *World Development Report*. New York: Oxford University Press, 1989.

WORLD BANK. *World Development Report 1990—Poverty*. New York: Oxford University Press, 1990.

ZIMMERMAN, C. *Spotlight on Brazil: Banking on change.* *Tobacco Reporter* 38–50, April 1990.

British Territories: Anguilla, Bermuda, British Virgin Islands, Cayman Islands, and Turks and Caicos Islands

General Characteristics

Anguilla, Bermuda, the British Virgin Islands (BVI), the Cayman Islands, and the Turks and Caicos Islands are five British territories having internal self-government in the Caribbean subregion (Pan American Health Organization [PAHO] 1990). In each of these territories, the Government of the United Kingdom is responsible for security and external affairs and is represented locally by a Governor. The system of internal government is bicameral, consisting of a Legislature and an Executive Council or Senate. Some members of these bodies are elected representatives; the remainder are appointed by the Governor.

Anguilla is a small island in the northern Lesser Antilles. The BVI are due east of Puerto Rico and encompass 148 km². The Cayman Islands are about 280 km south of Cuba and consist of a group of three islands that cover 250 km². Bermuda is situated in the Atlantic Ocean approximately 970 km due east of Cape Hatteras, North Carolina, and has an area of 54 km². The Turks and Caicos Islands consist of eight islands about 144 km north of Haiti and extend over an area of 502 km².

The economies of these islands are based on tourism and on international business, mainly off-shore banking and insurance (PAHO 1990). Per capita gross domestic product ranged from $US2,470 in Anguilla to $US23,640 in the Cayman Islands (Table 1). For Anguilla, the level during 1987 and 1988 reflected a 44 percent increase over the previous 3-year period (PAHO 1990).

The populations of the BVI and Bermuda result from high fertility in BVI and low fertility in Bermuda, decreasing mortality for both island entities, and extensive immigration and emigration during the 1970s and 1980s. The populations of Anguilla (6,806), the BVI (12,240), and the Turks and Caicos (14,000) are younger overall than those of Bermuda (58,620) and the Caymans (25,900). More than one-third of the population of the former group was under 15 years of age in the 1980s compared with 20 percent in Bermuda and 23 percent in the Caymans (Bermuda Statistical Department 1988; CARICOM 1985; Cayman Islands Statistics Office 1990). Significant emigration of working-aged adults, a relatively constant birth rate, and a high infant mortality rate (25 per 1,000 live births in 1985 to 1987) characterize the population pattern in Anguilla. In Bermuda, the population pattern is shaped by a low birth rate and a significant immigration of older adults attracted by the high standard of living.

In both Anguilla and Bermuda, the proportion of the population 65 years and older is approximately 10 percent; in the BVI, the Caymans, and the Turks and Caicos these proportions are 5.9, 7.4, and 6.4 percent, respectively (PAHO 1990). These comparatively lower proportions may be attributed to immigration of young adults attracted by employment opportunities in the three island groups. For example, between 1979 and 1989 the non-Caymanian population tripled, from 3,200 to 9,800 (Cayman Islands Statistics Office 1990). In the BVI, 43 percent of persons employed in 1984 were foreign-born (BVI Statistical Division 1984). The for-

Table 1. Health and economic indicators in the British territories, late 1980s

Indicators	Anguilla	Bermuda	Br. Virgin Islands	Cayman Islands	Turks and Caicos Islands
Population	6,806	58,620	12,240	25,900	14,000
(year)	(1987)	(1988)	(1987)	(1989)	(1989)
Age structure (1980)					
Percent < 15	35	20	34	22.8	43.9
Percent ≥ 65	10.3	9.5	5.9	7.4	6.4
Birth rate (per 1,000)	26	15.9	22	17.2	23.1
Crude death rate (per 1,000)	NA	7.5	NA	4.4	6.1
Infant mortality rate					
(per 1,000 live births)	25	9.4	23.6	7.0	22
Per capita GNP	$US2,470	$US22,177	$US9,492	$US23,640	NA
(year)	(1988)	(1988)	(1987)	(1990)	
Life expectancy at birth	NA	73	70	77.1	66

Sources: PAHO, 1990b; Stout, 1990; Cann, 1990; Rogers, 1990; Cayman Islands Statistics Office, 1990; Bermuda Statistical Report, 1988; Williams, 1990.

eign-born proportion of the Turks and Caicos population is not known, but the growth of the population that occurred between 1979 and 1989 (from 6,000 to 8,000) is thought to be due to an influx of illegal aliens from the Dominican Republic and Haiti (PAHO 1990).

In 1988, crude death rates for Bermuda, Cayman Islands, and Turks and Caicos Islands were 7.5, 4.4, and 6.1 per 1,000 population, respectively (Table 1). Life expectancy at birth was 70 years or more in Bermuda, BVI, and the Caymans, and 66 years in the Turks and Caicos (PAHO 1990). Crude birth rates in Bermuda and the Caymans (1989) were similar (15.9 and 17.2 per 1,000 population, respectively) and both were lower than those in Anguilla, BVI, and the Turks and Caicos (26, 22, and 23.1 per 1,000 population, respectively) (PAHO 1990). Very low infant mortality rates were reported from the Cayman Islands and Bermuda in the 1980s (7.0 and 9.4 per 1,000 live births, respectively) (Cayman Islands Statistics Office 1990; Bermuda Statistical Department 1988). Single-year infant mortality rates for Anguilla, the BVI, and the Turks and Caicos Islands were two to three times higher than in the other two colonies (25, 23.6, and 22 per 1,000 live births, respectively) (PAHO 1990).

These population and vital statistics data must be interpreted with caution because the number of events that occurs annually in each population is small; thus, indicators for single years may be inaccurate. Nevertheless, the data presented suggest that these islands are at various stages of a demographic transition between a pattern of high birth and death rates to one in which death rates are very low and birth rates are sufficient to replace the population. This pattern is characteristic of the "epidemiologic transition" from a disease profile dominated by infectious diseases to one in which the causes of illness and death are related to aging and behavioral risk factors, such as smoking (Mosley 1990). In colonies such as Bermuda and the Caymans, the relative size of the aging population will be greater than that expected from fertility and mortality patterns because of the influx of middle-aged and older adults. Half (49.8 percent) of the 1989 population of Bermuda was 30 years or older and approximately 20 percent was aged 45 to 64 years.

Tobacco Industry

Tobacco is not grown, and no tobacco products are manufactured in any of the five British Caribbean colonies (Rogers 1990; Cann 1990; Stout 1990; Kumar 1990; Williams 1990).

The principal tobacco product imported into these territories is manufactured cigarettes. The major brands imported are manufactured in the United States and the United Kingdom; these include Marlboro, Salem, Winston, Benson & Hedges, Camel, 555, Rothmans, Kool, Dunhill, and Merit (Rogers 1990; Cann 1990; Stout 1990; Kumar 1990; Williams 1990). Marlboro is imported into all five territories, and each of the next three brands listed is imported by at least three of the five. In the BVI, the brands 555, Marlboro, Benson & Hedges, Kool, and Merit account for 28.5, 22, 17.2, 7.6, and 4.9 percent of the market, respectively (Stout 1990). Cigarettes are sold mainly in packs of 20 in all the colonies. There is no evidence of illegal trade in tobacco products in these colonies (Rogers 1990; Cann 1990; Stout 1990; Kumar 1990; Williams 1990).

There are no data on trade in tobacco products in four of the five colonies because much of the sale of tobacco occurs through duty-free outlets. During 1979 to 1989, Bermuda imported an average of 166,273 kg of tobacco products annually, 98 percent of which (162,687 kg) was manufactured cigarettes (Cann 1990). However, imports to Bermuda of unmanufactured tobacco declined by a net of 57 percent and of manufactured cigarettes by 54 percent during those 10 years (Figure 1).

The average retail price of the 20-cigarette pack varies from $US1.00 in the Cayman Islands to $US2.50 in Bermuda (Rogers 1990; Cann 1990; Stout 1990; Kumar 1990; Williams 1990). No taxes are levied on retail sales of tobacco products in any of the colonies, and no data are available on excise duties imposed on imported tobacco products.

Tobacco Use

Consumption

Of all tobacco sold in Anguilla, 5 percent is pipe tobacco, 3 percent is in cigars, and 2 percent is in the form of smokeless tobacco; imported cigarettes account for the remaining 90 percent (Rogers 1990). In the Turks and Caicos Islands, imported cigarettes account for 48 percent of all tobacco sales, cigars for 30 percent, pipe tobacco for 15 percent, fine-cut tobacco for hand rolled cigarettes for 5 percent, and smokeless tobacco for 2 percent (Williams 1990).

Annual cigarette imports and yearly popula-

Figure 1. Tobacco imports, in metric tons, Bermuda, 1979–1989

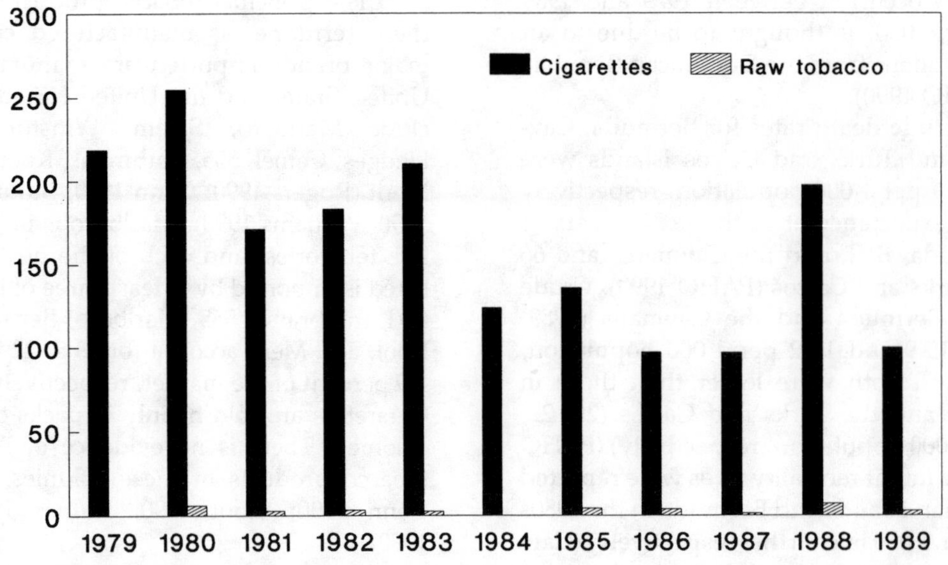

Source: Cann, 1990.

tion estimates were used to calculate per capita cigarette consumption for persons aged 15 years and older in Bermuda and the BVI (Cann 1990; Stout 1990; Bermuda Statistical Department 1988; BVI Statistical Division 1984; PAHO 1990). There was a 59 percent decline in the per capita tobacco consumption in Bermuda, from 5.3 kg in 1979 to 2.2 kg in 1989. Assuming that the conversion factor for manufactured cigarettes (1 cigarette = 0.865 grams of tobacco) can be applied, these data suggest that per capita cigarette consumption in Bermuda in 1989 (2,532) was less than that reported for the United States (3,000) (U.S. Department of Agriculture 1989) and similar to that for Canada (2,712) (Kaiserman and Allen 1990).

Domestic per capita tobacco consumption in the BVI was much lower than in Bermuda from 1979 to 1986. However, yearly per capita cigarette consumption among persons aged 15 years and older increased more than threefold from 1979 to 1982, from 680 cigarettes to 2,570. Reported consumption remained above 2,000 per person in 1983 and 1986 (Figure 2). The steep rise in per capita consumption in this colony may be due to an increase in the per capita income during the 1980s (BVI Statistical Division 1984; PAHO 1990). No data on cigarette consumption were available for 5 of the 11 years from 1979 to 1989. This absence of data suggests that official records may be unreliable and

that the observed increase in consumption from 1979 to 1986 may be in part artifactual.

The health implications of the consumption patterns presented above are unclear. Because all of these territories are major tourist destinations, the indicators for domestic cigarette consumption are likely affected by the large numbers of visitors who purchase cigarettes. For example, in 1980, Bermuda had a population of 54,050 residents and hosted 491,035 visitors (Bermuda Statistical Department 1988). It is impossible to separate tobacco consumption data for residents, nonresidents, and tourists.

Survey Data

Survey data may provide better information than consumption data for tobacco use in areas with significant tourist traffic. In 1990, a survey was conducted by the Health Department in Anguilla to determine the prevalence of cigarette smoking among a nonrandom sample of 59 males and 42 females aged 14 to 75 years (Rogers 1990). Sociodemographic data and information on cigarette smoking were collected through face-to-face interviews. Current, former, occasional, non-, and never smokers were classified according to the definitions of the World Health Organization (WHO 1983). Overall, the prevalence of current, former, and occasional smoking was only 5.9, 3.0, and 8.9

Figure 2. Per capita cigarette consumption,* British Virgin Islands, 1979–1986

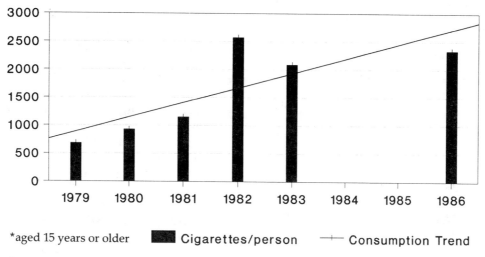

*aged 15 years or older ■ Cigarettes/person —⊢— Consumption Trend

Source: Stout, 1990.

percent, respectively; 82.2 percent of the respondents had never smoked (Table 2). The prevalence of any history of cigarette smoking was more than twice as high among males than among females (23.8 vs. 9.5 percent). The prevalence of current smoking was higher among those with no more than a primary education than among those with a secondary or tertiary education (27.3 vs. 3.3 percent) (Table 2). Among adolescents aged 10 to 19 years, prevalence of current, former, and occasional smoking was 2.2, 0.0, and 8.7 percent, respectively; 58.7 percent had never smoked cigarettes (Rogers 1990).

In 1985, the Advisory Sub-committee on Alcohol and Drug Abuse of the Cayman Islands sponsored a survey of students to assess attitudes,

knowledge, and behavior related to substances of abuse, including tobacco. The final survey sample included 2,063 students aged 10 to 17 years who attended school on January 23, 1985, and who completed a self-administered questionnaire (response rate = 99.8 percent). Smoking status of the respondents was stratified as ever smoker, current smoker, and never smoker. Ever smokers were defined as those who had used cigarettes on at least one occasion before the survey; current smokers were those who had smoked at any time during the month immediately preceding the survey; never smokers were those who had never smoked cigarettes (Kumar 1985). Of all respondents, 23.3 percent reported using cigarettes at least once, and 6.1 percent were current smokers; 76.7 percent had

Table 2. Prevalence (percent) of current, former, occasional, and never smoking among 101 adults aged 15–74 years, by sex and educational attainment, Anguilla 1990

	Smoking status				
	Current	Former	Occasional	Never	Sample size
Total	5.9	3.0	8.9	82.2	101
Men	10.2	5.1	8.5	76.2	59
Women	2.4	0.0	9.5	88.1	42
Educational attainment					
Primary/less	27.3	27.3	0.0	45.4	11
Secondary/tertiary	3.3	0.0	10.0	86.7	90

Source: Rogers, 1990.

Note: Ever smoking=history of smoking for 6 months or more in the past

Current smoking=at least once per day

Occasional smoking=less than daily smoking

Former smoking=not smoking occasionally or regularly at the time of the survey

Table 3. Age-specific prevalence (percent) of cigarette smoking among students aged 10–17 years, Cayman Islands, 1985

Age in years	Ever smoker	Current smoker*	Sample size
10	13.4	2.6	231
11	11.4	1.9	316
12	27.1	5.0	358
13	23.5	5.6	324
14	25.2	7.1	294
15	29.9	10.6	274
16	30.1	7.9	203
17	38.1	19.1	63
All boys	(NA)	7.9	998
All girls	(NA)	4.3	1065
Total	23.3	6.1	2063

Source: Kumar, 1985.
*Smoked at least once in the past month.
NA = Not available

never smoked (Table 3). Cigarette use was positively correlated with increasing age: approximately two of five 17-year-old students reported having smoked at least once compared with one in four 13-year-olds; current use was more than three times as common among 17-year-olds than among 13-year-olds (19.1 vs. 5.6 percent). As expected, more boys than girls were current smokers (7.9 vs. 4.3 percent). Of the 481 students who had ever smoked, only a small proportion did so on a daily or weekly basis (3.5 and 5.0 percent, respectively); the majority (88 percent) had used cigarettes only once or rarely. These data suggest that most regular smokers in the Caymans initiated this behavior shortly after reaching 14 years of age.

The survey also obtained information on reasons for starting to smoke cigarettes and on observed smoking by parents of the respondents. Curiosity (32.6 percent), peer pressure (12.0 percent), and enjoyment (11.2 percent) were most commonly cited as reasons for using cigarettes. Of all respondents, 44.6 percent reported having one or both parents who smoked. Current cigarette smoking was almost twice as common among the children of smokers than among those of nonsmokers (8.3 vs. 4.4 percent) (Kumar 1985). These data represent one of the most complete assessments of cigarette use among school-age youth in the Caribbean subregion.

Because no surveys of tobacco use have been performed among the adult populations of the Caymans, the BVI, or the Turks and Caicos, the true picture of tobacco use in the British territories is not known. Tobacco use among residents of Anguilla appears to be remarkably infrequent; data from face-to-face interviews are generally not as biased as self-administered questionnaires, but the small sample for this survey may not be representative of the entire island. Data collected from in-school students in the Caymans suggest that among those who are nearing the completion of high school, the prevalence of occasional and regular smoking may approach 20 percent, a rate similar to that in the United States and Canada (Kaiserman and Allen 1989; U.S. Department of Health and Human Services 1989a).

Smoking and Health

Vital statistics data provided to the Pan American Health Organization indicate that infectious diseases and diseases of children no longer contribute significantly to total mortality in any of the British territories (PAHO 1990). Currently, the principal causes of deaths in all of the territories are noncommunicable (mainly chronic) diseases, including coronary heart disease, cerebrovascular disease, cancer, and injuries (PAHO 1990).

Excluding Bermuda, fewer than 150 deaths occur each year in the territories collectively. In Bermuda, 1 (0.3 percent) of the 381 deaths among adults aged 35 years and older in 1988 was due to ill-defined conditions (Cann 1990). Six-year mortality data from the Cayman Islands Statistics Office indicate that only 2.8 percent of total deaths during 1984 to 1989 were classified as ill-defined conditions. Thus, mortality data are reliably recorded by cause of death, but the limited number of events precludes detailed analyses in these island entities.

The U.S. Surgeon General has reported smoking to be causally related to cancer of the lung, the larynx, trachea and bronchus, the oral cavity and lip, the esophagus, stomach and pancreas, the kidney and the bladder, as well as to coronary heart disease, cerebrovascular, peripheral vascular disease, and chronic obstructive lung disease (USDHHS 1989a). The small number of deaths each year in the British territories does not permit meaningful trend or attributable risk analyses of these causes of death in any of the five colonies. However, 6-year mortality data for the Caymans (1984 to 1989) (Cayman Islands Statistics Office 1989) and single-year mortality data for Bermuda (1988) (Cann 1990) were used to calculate proportionate mortality for several diseases that may be considered causally related to cigarette smoking.

Table 4. Number of deaths and proportional mortality (percent) due to smoking-related disease for men and women aged 35 years and over, Cayman Islands, 1984–89

Cause of death	Males No.	Males (%)	Females No.	Females (%)	Total No.	Total (%)
Ischemic heart disease (410–414)	50	(17.5)	53	(17.5)	103	(17.5)
Cerebrovascular disease (430–438)	36	(12.6)	45	(14.9)	81	(13.8)
Other heart disease (390–398, 401–405, 415–429)	34	(11.9)	40	(13.2)	74	(12.6)
Other circulatory disease (440–448)	5	(1.7)	8	(2.6)	13	(2.2)
C.O.P.D. (490–492, and asthma 496)	5	(1.7)	1	(0.3)	6	(1.0)
Other resp. dis. (010–012, 480–487, 493)	10	(3.5)	24	(7.9)	34	(5.8)
Cancer, lung (162)	22	(7.7)	3	(1.0)	25	(4.2)
Cancer, cervix (180)	—	(—)	7	(2.3)	7	(1.2)
Cancer, other (140–151, 157, 161, 188–189)	16	(5.6)	6	(2.0)	22	(3.7)
All other causes	108	(37.8)	116	(38.3)	224	(38.0)
All causes	286	(100.0)	303	(100.0)	589	(100.0)

Source: Kumar, 1990.

Of the principal causes of death among residents aged 35 years and older in the Cayman Islands during the 6-year period, coronary heart disease and cerebrovascular disease together accounted for 30.1 percent of total deaths among males and 32.4 percent among females. Proportionate mortality due to cancer of the lung was over seven times greater among males than among females (7.7 vs. 1.0 percent of total deaths). The principal smoking-related cancer in females was cancer of the cervix, accounting for 2.3 percent of all female deaths (Table 4).

Among Bermudians aged 35 years and older in 1988, cardiovascular disease (mainly coronary heart disease and cerebrovascular disease) accounted for approximately 34.4 percent among men and 35.7 percent among women of total deaths, respectively. Lung cancer was the single most significant cause of cancer death for both sexes; the proportionate mortality for lung cancer was 2.7 times higher for men than women (7.7 vs. 2.8 percent of total deaths) (Table 5).

Hypertension, diabetes mellitus, and obesity are prominent causes of morbidity in all of the island colonies (PAHO 1990). For example, one of every four patients attending clinics in the Cayman Islands is treated for hypertension, diabetes, or both (PAHO 1990). This information suggests that

Table 5. Number of deaths and proportional mortality (percent) due to smoking-related disease for men and women aged 35 years and over, Bermuda, 1988

Cause of death	Males No.	Males (%)	Females No.	Females (%)	Total No.	Total (%)
Ischemic heart disease (410–414)	55	(26.3)	49	(27.8)	104	(27.0)
Other heart disease (390–429)	17	(8.1)	10	(5.7)	27	(7.0)
Cerebrovascular disease (430–438)	17	(8.1)	14	(7.9)	31	(8.1)
Other circulatory disease (440–448)	7	(3.4)	7	(4.0)	14	(3.7)
C.O.P.D. (490–492, 496)	2	(1.0)	1	(0.6)	3	(0.7)
Other resp. dis.(010–012, 480–487, 493)	3	(1.4)	11	(6.3)	14	(3.7)
Cancer, lung (162)	16	(7.7)	5	(2.8)	21	(5.4)
Cancer, cervix (180)	—	(—)	4	(2.3)	4	(1.0)
Cancer, other (140–151, 157, 161, 188–189)	22	(10.5)	9	(5.1)	31	(8.1)
All other causes	70	(33.5)	66	(37.5)	136	(35.3)
All causes	209	(100.0)	176	(100.0)	385	(100.0)

Source: Cann, 1990.

the major risk factors for cardiovascular disease and cancer, other than tobacco use, are already common among residents of the colonies, even among the islands with younger population structures. If the prevalence of smoking noted among the parents of students in the Cayman Islands is typical of the smoking behavior among adults in the other territories, then the incidence of cardiovascular diseases and cancers attributable to smoking can be expected to increase as the large cohort of young adults ages. Moreover, it may be assumed that many of the foreign-born residents immigrating to the territories will be nearing retirement age, and many of these persons may have a history of tobacco use. For example, among U.S. citizens, the prevalence of cigarette smoking among men and women aged 45 to 64 years was 33.5 percent and 28.6 percent, respectively, in 1987 (USDHHS 1989b). Thus, an increasing burden of smoking-related diseases among the general population might be expected in the next several decades.

Tobacco Use Prevention and Control Activities

No official (written) Government policy on tobacco and health exists in any of the territories except Bermuda and the Cayman Islands (Rogers 1990; Cann 1990; Stout 1990; Kumar 1990; Williams 1990). Tobacco products are not subject to sales taxes in any of the islands, so relatively cheap cigarettes are readily available to residents and tourists alike.

In Bermuda, the Government currently is developing a policy to restrict smoking at all Government facilities, and a group of major employers is considering similar restrictions on worksite smoking (Cann 1990).

In April 1991, the Cayman Islands Government established a Health Promotion Council to address the leading cause of death, heart disease. In June 1991, the Heartbeat Cayman project was launched to reduce morbidity and mortality due to heart disease, and reduction of smoking was a key element of this campaign (Cayman's Health Promotion Programme 1991).

Bermuda has taken several legislative actions on tobacco-related policies. The Tobacco Products (Public Health) Act of 1987: No.2 became effective on April 1, 1988 (Government of Bermuda 1988). This Act requires that both a health warning and a statement of the tar content must be displayed on all packages of cigarettes and other tobacco products and in print media advertisements for tobacco. The Tobacco Products (Public Health) Regulations of 1988 specify that the health warning required in Bermuda is that required for domestic consumption of tobacco products either by the country of origin or by the country from which these products were exported. The Regulations also stipulate that the following standard health warning is to be used in any printed tobacco advertisement:

"HEALTH WARNING. SMOKING IS HAZARDOUS TO YOUR HEALTH"

Other national legislation in Bermuda forbids smoking in theaters, cinemas, and elevators, but there are no laws restricting the access of minors to tobacco products (Cann 1990).

In the Cayman Islands, a health warning is required by law to be displayed in all advertisements for tobacco products (Cayman Islands Government 1986). However, this requirement does not apply to advertisements appearing in any documents published outside the Cayman Islands. The warning reads:

"WARNING: SMOKING CAN SEVERELY DAMAGE YOUR HEALTH"

There is no antitobacco legislation of any type in any of the three other colonies (Rogers 1990; Stout 1990; Williams 1990). Although health warnings are printed on most packs of cigarettes imported to these islands from the United States and the United Kingdom, many cigarettes produced in the United States specifically for export are marked "Tax Exempt" and do not carry any warning messages (Rogers 1990; Stout 1990; Kumar 1990; Williams 1990). Voluntary restrictions on smoking in public places are quite common in the Cayman Islands, specifically in patient-care areas in the hospital, in Government buildings, and in some restaurants. Smoking has been banned on Cayman Airways since 1989 (Kumar 1990). Administrative restrictions on smoking are also in effect in many public places in the BVI and the Turks and Caicos, including health-care facilities, schools, business places, restaurants, and buses (Stout 1990; Williams 1990).

Bermuda and the Cayman Islands have specific legal restrictions on advertising of tobacco products. In Bermuda, no television or radio advertising of tobacco is permitted before 11:00 p.m., but point of purchase advertising, and sports promotions and corporate donations by tobacco companies have been reported (Cann 1990). In the BVI, tobacco advertising is permitted and used on radio, television (although no television station is located in the colony), and preceding movies. In the Cayman Islands, tobacco advertising is not permitted on media broadcast from within the islands or at any movies. However, advertising is permitted and used in print media and on billboards.

Because of the proximity to the United States and because of the increasing availability of cable television in the Caribbean, antitobacco messages via this medium are easily available to residents of all the British colonies. In the BVI in particular, print media messages about the risks of tobacco for cardiovascular disease (the most common cause of death in the islands) have been common. These are often based on information in the U.S. media. In the Caymans, antitobacco radio messages have been aired through the Government Information Service and Radio Cayman resources.

Tobacco-use prevention education has been integrated into the Family Life Education curriculum in all public schools in Bermuda and into the Health Studies curriculum for high school students in the BVI (Cann 1990; Stout 1990). The BVI Department of Health ("Family Tree Unit") distributes materials to marriage licensees that emphasize the dangers of smoking to the unborn fetus and newborn baby (Stout 1990).

In the BVI and Caymans, the local medical societies have demonstrated leadership in public education activities, including the posting of no smoking signs in medical facilities and worksites and in conducting community seminars. World No-Tobacco Day has been a focus of health department and medical society campaigns (Centers for Disease Control 1991). In addition, the Business and Professional Women's Association and the Caymans Against Substance Abuse are associated with the antismoking campaign in the Cayman Islands. In all of the colonies, church groups, especially the Seventh Day Adventist (SDA) Church, are modestly active in tobacco-related education. The SDA Church sponsors some of the rare cessation clinics in the colonies (Bermuda, Caymans, BVI). One private smoking cessation program operates in the Caymans (Kumar 1990).

Because of the administrative connection with the United Kingdom, some antitobacco education is provided to the territories from the Health Department of the United Kingdom. In the BVI, standard curricular materials for schools and additional public information materials produced in the United Kingdom have been used (Stout 1990). In the Cayman Islands, antismoking education is included in the schools' social education curriculum, intensifying around World No-Tobacco Day.

Summary and Conclusions

Anguilla, Bermuda, the British Virgin Islands, the Cayman Islands, and the Turks and Caicos Islands are five of the seven British territories still found in the Region of the Americas. The economies of all these islands are based primarily on tourism and off-shore business ventures such as banking and insurance. All of these islands are exposed to constant contact with tourists and media messages, primarily from North America, and thus, behaviors such as smoking and smoking cessation may be increasingly influenced by this cultural exposure. The tobacco industry in these territories is confined to trade in tobacco products, mainly cigarettes, that are manufactured in the United States and in the United Kingdom. The Governments derive excise tax revenue from this trade, but no sales taxes are levied on tobacco products, so relatively cheap cigarettes are available to both residents and tourists.

Data on domestic tobacco consumption are sparse. During 1979 to 1989, per capita consumption in Bermuda declined by 5.8 percent per year to 2.2 kg per person 15 years or older in 1989. The 1989 level was equivalent to 2,532 cigarettes per person, similar to that reported for Canada. The observed decline may reflect in part a decreasing demand for cigarettes by the large number of North American visitors. Per capita consumption in the BVI, though very much lower than in Bermuda during 1979 through 1986, increased threefold during the same period and is now similar to that in Bermuda. However, the increase observed may be related to increasing disposable income, unreliable official records, or to a combination of these and other factors. The available data are further limited in that it is not possible to estimate cigarette consumption for residents and tourists separately.

Data on adult tobacco use are available from one survey in Anguilla but from no other surveys of these territories. A relatively low prevalence of smoking among respondents to a school-based survey in the Caymans has been reported, and this may provide an opportunity for interventions aimed at preventing cigarette use. However, 44 percent of adolescents in the Cayman Islands also report that one or both of their parents are smokers.

Although specific evaluations on tobacco-related educational activities are not available, it appears that several channels for tobacco prevention and cessation information have been opened in the British territories. These include health-care providers, schools, licensing agencies, and churches. As with many other countries in the region, the SDA Church has provided cessation services to the public. In addition, school education has addressed tobacco use within the curriculum for at least two of the colonies. In the Cayman Islands, the Heartbeat Cayman project may provide a stimulus for more direct tobacco prevention and control activities.

Based on the data presented in this report, the following conclusions can be drawn:

1. Tobacco use behavior of the resident populations of the British territories should be monitored systematically by the use of regular household surveys. These surveys should form part of a surveillance system for behavioral risk factors for smoking-related and other chronic diseases.
2. Steps should be taken to enact and enforce legislation and regulations to prohibit or restrict the use of tobacco. These include restricting access of minors to tobacco, requiring labeling and health warnings on cigarette packages and advertisements, banning tobacco advertisements, and prohibiting smoking in public places. Consideration should be given to the possibility of adopting legislation already in effect in the United Kingdom.
3. Policies on health promotion should be formulated in all the territories. These policies should be multisectoral in approach and should include the development and distribution of antismoking health education and health promotion materials relevant to the local populations.
4. Nongovernmental and professional organizations should collaborate with each other and with Government agencies to maximize the impact of their activities aimed at prevention and cessation of tobacco use. Large Government-funded intervention programs may not be necessary in these small island entities, but existing resources should be coordinated more systematically by the health departments.

References

BERMUDA STATISTICAL DEPARTMENT. Bermuda Digest of Statistics 1988. No. 12. Ministry of Finance. Hamilton, Bermuda. 1988.

BRITISH VIRGIN ISLANDS STATISTICAL DIVISION. Chief Minister's Office. Tortola, British Virgin Islands. 1984.

CANN, J. Country Collaborator's Report, Bermuda, unpublished data, PAHO, 1990.

CARICOM. Population Census of the Commonwealth Caribbean—B.V.I., Volumes I & II. 1985.

CAYMAN ISLANDS STATISTICS OFFICE. *Population and Vital Statistics of the Cayman Islands*. Cayman Islands. 1990

CAYMAN ISLANDS GOVERNMENT. The tobacco product and intoxicating liquor advertising law (Law 21 of 1986). 1986.

CAYMAN'S HEALTH PROMOTION PROGRAMME. Heartbeat Cayman (1991–1996). Brochure, Health Services Department. 1991.

CENTERS FOR DISEASE CONTROL. World No-Tobacco Day. *Morbidity and Mortality Weekly Report* 40:341–342. 1991.

GOVERNMENT OF BERMUDA. The Tobacco Products (Public Health) Act, 1987.

KAISERMAN, M.J., ALLEN, T.A. Trends in Canadian tobacco consumption, 1980–1989. *Chronic Diseases in Canada* 11(4):54–55, July 1990.

KUMAR, A.K. Knowledge, Attitudes and Practices of Teenagers Towards Use of Alcohol and Drugs in the Cayman Islands. Advisory Subcommittee on Alcohol and Drug Abuse, Cayman Islands, 1985.

KUMAR, A.K. Country Collaborator's Report, Cayman Islands, unpublished data, PAHO, 1990.

MOSLEY, W.H., JAMISON, D.T., HENDERSON, D.A. The health sector in developing countries: problems for the 1990s and beyond. *Annual Review of Public Health*. 11:335–358, 1990.

PAN AMERICAN HEALTH ORGANIZATION. *Health Conditions in the Americas, 1990 Edition*. Pan American Health Organization. Scientific Publication No. 524, 1990.

THE READER'S DIGEST ASSOCIATION LIMITED. *The Reader's Digest Great World Atlas*. First Edition (Second Revise), 1964.

ROGERS, S. Country Collaborator's Report, Anguilla, unpublished data, PAHO, 1990.

STOUT, C. Country Collaborator's Report, British Virgin Islands, unpublished data, PAHO, 1990.

U.S. DEPARTMENT OF HEALTH AND HUMAN SERVICES. *Reducing the Health Consequences of Smoking: 25*

Years of Progress. A Report of the Surgeon General. U.S. Department of Health and Human Services, Public Health Service, Centers for Disease Control, Center for Chronic Disease Prevention and Health Promotion, Office on Smoking and Health. DHHS Publication No. (CDC) 89–8411, 1989a.

U.S. DEPARTMENT OF HEALTH AND HUMAN SERVICES. *Health United States 1988.* U.S. Department of Health and Human Services, Public Health Service, Cen-

ters for Disease Control, National Center for Health Statistics. DHHS Publication No. (PHS) 89–1232, 1989b.

WILLIAMS, J. Country Collaborator's Report, unpublished data, PAHO, 1990.

WORLD HEALTH ORGANIZATION. *Guidelines for the Conduct of Tobacco Smoking Surveys of the General Population.* Report of a WHO meeting held in Helsinki, Finland, November 29–December 4, 1982. WHO/SMO/83.4, 1983.

Canada

General Characteristics

The Tobacco Industry
    Agriculture
        Nature and extent
        Recent trends in production
        Government role
    Manufacturing
    Marketing
        Advertising and packaging
        Pricing and taxation
        Domestic and international trade

Tobacco Use
    Tobacco sales and consumption
        Trends, 1980–1989
    Population surveys
        Adult cigarette smoking
        Adolescent cigarette smoking
        Other forms of tobacco use
        Knowledge, attitudes, and opinions

Smoking and Health
    Overview of the health consequences
    Costs of smoking

Tobacco Use Prevention and Control Activities
    Government activities
        Restrictions on advertising
        Restrictions on purchasing
        Restrictions on consumption
        Education and health promotion
    Voluntary and private sector activities
        Influences on purchasing
        Influences on consumption
        Education and health promotion
        Nature of the control effort

Summary and Conclusions
    Trends in tobacco use and disease
    Progress toward national short-term objectives
    The balance sheet for tobacco use

References

General Characteristics

Canada is the northernmost country in the Americas, stretching from 42°N almost to the North Pole (85°N), and extending in breadth across six time zones. At 9,976 million km² in overall area, the country ranks as the second largest in the world. The population density is low, however: approximately 3 persons/km². Over three-quarters of the population lives in urbanized areas, and the vast majority of these people live in a relatively narrow strip in the southern regions of Canada, within 150 km of the U.S. border (Encyclopedia Britannica 1990).

Although the wealth of Canada historically has been based on natural resources derived from minerals in the Canadian Shield area and petroleum under the interior plains, the country's economy is now primarily service-oriented (Statistics Canada 1986a). Agriculture accounts for only a small part of economic activity: 3 percent of the gross domestic product (GDP) and 4 percent of the labor force (Statistics Canada 1991a). Tobacco production was 63,000 MT in 1988, far behind the major crops of wheat (26.3 million MT), barley (14.4 million MT), and corn (7.0 million MT) (Encyclopedia Britannica 1990).

In 1990, Canada's gross national product (GNP) was $C474 billion, or $C17,309 per capita (Encyclopedia Britannica 1990). The real growth rate in GNP between 1980 and 1988 was 3.4 percent, while the per capita growth in GNP for this period was 2.3 percent (World Bank 1989).

Canada and the United States have been major trading partners for many years. Since 1990, Canada has been a participant with the United States in a free-trade agreement that eventually will eliminate all remaining tariffs on trade between the two countries. Negotiations are currently underway to extend this agreement to include Mexico. Canada also concluded the Caribbean agreement in 1986 to permit tariff-free importation of many products from the Commonwealth countries and territories of the Caribbean (Wilkinson 1988).

Canada is a Federal parliamentary State with a central Government based in Ottawa. Ten provinces share responsibility with the Federal Government for health. The Federal role in health is to provide funding and set national standards for programs, which are administered at the provincial level. The provinces of Canada have primary responsibility for the organization and delivery of health care services and health promotion, but the Federal Government also participates in health promotion and is largely responsible for health protection. Thus, the three legislative acts that affect tobacco purchasing, marketing, and consumption are Federal (see "Prevention and Control Measures"). The shared, and sometimes overlapping, nature of jurisdiction in the health field means that federal-provincial cooperation is essential for any effort such as combating tobacco use.

Internationally, Canada shares common membership with other nations in the Americas in a number of multilateral bodies, most notably the Organization of American States, the Commonwealth, the Pan American Health Organization, and La Francophonie.

The 1990 population of Canada was an estimated 26,584,000 (Statistics Canada 1990c). At only 0.8 percent, the annual growth rate is the lowest in Canada's modern history. Canada is a relatively young nation compared to the industrialized societies of Europe. However, the Canadian population is older now than at any other time in the country's history, and is aging at a rate more rapid than that of other industrialized countries, including the United States (Dumas 1990). This aging trend is caused by both a very low fertility rate (currently 1.7 births per woman) and a steadily increasing life expectancy (from 73 years in 1970 to 77 years in 1988) (World Bank 1989). The number of persons aged 75 years and older increased by 140 percent between 1976 and 1986. Canadians aged 65 and over now account for more than 10 percent of the total population (Dumas 1990).

The crude death rate in Canada has stabilized at 7.0/1,000 persons, even though the population has aged (Dumas 1990). The infant mortality rate in 1989 was 7.5/1,000, a significant improvement over the 1981 rate of 9.6 (Statistics Canada 1991e). The major causes of death are cardiovascular disease and cancer (43 percent and 26 percent of the total, respectively). Lung cancer is the major site for cancer among males and the second leading site for female cancers. Chronic obstructive lung disease accounts for about 4 percent of all deaths (Bisch et al. 1989).

Lung cancer is expected to begin declining for both sexes within the next 5 years, as the heaviest-smoking cohorts age and die (Semenciw et al. 1989). This outcome assumes continued declines in the prevalence of smoking and the daily consumption by smokers. While these are reasonable assumptions, their impact may be offset by the aging of the "baby boomers." The result is likely to be a decline in the age-standardized mortality rate, although there may be a transient increase in the actual number of smoking-attributable deaths.

A general aging of the population, combined with sharp increases in health care costs, has renewed the priority attached to promotion and protection efforts (Epp 1986; Task Force on Health Promotion 1986; Spasoff 1987). With most provincial governments in Canada facing substantially increased debt in recent years, the sense of urgency about these pressures has increased.

The unexpectedly poor showing of Canadian adults on a recent literacy survey has generated a considerable amount of remedial activity by employers and the voluntary sector as well as Governments. In addition to the obvious relevance of literacy for the economic well-being of society, it is also apparent that a health strategy relying upon educational approaches to promotion and prevention requires a literate populace. While the true literacy rate will not change quickly, at least the problem is being addressed.

There is now considerable sentiment, although no consensus, among many of the provinces that the Federal Government should curtail its role in the health field, and provide the provinces with more latitude to organize and deliver health services. Despite a growing feeling among the general population that the Government is inefficient and wasteful, there is no apparent public support for reducing the regulatory role of the Government in certain areas, such as tobacco use. Many of the provinces prioritize health promotion in general and the curbing of tobacco use in particular (e.g., Task Force on Health Promotion 1986; Spasoff 1987). The National Strategy to Reduce Tobacco Use is endorsed by all the provinces as well as the Federal Government.

The Tobacco Industry

Agriculture

Nature and extent

The cultivation of tobacco in Canada has a long history, being well established by native peoples when the first European settlers arrived in New France (later Quebec) in the 1600s. The French colonists began trading tobacco as early as 1652, but cultivation was not regular until 1735 when the French Government first encouraged production (Seymour 1988).

The early tobacco crops were air cured and grown mostly in Quebec. Production in 1870 was 724,000 kg; this increased more than tenfold to 7,938,000 kg in 1910 (Seymour 1988). By then, skilled U.S. growers had been brought to southern Ontario by a predecessor of Imperial Tobacco. Production then turned to flue-cured tobacco and Ontario became the primary producing area in Canada. In 1989, Ontario produced 88 percent of the tobacco grown in Canada (Statistics Canada 1990d). Other production areas are Quebec (8 percent of the total) and Prince Edward Island (4 percent).

In 1989, Canadian farmers produced 75,573 MT (green weight) of tobacco on 31,140 ha (Statistics Canada 1990d), which accounted for 0.05 percent of all land under cultivation in the country (Statistics Canada 1987a). That year, there were 1,441 tobacco producers (Canadian Tobacco Manufacturers' Council 1990), representing about 4 percent of the total farming population (Agriculture Canada 1990). These tobacco farmers earned a total of $C297.4 million for their crops in 1989 (Statistics Canada 1990e), averaging $C22,579 per producer.

Recent trends in production

Total 1990 flue-cured tobacco production of 62,142 MT in Canada (Canadian Tobacco Manufacturers' Council 1991) was well above the value of 58,341 MT for 1988 (Statistics Canada 1990d), which was the lowest in 13 years. Despite increases in 1989 and 1990, current production is considerably below the record 113,290 MT of 1978 (Statistics Canada 1990d). These decreases are due both to declines in the prevalence of smoking (see Section III) and a reduction in the amount of tobacco per cigarette (Statistics Canada 1973, 1984).

Government role

Historically, the federal and provincial departments of agriculture have encouraged tobacco cultivation and have carried out research in attempts to improve crop yields.

An example of industry support can be found in the membership of the Canadian and Ontario Governments on the Tobacco Planning Advisory Committee. The committee was established in 1986 by the Ontario Ministry of Agriculture and Food to strengthen the province's tobacco industry and help it cope with declining demand. Other committee members are the domestic manufacturers of tobacco products, leaf dealers, and the Ontario Flue-cured Tobacco Growers Marketing Board (Price Waterhouse 1989). This last-mentioned group is an organization of growers who practice supply management aimed at stabilizing prices.

A relatively new Government activity is the Tobacco Diversification Plan, a program of the Federal department of agriculture that assists in the orderly downsizing of the Canadian tobacco industry by providing incentives to farmers to cease tobacco production and develop alternate crops for tobacco lands (Agriculture Canada 1990). However, another goal of the program is to improve the economic viability of those farmers who choose to continue in tobacco production. The plan was developed in response to decreased demand for tobacco products and, in consequence, Canadian leaf tobacco.

The Tobacco Diversification Plan has two components: a Tobacco Transition Adjustment Initiative ($C69.5 million) and an Alternate Enterprise Initiative ($C15 million). An evaluation conducted after 3 years of operation indicated that the Tobacco Transition Adjustment Initiative did assist significant numbers of farmers to cease production. However, half the program participants acknowledged that they would have quit even without the program, citing reduced crop sizes and returns, lack of confidence in the industry, and the influence of Government antismoking policies (Agriculture Canada 1990).

The Tobacco Transition Initiative clearly succeeded in reducing the number of tobacco farmer-entrepreneurs. However, 24 percent of program participants continue to work in tobacco farming as employees rather than as entrepreneurs (Agriculture Canada 1990).

The success of the Alternate Enterprise Initiative has been even more qualified, according to this evaluation. Available funds were not utilized for a variety of reasons, including a good crop in 1989 and the unwillingness of tobacco farmers to leave a well-established, high-income crop for a riskier lower-income one (Agriculture Canada 1990). Income per hectare derived from tobacco was much higher than most potential alternatives except strawberries and carrots (Ontario Ministry of Agriculture and Food 1984).

Manufacturing

The manufacture of tobacco products in 1990 occupied 4,404 employees whose earnings totaled $C261 million (Canadian Tobacco Manufacturers' Council 1990). This amounted to 0.03 percent of the Canadian work force and 0.06 percent of Canadian wage-earners (Statistics Canada 1990f). In addition, tobacco manufacturers spent about $C85 million on advertising in 1988 (Fennell 1988b).

Total cigarette production in 1989 was 50.3 billion cigarettes and 7.75 million kg of fine-cut tobacco (Canadian Tobacco Manufacturers' Council 1990), placing Canada 15th among the world's tobacco producing countries (Kaiserman and Collishaw 1991) (Table 1). From 1971 through 1981, cigarette production grew at an average annual rate of 2.8 percent. From 1982 through 1988, the average annual number of cigarettes produced declined by 3.7 percent. In contrast, the volume of fine-cut tobacco began to increase in 1981, and annual production grew by 7.4 percent through 1988 (Imperial Tobacco 1989a). At present, there are only three manufacturers, all of which are foreign-controlled (Table 2).

The dominant position of Imperial Tobacco may be due to its association with the Imasco family of companies. Based in Montreal, Imasco was ranked 14th in profit among all Canadian companies in 1989 (Report On Business 1990). Three of Imasco's other operating companies provide almost 1,200 retail sales outlets for Imperial's products.

All of these producers of tobacco products are vertically integrated; that is, they are involved in all stages of production, from the processing of tobacco leaf, through manufacture of various tobacco products, to wholesaling. In the 1960s, the tobacco companies formed an industry lobbying association, the Canadian Tobacco Manufacturers' Council, to represent their interests before the Government against the Canadian antismoking movement.

Table 1. Domestic production, importation, and exportation of tobacco products, Canada, 1990

	Domestic		Imported		Exported
Cigarettes (millions)	47,600	(−7%)	445	(−32%)	2,700 (+30%)
Cigars (millions)	222	(−7%)			
Fine-cut ('000 kg)	7,750	(−4%)			
Pipe tobacco ('000 kg)	18.5	(−21%)	305	(−37%)	

Source: Kaiserman and Collishaw, 1991.

Table 2. Market share of major Canadian tobacco manufacturers

Company	Market share (%) 1989	1971
Imperial Tobacco	57	39
Rothmans/Benson & Hedges	26	38
RJR-MacDonald	17	24

Source: Imperial Tobacco, 1989a.

Marketing

Advertising and packaging

Advertising expenditures peaked in 1980 when the three tobacco companies spent a total of $C57 million on cigarette advertising (Imperial Tobacco 1990a). In 1988, advertising was 91 percent of the 1981 amount (after inflation), and in 1989 it was estimated to fall even lower in real dollar terms (Imperial Tobacco 1990a). Prior to the introduction of legislation banning advertising in 1989, these declines resulted from a voluntary agreement to limit the increase in advertising expenditures to 75 percent of the rate of inflation (Canadian Tobacco Manufacturers' Council 1989b). However, true advertising expenditures may have increased at a faster rate in unreported categories.

Advertising of tobacco products is regulated by the 1988 Tobacco Products Control Act, which prohibits advertising in all forms, including electronic and print media, signs, and billboards, and restricts the use of brand names in sponsorship of sports or cultural events and the display of tobacco trademarks on nontobacco products. Radio and television in Canada had carried no cigarette advertising since 1972, when the tobacco industry adopted several voluntary restrictions in response to the threat of a legislated advertising ban.

Internal advertising strategies devised by Imperial Tobacco cast doubt on their publicized commitment to target established adult smokers only:

"The activity shown should be one which is practiced by young people 16 to 20 years old, or one that those people can reasonably aspire to in the near future" (Imperial Tobacco 1989b).

"To position the campaign against the target market on a demographic structure with a bias to [age] 15–35 and with equal male/female emphasis" (Spitzer 1989).

Table 3. Relative emphasis on target groups for 1981 advertising campaign by Imperial Tobacco

	English language	French language
Weight 1.0	Age 12–24 (M & F)	Age 18–24 (M)
Weight 0.9		Age 18–24 (F)
Weight 0.8		Age 12–17 (M)
Weight 0.7	Age 25–34 (M & F)	Age 12–17 (F)
Weight 0.6		Age 25–34 (M)
Weight 0.5		Age 25–35 (F)
Weight 0.0	Age 35+ (M & F)	

Source: Imperial Tobacco Ltd., 1989a.

Media plans for Imperial Tobacco for 1981 identified target age groups and their respective "weights" or emphasis for the Player's Light brand (Imperial Tobacco 1989a), as shown in Table 3.

In addition to advertising, other forms of marketing development consumed significant funds. In 1987, for example, Imperial Tobacco spent $C1.3 million to develop packaging and another $C1.7 million on market research (Imperial Tobacco 1990a). Part of this latter expenditure was for monthly surveys of consumer behavior and attitudes.

Pricing and taxation

The average retail price of domestically manufactured cigarettes in Canada is $C42.00 for a carton of 200 cigarettes ($C5.24 for a pack of 20 king size), while a 200–g tin of fine-cut tobacco now costs about $C38.00 (Department of Finance 1991). It thus requires about 20 minutes labor at the average industrial wage to purchase one pack of cigarettes, and 15 minutes to buy the equivalent fine-cut tobacco. The only significant variation in price is due to different rates of taxation in the provinces, which on average account for 77 percent of the retail price (Department of Finance 1991).

The taxation rate on fine-cut tobacco in Canada has lagged considerably behind that of cigarettes. Tax increases introduced during 1989 brought the rate on fine-cut tobacco to two-thirds of the rate for manufactured cigarettes (Department of Finance 1989). This differential was maintained with the tax increases in the Federal budget of February 1991 (Department of Finance 1991). However, cigarette-making kits using fine-cut tobacco pre-rolled into tobacco sticks, a growing market segment, are now taxed on a per-cigarette basis rather than by weight, in effect creating a third intermediate tax incidence category. Moreover, the province of Ontario, with one-third of the country's population, has recently removed the tax advantage of purchasing fine-cut tobacco. The latest increase of $C0.03 per cigarette is only the most recent in a series of increases by provincial governments. Since the 1989 Federal budget, the Government effort to discourage smoking has been cited as an additional reason for raising tobacco taxes. The real tobacco price index, the price of tobacco products adjusted for inflation, more than doubled from 1980 to 1990 (Kaiserman and Collishaw 1991).

Domestic and international trade

In 1985, there were 137 wholesalers, 90,000 retailers, and 23,000 vending machines. Tobacco sales were said to account for an estimated 22,000 jobs (Seymour 1988).

Although the export trade is rather small (6 percent of production), it grew 30 percent from 1988 to 1989. Most of these exports were probably cigarettes that were smoked by Canadians in the United States or the Caribbean, or that found their way back into Canada as either legitimate duty-free cigarettes or as illegal re-imports.

The high rate of taxation provides considerable temptation to smuggle tobacco into Canada, and there are several regions of the country where smuggling does occur fairly consistently, such as through an Indian Reserve straddling the Canada-United States borders. An estimated 8 million cartons annually change hands illegally in one reservation alone (KPMG Peat Marwick Thorne 1990). Another noteworthy location of smuggling activity is between the French islands of St. Pierre et Miquelon and neighboring Newfoundland. Overall, about 70 percent of the smuggled cigarettes are manufactured in Canada, exported legally, and re-imported illegally; the balance is mostly U.S.-manufactured cigarettes (KPMG Peat Marwick Thorne 1990).

Imports of cigarettes are insignificant compared to domestic production. Imported pipe tobacco, however, predominates over the domestic variety. Nevertheless, the total sales of pipe tobacco and cigars is extremely low at 0.6 percent of the market (Kaiserman and Allen 1990).

In 1989, Imperial Tobacco, with 58 percent of the market, had gross revenues of $C2.385 billion. Tax revenues for Federal and provincial governments from cigarette sales are significant. In 1989,

the total estimated value was $C5.5 billion (Canadian Tobacco Manufacturers' Council 1990), or two-thirds of total consumer expenditures of $C8.2 billion in the same year. The tax increases in the 1991 budget will increase Federal revenues by $C1.4 billion in 1991 and 1992 (Department of Finance 1991). Tobacco tax revenues account for 2 percent of all Federal and provincial revenues. The major significance of the tobacco industry in Canada is from the tax revenue it produces for the Government. Tobacco is of relatively minor and declining importance as an agricultural commodity, although it remains the third largest cash crop in Ontario.

Tobacco Use

Tobacco Sales and Consumption

Trends, 1980–1989

In 1989, there were 51,309 MT of tobacco products, including 56,190 million cigarettes, sold in Canada—the lowest amounts in well over a decade (Kaiserman and Allen 1990). The retail value of these sales was $C8.2 billion (Canadian Tobacco Manufacturers' Council 1990). For the 6.49 million smokers aged 15 and older (see next section), this represents an average of 23.7 cigarettes each day, or 2,712 cigarettes per year for all persons.

As shown in Table 4, cigarettes made up 81 percent of total sales by weight. The only other form of tobacco of any significance was fine-cut (15 percent); cigars accounted for less than 2 percent, and pipe and smokeless tobacco were each less than 1 percent of the total sales by weight (Kaiserman and Allen 1990).

Tobacco sales in 1989 declined 6.8 percent from a year earlier; this was the largest decline in a decade of steadily decreasing sales (Kaiserman and

Table 4. Sales of tobacco products, Canada, 1989

Form	Tonnes	Pieces
Cigarettes	41,621	48,047 million
Fine-cut	8,143	8,143 million
Cigars	847	228 million
Smokeless	371	—
Pipe	327	—
TOTAL	51,309	56,190 million*

Source: Statistics Canada, 1989b.
*Cigarettes + fine-cut, assuming 1 g/cigarette for the latter.

Figure 1. Purchases of cigarettes and fine-cut tobacco, in billions of units and tonnes, Canada, 1980–1990

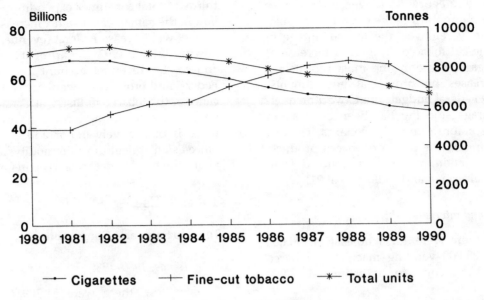

Source: Statistics Canada (annual), Catalogue No. 65-007.

Allen 1990) (Figure 1). Compared to 1980, sales by weight were down 21 percent overall, and down 29 percent in weight per capita (age 15 years and older). Manufactured cigarette sales per capita were down 30 percent (Kaiserman and Allen 1990), while the consumption per smoker was 13 percent less than the 1980 level of 27.2 cigarettes daily (see next section).

Sales of fine-cut tobacco increased steadily through the 1980s, presumably because of its relatively favorable tax treatment. Sales of this form of tobacco did not begin to decline until 1989, considerably later than for manufactured cigarettes (Figure 1).

Population surveys

Tobacco use in Canada has been monitored by population surveys on a regular basis since 1965. Most surveys were carried out for the Department of National Health and Welfare by Statistics Canada, the national statistics agency. Response rates of these surveys have exceeded 90 percent and sample sizes average 30,000. Findings reported below for 1989 are from a national telephone survey of 11,634 adults on alcohol and illicit drug use as well as tobacco (Eliany et al. 1990).

Few national surveys have covered smoking among Canadians younger than age 15, but a series of Gallup polls in the 1980s, as well as limited other sources, provides some insight into smoking behavior by adolescents.

Adult cigarette smoking

Thirty-two percent of Canadians aged 15 and older were smokers in 1989 (Stephens and Taylor 1991). Virtually all of the smokers were daily smokers, and the largest proportion of these smoked 11 to 25 cigarettes daily (Table 5). The highest rates of smoking (38 percent) were found among women aged 20 to 24 and men aged 25 to 44.

After a steady decline from 50 percent in 1965 to 34 percent in 1985, the rate of decline slowed (Figure 2). A large national survey in 1990 found that 41 percent of current smokers intended to quit or at least reduce their smoking.

In 1989, one-quarter of adult Canadians were former smokers. However, this is 44 percent of persons who have ever smoked. Thus, almost half of Canadians who have ever smoked had quit by 1989 (Stephens and Taylor 1991).

Two-thirds of smokers consume 11 to 25 cigarettes daily and 10 percent smoke more than a pack (more than 26 cigarettes) each day. Men are heavier smokers than are women overall (Stephens and Taylor 1991).

The fairly constant proportion of Canadians smoking in recent years (Figure 2) seems to contradict the fact that tobacco sales continue to decrease.

Table 5. Number of smokers, prevalence of cigarette smoking, and amount smoked daily, by age and sex, Canada, 1989

	Est'd '000	Type of cigarette smoker				Cigarettes daily		
		Never	Former	Occas.	Regular	1–10	11–25	26+
TOTAL	20,285	42%	26%	1%	31%	8%	20%	3%
15+ M	9,920	37	30	1	33	7	21	4
F	10,365	48	22	1	29	9	18	2
15–19 M	956	66	12	—	21	9	12	—
F	910	64	12	—	22	13	9	—
20–24 M	1,027	51	12	—	36	8	24	3
F	1,007	44	18	—	38	13	24	—
25–44 M	4,289	35	27	—	37	7	25	5
F	4,343	41	24	—	34	10	23	—
45–64 M	2,486	28	38	—	34	7	21	6
F	2,549	45	23	—	30	8	20	2
65+ M	1,162	24	54	—	21	6	12	—
F	1,557	63	21	—	16	6	9	—

Source: Stephens and Taylor, 1991.

The explanation is the reduced daily consumption by smokers, and the reduced quantity of tobacco per cigarette. In 1985, 20 percent of smokers consumed 1 to 10 cigarettes daily; in 1989, this figure was 26 percent. Almost every age and sex group showed a decline in daily consumption from 1985 to 1989 (Stephens and Taylor 1991). There has also been a switch to lower-tar-yield brands in Canada. From 1977 to 1986, the proportion of regular smokers in the lowest tar category (0 to 9 mg) doubled from 11 to 24 percent for women, and from 7 to 16 percent for men (Stephens 1988).

As in earlier surveys in Canada, the findings for 1989 show a clear association between smoking and educational attainment for all age and sex groups (Stephens and Taylor 1991). The prevalence of smoking is lowest among university graduates, regardless of age.

Figure 2. Current smoking prevalence (percent) among adults aged 15 and older, Canada, 1965–1990

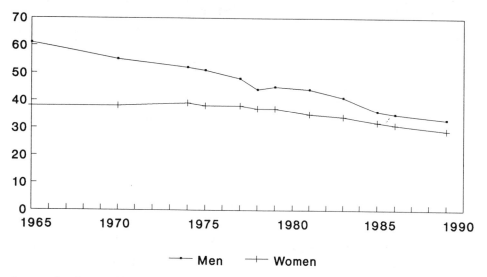

Source: Stephens, 1991.

Consistent differences among ethnic groups in Canada are evident. French speakers are more likely to be smokers than are English speakers, who in turn have a higher prevalence of smoking than speakers of other languages (Létourneau 1989). However, foreign-born individuals were less likely to smoke than were Canadian-born members of the same ethnic group (Millar 1991).

Adolescent cigarette smoking

Annual Gallup polls of 2,000 persons per year from 1983 through 1986 report that on average 9 percent of 12- to 14-year-olds were current smokers and that there was no change from year to year (Stephens 1988).

Although Native people constitute a small proportion of the Canadian population, the rate of smoking among Native youth is noteworthy. Among 5- to 9-year-old Indians and Inuits, 14 percent were occasional smokers in 1987 (Millar and Peterson 1989). Among 10- to 14-year-olds, 27 percent were occasional smokers and 10 percent were daily smokers. Only a minority (33 percent) of 15- to 19-year-olds were nonsmokers (Millar and Peterson 1989).

For most Canadians, smoking appears to begin during ages 15 to 19 years; 22 percent of this age group were smokers in 1989 (Table 5). Among this group, however, there has been a substantial de-cline in the prevalence of smoking since 1979, from 47 to 22 percent among males and from 46 to 24 percent among females (Stephens and Taylor 1991) (Figure 3). It is important to note that the rate for females has declined at the same rate as that for males, and while adolescent females were more likely than their male counterparts to smoke during the mid-1980s, this is no longer the case (Stephens and Taylor 1991). The age of onset declined steadily during the 20th century (Ferrence 1990). However, since the most recent data are from 1984, it is not possible to say whether recent interventions have had any impact on age of onset.

A majority of Canadian children (54 percent) live in households with at least one smoker, and such youth are twice as likely to be regular smokers as those who do not live with a smoker (Millar and Hunter 1991). Although this holds true for all socioeconomic levels, youth in low socioeconomic families are more likely to be exposed to smokers (Millar and Hunter 1990, 1991).

Other forms of tobacco use

Less than 2 percent of adult men smoke only a pipe or cigar, and the highest rate of such use (5 percent) is by men aged 65 and older (Millar 1988b). Smokeless tobacco use is rare in Canada, except among certain subpopulations. In 1986, use of both snuff and chewing tobacco was confined to males,

Figure 3. Current smoking prevalence (percent) among youth, Canada, 1979–1989

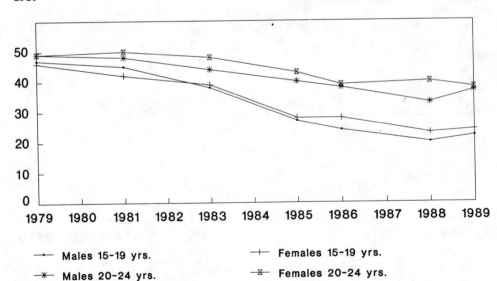

Source: Stephens and Taylor, 1991.

and the overall prevalence of use was under 1 percent (Millar 1989). Use among Native populations is much higher, however. In 1987, 12 percent of Indian males and 19 percent of Inuit males aged 10 to 19 used chewing tobacco in the Northwest Territories. Female rates were somewhat lower, but still significant, and there was use reported by 5- to 9-year-olds (Millar and Peterson 1989). Among Indian boys aged 5 to 9 years, 29 percent used snuff.

Knowledge, attitudes, and opinions

Preliminary findings from the 1990 Health Promotion Survey, a telephone survey of almost 14,000 persons aged 15 and older, indicate that 49 percent identify smoking as the main cause of heart disease (Statistics Canada 1991d). When respondents were asked to identify the health hazards of smoking on another survey, 44 percent specified lung cancer, 34 percent mentioned cancer in general, and 20 percent each indicated heart disease and emphysema. Only 1 percent failed to identify any health hazards. Smokers and nonsmokers were equally well-informed (Environics 1990a).

Public support for Government action on smoking was high in 1985 (Rootman et al. 1988) and has increased since. In 1990, 39 percent of adults felt it was ''very important'' for Government to deal with smoking as a health issue (Statistics Canada 1991d); in the 1985 survey, this figure was 33 percent. These attitudes may help explain the support for increased tobacco taxes: 46 percent of Ontario adults strongly supported a 10-percent cigarette tax increase (Environics 1990b). The level of support increases when the tax revenue is earmarked for research into smoking-related diseases (65 percent) or for prevention among young people (64 percent). Not surprisingly, only 17 percent of smokers were strongly in favor of a tax increase, but if the increased revenue was to be used to help people quit smoking, 53 percent of smokers were strongly supportive.

The 1985 Health Promotion Survey (Rootman et al. 1988) reported that 70 percent of adults were aware that children are more likely to smoke if their parents smoke, and 91 percent reported that women should not smoke during pregnancy. Most Canadians were also aware that smoking cessation reduces the risk of smoking-related disease, even after 10 years of smoking. One-third thought such risk would be reduced ''a great deal,'' while another 30 percent thought the risk reduction would be ''a moderate amount.''

In summary, substantial declines in tobacco consumption are evident in Canada, whether measured by sales, the prevalence of smoking, or the daily amount smoked. As the population ages, cohorts with relatively low smoking prevalence are being replaced by those with higher smoking prevalence. A substantial decline in the proportion of smokers under age 25 suggests that long-term declines in smoking prevalence are likely. These declines are coincident with the introduction of antismoking measures including taxation policy, advertising restrictions, and mass media promotion. The only noteworthy exception is the increased sales in fine-cut tobacco for hand-made cigarettes. The relatively favorable tax treatment of such tobacco, compared to ready-made cigarettes, may be the cause of this pattern.

Smoking and Health

Overview of the Health Consequences

Deaths in Canada attributable to smoking have been documented since the 1960s (Best et al. 1961), and this information has contributed greatly to the public debate about prohibitions on advertising, selling, and consuming tobacco (see next section). In 1989, smoking was responsible for an estimated 38,000 deaths (Collishaw and Leahy 1991), or 20 percent of all deaths in that year (Table 6). For men aged 35 years and older, the age-standardized mortality rate (ASMR) was 474.5/100,000, and for women, 165.2/100,000.

Smoking is estimated to account for 271,497 years of potential life lost (PYLL) before age 75. This is 3,543 PYLL for 100,000 man-years and 1,248 PYLL for 100,000 woman-years (Collishaw and Leahy 1991).

Based on data from a 7-year mortality followup of the 1978 and 1979 Canada Health Survey, Mao and colleagues (1988) compared the risk of dying among four hypothetical cohorts: male and female smokers and never-smokers. Over half the male smokers are expected to die before age 70, almost double the rate of the male nonsmokers. Among women, 27 percent of smokers and 17 percent of nonsmokers are predicted to die by age 70. For both sexes, smoking is expected to cause seven to eight times the number of early deaths due to traffic accidents, suicide, murder, AIDS, and drug abuse combined (Mao et al. 1988).

From the point of view of causes of death, smoking-related diseases account for the top-

Table 6. Relative risks[a] (RR) for death attributed to tobacco use and smoking-attributable mortality (SAM) for current and former smokers, by disease category and sex, Canada, 1989

Disease category	(ICD-9)	Males RR Current smokers	Males RR Former smokers	Males SAM	Females RR Current smokers	Females RR Former smokers	Females SAM	Total SAM
Adult diseases (> =35 years of age)								
Neoplasms								
Lip, oral cavity, pharynx	(140–149)	27.5	8.8	637	5.6	2.9	143	780
Esophagus	(150)	7.6	5.8	521	10.3	3.2	164	685
Pancreas	(157)	2.1	1.1	329	2.3	1.8	317	646
Larynx	(161)	10.5	5.2	300	17.8	11.9	61	361
Trachea, lung, bronchus	(162)	22.4	9.4	8,508	11.9	4.7	2,911	11,419
Cervix uter	(180)	N/A	N/A	0	2.1	1.9	116	116
Urinary blades	(188)	2.9	1.9	367	2.6	1.9	91	458
Kidney, other urinary	(189)	3.0	2.0	316	1.4	1.2	40	356
Cardiovascular diseases								
Rheumatic heart disease	(390–398)	1.9	1.3	47	1.7	1.2	49	96
Hypertension	(401–404)	1.9	1.3	119	1.7	1.2	74	193
Ischemic heart disease	(410–414)							
Ages 35–64		2.8	1.8	3,029	3.0	1.4	697	3,726
Ages 65+		1.6	1.3	3,934	1.6	1.3	1,817	5,751
Pulmonary heart disease	(415–417)	1.9	1.3	112	1.7	1.2	55	167
Other heart disease	(420–429)	1.9	1.3	1,048	1.7	1.2	463	1,547
Cerebrovascular	(430–438)							
Ages 35–64		3.7	1.4	425	4.8	1.4	384	809
Ages 65+		1.9	1.3	1,164	1.5	1.0	384	1,548
Artherosclerosis	(440)	4.1	2.3	467	3.0	1.3	281	748
Aortio aneurysm	(441)	4.1	2.3	730	3.0	1.3	153	883
Other arterial disease	(442–448)	4.1	2.3	261	3.0	1.3	106	367
Respiratory diseases								
Respiratory tuberculosis	(010–012)	2.0	1.6	23	2.2	1.4	8	31
Pneumonia/influenza	(480–487)	2.0	1.6	921	2.2	1.4	510	1,431
Bronchitis/emphysema	(491–492)	9.7	8.8	907	10.5	7.0	334	1,241
Asthma	(493)	2.0	1.6	66	2.2	1.4	65	131
Chronic airways obstruction	(496)	9.7	8.8	3,006	10.5	7.0	1,211	4,216
Pediatric diseases (< 1 yr of age)								
Low birth weight	(765)	1.8	1.8	27	1.8	1.8	20	47
Respiratory distress syndrome	(769)	1.8	1.8	34	1.8	1.8	22	56
Respiratory condition-newborn	(770)	1.8	1.8	21	1.8	1.8	16	37
Sudden infant death syndrome	(798)	1.5	1.5	36	1.5	1.5	21	57
Fire deaths[b]				81			38	119
Passive smoking death[c]				65			268	333
TOTAL				27,537			10,820	38,357

Source: Collishaw and Leahy, 1991a.

[a]Relative to never smokers.

[b]Data from Reference 9.

[c]Deaths among nonsmokers from lung cancer attributable to passive smoking.

Table 7. Years of potential life lost (YPLL) rates and age-standardized mortality rates (ASMR) due to selected smoking-related diseases, Canada, 1987–88

Cause of death	YPLL before age 75 per 100,000 p-y (1987–88)			ASMR per 100,000 persons (all ages) (1988)		
	Rank	M	F	Rank	M	F
CHD	1	1,355	375	1	187.8	90.1
Lung cancer	4	597	268	2	63.9	22.0
Stroke	6	203	159	3	41.4	35.7
COPD	8	147	75	4	35.2	11.3
Bladder cancer	21	27	7	>15	5.9	1.7

Sources: Wilkins and Mark, 1991; Hum and Semenciw, 1991.

ranked four among all causes when both males and females are combined. When years of potential life lost, which put more emphasis on early death, are considered, four of these smoking-related illnesses still rank among the top 10 (Table 7).

Death rates due to both coronary heart disease (CHD) and stroke dropped substantially between 1959 and 1988 for both men and women (Figures 4 and 5). For the most recent period (1979 to 1988), the average annual rate of decline in CHD and stroke for both men and women was greater than during the earlier periods of 1969 to 1978 or 1959 to 1968. Thus the decline in cardiovascular dis-

ease (CVD) mortality appears to be accelerating, now averaging approximately a 3.5-percent loss yearly (Hum and Semenciw 1991).

Despite these significant improvements in mortality in the last three decades, CHD and stroke have maintained their positions among the top three causes of death in Canada for each sex. CHD in particular accounts for almost three times as many deaths as the second-ranked cause for either sex. Smoking is clearly implicated in much of this premature mortality, accounting for an estimated 8 percent of male deaths and 2 percent of female deaths before age 70 due to cardiovascular disease

Figure 4. Age-standardized mortality rates, coronary heart disease and lung cancer, among men aged 25–74, Canada, 1951–1989

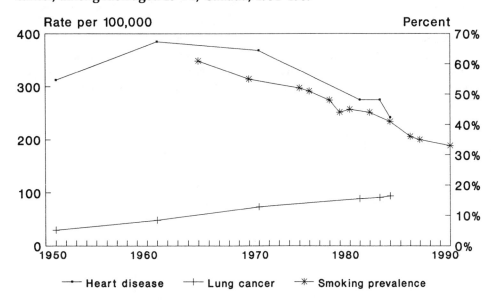

Source: Statistics Canada, 1991.

Figure 5. Age-standardized mortality rates, coronary heart disease and lung cancer, among women aged 25–74, Canada, 1951–1989

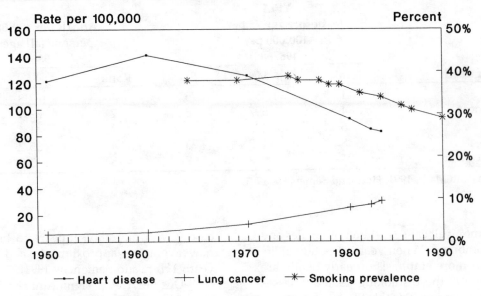

Source: Statistics Canada, 1991.

(Mao et al. 1988). Declines in the prevalence of smoking underlie some of the declines in death due to cardiovascular disease.

Lung cancer is the second leading cause of death for men in Canada, and the fourth leading cause for women (Hum and Semenciw 1991). In 1990, there were 113 new smoking-related cancers/100,000 men in Canada and 38/100,000 women (National Cancer Institute 1990) (Table 8). In comparison to lung cancer, cancers of the bladder, mouth, lip, and pharynx are both less common and more amenable to treatment.

In contrast to CVD, lung cancer death rates have been increasing over the last three decades in Canada (Figures 4, 5).

For men, the increase during the 1980s (annual average of 1.2 percent) was much lower than in the periods 1959 to 1968 (5.0 percent) or 1969 to 1978 (3.1 percent) (Hum and Semenciw 1991). Male rates were projected to begin a downturn in the early 1990s (Semenciw et al. 1989), and it appears that this projection may be accurate. For women, the trends in lung cancer are less encouraging. The period of greatest annual increases (7.1 percent) was relatively recent compared to men (1969 to 1978), and the increases for the period 1979 to 1988 were still significant (5.7 percent) (Hum and Semenciw 1991). As a consequence, lung cancer rates for women are not expected to plateau until the end of the century (Semenciw et al. 1989). Smoking is

Table 8. Incidence of new cases and deaths, and survival rates for selected smoking-related cancers, Canada, 1990

Site	New cases per 100,000 persons (1990)		ASMR per 100,000 persons (all ages) (1990)		Five-year survival (age 65+)	
	M	F	M	F	M	F
Lung	77	28	58	21	8%	12%
Bladder	23	6	5	1	63%	61%
Oral	13	4	5	1	77%	58%

Source: National Cancer Institute, 1990.

estimated to be responsible for 10 percent of cancer deaths before age 70 in males and 6 percent in females (Mao et al. 1988). An estimated 333 deaths in 1989 were due to lung cancer caused by passive smoking (Wigle et al. 1987; Collishaw and Leahy 1991).

In 1988, chronic obstructive pulmonary disease (COPD) was the fourth leading cause of death for men and the seventh for women in Canada (Hum and Semenciw 1991). COPD was responsible for 222 PYLL per 100,000 p-y in 1987 to 1988 (Table 7) (Wilkins and Mark 1991). COPD is projected to plateau in the early 1990s for men, and to be of steadily increasing importance into the next century as a cause of death for women (Semenciw et al. 1989).

Restrictions in normal activities, including work ("disability days"), are related to smoking status (Rogers 1985). Data from the 1978–1979 Canada Health Survey show a consistent positive relationship between disability days and smoking. Heavier smokers averaged one-fifth more disability than did never-smokers. When healthy smokers age 65 and older (the anomalous survivors) were excluded from the analysis, the disability rate of never-smokers averaged about half that of heavy smokers (Rogers 1985).

In 1991, a national survey revealed that 44 percent of the Canadian work force is exposed to second-hand smoke at work. Such exposure is inversely related to occupational status (e.g., 36 percent of managers and professionals vs. 54 percent of semiskilled and unskilled workers) (Canada Health Monitor 1991).

Costs of Smoking

The total direct costs (i.e., medical and hospital care, drugs, and research) of treating the three principal smoking-related illnesses in Canada in 1986 were $C9.3 billion, or almost one-quarter of total health care expenditures in Canada. The additional indirect costs of disability pensions and income lost due to premature death were twice this figure, bringing the total costs to an amount in excess of $C26 billion for the year (Table 9). However, only some of these costs are attributable to smoking (Wigle et al. 1991).

Estimates of some of the costs directly attributable to tobacco use have been calculated for 1989. These estimates were derived from Canadian data sources using the human capital approach (Schultz et al. 1991). In 1989, the health consequences of tobacco cost Canadians a total of $C9.5 billion in

Table 9. Costs ($C billions) of selected smoking-related diseases, Canada, 1986

Type of disease	Direct costs	Indirect costs	Total costs
Cardiovascular	5.0	8.5	13.5
Cancer (all)	1.9	7.2	9.1
Respiratory	2.4	1.4	3.8
TOTAL	9.3	17.1	26.4

Source: Wigle et al., 1991.

Table 10. Selected costs of tobacco use, Canada, 1989 ($C billion)

Costs	Age groups		Total
	35–64	65+	
Health costs			
Direct care	1.3	0.6	1.9
Premature mortality	4.1	2.7	6.8
Disability	0.6	0.1	0.7
Perinatal mortality			0.1
Property and forest fires			0.1
Retail expenditures on tobacco			
Tobacco taxes			5.5
Manufacturers' and trade margins			2.7
Total expenditures related to tobacco			17.8

Source: Collishaw and Leahy, 1991 (in preparation).

health care, premature mortality, and employment loss due to disability. In addition, smoking-related forest fires and property fires cost another $C.132 billion. In the same year, Canadians spent $C8.2 billion to purchase tobacco products, providing Federal and provincial Governments with $5.5 billion in excise, sales, and other taxes (Canadian Tobacco Manufacturers' Council 1990). Thus the personal and societal costs to Canadians for tobacco use in 1989 totaled $C17.8 billion (Table 10).

Tobacco Use Prevention and Control Activities

Government Activities

Prevention and control measures directed at tobacco use in Canada involve three levels of the Government and several different departments and agencies at each level. Advertising is governed by the Federal Tobacco Products Control Act; purchasing is affected by Federal and provincial taxation policies and municipal restrictions on vendors and machines; and consumption is restricted by the Federal Non-Smokers Health Act as well as provincial statutes and municipal by-laws. Federal and provincial Governments offer incentives to tobacco growers to cease production, and they provide the public with health education materials and information about smoking-cessation programs. All of these activities are included under the National Strategy to Reduce Tobacco Use, a framework developed and subscribed to by a broad spectrum of Government and national health agencies.

The National Strategy was initiated in May 1985 and is committed to the protection of nonsmokers, the prevention of smoking, and cessation by current smokers. As set out by the Steering Committee (1988) the goals and long-term objectives are:

Goal #1. To protect the health and rights of nonsmokers.

Objective: To decrease by the year 2000 the estimated proportion of nonsmokers exposed to smoke at home and/or at work from the current (1985) level of 60 to 86 percent to less than 40 percent. Short-term objectives involve increased restrictions on environmental tobacco smoke and parental awareness of the risk to children caused by tobacco smoke.

Goal #2. To help nonsmokers stay smoke-free.

Objective: To reduce by 30 percent by the year 2000, smoking onset among 12- to 19-year-olds, and by 20 percent among 20- to 29-year-olds. Short-term objectives are to establish nonsmoking as the norm in society, to control advertising and sales of tobacco products, and to aim effective public education programs at key target groups.

Goal #3. To encourage and help those who want to quit smoking.

Objective: By the year 2000, to increase by 50 percent the number of ex-smokers, and to reduce by 20 percent tobacco consumption per smoker. Short-term objectives involve the implementation of smoking cessation programs for high-risk groups and doubling the number of health professionals and employers promoting cessation.

Seven strategic directions identified in 1985 by the National program have been actively pursued since. These are: legislation, access to information, availability of services and programs, message promotion, support for citizen action, intersectoral

policy coordination, and research/knowledge development.

Legislative actions on tobacco have been described briefly above. Access to information involves the production and distribution of print, visual, and other educational resources to keep the public informed about new tobacco hazards. The National Clearinghouse on Tobacco and Health was established in February 1989. Among other activities, the Clearinghouse has compiled an extensive directory of Canadian agencies and individuals involved in the creation of a tobacco-free society, and distributes current information on smoking cessation programs and other select issues (National Clearinghouse on Tobacco and Health 1989).

The availability of services and programs, particularly for hard-to-reach groups, has been addressed through peer-assisted learning and community self-help groups. The Clearinghouse serves as an important information and networking resource for these activities.

Message promotion seeks to create greater acceptance of nonsmoking as positive, attractive, and socially desirable. Messages are aimed at target groups such as Native groups, women, and French speakers.

Support for citizen action under the National Strategy means that voluntary, community-based action—including research, advocacy, training, and networking—is encouraged and supported. Grants and contributions are provided for these purposes.

Intersectoral policy coordination is a fundamental component of the National Strategy; some aspects of it have already been cited. In addition to the efforts of health agencies to reduce smoking, this strategy extends to such measures as increased taxation on tobacco purchases, financial incentives to tobacco farmers to take up alternate crops, and enforcement by the Department of Labor of smoke-free workplaces. The national voluntary health organizations also play a role in the guidance of the National Strategy.

Research and knowledge development refers not only to continued and expanded monitoring of the prevalence of tobacco use, but also to improved understanding of the economics of the tobacco industry, the nature of tobacco addiction, and evaluation of prevention, promotion, and cessation efforts.

The National Strategy to Reduce Tobacco Use in Canada is now 6 years old. Work is underway as of the spring of 1991 to revise the Directional Paper, which is the key program document (Steering Committee 1988).

Restrictions on advertising

The key provision of the Tobacco Products Control Act, which covers advertising and promotion in all forms including sponsorships, is that "No person shall advertise any tobacco product offered for sale in Canada" (Health and Welfare Canada 1988).

The new law came into force in January 1989. Previously, broadcast advertising in Canada had been forbidden voluntarily since 1972, and print advertising was supposed to be limited in terms of dollar expenditures and minimum ages targeted. The tobacco industry adopted these voluntary restrictions to persuade the Federal Government that legislation was not necessary. However, it was clear by the mid-1980s that the voluntary approach was not working, and the new law was passed in 1988.

The major provisions of the Tobacco Products Control Act and its regulations (Health and Welfare Canada 1989a, 1989b) are as follows:

- no advertising in the electronic or print media
- no billboards or transit posters after January 1993
- no contests or free distribution of cigarettes
- no use of trademarks other than on tobacco products
- sponsorship of cultural and sporting events limited to their 1987 dollar value, and no use of tobacco product names in association with the sponsored events
- health warnings and toxic components to be clearly marked on all packages, with leaflets inserted in undersize packages
- four health warnings to be rotated on cigarette packages:
  — SMOKING REDUCES LIFE EXPECTANCY
  — SMOKING IS THE MAJOR CAUSE OF LUNG CANCER
  — SMOKING IS A MAJOR CAUSE OF HEART DISEASE
  — SMOKING DURING PREGNANCY CAN HARM THE BABY
- two health warnings to be rotated on cigar and pipe tobacco packages:
  — THIS PRODUCT CAN CAUSE CANCER
  — THIS PRODUCT IS NOT A SAFE ALTERNATIVE TO CIGARETTES
- a health warning to be on all smokeless tobacco packages:
  — THIS PRODUCT CAN CAUSE MOUTH CANCER
- mandatory reporting to Government of:
  — the constituents of all tobacco products and

their smoke, whether manufactured or imported
— the volume of all tobacco products manufactured or imported
— the monetary value of sponsorships

Although the new law required the warnings to be "legible and prominently displayed in contrasting colors" (Health and Welfare Canada 1989a), Imperial Tobacco, the largest of the three tobacco manufacturers operating in Canada, spent $C10 million in 1989 to design with the least impact possible new packages for cigarettes incorporating these health warnings (Imasco 1990). Proposed new regulations will require the messages to be black-on-white and white-on-black, regardless of the package colors (Health Protection Branch 1990).

Almost immediately after passage of the Tobacco Products Control Act, all three major manufacturers launched lawsuits against the Act. On July 26, 1991, Mr. Justice Jean-Jude Chabot of the Superior Court in the Province of Quebec, declared the Act to be "ultra vires the Canadian Parliament in that it infringes on provincial jurisdiction" (Quebec Superior Court 1991a). In addition, he declared the Act to be contrary to Canadian Charter of Rights and Freedoms and consequently null and void (Quebec Superior Court 1991a). The Government of Canada, represented by the Attorney General of Canada, appealed this decision citing 38 instances of errors and omissions (Quebec Superior Court 1991b). It is anticipated that the Supreme Court of Canada will eventually have to rule on this issue. Nevertheless, until such time as the appeal process is complete, the Tobacco Products Control Act remains in force.

Restrictions on purchasing

Under the Federal Tobacco Restraint Act (1908), it is an offense for anyone under the age of 16 to possess tobacco. Even if this Act were enforced, penalties would be of little deterrence as they have not changed since they were set in 1908. In certain provinces, statutes set higher ages for the purchase of tobacco. In Ontario, for example, the minimum age is 18 years. The City of Ottawa passed a by-law in 1990 requiring the licensing of all tobacco retailers, including vending machine operators (Ottawa 1989). These measures are indicative of growing community interest in restricting sales to minors.

A far more significant restraint on the purchase of tobacco arises from taxation policy. Ciga-

Figure 6. Per capita cigarette consumption* and tobacco prices, Canada, 1980–1991

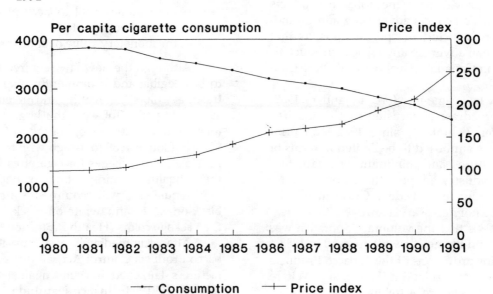

* Persons aged 15 and older. 1991 data are estimated.

rettes are highly taxed in Canada (77 percent of total price). The most recent Federal budget increased the tax per cigarette by $C0.03 (Department of Finance 1991). This increase was described explicitly by the finance minister as a public health measure. Previous increases had been treated as ways to raise revenue. Despite proportional tax increases for fine-cut tobacco, the tax is two-thirds the level of manufactured cigarettes (Department of Finance 1991). The Province of Ontario closed this gap with its changes to the tobacco tax in 1990 (Canadian Cancer Society et al. 1991).

For adults, the decline in consumption is proportionally less than the increase in taxes (Ferrence et al. 1991) (Figure 6); however, for Canadian adolescents, the decline in smoking is proportionally greater. In fact, Ferrence and colleagues (1991) concluded that "a ten percent increase in the relative price of cigarettes (over and above inflation) would likely result in a seventeen percent decrease in cigarettes consumed per capita by 15–19 year olds, a fourteen percent decrease in smoking, and a six percent decrease in consumption per smoker."

Tobacco taxes in Canada recently have risen much faster than has real disposable income. The "effective price" index of tobacco was 78.5 in 1991, about the same level as in the mid-1950s when the tobacco epidemic approached its zenith, but considerably higher than the all-time low effective price index of 34.6 reached in 1980 (Canadian Can-

cer Society et al. 1990). As of June 1991, taxes for a carton of 200 cigarettes ranged from $C32.75 to $C43.42.

Over 80 percent of those people surveyed in the fall of 1989 supported a tax increase if it could be shown to reduce greatly smoking among young people. Smokers as well as nonsmokers were more likely to support than to oppose increases in tobacco taxes (Canadian Cancer Society et al. 1990). Notwithstanding the public support for increased taxes, the tobacco industry began a campaign of protest in the spring of 1991. This took the form of encouraging smokers to complain to the Prime Minister about the "unfair taxes"; the tobacco companies provided for the purpose postcards printed on the inside of 25 million cigarette packages.

Restrictions on consumption

In 1988, Parliament passed the Non-smokers' Health Act to provide under Federal jurisdiction a smoke-free environment to all workplaces. A revised, strengthened, and more enforceable amended law came into effect in January 1990. Coverage includes not only the Federal public service, but also Crown corporations and federally regulated industries such as banking, insurance, trucking, and broadcasting. If a workplace chooses to permit smoking, it must be restricted to smoking rooms only. Many workplaces, including the

215,000–strong Federal public service, have chosen to ban smoking entirely. The Minister of Labor enforces this ban. Both tobacco consumption and worker complaints about smoke dropped substantially after a 1986 ban on smoking in Federal Government buildings (Millar 1988), and the quality of indoor air improved (Collishaw 1990).

Smoking is banned on all Canadian airline flights of up to 6 hours, and it is being phased out of longer international flights, with a complete ban to be in place by July 1993. Air Canada already had banned smoking on all its flights effective October 1, 1990. Smoking is prohibited on intercity buses, and it is restricted to one-third of the seats on trains and ships (Non-Smokers' Health Act 1988; Non-Smokers' Health Act-Amendment 1989; Non-Smokers' Health Regulations 1989; Non-Smokers' Health Regulations-Amendment 1990).

Most provinces in Canada restrict smoking in Government buildings (Ontario Government 1989) and the province of Ontario has extended these restrictions to the private sector (Bill 194). In many cases, however, smoking is permitted in designated areas with no requirement that they be separately ventilated (Mahood 1989).

As of mid-1988, two-thirds of Ontario's residents lived in municipalities with no-smoking laws (Ontario Interagency Council on Smoking and Health 1988). A survey in 1988 also revealed that 114 Canadian municipalities had smoking by-laws at that time—an increase of 56 percent over 1987, and of 192 percent over 1986 (Calgary Health Services 1988). In mid-1988 (prior to the passage of the Ontario legislation), 22 municipalities included the workplace in their by-laws restricting smoking.

The self-governing nature of educational institutions means that they are not often covered by municipal restrictions on smoking. A survey of schools in 1990 revealed that 58 percent have total bans on smoking and another 39 percent have partial bans (Health Promotion Directorate n.d.). Sixty percent of schools conduct special education programs regarding tobacco use.

Education and health promotion

Three parts of the National Strategy emphasize educational approaches. They are: access to information, message promotion, and availability of services/programs (Steering Committee 1988). The first two of these strategies are directed at the general public; the last is concerned with identifying and reaching high-risk groups. Some examples of education and health promotion activities are:

- *National Non-smoking Week.* An annual event to heighten awareness of smoking and to encourage cessation on "Weedless Wednesday." In recent years, themes have focused on high-risk groups such as women (1988) and children (1989 and 1990).

- *"Smoke Free: For a New Generation of Non-smokers."* An educational resource for educators of children aged 3 to 6 years; developed jointly by the Federal Department of Health and the Canadian Cancer Society.

- *"Break-Free All Stars" Program.* Under development by the Federal Health Department as an educational resource for coaches and other sports leaders of 8- to 10-year-old children.

- *PAL Smoking Prevention Program.* A peer-assisted learning resource for 11- to 13-year-olds to discourage uptake and encourage cessation of smoking.

- *"Break-Free" Advertising Campaign.* A national program of radio and television advertising aimed at 10- to 17-year-olds.

- *"Kids Decide but Parents Can Tip the Scales."* An information pamphlet for parents; stressing the addictive properties of tobacco and the importance of parents as role models.

- *Smoking Cessation Resource Guides.* Information on selecting a smoking cessation program; intended for employers and for the general public.

- *Francophone Consultation.* A workshop on the high prevalence of tobacco use by French-speaking Canadians.

Education is a provincial responsibility, and most Canadian children receive some health education, including information about the hazards of tobacco and other substances. However, not all children are exposed to health education at a sufficiently young age to discourage smoking uptake; 61 percent are exposed to health education in grades 1 through 7 while only 35 percent study health in grade 8 (age 12 to 13) (Trottier 1987).

The impact of the two main federal legislative Acts, the Nonsmokers' Health Act and the Tobacco Products Control Act, cannot yet be assessed comprehensively, but some observations are possible (Collishaw 1990). Tobacco cultivation continues to decline, but the number of farmers is decreasing at a faster rate than is the area farmed, leaving fewer and larger tobacco farms. Imported cigarettes (mainly American) still claim about 1 percent of the Canadian market, contrary to fears expressed by Canadian manufacturers during the legislative hearings. This may be because Canadian smokers prefer their usual brands, or because American manufacturers did not wish to divulge their cigarettes' constituents to the Canadian Government as required. Sponsorship of cultural and sports events continues, while publishers and advertising agencies appear to have found other advertisers. Considering that many Canadian newspapers voluntarily had ceased to accept tobacco advertising well before the ban was enforced, the impact of the lost advertising revenue is probably less than was feared by many.

Voluntary and Private Sector Activities

As noted above, a close working relationship exists in Canada involving the Federal Government, provincial health departments, and voluntary groups. Prominent among the latter is the Nonsmokers' Rights Association. Two umbrella organizations are the Canadian Council on Smoking and Health and the Ontario Interagency Council on Smoking and Health, both of which have member agencies from Government and the voluntary sector. In addition, there is close cooperation between public and voluntary sectors in the National Strategy to Reduce Tobacco Use in Canada. The participating agencies are:

- Canadian Cancer Society
- Canadian Council on Smoking and Health
- Canadian Lung Association
- Canadian Medical Association
- Canadian Nurses Association
- Canadian Pharmaceutical Association
- Canadian Public Health Association
- Heart and Stroke Foundation of Canada
- Physicians for a Smoke-Free Canada.

As nongovernmental bodies with their own status in the professional community, such groups can and do pressure Government to reinforce its antitobacco measures. For example, the Federal and Ontario ministers of finance both received detailed submissions supporting increased tobacco taxes in their latest budgets (Canadian Cancer Society et al. 1990, 1991).

Influences on purchasing

Two major nongovernmental influences on tobacco-purchasing behavior have been the move

to ban cigarette sales in pharmacies and the refusal of many influential newspapers (before the passage of the Tobacco Products Control Act) to accept tobacco advertising.

In 1988, approximately 22 percent of cigarettes were sold in drug stores (ERC Statistics International 1988). The Canadian Pharmaceutical Association began to encourage pharmacists to discontinue sales, with the first phase-out scheduled for the province of Quebec in April 1991 (Canadian Press 1991), followed by Manitoba. Ontario is scheduled to phase out pharmacy sales of tobacco products in 1993 (Sutter 1991). If adopted and enforced by Ontario and Quebec, this regulation would mean that more than two-thirds of Canadian smokers would be reminded further of the incompatibility of smoking and health. Canada's largest drug store chain, Shoppers' Drug Mart, is opposed to such a ban; it is owned by the parent company of Imperial Tobacco (Imasco 1990).

Other measures promoted by the Canadian Medical Association include an increase in the legal minimum age for purchasing tobacco, a ban of all vending machines, a prohibition on the sale to minors of candy cigarettes or other items resembling tobacco products, and increased fines and enforcement for selling tobacco to minors (Canadian Medical Association 1991b). Physicians for a Smoke-free Canada has advocated tougher regulations and more enforcement of the Tobacco Products Control Act, higher tobacco taxes, and a toughening of the Tobacco Restraint Act (Pipe et al. 1991).

Influences on consumption

The Canadian Medical Association has cautioned the health community against complacency in the wake of passage of the two Acts in 1988, and has urged the establishment of clear objectives for reduction of smoking (Walters 1991). It is the view of the Physicians for a Smoke-free Canada that "political, not clinical, activity will be more successful in conquering tobacco-related diseases" (Pipe et al. 1991, pp. 138–9). As an example of its innovative approach to discouraging tobacco consumption, this association has urged that leases with restaurants and stores in physician-owned buildings prohibit smoking (Pipe et al. 1991).

The Canadian Medical Association advises physicians to prohibit smoking in patient areas and to discourage smoking by patients in hospital; it supports extended protection for nonsmokers from environmental tobacco smoke, and it has banned smoking at its own official and social functions (Canadian Medical Association 1991b). A larger physician role in helping patients to stop smoking is also advocated (Walters 1991).

The vast majority of life insurance companies continue their long-standing practice of offering favorable rates to nonsmokers. For example, a 45-year-old nonsmoker pays an average premium of about 30 percent less for whole life insurance compared to a smoker of the same age.

Education and health promotion

Although the health coalition in Canada has shown considerable innovation in the measures it has taken to discourage tobacco use, it is still actively involved in "traditional" public education and health promotion. Often this takes the familiar form of distributing pamphlets and booklets describing the dangers of smoking. However, there is also a wide variety of activities which require greater involvement than simply reading. Among the more novel projects are:

- *The "Quit Line."* A toll-free number with accompanying publicity at the time of National Non-smoking Week to provide information and basic counseling on cessation (Canadian Council on Smoking and Health).

- *"Smoke Free Spaces."* A program initially directed at schools and subsequently expanded to other locales, to encourage and recognize a completely smoke-free environment (Heart and Stroke Foundation of Canada).

- *"Jump Rope for Heart."* A fund-raising group activity to encourage aerobic activity and healthy lifestyles among youth (Heart and Stroke Foundation of Canada).

- *"Charagraf."* An antismoking poster contest for Quebec students in collaboration with Musique Plus (Much Music).

Nature of the control effort

The two essential features of the Canadian effort to control tobacco use are the comprehensive nature of the National Strategy and its intersectoral quality.

The claim to comprehensiveness is justified on the grounds that the Strategy simultaneously includes cultivation, advertising, purchasing, and consumption of tobacco. Only the manufacturing process itself is not affected directly by the National Strategy to Reduce Tobacco Use. However, the vigorous and incessant lobbying efforts on behalf of

manufacturers of tobacco products suggest that there are at least strong indirect impacts on this aspect as well.

The variety of measures to combat tobacco use also supports the claim to a comprehensive program: incentives to farmers to cease production of tobacco, a legislated ban on advertising and restrictions on sponsorships, heavy increases in taxation in the last two Federal budgets, mandatory restrictions on consumption in public places and many private worksites, health education and promotion for both the public at large and high-risk groups, cessation programs for smokers, support for a social climate which disapproves of smoking, development of a network and information resources to sustain the antismoking campaign, vigorous and consistent lobbying of Government by the major voluntary health associations, reduction in the number of tobacco outlets, and research and knowledge development.

The comprehensiveness of the approach is also seen in the variety of players working toward the goals of the National Strategy to Reduce Tobacco Use: several Federal and provincial departments in addition to those responsible for public health, municipalities, voluntary health associations, professional associations, and private employers. Most of these explicitly endorse the goals of the National Strategy; many are directly involved in the Strategy's guidance. Thus their efforts are both complementary and mutually reinforcing. This was seen most clearly during the debate on the Tobacco Products Control Act and the Non-smokers' Health Act: the health coalition was united and consistent in its presentations and its lobbying in general (Kyle 1989).

The comprehensive and multifaceted nature of the tobacco control effort also makes it difficult to identify the effectiveness of any single measure. Nevertheless, many relevant observations are possible about impacts, as well as some inferences about probable causes.

Manufacturing. Cigarette production grew at an annual rate of 2.8 percent from 1971 to 1981, and then declined at an average rate of 3.7 percent annually through 1988. In contrast, fine-cut tobacco manufacturing began to grow in 1981; this trend has now been reversed. Manufacturing trends since the introduction of the Federal legislation at the beginning of 1989 indicate that cigarette production fell by 9 percent in 2 years. Once advertising was banned, tobacco company profits rose as expected (Collishaw 1990), but this is likely to be a short-lived phenomenon.

Advertising. In contrast to the era of voluntary controls on advertising (1972 to 1988), tobacco products now have much less visibility in the Canadian media, and there are relatively few concerns about marketing efforts directed at under-age youth, although such concern does remain. Sponsorships for tobacco products continue, but with somewhat less visibility, since these must not appear in the advertising for the event. However, many events are sponsored by newly formed companies that bear the same name as the tobacco products they sell, which circumvents the spirit, if not the letter, of the Tobacco Products Control Act. The recession of 1990 and 1991 has reduced corporate philanthropy in all forms, making it difficult to assess the impact of the sponsorship restrictions on the viability of sports and cultural groups.

Consumption. Tobacco sales in 1990 were the lowest in a decade, as was the number of cigarettes both per smoker and per capita. The decline in 1989 cigarette sales (7.8 percent) was the largest annual drop to date. These figures are consistent with the manufacturing trends and with the findings from population surveys. They also coincide with the introduction of the advertising ban and the restrictions on consumption (January 1, 1989). These drops in tobacco consumption occur near the end of a decade of steady increases in the effective price of tobacco, even though they precede the large jumps in taxation in the Federal budgets of 1990 and 1991. Tobacco tax revenues are higher than ever (an estimated $C6.5 billion in 1991) (Department of Finance 1991), but these are expected to decline as consumption continues to decrease.

Environmental quality. The ban on smoking in Federal Government office buildings in January 1987 and the more widespread restrictions in January 1989 were both followed by improvements in measured air quality (Millar 1988; Collishaw 1990). Improvements in absenteeism and productivity could be expected to follow, but this question has not yet been investigated. According to preliminary data from the 1990 Health Promotion Survey (the year after new restrictions on smoking in public places were initiated), 57 percent of smokers claimed they faced restrictions on where or when they could smoke and 88 percent of these persons reported that the effect of these restrictions was that they smoked less each day (Statistics Canada 1991d).

Public attitudes. Despite generally negative attitudes toward ever-increasing taxation, the Canadian public has indicated a high level of support for increased tobacco taxes (Canadian Cancer Society et al. 1990). The Ontario public has also demonstrated approval of the lobbying efforts of agencies such as the Heart and Stroke Foundation. In a survey conducted in early 1990, 66 percent of Ontario adults said it was a "very important" role of the Foundation to "pressure Government and business to make changes to reduce people's chances of having heart problems or stroke"; another 23 percent said it was at least "somewhat important" (Stephens 1990). Surveys have also revealed a high level of awareness of public education campaigns conducted by the Federal Government.

Despite this apparent success, there remain some areas where further action, particularly of a regulatory nature, is needed. Many of these areas are being debated (Pipe et al. 1991; Mahood 1989), and as noted, the Directional Paper for the National Strategy is being updated.

Sales to minors. Further restrictions are needed, including an increase in the minimum age to 18 years in all jurisdictions, along with licensing of vendors, enforcement, meaningful penalties for under-age sales and sales of single cigarettes, and controls on vending machines.

Warning labels. More explicit regulations would ensure that warnings on cigarette packages are highly visible. Additional messages about the addictive properties of tobacco and the hazardous nature of second-hand smoke are also called for.

Tax treatment. Increases in Federal and provincial taxes in future budgets should match the magnitude of those in the 1990 and 1991 budgets, with some of the revenue allocated to control of smuggling. The preferential tax treatment of fine-cut tobacco by the Federal Government should be eliminated.

Workplace consumption. In 1986 at the national level, 53 percent of the working population of Canada reported that smoking was permitted in their immediate work area. The prevalence of the right to smoke in the immediate work area ranged from 39 percent among professional workers to 67 percent among transportation workers. Large percentages of both the working population (81 percent) and smokers (65 percent) favor restrictions on smoking in the workplace (Millar and Bisch 1989). The present restrictions in Ontario on workplace smoking need to be strengthened. As Canada's largest province, this would not only mean coverage with a single measure for one-third of the population, but it would also provide a positive example to other provinces.

Summary and Conclusions

Trends in Tobacco Use and Disease

Tobacco continues to have a devastating impact on Canadians. Smoking accounts for 20 percent of all deaths. The most important causes of both death and lost productivity are smoking related, and the costs of health care, premature death, and property damage amount to $C9.6 billion each year. This situation is unlikely to change dramatically in the near future. Cardiovascular disease, cancer, chronic obstructive pulmonary disease, and other chronic diseases have been the principal causes of death in Canada for some generations, and there is little to suggest that this will change, even with the prospect of increased deaths due to AIDS. Coronary heart disease is expected to continue to decline, presumably reflecting decreases in the prevalence of smoking as well as improvements in diet and more frequent physical activity (Stephens and Craig 1988). Lung cancer already may have started to decline for men as predicted (Semenciw et al. 1989), but there is as yet no sign that it has reached its peak for women. These gender differences are usually attributed to the earlier peak in smoking by men than by women. The fact that smoking prevalence among Canadian women began to decline later is well recognized; that the cutback by men was steeper than by women is sometimes overlooked.

Projections of the prevalence of smoking to 2010, based on 15 years of very consistent trends, suggest that within the next few years, smoking will be more common among women than men, and that the gender gap will widen considerably as time passes. These projections, which assume a continuation of past trends, indicate that almost 20 percent of adult women in Canada will still be smokers 20 years from now. It is conceivable that these projections are too pessimistic, since they are based on behavior exhibited during a period when tobacco companies focused their advertising attention on young people of both sexes. Such advertising has been banned by law for more than 2 years, but it is still too early to assess impact of the ban on smoking behavior. Some other measures to discourage smoking, implemented under the umbrella of the National Strategy to Reduce Tobacco Use in Canada, are also too recent to have had a discernible impact on trends in consumption.

The comprehensive, multifaceted and intersectoral quality of Canada's National Strategy to Reduce Tobacco Use makes rigorous assessment of individual measures very difficult. Tobacco taxes have been steadily rising in Canada for a decade, while tobacco consumption has been falling (Figure 6). It is difficult to review this evidence without concluding that there is a strong causal relationship underlying it: (a) the declines follow the tax increases, (b) there is sometimes a brief resumption of smoking as smokers get used to the new tax, (c) the tobacco manufacturers bitterly oppose new taxes, (d) there appears to be a "dose-response" relationship in that the declines in smoking are proportional to the increases in tax, (e) consumption patterns for different forms of tobacco have changed in response to different tax rates, and (f) new quitters credit (or blame) the new taxes for their change in habit.

These tax increases have been strongly supported by the major voluntary and professional health associations. In the 1991 Federal budget, the increases were described as a public health measure for the first time. Survey evidence and even, under certain circumstances, the support of smokers were cited to indicate broad public support for these taxes. It is apparent that the public opposes smoking in public places and supports further Government restrictions. It is not yet apparent that the public realizes the economic cost to society of tobacco consumption. In the present climate, it is likely that such a realization would lead to calls for further curtailment of smoking, in private as well as public settings.

The important policy question at this time concerns the impact of further tax increases. While a continued decline in consumption is likely, its rate in proportion to the tax hikes may diminish if the remaining smokers become an increasingly intransigent group of the most addicted tobacco users. However, even if this prediction holds, future tax increases are likely to be as effective as past ones in discouraging potential new smokers. For this reason alone, future increases are justified, although it may take many years before they achieve the intended effect of eliminating smoking, if current smokers continue to adapt as have smokers in the past.

In the meantime, it may be politically both prudent and effective to direct some additional tax revenues toward cessation programs. This may have the effect of blunting the opposition of existing smokers to new taxes, while at the same time making a substantive contribution to reducing the overall prevalence of smoking. It may also be necessary to direct a proportion of tax revenues to increased monitoring of sales infractions and smuggling.

Progress toward National Short-term Objectives

Increase restrictions on environmental tobacco smoker. The Non-smokers' Health Act effectively restricted smoking in federally governed workplaces as of 1989, but the vast majority of the working population is not covered by this legislation. Provincial statutes and municipal by-laws are either weak or nonexistent, and the extent of enforcement is unknown.

Establish nonsmoking as the social norm. As less than one-third of the adult population smokes, it is clear that nonsmoking is at least the statistical norm. No national data exist to describe whether the population is aware of this fact, but widespread public support for restrictions on smoking indicates that the population at least adopted the norm of nonsmoking in public. There is no evidence available to suggest that the public opposes all smoking, or that the cost to the public treasury is appreciated.

Control advertising and rates. Passage of the Tobacco Products Control Act and its regulations has clearly changed the face of tobacco advertising in Canada. Although certain restrictions will not be phased in for another 2 years, the most visible forms of advertising have already disappeared from public view. It remains to be seen whether or not sponsorship of cultural and sporting events will increase with the end to the current economic recession. Progress on control of sales, particularly to minors, has been much less visible; this clearly calls for strengthening of the Tobacco Restraint Act, now under consideration by the Federal Government.

Direct education at key targets. Youthful non-smokers, women, Native people, and French-speaking Canadians have all been identified as target groups for the National Strategy to Reduce Tobacco Use. A number of innovative programs to reach youth through their peers, teachers, and coaches have been devised by both Government and the voluntary sector, but programs developed for the other target groups remain an exception rather than the norm.

Provide cessation programs for high-risk groups. Resource guides and other materials for encouraging cessation are now readily available to employers and others through the federally supported National Clearinghouse on Tobacco and Health and the Canadian Council on Smoking and Health.

There are evidently still difficulties in reaching high-risk groups, however, considering the extent of exposure to second-hand smoke by workers in service jobs and manual labor.

Double the promotion of cessation. No trend data are available to assess progress on the objective of doubling the number of health professionals and employers promoting smoking cessation, but the active antismoking stance of the Canadian Medical Association and other professional associations, as well as the demand for the smoking cessation resource materials, suggests an increased promotion of cessation.

The Balance Sheet for Tobacco Use

The health and property damage costs in Canada of tobacco use that can be quantified totaled $C9.6 billion in 1989. This very substantial sum is a conservative estimate, however, as it omits several significant costs which cannot be readily estimated. These are health care for diseases arising from exposure to environmental tobacco smoke, lost productivity due to exposure to smoking by co-workers and family members, property damage and maintenance needs due to tobacco smoke, enforcement and tax collection, and monitoring of smoking and research on its consequences by Government and the voluntary sector.

Although $C9.6 billion understates the health and property damage costs of smoking in Canada, it is a cost that is covered only partially by tax revenues. In 1989, smokers spent $C8.2 billion on their habit, generating in the process $C5.5 billion in tobacco taxes. When the income and property taxes of the tobacco manufacturers are included (Table 11), the total of $C5.6 billion is sufficient to cover only 58 percent of the identified societal costs of

Table 11. Costs and taxes due to smoking, Canada, 1989

Costs		$C9.6 billion
Health costs and related	9.5	
Property damage	0.1	
Manufacturers', wholesalers', and retailers' share of consumable expenditures on tobacco		$C2.7 billion
Taxes		$C5.6 billion
Tobacco taxes from smokers	5.5	
Income and property taxes from manufacturers	0.1	

smoking, a shortfall of $C4 billion. Even with the latest tax increases, and assuming no change in the costs of smoking, the shortfall in 1991 would be $C3.2 billion.

The net cost of smoking has received little public discussion or debate in Canada because many of the key costs were previously unknown. Such knowledge, in the face of rising health care costs, budgetary deficits, and resistance to general tax increases, is likely to lead to support for further strong measures to curtail smoking in Canada.

In summary, Canada enjoys one of the most comprehensive, and arguably the most effective, national tobacco-use prevention and control programs in the world. Several gaps in the program have been identified, but legislative, policy, and educational programs currently in place can serve as a substrate on which to build additional effective strategies. The future disease impact of smoking will be an important outcome measure to test the effectiveness of interventions currently addressed in good faith but without strict experimental evidence of effectiveness. In many ways, Canada serves as the world's laboratory for demonstrating the effectiveness of the multiple activities that constitute the state-of-the-art in the public health practice of tobacco use prevention and control.

References

AGRICULTURE CANADA. *Evaluation of the Tobacco Diversification Plan (Tobacco Transition Adjustment Initiative and Alternative Enterprise Initiative) Executive Report.* Ottawa: Agriculture Canada, Audit and Evaluation Branch, Program Evaluation Division, December 6, 1990.

ARRAIZ, G.A. Mortality patterns from 1931 to 1986 of Canadians aged 35 to 64. *Chronic Diseases in Canada* 10(2): 25–27, 1989.

ARRAIZ, G.A., WONG, T. Recent incidence and mortality trends of some diseases among females in Canada. *Chronic Diseases in Canada* 11(2):22–24, 1990.

BEST, E.W.R., JOSIE, G.H., WALKER, C.B. A Canadian study of mortality in relation to smoking habits—A preliminary report. *Canadian Journal of Public Health* 52: 99–106, 1961.

BISCH, L., LEE, K., MARK, E. Major causes of death, Canada, 1989. *Chronic Diseases in Canada* 10(2):22–24, 1989.

BODDEWYN, J.J. Evidentiary submission of Jean J. Boddewyn, Ph.D., Professor of Marketing/International Business before the Legislative Committee of the House of Commons considering Bill C-51 on behalf of the Canadian Tobacco Manufacturers' Council. January 20, 1988.

CALGARY HEALTH SERVICES. *Smoking By-laws in Canada 1988.* Calgary, Alberta: City Health Department, 1988.

CANADA HEALTH MONITOR. *Highlights Report, Survey #5.* Toronto: Earl Berger/Price Waterhouse, 1991.

CANADIAN CANCER SOCIETY (ONTARIO DIVISION), CANADIAN ONCOLOGY SOCIETY, HEART AND STROKE FOUNDATION OF ONTARIO, ONTARIO LUNG ASSOCIATION, NON-SMOKERS' RIGHTS ASSOCIATION, ONTARIO COUNCIL ON SMOKING AND HEALTH, PHYSICIANS FOR A SMOKE-FREE CANADA. *Health-Oriented Policy Options on Tobacco Tax in the 1991 Ontario Budget.* A submission to the Treasurer of Ontario, the Honourable Floyd Laughren. January 1991.

CANADIAN CANCER SOCIETY, CANADIAN COUNCIL ON SMOKING AND HEALTH, CANADIAN MEDICAL ASSOCIATION, HEART AND STROKE FOUNDATION OF CANADA, NON-SMOKERS' RIGHTS ASSOCIATION, PHYSICIANS FOR A SMOKE-FREE CANADA. *Sustaining a Successful Policy: The Treatment of Tobacco Taxation in the 1991 Federal Budget.* A submission to the Minister of Finance, the Honourable Michael Wilson. December 1990.

CANADIAN COUNCIL ON SMOKING AND HEALTH. Tobacco Regulations. *CCSH Smoking or Health Update,* Spring 1989.

CANADIAN MEDICAL ASSOCIATION. OMA throws support behind pharmacies that ban tobacco. *Canadian Medical Association Journal* 144 (6):742, 1991a.

CANADIAN MEDICAL ASSOCIATION. Smoking and health: 1991 Update (CMA Policy Summary). *Canadian Medical Association Journal* 144 (2):232a–b, 1991b.

CANADIAN PRESS. Québec drugstores move to ban tobacco. *The Globe and Mail,* February 20, 1991.

CANADIAN TOBACCO MANUFACTURERS' COUNCIL. *Correspondence between Health and Welfare and the Tobacco Manufacturers.* From RJR-MacDonald Inc. vs the Attorney General of Canada, Quebec Superior Court, vol 23, November 23, 1989, Exhibit AG-75.

CANADIAN TOBACCO MANUFACTURERS' COUNCIL. *Tobacco in Canada 1989.* Ottawa: Canadian Tobacco Manufacturers' Council, April 1990.

CANADIAN TOBACCO MANUFACTURERS' COUNCIL. *Tobacco in Canada 1990.* Ottawa: Canadian Tobacco Manufacturers' Council, April 1991.

COLLISHAW, N.E. *Monitoring Effectiveness of Canada's Health-oriented Tobacco Policies.* Presented to the National

Workshop on Smoking and Health, Halifax, Nova Scotia, September 21, 1990.

COLLISHAW, N.E., LEAHY, K. Mortality attributable to tobacco use in Canada, 1989. *Chronic Diseases in Canada* 12(4):46–49, 1991.

CONSULTATION, PLANNING AND IMPLEMENTATION COMMITTEE. *Directional Paper of the National Program to Reduce Tobacco Use in Canada.* Ottawa, June 1987.

DEPARTMENT OF FINANCE. Budget Speech, delivered in the House of Commons by the Honourable Michael H. Wilson, Minister of Finance, April 1989.

DEPARTMENT OF FINANCE. The Budget—tabled in the House of Commons by the Honourable Michael H. Wilson, Minister of Finance, February 26, 1991.

DUMAS, J. *Report on the Demographic Situation in Canada 1989. Current Demographic Analysis.* Statistics Canada Catalogue No. 91–209E, 1990.

ELIANY, M., GIESBRECHT, N., NELSON, M., WELLMAN, B., WORTLEY, S. (eds.). *National Alcohol and Other Drugs Survey 1989: Highlights Report.* Health and Welfare Canada, Catalogue No. H39–175/1990E, 1990.

ENCYCLOPEDIA BRITANNICA. *Encyclopedia Britannica World Data Annual 1990.* Chicago: Encyclopedia Britannica, 1990.

ENVIRONICS RESEARCH GROUP LTD. *Awareness of Health Hazards Due to Smoking.* Report prepared for the Canadian Council on Smoking and Health, 1990a.

ENVIRONICS RESEARCH GROUP LTD. *Public Attitudes toward a New Tobacco Tax.* Report prepared for the Canadian Council on Smoking and Health, 1990b.

EPP, JAKE. *Achieving Health for All: A Framework for Health Promotion.* Ottawa: Department of National Health and Welfare, 1986.

ERC STATISTICS INTERNATIONAL LIMITED. *The World Cigarette Market—The 1988 International Survey.* Volume 1, 1988.

FENNELL, P.J. Opening Statement to the Legislative Committee on Bill C-51 by P.J. Fennell, President and C.E.O., Rothmans, Benson & Hedges Inc., and Chairman, Canadian Tobacco Manufacturers' Council. January 20, 1988a.

FENNELL, P.J. *Proceedings of the Standing Senate Committee on Social Affairs,* Science and Technology, Senate of Canada, 33rd Parliament, 2nd Session, June 22, 1988b.

FERRENCE, R.G. *Trends in Tobacco Consumption in Canada 1900–1987.* From RJR-MacDonald Inc. vs the Attorney General of Canada, Quebec Superior Court, vol 46, March 14, 1990, Exhibit AG-188.

FERRENCE, R.G., GARCIA, J.M., SYKORA, K., COLLISHAW, N.E., FARINON, L. Effects of Pricing on Cigarette Use among Teenagers and Adults in Canada 1980–1989. (mimeo) February 1991.

FIRE COMMISSIONER OF CANADA. *Fire Losses in Canada: 1989 Annual Report.* Ottawa: Supply and Services Canada, Catalogue No. W51–1989, 1989.

GALLUP CANADA, INC. *Final Report on a Survey of Canadians' Knowledge of and Attitudes toward the Harmful Effect of Smoking.* Prepared for the Canadian Cancer Society, October 20, 1988.

GOLDFARB CONSULTANTS. *Public Attitudes towards Bill C-51.* March 1988.

HARRIS, J.E. *Supplementary Report by Dr. Jeffrey E. Harris, M.D., Ph.D.,* March 11, 1990. From RJR-MacDonald Inc. vs the Attorney General of Canada, Quebec Superior Court, vol. 52, March 27, 1990, Exhibit AG-197.

HEALTH PROMOTION DIRECTORATE, HEALTH AND WELFARE CANADA. *Survey of Smoking Policies in Canadian Schools.* Fact Sheet, n.d.

HEALTH PROMOTION STUDIES UNIT. *Evaluative Summaries for the 1983–84 Health Promotion Directorate Media Campaigns.* Ottawa: Health and Welfare Canada, 1985.

HEALTH PROTECTION BRANCH. Proposed amendments to the tobacco products control regulations. *Information Letter* No. 776, March 1, 1990.

HEALTH AND WELFARE CANADA. *Tobacco Products Control Act: 35–36–37, Elizabeth II,* Ch. 20. June 28, 1988.

HEALTH AND WELFARE CANADA. Tobacco products control regulations. *Canada Gazette* Part II, Vol. 123, No. 2, SOR 89–21, January 18, 1989a.

HEALTH AND WELFARE CANADA. Tobacco products control regulations—Amendment. *Canada Gazette* Part II, Vol. 123, No. 11, SOR 89–248, May 24, 1989b.

HEALTH AND WELFARE CANADA. *Report of the Canadian Blood Pressure Survey.* Ottawa: Minister of Supply and Services, 1989c. (Catalogue No. H39–143/1989E).

HEALTH AND WELFARE CANADA. *National Health Expenditures in Canada, 1975–1987.* Ottawa: Health and Welfare Canada, Catalogue No. H21–99/1990E, 1990.

HOOVER, J., MCDERMOTT, R., HARTSFIELD, T. The prevalence of smokeless tobacco use in native children in northern Saskatchewan. *Canadian Journal of Public Health* 81:350–352, 1990.

HUM, L., SEMENCIW, R. Mortality patterns in Canada, 1988. *Chronic Diseases in Canada* 12(2):16–19, 1991.

IMASCO LIMITED. *Annual Report 1989.* Montreal: Imasco Limited, 1990.

IMASCO LIMITED. *Annual Report 1990.* Montreal: Imasco Limited, 1991.

IMPERIAL TOBACCO LIMITED. *Fiscal '80 Media Plans—Phase I.* From RJR-MacDonald Inc. vs the Attorney General of Canada, Quebec Superior Court, vol 6, October 2, 1989a, Exhibit ITL-13.

IMPERIAL TOBACCO LIMITED. *Player's Filter '81 Creative Guidelines.* From RJR-MacDonald Inc. vs the Attorney General of Canada, Quebec Superior Court, vol 8, October 4, 1989b, Exhibit AG-35.

IMPERIAL TOBACCO LIMITED. *Domestic Operating Expense Summary. Fiscal Years (Apr-Mar) 1982 through 1987.* From RJR-MacDonald Inc. vs the Attorney General of Canada, Quebec Superior Court, vol 65, June 8, 1990a, Exhibit AG-30b.

IMPERIAL TOBACCO LIMITED. *The Canadian Tobacco Market at a Glance, 1989.* From RJR-MacDonald Inc. vs the Attorney General of Canada, Quebec Superior Court, vol 65, June 8, 1990b, Exhibit AG-31.

IMPERIAL TOBACCO LIMITED. *Domestic Advertising Expense Summary.* Fiscal years (Apr-Mar) 1982 through 1987. From RJR-MacDonald Inc. vs the Attorney General of Canada, Quebec Superior Court, vol 65, June 8, 1990c, Exhibit AG-30a.

INDOORAIR *Newsletter.* Fall 1988.

KAISERMAN, M.J., ALLEN, T.A. Trends in Canadian tobacco consumption, 1980–1989. *Chronic Diseases in Canada* 11(4):54–55, 1990.

KAISERMAN, M.J., COLLISHAW, N.E. Trends in Canadian tobacco consumption, 1980–1990. *Chronic Diseases in Canada* 12(4):50–52, 1991.

KAISERMAN, M.J., DUCHARME-DANIELSON, C. Global per capita consumption of manufactured cigarettes—1989. *Chronic Diseases in Canada* 12(4):56–60, 1991.

KOZLOWSKI, L.T., COAMBS, R.B., FERRENCE, R.G., ADLAF, E.M. Preventing smoking and other drug use: let the buyers beware and the interventions be apt. *Canadian Journal of Public Health* 80(6):452–456, 1989.

KPMG PEAT MARWICK THORNE. The smuggling of U.S. manufactured and Canadian duty-free cigarettes into Canada and inter-provincial smuggling. Mimeo, March 5, 1990.

KPMG PEAT MARWICK THORNE. The smuggling of U.S. manufactured and Canadian duty-free cigarettes into Canada and inter-provincial smuggling: An update. Mimeo, March 20, 1991.

KYLE, K. *Beyond the Medical Model—Reflections on Public Health Advocacy in Canada.* Presented to the First National Conference on Chronic Diseases in Canada, Toronto, April 1989.

LACASSE, F., RAYNAULD, A. The economic analysis of advertising—the economic impact of Bill C-51. Mimeo, December 1987.

LETOURNEAU, G. *Francophones and Smoking.* Ottawa: Health and Welfare Canada, Catalogue Number H39–157/1989E, 1989.

LIBRARY OF PARLIAMENT. *Bill C-51, The Tobacco Products Control Act—Summary of Evidence and Submissions,* Ottawa, 1988.

MAHOOD, G. Ontario's bill to control smoking in the workplace worthless. *The London Free Press* June 9, 1989.

MAO, Y., MORRISON, H., NICHOL, R., PIPE, A., WIGLE, D. The health consequences of smoking among smokers in Canada. *Canadian Journal of Public Health* 79: 388–391, 1988.

MILLAR, W.J. Smoking prevalence among Canadian adolescents: a comparison of survey estimates. *Canadian Journal of Public Health* 76:33–37, 1985.

MILLAR, W.J. Evaluation of the impact of smoking restrictions in a government work setting. *Canadian Journal of Public Health* 79(5):379–382, 1988a.

MILLAR, W.J. *Smoking Behaviour of Canadians 1986.* Ottawa: Health and Welfare Canada, Catalogue number H39–66/1988E, 1988b.

MILLAR, W.J. The use of chewing tobacco and snuff in Canada, 1986. *Canadian Journal of Public Health* 80:131–135, 1989.

MILLAR, W.J. *Smoking Behaviour of Canadian Ethnic Groups.* Statistics Canada, Canadian Centre for Health Information. A report submitted to Health and Welfare Canada.

MILLAR, W.J., BISH, L. Smoking in the workplace 1986: Labour Force Survey estimates. *Canadian Journal of Public Health* 80:261–265, 1989.

MILLAR, W.J., HUNTER, L. The relationship between socioeconomic status and household smoking patterns in Canada. *American Journal of Health Promotion* 5(1):36–43, 1990.

MILLAR, W.J., HUNTER, L. Household context and youth smoking behaviour: Prevalence, frequency and tar yield. *Canadian Journal of Public Health* 82:83–85, 1991.

MILLAR, W.J., PETERSON, J. *Tobacco use by youth in the Canadian Arctic.* Ottawa: Health and Welfare Canada, Catalogue Number H39–140/1989E, 1989.

NATIONAL CANCER INSTITUTE OF CANADA. *Canadian Cancer Statistics 1990.* Toronto: National Cancer Institute, 1990.

NATIONAL CLEARINGHOUSE ON TOBACCO AND HEALTH. *Fact Sheet Series: Children and Tobacco*, Nov. 1989.

NON-SMOKERS' HEALTH ACT. 35–36–37 Elizabeth II, Ch. 21. June 28, 1988.

NON-SMOKERS' HEALTH ACT—AMENDMENT. 38 Elizabeth II, Ch. 7. June 29, 1989.

NON-SMOKERS' HEALTH REGULATIONS. *Canada Gazette Part II*, 124 (1), SOR/90–21, December 14, 1989.

NON-SMOKERS' HEALTH REGULATIONS AMENDMENT. *Canada Gazette Part II*, 124 (13), SOR/90–335, June 8, 1990.

NON-SMOKERS' RIGHTS ASSOCIATION. *A Catalogue of Deception: The Use and Abuse of Voluntary Regulation of Tobacco Advertising in Canada*. A report for submission to the Honourable Jake Epp, January 1986. From RJR-MacDonald Inc. vs the Attorney General of Canada, Quebec Superior Court, vol 28, November 23, 1989, Exhibit AG-74.

NON-SMOKERS' RIGHTS ASSOCIATION. *Canadian Tobacco Taxes per 200 grams of Fine-Cut Tobacco*, June 1991.

ONTARIO FLUE-CURED TOBACCO GROWERS' MARKETING BOARD. *1990 Annual Report*. 1990.

ONTARIO GOVERNMENT. A comparative overview of smoking restriction policies in Canadian provincial and territorial jurisdictions. Ontario Government Press Release, 1989.

ONTARIO INTERAGENCY COUNCIL ON SMOKING AND HEALTH. Non-smoking bylaws in Ontario: a survey. *Ontario Interagency Council on Smoking and Health* Fall/Winter, 1988, p. 1.

ONTARIO MINISTRY OF AGRICULTURE AND FOOD. *Agricultural Handbook*. Toronto: Ministry of Agriculture and Food, 1984.

ONTARIO PUBLIC HEALTH ASSOCIATION. OPHA writes to Ontario College of Pharmacists. *OPHA News* 3 (3), 1991.

OTTAWA (CORPORATION OF THE CITY OF). *Retail Sale of Tobacco, Cigars or Cigarettes*. By-law No. L-6, Schedule 26, October 1989.

PIPE, A., WALKER, J., ESDAILE, D. Canadian physicians and tobacco. *Canadian Medical Association Journal* 144 (2):137–139, 1991.

POIRIER, P. Tobacco thefts likely to rise, police predict. *Globe and Mail*, February 18, 1991.

PRICE WATERHOUSE PROJECT TEAM. Quota Subcommittee of the Tobacco Advisory Committee, *Tobacco Quota Study—Final Report*. Ottawa: Price Waterhouse, November 21, 1989.

QUEBEC SUPERIOR COURT. RJR-Macdonald vs. the Attorney General of Canada and the Attorney General of Quebec. #500-05-009755-883, 1991a.

QUEBEC SUPERIOR COURT. The Attorney General of Canada vs RJR-Macdonald Inc. #500-05-009755-883, 1991b.

ROGERS, B. Reported disability experience in relation to cigarette smoking on the Canada Health Survey (1978–79). *Chronic Diseases in Canada* 5(4):83–85, 1985.

ROOTMAN, I., WARREN, R., STEPHENS, T., PETERS, L. (eds.). *Canada's Health Promotion Survey Technical Report*. Ottawa: Health and Welfare Canada, Catalogue Number H39–119/1988E, 1988.

SCHULTZ, J.M., NOVOTNY, T.E., RICE, D.P. Quantifying the disease impact of cigarette smoking with SAMMEC II software. *Public Health Reports* 106 (3):326–333, 1991.

SEMENCIW, R., HILL, G., MAO, Y., WIGLE, D. Chronic disease mortality trends to the year 2000. *Chronic Diseases in Canada* 10(3):44–49, 1989.

SEYMOUR, C.M. Tobacco-products industry. In Marsh, J.H. (ed.). *The Canadian Encyclopedia*, 2nd Edition, Edmonton: Hurtig Publishers, 1988.

SPASOFF, R.A. (Chairman, Panel on Health Goals for Ontario). *Health for All Ontario*. Toronto: Ontario Ministry of Health, 1987.

SPITZER, MILLS & BATES LTD. *The Player's Family—A Working Paper*, prepared for Imperial Tobacco Ltd., March 25, 1977. From RJR-MacDonald Inc. vs the Attorney General of Canada, Quebec Superior Court, vol 8, October 4, 1989, Exhibit AG-33.

STATISTICS CANADA. *Tobacco Products Industries*, Statistics Canada, Cat. No. 32–225 Annual, 1973.

STATISTICS CANADA. *Tobacco Products Industries*, Statistics Canada, Cat. No. 32–225 Annual, 1984.

STATISTICS CANADA. *Canada Handbook*. Statistics Canada, Catalogue No. CS11–403–1986E, 1986a.

STATISTICS CANADA. *Longevity and Historical Life Tables, 1921–1981 (Abridged), Canada and the Provinces*. Statistics Canada, Catalogue No. 89–506, 1986b.

STATISTICS CANADA. *Agriculture Census, Canada 1986*. Statistics Canada, Catalogue No. 96–102, 1987a.

STATISTICS CANADA. *Summary of Canadian International Trade*. Statistics Canada, Catalogue No. 65–001, 1987b.

STATISTICS CANADA. *Agriculture Economic Statistics.* Statistics Canada, Catalogue No. 21-603, 1987c.

STATISTICS CANADA. Hospital Morbidity. *Health Reports* 1 (2) Supplement. Statistics Canada, Catalogue No. 82-003S, 1989a.

STATISTICS CANADA. *Production and Disposition of Tobacco Products.* Statistics Canada, Catalogue No. 32-022 monthly, 1989b.

STATISTICS CANADA. *Farm Cash Receipts.* Statistics Canada, Catalogue No. 21-001, 50(4), March 1990a.

STATISTICS CANADA. Survey of literacy skills used in daily activities. *Statistics Canada Daily,* Catalogue No. 11-001, May 30, 1990b.

STATISTICS CANADA. *Postcensal Annual Estimates of Population by Marital Status, Age, Sex and Components of Growth for Canada, Provinces and Territories,* June 1, 1990. Statistics Canada, Catalogue No. 91-210, 1990c.

STATISTICS CANADA. *Fruit and Vegetable Production.* Statistics Canada, Catalogue No. 22-003 Seasonal, August 1990d.

STATISTICS CANADA. *Farm Cash Receipts.* Statistics Canada, Catalogue No. 21-001, 51(3), November 1990e.

STATISTICS CANADA. *Canadian Economic Observer.* Statistics Canada, Catalogue No. 11-010, 3(12) Monthly, December 1990f.

STATISTICS CANADA. *Education in Canada 1988/89.* Statistics Canada, Catalogue No. 81-229, 1990g.

STATISTICS CANADA. *Canada: A Portrait.* Statistics Canada, Catalogue No. 11-403, 1991a.

STATISTICS CANADA. Control and sale of alcoholic beverages. Unpublished tabulations, 1991b.

STATISTICS CANADA. *Employment, Earnings and Hours.* Statistics Canada, Catalogue No. 72-002, February 1991c.

STATISTICS CANADA. Health Promotion Survey 1990, Weighted and Unweighted Counts. Mimeo, 1991d.

STATISTICS CANADA. National Mortality Database. Canadian Centre for Health Information, unpublished tabulations, 1991e.

STEPHENS, T. *A Critical Review of Canadian Survey Data on Tobacco Use, Attitudes and Knowledge.* Tobacco Programs Unit, Health and Welfare Canada, April 1988.

STEPHENS, T. *Public Awareness of the Heart and Stroke Foundation of Ontario.* A report on a survey conducted for the Foundation in January 1990.

STEPHENS, T., CRAIG, C.L. *The Well-Being of Canadians.* Ottawa: Canadian Fitness and Lifestyle Research Institute, 1988.

STEPHENS, T., TAYLOR, L. Smoking in Canada—1989: Down but not out. *Chronic Diseases in Canada* 12(4):63–64, 1991.

SUTTER, S. Ontario drugstore tobacco ban put off. *Ontario Addiction Journal,* June 24, 1991.

TASK FORCE ON HEALTH PROMOTION. *Objective: A Health Concept in Québec.* Ottawa: Canadian Hospital Association, 1986.

TOBACCO RESTRAINT ACT.: 35-36-37 Elizabeth II, Ch.T-9, 1908.

TROTTIER, A. Results of a national survey on physical education in the provinces. *CAHPER Journal* 53(6):8–9, 1987.

WALTERS, D.J. The gathering momentum against tobacco: Action by physicians is needed on all fronts. *Canadian Medical Association Journal* 144(2):134–136, 1991.

WIGLE, D.T., COLLISHAW, N.E., KIRKBRIDE, J., MAO, Y. Deaths in Canada from lung cancer due to involuntary smoking. *Canadian Medical Association Journal* 136: 945–951, 1987.

WIGLE, D.T., MAO, Y., WONG, T., LANE, R. Economic burden of illness in Canada, 1986. *Chronic Diseases in Canada* 12(3), Supplement, 1991.

WILKINS, K., MARK, E. Potential years of life lost, Canada, 1987–1988. *Chronic Diseases in Canada* 12(2):12–15, 1991.

WILKINS, R. Measuring health status and consequences of health problems: Disability. Proceedings of the Workshop on *Measuring the Health of Canadians Using Population Surveys,* Ottawa, Sept. 13-14, 1991.

WILKINSON, B.W. International trade. In MARSH, J.H. (ed.). *The Canadian Encyclopedia,* 2nd Edition. Edmonton: Hurtig Publishers, 1988.

WONG, T., ARRAIZ, G. Smoking-attributable mortality and the years of potential life lost in Canada, 1986. *Chronic Diseases in Canada* 11(1):11–12, 1990.

WORLD BANK. *The World Bank Atlas 1989.* Washington, D.C.: International Bank for Reconstruction and Development/The World Bank, 1989.

Chile

General Characteristics

Chile is a republic of more than 13 million inhabitants located on the Pacific coast of South America (Centro Latinoamericano Demográfico [CELADE] 1990). It ranks tenth in geographic size (756,626 km²) among countries of the Americas. The population is mainly urban (85 percent), with 39 percent of all inhabitants living in the greater Santiago area. Chile's population has shown a steady increase in the proportion of persons aged 15 and older, from 61 percent in 1965 to 67 percent in 1988 (Table 1). With a 1988 per capita gross national product (GNP) of $US1,150, Chile is ranked by the World Bank among "lower middle income countries"; the annual rate of growth (0.2 percent between 1965 and 1987) improved after democratization in 1989 (World Bank 1990). Health and economic indicators for Chile are among the best of all Latin American countries (CELADE 1990; World Bank 1990) (Table 1). Unlike the trends shown by most other countries of Latin America, the annual rate of inflation declined during the 1980s. Between 1965 and 1980, inflation averaged 129.9 percent per year; between 1980 and 1987, average annual inflation was 20.6 percent. In 1987, the foreign debt was $US21 billion, equivalent to 103.6 percent of the GNP.

The Tobacco Industry

Agriculture

Chile has produced tobacco for many years. Approximately 1,200 tobacco farmers (Misdorp 1990) work on 2,500 ha of tobacco farmland, or 0.16 to 0.19 percent of the country's total arable land.

Tobacco agriculture is concentrated in Chile's fertile central valley. Approximately 3,760 persons (0.4 percent of the agricultural workforce) are involved in tobacco agriculture at least part-time (Agro-Economic Services and Tabacosmos, Ltd. 1987). Chiletabacos (a domestic tobacco subsidiary of British American Tobacco, Ltd. [BAT]) provides technical and financial assistance through contracts with tobacco farmers who each farm on average 20 ha (Misdorp 1990).

Data reported by both the U.S. Department of Agriculture (USDA) and the Chilean Ministry of Agriculture indicate that tobacco production declined from approximately 7,500 in 1979 to 4,780 MT in 1983. By 1989, tobacco production had increased to more than 9,000 (Table 2). Tobacco production is expected to increase by 50 percent over the next 5 years; this increase is directed mainly toward the export market (U.N. Food and Agriculture Organization 1990). In 1988, tobacco represented approximately one percent of all agricultural exports. Exports increased 15 percent between 1988 and 1989 (USDA 1990, Table 2). Between 1980 and 1989, imports decreased by almost 75 percent. Tobacco industry sources report that the United States imported 2,000 MT and Japan imported 500 MT of tobacco from Chile in 1989 (Misdorp 1990). The increase in tobacco exports has coincided with a major improvement in Chile's overall foreign trade situation (Pan American Health Organization [PAHO] 1990).

Manufacturing, Trade, and Taxes

In 1989, three cigarette-manufacturing companies provided employment for 1,945 persons (0.4 percent of the industrial workforce) in Chile (Max-

Table 1. Health and economic indicators, Chile, 1980s

Indicator	1965	1988
Population	7,614,000	12,800,000
Percent <15 years	39.4	33.4
Percent urban	72	85
Crude birth rate (per thousand persons)	34	23
Crude mortality rate (per thousand persons)	11	6
Life expectancy at birth		
Men	55.3	67.5
Women	60.9	74.5
Infant mortality rate (per thousand live births)	101	20
Average annual inflation rate (1980–1988) (percent)		20.8
Percent literate (age 12 and older)		94.4
Per capita gross national product (US$)		1,510

Sources: CELADE, 1990; PAHO, 1990; World Bank, 1990.

Table 2. Unmanufactured tobacco production, exports, imports, and total domestic consumption, in metric tons, Chile, 1979–1989

Year	Production	Exports	Imports	Total domestic consumption
1979	7,508	0	1,357	10,300
1980	5,256	0	2,281	13,707
1981	5,608	110	3,300	8,009
1982	4,910	1,109	2,540	5,940
1983	4,780	980	1,010	6,530
1984	7,280	1,720	340	6,800
1985	6,230	1,357	310	5,712
1986	6,450	1,100	560	6,530
1987	7,219	1,894	272	6,468
1988	8,019	2,080	979	6,988
1989	9,277	2,400	600	7,104

Source: USDA, 1990.

well 1990). La Compañía Chile de Tabacos (Chiletabacos, S.A.) is a subsidiary of BAT. Two smaller companies also operate in Chile: Facil is a subsidiary of the Philip Morris Company and R.J. Reynolds operates as a subsidiary of the multinational of the same name (Sepúlveda 1990). Chiletabacos, S.A. dominates the domestic market with over 90 percent of reported sales (Tobacco Merchants Association [TMA] 1989). The tobacco manufacturing industry demonstrates a moderate degree of vertical integration, with subsidiaries for distribution and for production of packaging material. Cigarette production varied between seven and 10.5 billion per year (Table 3) and accounted for approximately two percent of the gross domestic product in the 1980s.

The average price of a pack of 20 cigarettes was 140 pesos in 1990 (Sepúlveda 1990). Cigarette prices increased 16.2 percent overall in 1989, whereas the cost of living increased 21.4 percent during the same period (Misdorp 1990). Federal excise tax accounted for approximately 70 percent of the retail price of cigarettes and represented 5.2 percent of the total Government tax revenue in 1989 ($US200 million) (Sepúlveda 1990).

Cigarette vending machines are not used in

Table 3. Manufactured cigarettes, production, exports, imports, and total domestic consumption (in millions), and per capita consumption for persons age 15 and older, Chile, 1979–1989

Year	Production	Exports	Imports	Total domestic consumption	Per capita consumption (age ≥ 15)
1979	9,988		400	10,028	
1980	10,500		526	11,026	1,403
1981	10,700		800	11,500	1,200
1982	7,800		1,100	8,900	980
1983	7,900		300	8,200	961
1984	8,220		157	8,377	1,014
1985	8,260		120	8,380	1,019
1986	8,260	30	170	8,400	1,005
1987	8,630	40	107	8,697	1,079
1988	9,353	39	63	9,377	1,080
1989	9,718	40	60	9,738	1,075

Sources: USDA, 1990; TMA, 1989.
NA = not available.

Chile. There is no evidence of an extensive illegal trade in cigarettes in Chile. Imports represented approximately 1.5 percent of total domestic cigarette consumption in 1987 and 1988.

Advertising and Marketing

All types of tobacco advertising including that in the electronic media are permitted and used in Chile. However, by regulation of the National Television Council, no tobacco advertisements may be broadcast on television before 9:30 p.m. The total annual spending on all types of cigarette advertising was $US1.5 million for 1984 and 1985. Of this total, 69 percent was for television advertising, 20 percent for magazine advertising, and 11 percent for newspaper advertising. The total tobacco advertising budget accounted for less than one percent of spending on advertising for all consumer products (PAHO 1986). Among the 10 leading Chilean advertisers in 1987 and 1988, one was a cigarette company; the advertising budget for this company (Chiletabacos, S.A.) was six percent of total operating expenditures.

In 1986, Chiletabacos, S.A. established a new tobacco factory. In conjunction with this endeavor, the company also established a health clinic and heavily promoted both through the media. The tobacco companies have been effective in limiting warnings in television advertisements, and succeeded in stopping the distribution of an anti-smoking postage stamp in 1987 (Sepúlveda 1990).

Tobacco Use

Consumption Data

Tobacco consumption data are available from three sources, including the TMA (1989), the USDA (1990), and the Instituto Nacional de Estadísticas (Sepúlveda 1990). The data for the TMA and USDA use similar sources (TMA 1989). The data compiled by the Chilean Government differ slightly from those of the previous two data sets, but because more complete data were provided by the USDA and because comparisons with other countries are made, USDA data will be reported primarily.

In the 1970s, the average annual adult (aged 15 and older) per capita cigarette consumption increased 4.6 percent (TMA 1989). Except for 1984, the annual per capita cigarette consumption declined by 4.0 percent per year during the 1980s (TMA 1989) (Table 3). Estimated adult per capita consumption in 1989 was 1,075, almost one-third that in the United States (2,900) (USDA 1990). An estimated two to three percent of all tobacco consumed is used for pipes, while another one to two percent is used for cigars; cigar consumption fell an average of 6.6 percent per year in the 1980s (Sepúlveda 1990). The proportion of unfiltered cigarettes consumed remained at approximately one percent during the 1980s (TMA 1989).

Behavioral Surveys

Several different surveys of adults have been performed in Chile, and some important trend analyses are possible using selected data from these surveys (Table 4). Santiago was included in the 1971 PAHO survey of tobacco use among adults aged 15 to 74 years in eight Latin American cities (Joly 1977). Subsequently, Medina surveyed 998 Santiago adults in 1984 (Medina 1986) and 2,700 adults in 12 different Chilean cities in 1985 (Medina 1985). In a survey sponsored by PAHO, Berrios and colleagues surveyed 1,800 Santiago adults in 1986 for chronic disease risk factors (Berrios 1987). In addition, data from Santiago residents are available from the 1988 Gallup survey of urban adults aged 18 years and older in 12 Latin American cities; the study was sponsored by the American Cancer Society (Gallup 1988).

The Joly survey was a multistaged, randomized household survey of 1,975 individuals. Data from the different Latin American cities surveyed by Joly may be compared although the data cannot be generalized from each survey city to the populations of their respective countries. The overall prevalence of current smoking (which includes both occasional and daily smoking) in 1971 was similar in the three survey cities of the Southern Cone subregion (35.7 percent in Santiago, Chile; 36.2 percent in La Plata, Argentina; and 36.0 percent in São Paulo, Brazil). Significant differences between these study populations appear when stratified by sex and age: the prevalence of current smoking among men was less in Santiago (47.1 percent) than that among men in La Plata (54.4 percent) and São Paulo (53.8 percent). Among women, 26.2 percent were current smokers in Santiago, compared with 20.0 in La Plata and 20.2 percent in São Paulo in 1971. Current smoking prevalence was highest (52.5 percent) among men aged 25 to 39 years. The prevalence of smoking among women in this age group was 30 percent (Table 5).

The Joly survey also asked about the age of initiation of smoking. Most adult smokers (73.6 percent of men and 61.4 percent of women) began to smoke before age 20. Further, 38.0 percent of

Table 4. Surveys on smoking and prevalence (percent) of current smokers by sex, Chile, 1971–1988

Survey	Date	Sample	Age group	Men	Women	Both
Adults						
Joly 1977	1971	Santiago N=1778	15–74	47.1	26.2	35.7
Medina 1986	1984	Santiago N=998	15+	33.5	27.6	30.1
Medina 1985	1985	12 Cities N=2,700	15+			31.0
Sepúlveda 1987	1986	Health N=915	20–60	34.8	30.2	
Berrios 1987	1986	Santiago N=1,800	15+	36.0	31.9	33.3
Gallup 1988	1988	Santiago N=600	18+	41	37	39
Adolescents						
Salas 1980	1979	High school N=312	18–20	69.2	65.0	66.7
Reyes 1982	1981	High schools Santiago area N=2,172	15–22	58.8	52.9	56.5
Sobarzo 1987	1986	Rural students N=415	18–20	37.2	28.4	34.0
Sepúlveda 1986	1986	High school N=761	Mean age 17			
Valenzuela	1988	Santiago N=1,665	15–24	53.3	41.0	50.9

men and 27.2 percent of women reported that they began smoking before age 16 years.

In 1971, approximately one-fifth of Santiago smokers were heavy smokers (22.8 percent of men and 18.0 percent of women) (Table 5). Conversely, 44.3 percent of men smoked fewer than 10 cigarettes per day, and 59 percent of women smoked fewer than 10 cigarettes per day. This tendency to-

ward lighter smoking is in contrast to that observed for male smokers in the other two countries of the subregion. Among residents of La Plata, 38.2 percent of men and 17.5 percent of women smoked more than 20 cigarettes per day. In São Paulo, 51.5 percent of men and 18.5 percent of women were heavy smokers.

Respondents to the Joly survey reported

Table 5. Prevalence (percent) of never, current,* and ex-smokers, and number of cigarettes smoked per day, Santiago, 1971

Sex	Age group	Never smokers	Current* smokers	Ex-smokers	1–9	10–19	20+
			Prevalence			Cigarettes per day	
Men	15–74	43.0	47.1	9.9	44.3	30.5	22.8
	15–24	45.0	49.8	5.2			
	25–39	38.6	52.5	8.9			
	40–54	44.3	46.7	9.0			
	55–74	45.9	28.1	26.0			
Women	15–74	68.4	26.2	5.4	59.0	22.8	18.0
	15–24	67.9	30.0	2.2			
	25–39	65.4	30.0	4.5			
	40–54	66.5	25.6	8.1			
	55–74	79.0	11.0	10.0			
Both	15–74	56.8	35.7	7.5			
	15–24	57.2	39.3	3.6			
	25–39	53.0	40.4	6.6			
	40–54	56.7	34.8	8.5			
	55–74	64.5	18.5	17.0			

Source: Joly, 1977.

* Includes occasional and daily smokers.

Table 6. Prevalence (percent) of current, occasional, and nonsmokers among adults, aged 15 and older, by sex and age group, Santiago, 1984

Sex	Age group	Current smokers	Occasional smokers	Nonsmokers	N
Men	≥ 15 Years	33.5	10.4	56.1	412
Women	≥ 15 Years	27.6	11.6	61.1	586
Both	≥ 15 Years	30.1	10.9	59.0	998
	< 30	34.6	15.0	50.4	260
	30–49	33.6	11.6	51.7	327
	50+	18.7	5.3	75.9	411

Source: Medina, 1986.

smoking tabaco negro at rather high rates (33.6 percent among male smokers and 30.5 percent among female smokers). Compared to the other eight cities in the Joly survey, only smokers in Bogotá, Colombia, reported smoking tabaco negro more frequently (58.9 percent among men and 42 percent among women).

The 1984 data from a population-based survey of Santiago residents aged 15 and older (Medina 1986) suggest that the prevalence of current and occasional smoking (together) among men (43.9 percent) declined somewhat and that the prevalence of current and occasional smoking (together) among women (39.1 percent) increased substantially over the previous 13 years. The prevalence of smoking (34.6 percent) among persons under 30 was higher than those aged 30 to 49 years (33.6 percent) or 50 and older (18.7 percent) (Table 6).

Medina subsequently surveyed populations from 12 other Chilean cities: Iquique, Antofagasta, Coquimbo, Serena, Valparaíso, Viña del Mar, Rancagua, Talca, Chillán, Concepción, Talcahuano, and Coronel (Medina 1985) (Table 7). Overall, the proportion of adults in these cities who were current smokers in 1985 (31 percent) was similar to the proportion in Santiago during 1984. The prevalence of current smoking was higher among those with the highest socioeconomic status compared with those of low socioeconomic status (40.4 vs. 19.8 percent) (definition not provided). Similarly, the prevalence of smoking was positively related to educational attainment: 23.6 percent among persons with primary education; 32.6 percent among persons with secondary education; and 33.6 percent among persons with tertiary education. The prevalence data for the category "occasional smoking" are not available for this survey and therefore the data cannot be directly compared with the 1971 Joly survey.

In 1986, primary health care personnel in Metropolitan Santiago aged 20 to 60 years of age were

Table 7. Prevalence (percent) of current smokers and nonsmokers among urban adults aged 15 years and older from 12 cities (Iquique, Antofagasta, Coquimbo, Serena, Valparaíso, Viña del Mar, Rancagua, Talca, Chillan, Concepcion, Talcahuano, Coronel), by socioeconomic status and educational attainment, Chile, 1985

Category	Current smokers	Non-smokers	N
Total	31	69	2,700
Socioeconomic level			
Lowest	19.8		
Highest	40.4		
Educational level			
Primary	23.6		
Secondary	32.6		
Tertiary	33.6		

Source: Medina, 1985.

surveyed as to tobacco use (Sepúlveda 1987). The prevalence of current daily smoking among men (34.8 percent) was similar to that among Santiago men surveyed by Medina in 1984, but the prevalence of smoking among women (30.2 percent) was substantially higher (Table 8). A high proportion of former smokers was noted in this sample (38.0 percent among men and 32.9 percent among women), suggesting that the prevalence of smoking was much higher among these subjects in the past. This finding is consistent with the Medina data that showed a higher current smoking prevalence among persons with high socioeconomic and educational status. As health professionals, these persons now may be quitting as a result of their concern about the health effects of smoking.

Residents of Santiago and five other Latin

Table 8. Prevalence (percent) of daily smokers, occasional smokers, and ex-smokers among primary health care personnel, by sex, Santiago Metropolitan Region, 1986

Category	Daily smokers	Occasional smokers	Ex-smokers	N
Men	34.8	17.4	38.0	184
Women	30.2	17.5	32.9	731

Source: Sepúlveda, 1987.

American cities (Porto Alegre, São Paulo, Caracas, Havana and Piedras Negras) were surveyed on behalf of PAHO for chronic disease risk factors in 1986 (Berrios 1987). This two-stage, stratified household sample of 1,800 persons aged 15 years and older in Santiago was comparable to other cities in the survey. The overall proportion found of current daily smokers for both sexes was similar to that in previous surveys of Santiago residents (33.3 percent) (Table 9). The prevalence of current daily smoking among women was relatively high (32.3 percent) and similar to that for men (34.9 percent). Again, there appears to be a relationship between high socioeconomic and educational status and higher smoking prevalence. Berrios found that male San-

tiago smokers smoked an average of 12.7 cigarettes per day and that female smokers smoked only an average of 8.6 cigarettes per day. She also found that the age of smoking initiation may have decreased since the Joly survey in 1971. In 1986, 83.7 percent of men and 76.5 percent of women began smoking before age 20. When compared with the 1971 Joly survey, the combined daily and occasional smoking prevalence among men (50.8 percent) and among women (44.8 percent) were again higher in 1987.

Residents of Santiago were again surveyed by the Gallup Organization on behalf of the American Cancer Society in 1988 (Gallup 1988) (Table 10). Scant methodological information is available for this survey. The prevalence of current smoking, which presumably includes occasional smoking, was somewhat higher among respondents to this survey than was found in previous surveys (41 percent among men and 37 percent among women; 39 percent overall). In general, the data show a similar relationship between higher socioeconomic level and higher smoking prevalence (41 percent among persons with high socioeconomic status and 35 percent among persons with low socioeconomic status; no definition provided).

Table 9. Prevalence (percent) of current smokers, ex-smokers, and occasional smokers, by sex, socioeconomic level, educational attainment, and occupation, Santiago, 1986

Category	Current smokers	Ex-smokers	Occasional smokers	N
Men	34.9	17.7	15.8	475
Women	32.3	12.5	11.1	728
Both	33.3	14.6	13.0	1,203
Socioeconomic level				
Highest	32.5	13.8	14.9	543
Lowest	34.7	15.8	10.0	329
Educational attainment				
Primary	46.4	29.0	24.2	252
Secondary	59.4	20.6	20.1	394
Higher	57.5	24.1	18.4	87
Occupation				
Private	56.1	23.1	20.8	264
Independent	51.0	27.6	21.4	98
Military	50.0	33.3	16.7	6
Retired	33.3	56.7	10.0	30
Unemployed	63.5	21.2	15.4	52
Housekeeping	56.5	22.3	21.0	186
Student	60.7	8.2	31.2	61
Other	41.7	27.8	27.8	36

Source: Berrios, 1987.

Table 10. Prevalence (percent) of current smokers and ex-smokers among adults, aged 18 years and older, by sex, age group, and socioeconomic status, Santiago, 1988 (N=600)

Category	Current smokers	Ex-smokers
Total	39	14
Men	41	17
Women	37	11
Age group		
Men		
18–29	51	7
30–49	46	11
50 and older	23	33
Women		
18–29	50	8
30–49	35	18
50 and older	25	8
Socioeconomic status		
High	41	18
Low	35	12

Source: Gallup, 1988.

Prevalence of Smoking among Adolescents

Five surveys of smoking among Chilean adolescents have been reported since 1980 (Table 11). In 1981, 330 students (15 to 20 years old) from one class of a Santiago secondary school were surveyed using a self-administered questionnaire (Salas 1980). The prevalence of current smoking among those 15 to 16 years old and those 17 to 20 years old was very high (55.1 and 64.5 percent, respectively); the prevalences for men and women were similar.

Reyes (1982) surveyed 2,172 secondary students aged 13 to 20 years living in the western part of Santiago. The prevalence of ever smoking was quite similar among men and women (58.8 percent and 53.0 percent overall). Female respondents reported a lower age of initiation than did male respondents: 15.8 percent of female smokers reported that they began smoking between ages 10 and 12 years; 9.1 percent of male smokers began smoking during these ages. Almost all smokers smoked fewer than 10 cigarettes per day (94.4 percent of men and 97 percent of women). Additional data for alcohol use were reported from this survey: 23 percent of respondents were nonsmokers and nonusers of alcohol; 16 percent were smokers only; 21 percent used alcohol only; and 40 percent used both alcohol and tobacco.

Table 11. Prevalence (percent) of smoking among adolescents, various surveys, by age and sex, Chile, 1979–1989

Salas 1980 (Secondary school, N=312)

Age group	Male	Female	Both
15–16	51.6	56.6	55.1
17–20	65.0	64.2	64.5

Reyes 1982 (Secondary schools in Santiago, N=2,172)

Age	Male	Female	Both
14	42.8	17.0	35.0
15	40.0	39.3	39.7
16	54.1	48.4	51.8
17	61.5	50.6	57.5
18	65.1	63.5	64.5
19	51.6	69.5	48.2
20	85.0	22.2	73.1
Total 14–20	58.8	52.9	56.5

Sepúlveda 1986a (Secondary school, N=76)

Age group	Both
15	48.3
16	51.0
17	58.0
18	57.1
19–20	50.9

Sobarzo 1987 (Rural students, N=415)

Age group	Male	Female	Both
<14	37.5	14.2	26.7
14–15	37.9	14.1	25.7
16–17	34.8	19.4	26.2
>17	37.2	28.4	34.0

Valenzuela 1989 (Santiago young adults, aged 15–24, N=1,665)

Age group	Male	Female
15–17	46.0	33.9
18–19	60.1	44.0
20–21	55.2	36.0
22–24	56.2	42.1
All ages	53.3	41.0

In 1986, 761 secondary students aged 16 to 20 years from two municipal schools in Santiago communities surveyed for tobacco use reported a relatively high prevalence of current smoking (approximately 50 percent overall [exact data unavailable]) (Sepúlveda, 1986).

In 1988, 458 rural secondary students aged 13 to 20 years were surveyed by means of a self-administered questionnaire (Sobarzo 1987). The prevalences of current smoking among both men (37.2 percent) and women (28.4 percent) aged 17 to 20 were much less than those of Santiago students of the same age range reported by Sepúlveda.

However, in 1988, the U.S. Centers for Disease Control (CDC) and the University of Chile School of Public Health surveyed 1,665 young adults (aged 15–24) in Greater Santiago (Valenzuela 1989). This carefully conducted survey reported a much higher prevalence of smoking among men (53.3 percent) and women (41.0 percent) (Table 11). The prevalence of current smoking increased with higher education for women and decreased with higher education for men. Approximately 90 percent of women and 80 percent of men smoked one-half pack of cigarettes or less.

The prevalence of smoking among young persons, rural and urban, is remarkably high in Chile, even though differences in methodology and definitions for "current smoker" among the surveys preclude reliable comparison. The tendency toward a declining age of initiation, observed in the Joly and Berrios surveys, is disturbing. For those surveys reporting prevalence by age and sex, smoking prevalence is higher in the younger age groups. Thus, a cohort of aging persons with high smoking prevalence will likely emerge over the next few decades in Chile. These smokers will begin to display excess morbidity and mortality due to smoking-related diseases unless widespread cessation, as indicated by the 50-percent quit rates (defined as the proportion of ex-smokers among all persons who had ever smoked) in Santiago health workers (Sepúlveda 1987), is assured. Young, urban, well-educated persons seem to be the group at highest risk for tobacco use in Chile. This pattern is reminiscent of that observed in developed nations during the 1950s and 1960s, before knowledge about the health consequences of smoking was widespread. Tobacco use among women is particularly problematic in Chile; because of high prevalence rates in the past and a well-documented increase in present rates, the disease impact of smoking among women may be substantial in the near future.

Smoking and Health

Mortality data in Chile are of a particularly high quality, with less than 10 percent of causes of death classified as ill defined (ICD 780–789) (PAHO 1990). Cardiovascular disease and malignant tumor are the two leading causes of death in Chile. The incidence of both of these broad disease categories may be closely related to historically high rates of tobacco use in the Chilean population. More than half (57.6 percent) of all deaths in persons aged 35 and older are caused by smoking-related diseases (cardiovascular disease, lung cancer, other smoking-related cancers, and lung disease) (Sepúlveda 1990). In 1983, Sepúlveda and Naveillan (1986) estimated that of 74,428 registered deaths, 5,316 (7.1 percent) were attributable to smoking. In comparison, smoking accounted for approximately 15 percent of all deaths in the United States in 1984 (Centers for Disease Control 1987).

Lung cancer mortality may be considered an indicator of the population effects of smoking. In Chile, the mortality rate for lung cancer has increased by factors of 16 among men and 10 among women since 1935. In 1988, lung cancer accounted for 2.5 percent of all deaths among men and 1.2 percent of all deaths among women aged 35 or older (World Health Organization 1988).

The overall age-adjusted mortality rate declined by 48 percent among men and by 54 percent among women between 1968 and 1987 (Table 12). The overall age-adjusted mortality for all causes of cancer has also decreased, by 14 percent for men and by 21 percent for women. However, the age-adjusted lung cancer mortality rates increased between 1968 and 1987, by 18 percent for men and by 23 percent for women. These data support the notion of an improving overall health status for Chileans with an increasing effect of historically high smoking prevalence rates. These have provoked an

Table 12. Changes in mortality rates (per 100,000 persons), by sex and age group for all causes of death, all cancers, and lung cancer, Chile, 1968–1987

Sex and category	Age group 25–44	Age group 45–64	Age group 65+	Age-adjusted
Male				
All causes	−0.57	−0.45	−0.11	−0.48
All cancers	−0.35	−0.23	−0.01	−0.14
Lung cancer	−0.35	+0.11	+0.37	+0.18
Female				
All causes	−0.64	−0.44	−0.21	−0.54
All cancers	−0.31	−0.21	−0.13	−0.21
Lung cancer	−0.40	+0.06	+0.60	+0.23

Source: Unpublished tabulations, PAHO Mortality Data Bank, 1991.

increasing mortality rate for lung cancer. In particular, the effects of smoking among women in Chile are evident in the higher rate of increase in age-adjusted lung cancer mortality as compared with that for men. The age-adjusted lung cancer mortality among men is still two to three times higher than that among women in Chile.

Tobacco Use Prevention and Control Activities

Government Action: Executive Structure and Policies

Since 1985, a tobacco control program has been active within the Health of Adult program of the Ministry of Health. The annual budget for this activity is approximately $US15,000. Activities have included a smoking prevention education project in 1987 for municipal high schools in three Santiago-area communities; this project was extended to three other communities in 1988. The baseline prevalence among students 13 years and older in the study communities was 34 percent, with 5 percent reporting daily smoking. By 1990, this project had involved 10,000 students, and educational activities included parents and guardians in the communities. The project is a collaborative effort among the Ministries of Health and Education, the Public Health Service, the provincial departments of education, and municipal corporations of health and education. An evaluation study has been performed comparing intervention groups and control groups; preliminary results suggest a significant difference in the initiation of tobacco use in the intervention groups compared with controls (3.2 vs. 10 percent) during the education program. Six months after the intervention, no additional new smokers were reported in the intervention group, and 20 percent of the nonsmokers in the control group had begun to smoke. For those students in the intervention group who were already smokers, no effect of the educational program was observed. Thus, prevention education is effective prior to the uptake of smoking. When students become dependent on tobacco, education has little effect on their behavior. Additional plans have been made to include the tobacco use prevention program as an integrated part of the school health curriculum (Latin American Coordinating Committee on Smoking Control 1990).

The tobacco program published a document aimed at promoting and providing guidance for an-

tismoking activities entitled, "Fundamentals and Basic Strategies for the Control of Smoking in Chile" (Ministry of Health 1986). In addition, the program regularly provides information, references, and resources to groups wishing to institute tobacco prevention and control activities (Sepúlveda 1990).

In 1986, a Government decree was issued creating the National Commission to Control Smoking (Chapman 1990), a multisectoral organization made up of representatives from various Government ministries, the Association of Environmental Journalists, the National Cancer Society, the Chilean Association of Respiratory Diseases, the Catholic University Faculty of Medicine, the Consumer Protection Association, the Adventist Church, and other volunteer agencies. The commission's purpose was to help plan tobacco-related education, to compile tobacco-related data, to advise the Government on tobacco policies, and to establish international linkages (Sepúlveda 1990).

Public Information Activities

The tobacco program and voluntary groups have had extensive media contact in Chile through interviews, articles in journals and magazines, and advertisements. These activities have been directed primarily toward youth and women. The Women and Children's Health Plan includes antismoking goals and objectives (Sepúlveda 1990). Both radio and television programming include regular antitobacco messages. World No Tobacco Day is actively celebrated throughout Chile, with diverse programs within the Health Service, city Governments, and other public and private institutions.

In 1981, the daily newspaper "El Mercurio" sponsored in its Sunday supplement an antismoking campaign directed at middle- and high-socioeconomic-status readers. This campaign served to elevate debate on laws limiting tobacco advertising and provoked a strong reaction by tobacco companies in Chile (Sepúlveda 1990).

Legislation and Policies on Tobacco

Moderate legislative actions against tobacco advertisement are evident in Chile. Advertisements and cigarette packs must bear the following health warning:

"Tobacco may cause cancer"

This warning must occupy 10 percent of the advertisement surface and must be included on all cigarette packages manufactured in Chile (Decree 106,

April 8, 1981, supplemented by Decree 156, June 2, 1981). Cigarette advertisements on television are prohibited before 9:30 p.m. (Rodríguez 1986).

In 1986, a draft law that would have prohibited all forms of tobacco promotion was submitted to the legislature. The bill was not passed because of Ministry of Health opposition. A second proposal to ban the use of images and allow only text in tobacco advertisements was also unsuccessful. A new antitobacco initiative was developed in 1990 by the Senate Health Commission that would restrict tobacco advertising, smoking in public places, and sales of tobacco to minors (Sepúlveda 1990).

Several administrative and legal restrictions on smoking in public places are reported in Chile, but the extent to which these restrictions are enforced is unknown. The Ministry of Health restricts the use of tobacco at all health service facilities (internal memoranda, December 11, 1981 and June 1982). Smoking is restricted in public schools through administrative order (May 11, 1981). Transportation Law Number 18.250 (February 7, 1985) bans smoking on all buses. No enforcement sanctions for any of these restrictions are reported (Sepúlveda 1990).

There is no legislative requirement to report tar and nicotine levels of cigarettes produced in Chile. In 1982, Chiletabacos analyzed five filtered brands for tar and nicotine (Table 13). Tar levels ranged from 9 to 18 mg per cigarette, and nicotine levels ranged from 0.7 to 1.2 mg per cigarette. These levels are in the middle range for tar and nicotine content. For example, the 10 lowest tar cigarette brands reported by the U.S. Federal Trade Commission (USFTC) range from 0.5 to 2 mg per cigarette, and the 10 highest brands range from 24 to 26 mg per cigarette (USFTC 1991).

There are no laws or regulations regarding mandatory antitobacco school education or access to tobacco by minors. It is estimated that 18 percent of all cigarettes sold commercially are sold as single cigarettes (Rodríguez 1986).

Table 13. Tar and nicotine yield (in mg per cigarette) of the five most popular brands sold in Chile, 1982

Brand	Tar	Nicotine
Advance	9.0	0.7
Derby	16.0	1.2
Viceroy lights	13.0	1.0
Belmont	17.0	1.2
Life king size	18.0	1.1

Source: Chiletabacos, S.A., 1982.

Action by Nongovernmental Agencies

Nongovernmental agencies have been very active in tobacco prevention and control in Chile. For example, the Chilean Society of Respiratory Diseases (CONAC) produced television messages in 1989 in cooperation with a pharmaceutical company. The Association of Laryngectomy Patients (CONALACH) organized a mobile show for presentations at schools, offices, and worksites. The Consumer Protection Association (ACHICO) is planning new antitobacco activities. Community programs targeting drug and alcohol use among adolescents include tobacco use. The National Cancer Society is very active in presenting prevention messages in the electronic and print media, as well as in training schoolteachers to help prevent smoking among their students (Sepúlveda 1990; Rodríguez 1986).

Cessation and Information Programs

Several treatment and information programs on tobacco addiction are reported in Chile (Sepúlveda 1991). These include the following:

- The Institute for Respiratory Diseases and Thoracic Surgery has been operating treatment services for patients who wish to quit smoking since 1988.
- Health services facilities have been targeted by the tobacco control program through information on tobacco and cessation in clinical meetings and lectures.
- Educational programs have been provided by the tobacco control program for employees in the Ministry of Justice, the Ministry of Transportation, and the Ministry of Health.
- Primary health care staff have received special training and information with regard to high-risk patients (i.e., pregnant women, chronic disease patients, and women who use oral contraceptives).
- Tobacco program educational activities have targeted workers in both the private and public sectors.
- Several private physicians and clinics offer smoking cessation programs (details unavailable).
- The Seventh Day Adventist Church offers to the general public a three day group program to quit smoking.

Summary

Chile demonstrates relatively good general health and economic indicators when compared with other countries in Central and South America. The country has recently returned to a democratic system of Government, and its plans for economic recovery appear to be succeeding. It produces, exports, and imports both tobacco and cigarettes. Exports, which began in the 1980s, are increasingly important in the Chilean economic recovery, while the importance of imports and domestic per capita consumption is declining.

The prevalence of smoking among urban Chilean men has declined since 1971, but the prevalence of smoking among women has increased so that the proportion of urban women who smoke is nearly identical to that for urban men. Most smokers smoke fewer than 10 cigarettes per day. The age of initiation of smoking has declined over the last two decades in Santiago.

The mortality profile of Chile is characterized by the dominance of chronic diseases as causes of death. Over half of all deaths in 1988 may be at least partially related to smoking, and at least seven percent of all deaths in 1983 were caused by smoking. The rate of increase in lung cancer mortality among Chilean women is remarkable in that it is increasing at a faster rate than among Chilean men and is higher than that for women in other countries of the subregion. This pattern reflects the change in smoking prevalence among Chilean women in the last two decades and suggests that future mortality patterns among women will be dominated by smoking-related diseases.

Moderate restrictions on tobacco product advertising have been in place since 1981 and include restrictions on when these ads can be shown on television. Warnings must appear on cigarette packs and in advertisements. Smoking is prohibited by law on buses. Restrictions on smoking in public places are limited to internal regulations at schools and health services.

Chile has an official infrastructure in place for the prevention and control of tobacco. Tobacco prevention and control activities have been implemented under the Ministry of Health's Health of Adult Program and the Women's Health Program. Nongovernmental organizations have been active in tobacco control in Chile.

Conclusions

1. Tobacco use has caused a substantial increase in lung cancer mortality in Chile between the 1960s and 1980s. Of most concern is the higher rate of increase in lung cancer mortality among women compared with men.

2. In 1986, the prevalence of current daily smoking among urban Chilean women and men was very similar (34.9 percent and 32.3 percent, respectively). However, the prevalence of daily and occasional smoking combined among urban men declined somewhat from 47.1 percent in 1971 to 43.9 percent in 1984, and the prevalence among women increased substantially from 26.3 percent in 1971 to 39.1 percent in 1984.

3. Higher prevalences of smoking are observed for persons with high socioeconomic status and educational attainment compared with persons of low socioeconomic status and minimal education.

4. A substantial governmental and nongovernmental infrastructure to prevent and control tobacco exists in Chile. Evaluation of tobacco prevention activities shows that education can prevent smoking initiation but has no effect on cessation among young persons.

5. Modest legislative and policy interventions against tobacco advertising and smoking in public places are developing in Chile. However, the tobacco industry appears to be effective in curbing such legislation through political pressure and economic influences.

References

AGRO-ECONOMIC SERVICES AND TABACOSMOS, LTD. *The Employment, Tax Revenue and Wealth that the Tobacco Industry Creates.* September 1987.

BERRIOS, X. *Estudio de factores de riesgo suceptibles de intervención para la prevención de las enfermedades crónicas del adulto 1986–1987.* Washington, D.C.: Pan American Health Organization, 1987.

CENTRO LATINOAMERICANO DE DEMOGRAFIA. *Boletín Demográfico,* Año XXIII, No. 45. Santiago de Chile, enero de 1990.

CENTERS FOR DISEASE CONTROL. Smoking-attributable mortality and years of potential life lost—United States, 1984. *Morbidity and Mortality Weekly Report* 36(42):694–697, 1987.

CHAPMAN, S., WONG, W.L. *Tobacco Control in the Third World. A Resource Atlas.* Penang: International Organization of Consumers Unions, 1990.

EUROMONITOR CONSULTANCY. *The World Market for Tobacco: Strategy 2000,* Volumes I–II. August 1989.

GALLUP ORGANIZATION, INC. *The Incidence of Smoking in Central and Latin America*. Princeton, N.J.: Gallup Organization, Inc., 1988.

JOLY, D.J. *Encuesta sobre las características del hábito de fumar en América Latina*. Washington, D.C.: Organización Panamericana de la Salud, Publicación Científica No. 337, 1977.

LATIN AMERICAN COORDINATING COMMITTEE ON SMOKING CONTROL. *Report of the Sixth Annual Meeting*. Quito, January 25–27, 1990.

MAXWELL, J.C. *The Maxwell Consumer Report: International Tobacco 1989, Part Three*. Richmond, Virginia: Wheat First Securities/Butcher & Singer, Inc. WFBS-5685, October 30, 1990.

MEDINA, E. Encuesta de tabaquismo en la población general de Santiago. *Revista Medicina de Chile* 114:257–262, 1986.

MEDINA, E. *Tabaquismo en doce ciudades chilenas*. Gallup, Chile, 1985.

MINISTRY OF HEALTH. *Fundamentos y estrategias para el control del hábito de fumar en Chile*. Santiago, 1986.

MISDORP, S. Chile's burley excellent; U.K. buys Argentine; Paraguay wanes. *Tobacco International* 39:22–24, August 15, 1990.

PAN AMERICAN HEALTH ORGANIZATION. *Health Conditions in the Americas—1990 Edition*. Scientific Publication No. 524. Washington, D.C.: Pan American Health Organization, 1990.

REYES, F.C., REX, C.S., BRAVO, I.L., OYARZUN, R.V. El hábito de fumar en estudiantes de educación media, en Santiago, Chile. *Boletín Oficina Sanitaria Panamericana* 93(6):533–540, 1982.

RODRIGUEZ, H. Chile Report. In: *Control del Hábito de Fumar—Taller Subregional para el Cono Sur Y Brasil, Buenos Aires, Argentina, November 1985*. Cuaderno Técnico No. 2, Washington, D.C.: Pan American Health Organization, 1986.

SALAS, I. Prevalencia de tabaquismo en alumnos de enseñanza media de las comunas de Providencia y Las Condes. *Revista Medicina de Chile* 108:453, 1980.

SEPULVEDA, C. Country Collaborator's Report, Chile (unpublished data), Pan American Health Organization, 1990.

SEPULVEDA, C. Estudio del hábito de fumar en estudiantes de grado medio comunidad Nunoa y Conchali de Santiago, unpublished, 1986.

SEPULVEDA, C. Prevalencia del hábito de fumar en personal de salud de atención primaria de la region metropolitana. *Boletín Epidemiología de Chile* 14(2):40–49, 1987.

SEPULVEDA, C., NAVEILLAN, C. Mortalidad y morbilidad imputables al hábito de fumar. *Boletín Vigilancia y Epidemiología* 33(4):1986.

SOBARZO, A.P., MUNOZ, J., et al. Tabaquismo en estudiantes de enseñanza media de una comunidad rural. *Revista Medicina de Chile* 115:167–171, 1987.

TOBACCO MERCHANTS ASSOCIATION OF THE UNITED STATES, INC. *Production and consumption of tobacco products for selected countries 1979–1988*. Special Report 89-3, September 28, 1989.

U.S. DEPARTMENT OF AGRICULTURE. Tobacco, Cotton, and Seeds Division, Foreign Agricultural Service (unpublished data), Washington, D.C., 1990.

U.S. FEDERAL TRADE COMMISSION. *Tar, Nicotine, and Carbon Monoxide of the Smoke of 475 Varieties of Domestic Cigarettes*. Washington, D.C., 1991.

U.N. FOOD AND AGRICULTURE ORGANIZATION. *Tobacco: Supply, Demand, and Trade Projections, 1994 and 2000*. Rome: Food and Agriculture Organization of the United Nations, FAP Economic and Social Development Paper 86, 1990.

VARGAS, N., CARRETO, A., SALOMON, V. Hábito de fumar en la población escolar urbana. *Rev Chil Pediatr* 51:379, 1980.

VALENZUELA, M.S., HEROLD, J.M., MORRIS, L. *Encuesta de salud reproductiva en adultos jóvenes. Gran Santiago 1988*. Informe Final Universidad de Chile, Departamento de Salud Pública, División Ciencias Médicas Occidente. U.S. Public Health Service, Centers for Disease Control, Atlanta, Georgia, 1989.

WORLD BANK. *World Development Report–1990—Poverty*. New York: Oxford University Press, 1990.

WORLD HEALTH ORGANIZATION. Trends in mortality for selected causes of death, 1950–54 to 1980–84. In: *1988 Health Statistics Annual*. Geneva: World Health Organization, 1988.

Colombia

General Characteristics

The Tobacco Industry
   Agriculture
   Manufacturing
   Cigarette production and illegal trade
   Advertising and promotion

Tobacco Use
   Per capita consumption
   Surveys
      Prevalence of smoking among adults
      Prevalence of smoking among adolescents
      Other surveys
      Other forms of tobacco use

Smoking and Health
   General mortality
   Morbidity and mortality due to lung cancer
   Morbidity and mortality due to other smoking-associated malignancies

Tobacco Use Prevention and Control Activities
   Government actions
      Executive structure and policies
      Legislation
      School-based education
      Public information campaigns
      Taxes
   Nongovernmental organizations

Summary and Conclusions

References

General Characteristics

Although Colombia has had an uninterrupted democratic system since 1957, several large social and political groups have been excluded from any real participation in political decision-making (Leal 1989). This situation along with rapid urbanization contributed to a culture of violence in Colombia. In 1960, 70 percent of the population was rural and 30 percent was urban; by 1990 these percentages had reversed. The emergence of powerful narcotics traffickers generated more violence, which in turn furthered the political and social conflict. During the late 1980s, Colombia had one of the highest rates of death from violent causes in the world: 62.8/100,000 inhabitants (Losada 1989).

In spite of the political and social turmoil, stable economic policies created moderate but sustained economic growth over the past few decades. The per capita gross domestic product (GDP) grew by 3.7 percent per year in the 1970s; in the 1980s, when most of Latin America suffered under severe economic recession, Colombia's GDP grew by 1 percent per year. As a result, public spending on education as a percentage of GDP increased from 1.7 percent in 1960 to 2.8 percent in 1986, and public spending on health increased from 0.4 percent of the GDP in 1960 to 0.8 percent of the GDP in 1986 (Programa de las Naciones Unidas para el Desa-rrollo 1990). Income distribution improved and real wages increased in the 1980s. However, more than 40 percent of Colombia's 31.7 million citizens (World Bank 1990) still live in poverty.

The infant mortality rate decreased from 86/1,000 live births in 1965 to 39/1,000 in 1988, and the crude birth rate decreased from 43 to 26 per 1,000 persons over the same interval. Declining fertility and a falling crude mortality rate (from 11 to 6 per 1,000 persons), will cause a continued decline in the proportion of Colombians under 15 years of age, along with an increased proportion aged 65 and older in the next few decades (World Bank 1990) (Table 1). Thus, chronic noncommunicable diseases will become increasingly important in Colombia's health situation in the near future.

Colombia, like other nations of Latin America, has begun to increase exports and accelerate its rate of growth. Tobacco has been important to the Colombian economy for hundreds of years, and its importance in international trade is becoming re-established.

The Tobacco Industry

Agriculture

Tobacco growing became very important to the Spanish colonies within 30 years of Columbus' first voyage to the New World. Initially, the State was the sole buyer of this product and remained so after liberation. From 1850, when free trade was permitted, until the end of the 19th century, tobacco was the principal export (Harrison 1952). *Tabaco negro* (dark tobacco) was the only variety grown until 1960, when *tabaco rubio* (light tobacco) production began. The historical and cultural importance of tobacco use since very early in the 20th century in Colombia bears directly on both current mortality patterns and the cigarette manufacturing industry in Colombia.

Colombia is the third largest producer of tobacco in Latin America, following Brazil and Cuba (Chapman 1990). Tobacco cropland increased from an average of 20,900 ha in the 1960s to an average of 28,200 ha in the 1970s (Kalmanovitz 1978); thereafter, land planted with tobacco declined to an average of 23,700 ha in the 1980s, totaling 18,500 ha in 1986. In 1983, the estimated tobacco cropland was only 0.7 percent of total arable land, an increase from 0.6 percent in 1971 (Agro-economic Services, Ltd. 1987) (Table 2).

This growth can be explained by an increased foreign demand for Colombian tobacco and promo-

Table 1. Health and economic indicators, Colombia, 1980s

Indicator	Year	Value
Population	1990	32,000,000
Percent urban	1990	70
Percent <15	1988	35.9
Percent ≥65	1988	4.3
Adult literacy rate	1985	12
Life expectancy at birth	1988	68
Crude mortality rate per 1,000 persons	1988	6
Crude birth rate per 1,000 persons	1988	26
Infant mortality rate	1988	39
Per capita gross national product (US$)	1988	1,180
Gross domestic product (million US$)	1988	39,070

Sources: United Nations Development Program, 1990; World Bank, 1990.

Table 2. Area cultivated (ha x 1,000), leaf tobacco production, imports, exports, and total domestic consumption (Metric tons x 1,000), Colombia, 1960 to 1990

Year	Area	Production	Exports	Imports	Total domestic consumption
1960	14	25	9	0.001	16.00
1961	14	28	10	0.006	18.01
1962	19	38	11	0.007	27.01
1963	22	42	16	0.004	26.00
1964	22	41	16	0.005	25.01
1965	25	40	11	0	29.00
1966	27	44	13	0	31.00
1967	21	38	12	0.001	26.00
1968	21	39	9	0.001	30.00
1969	24	44	13	0.001	31.00
1970	23	42	13	0.001	29.00
1971	23	39	15	0.001	24.00
1972	26	36	20	0	16.00
1973	na	na	na	1.3	na
1974	na	na	na	0.6	na
1975	31.6	49.1	17.4	0.3	32.00
1976	29.7	38.6	10.9	0.05	27.75
1977	33.3	58.3	26.8	0.3	31.8
1978	28.8	46.6	19.8	0.3	0.1
1979	30.6	51.5	11.9	0.3	39.9
1980	28.5	44.5	16.9	0.9	28.5
1981	30.1	50.1	9.6	0.8	41.3
1982	30.9	48.7	9.8	1.8	40.7
1983	28.8	47.8	9.2	3.7	42.3
1984	21.1	34.6	10.5	3.6	27.7
1985	17.6	27.2	12.7	4.2	18.7
1986	18.5	28.6	11.4	4.5	21.7
1987	21.1	34.9	8.4	3.0	29.5
1988	21.4	35.7	7.6	1.5	29.6
1989	19.0	31.1	na	3.2	34.3
1990	19.6	33.9	na	na	na

Sources: Kalmanovitz, 1978; National Planning Department, 1983; USDA, 1990.

tion of tobacco agriculture by the local cigarette manufacturing companies, which provide technical assistance to small growers to increase the yield of tobacco per hectare. In Colombia, the peasant farmer who grows tobacco essentially depends on the cigarette manufacturing industry because the industry sets the prices and loans money to these farmers for each new harvest's expenses (Departamento Nacional de Planeación 1983). In addition, Government credit agencies loaned the tobacco agricultural sector $US433,882 in 1987, representing 1.3 percent of all agricultural loans.

In 1983, the number of full-time agricultural workers associated with tobacco was estimated at 100,500, representing 23.2 percent of all agricultural employment (Chapman 1990). This obviously erroneous estimate was cited from an agricultural industry report (Agro-economic Services, Ltd. 1987). However, considering that each ha of tobacco cropland generates 500 employees, and that the 1986 tobacco cropland was only about 19,000 ha, the estimated full-time equivalent of workers should only be approximately 8,500, or less than 2 percent of total agricultural employment.

In summary, tobacco agriculture has been expanding slightly in Colombia, especially due to an increase in exports. However, its importance in the national economic context is minimal. The State

Figure 1. Percentage distribution of type of tobacco and types of cigarettes smoked, Colombia, 1969 to 1980

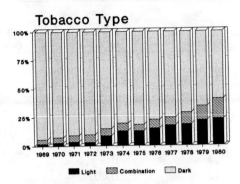

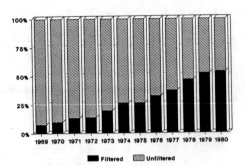

Source: National Planning Department, 1983.

supports this agricultural activity through the promotion of exports, the provision of loans, and the provision of agricultural research extension activities through the Colombian Agricultural and Livestock Institute (ICA).

Manufacturing

In 1987, 18 of the total 6,406 industrial enterprises in Colombia were cigarette- and cigar-manufacturers. Of these, two large cigarette companies were responsible for 92.4 percent of production. These companies are the Compañía Colombiana de Tabaco, S.A., (COLTABACO) with three factories, and the Productora Tabacalera de Colombia, S.A., (PROTABACO) with one factory; the latter manufactures brands of Liggett and Myers Tobacco, a multinational tobacco company. In 1986, a third company, Nacional de Cigarrillos, S.A., was absorbed by COLTABACO. The rest of the companies are small producers of hand-made leaf cigars and calillas (''thin'' cigars) in the Departments of Santander and Valle. In addition, in the tobacco-producing areas such as Sucre and Bolivar Departments, cigars and calillas for local consumption are made from tobacco that has been rejected for export purposes.

In 1980 the tobacco manufacturing industry employed 2,818 persons, or 0.6 percent of all industrial workers. The industry had stagnated between 1970 and 1980 and its contribution to the GDP decreased (Departamento Nacional de Planeación 1983). However, the industry appeared to shift to meet changing consumer tastes by increasing relative production of filtered *tabaco rubio* cigarettes (Figure 1). After this reorientation, real production of manufactured tobacco products increased by

56.6 percent, and employment in the tobacco manufacturing industry increased by 3.2 percent (Dirección de Impuestos Nacionales 1987).

Until the middle 1960s, the now extinct National Institute for Tobacco Promotion received a 1-percent tax on the value of cigarettes imported (Rodríguez 1960). After the middle 1960s, these tax revenues were directed toward the Colombian Agricultural and Livestock Institute to support research on tobacco. In 1970, the National Planning Department prepared a report entitled, ''Definition of a Policy for the Cigarette Industry,'' which described the tobacco manufacturing industry as ''dynamic.'' However, the health consequences of smoking were recognized by the Planning Department, and the report concluded that the tobacco industry could not be protected at the expense of others with greater social importance. It also stated that increased consumer prices might benefit tobacco growers and at the same time benefit health through reduced demand and consumption (Departamento Nacional de Planeación 1970). Unfortunately, this policy statement was never integrated with actions by the health sector; as a result, the tobacco-manufacturing industry actually became stronger in the 1970s.

Cigarette Production and Illegal Trade

Data from the U.S. Department of Agriculture (USDA) (1990) and from a 1983 study by the National Planning Department may be used to estimate cigarette production and trade in Colombia (Tables 3 and 4). From 1970 to 1980, the quantities of illegally imported cigarettes estimated by the tobacco companies were added to the estimates of the National Planning Department. Planning Depart-

Table 3. Manufactured cigarettes: production, imports, total domestic consumption, and per capita consumption (age ≥ 15), Colombia, 1969 to 1980

Year	Production	Imports	Exports	Total domestic consumption	Per capita consumption (age ≥ 15)
1969	20,049	1,313	—	21,362	1,911
1970	20,780	1,696	—	22,476	1,948
1971	20,528	2,234	—	22,762	1,911
1972	19,403	2,630	—	22,033	1,792
1973	21,065	2,539	1	23,603	1,859
1974	21,064	3,351	4	24,411	1,862
1975	22,809	3,355	2	26,162	1,932
1976	20,638	4,862	—	25,500	1,824
1977	21,877	5,258	—	27,135	1,880
1978	20,918	6,495	—	27,413	1,839
1979	18,246	8,778	—	27,024	1,755
1980	19,271	9,357	—	27,628	1,737

Source: National Planning Department, 1983.

ment data for these years also include those from small enterprises, but these data are not included in USDA estimates. After 1983, USDA data include estimates of illegal imports (Tobacco International 1989a). Thus, for 1981 and 1982, domestic cigarette consumption is underestimated. As noted earlier, cigarette production remained stable in the 1970s and increased in the 1980s.

Illegal importation of cigarettes from the United States has been extensive, with fewer illegal imports from Venezuela and Ecuador. The domestic cigarette industry has estimated that contraband supplies 35 to 43 percent of the domestic market (Tobacco International 1989b). However, the industry is using these data to criticize the State for not protecting the domestic industry. In addition, in 1990, a package of contraband cigarettes was 56 to 116 percent more expensive than the most popular domestic filter cigarettes and 254 percent more expensive than the most popular unfiltered dark tobacco cigarettes (Tobacco International 1989a).

The multinational tobacco companies through advertising have created a market for these imported brands in Colombia, and this alone may explain the high participation in the cigarette market among those persons with the most disposable income to spend on imported products such as U.S.-made cigarettes. Available surveys do not permit analysis of this supposition, however. Nevertheless, it is contradictory that the domestic cigarette industry boasts of prosperity and increased profits while at the same time projecting doom because of illegal imports (Tobacco International 1989b).

Advertising and Promotion

Since 1983, advertising of cigarettes on television has been prohibited until after 11 p.m. (Ministerio de Comunicaciones 1982). Tobacco product advertising is permitted on radio, in the print media, and on outdoor billboards. Albornoz (1989) reported that one of the two largest broadcasting networks in Colombia (Radio Cadena Nacional) transmitted 59 cigarette advertisements on one Friday, mostly during news broadcasts and sponsored sports programs. This is equivalent to one cigarette advertisement shown every 12 minutes during the 12 hours watched by the largest audience. The largest national newspaper (El Tiempo) daily carries cigarette advertising in its sports section; this newspaper features the most popular sports in Colombia: soccer and cycling. All of the nationally circulated variety, economic, and news magazines carry at least one page of cigarette advertising in color.

Despite a 1983 resolution by the Bogotá city council that prohibited billboard advertising in residential areas (Concejo de Bogotá 1983), the cigarette industry erected bus stops labeled with tobacco product advertising every 300 m throughout the entire city.

The cigarette companies aggressively support

Table 4. Production, imports, exports, total domestic consumption, and per capita consumption of manufactured cigarettes (age ≥ 15), Colombia, 1960 to 1989

Year	Production	Imports	Exports	Total domestic consumption	Per capita consumption (age ≥ 15)
1960	15,353	307	1	15,659	1,899
1961	16,443	355	2	16,796	1,969
1962	16,221	235	0	16,456	1,864
1963	17,753	152	0	17,905	1,957
1964	17,398	40	8	17,430	1,837
1965	20,000	27	12	20,015	2,032
1966	20,800	30	4	20,826	2,049
1967	17,694	24	0	17,718	1,689
1968	21,110	552	0	21,662	2,000
1969	19,568	1,003	0	20,571	1,841
1970	18,825	1,824	0	20,649	1,790
1971	20,918	571	0	21,489	1,804
1972	18,933	89	0	19,022	1,547
1973	21,086	152	1	21,237	1,673
1974	18,170	58	4	18,224	1,390
1975	18,904	70	2	18,972	1,401
1976	18,344	6	0	18,350	1,313
1977	18,520	900	0	19,420	1,345
1978	18,500	800	0	19,300	1,294
1979	20,600	1,500	0	22,100	1,435
1980	21,200	1,940	0	23,140	1,455
1981	19,800	1,600	180	21,220	1,293
1982	20,100	1,568	246	21,422	1,266
1983	22,525	10,633	94	33,064	1,894
1984	23,840	10,488	100	34,228	1,891
1985	24,050	10,540	100	34,490	1,856
1986	24,181	10,549	100	34,630	1,824
1987	21,987	12,933	100	34,820	1,794
1988	20,721	14,379	100	35,000	1,762
1989	20,200	14,920	100	35,020	1,722

Source: USDA, 1990.

sports. Such promotions include professional soccer championships (since 1989), the Radio Cadena Nacional cycling classic (1990) (the motto of this competition was, ''Do not smoke contraband cigarettes''), a horsemanship cup (since 1989), and popular musical concerts (1990). These promotions also facilitate legal and illegal tobacco product advertising on television through the promotion of these events. In addition, cigarette advertising proliferates in soccer stadiums, tennis courts, and theaters; in fact, the obstacles in horsemanship competitions replicate large packs of cigarettes. In 1991, distribution of free cigarettes by attractive young women began in Colombian urban centers (Ronderos-Torres 1991).

Cigarette advertising is ubiquitous in Colombia; the brands advertised include those which are sold only illegally in Colombia. In other nations of Latin America, multinational tobacco companies have promoted their products despite the illegality of those products in countries that were protecting their domestic tobacco industries. This promotion was temporally associated with an illegal trade in cigarettes and an eventual capitulation of those nations to permit either licensure of or acquisitions by multinational tobacco companies within their borders. In this respect, Colombia is unique in Latin America. The multinationals do not dominate the Colombian cigarette market. Whereas nearly all of the other Latin American national cigarette markets are controlled by multinational tobacco companies, only 49 percent of the Colombian market is multinational. Much of this market must reflect illegal imports, however, because the concessionaire producing one multinational brand in Colombia (PRO-TOBACO) has a much smaller market share than do the brands produced by the domestic company, COLTABACO.

Tobacco Use

Per Capita Consumption

Annual per capita cigarette consumption has fluctuated between 1,700 and 2,000 cigarettes in Colombia since 1960 (Table 3). Although the exact quantity of illegally imported cigarettes consumed is unknown, per capita consumption for 1975 to 1985 may be estimated through a household survey of consumer expenditures (including tobacco) in the 15 largest cities of the country (Departamento Administrativo Nacional de Estadísticas 1987). In constant 1975 prices, the household expenditure for tobacco increased 10 percent from 1975 to 1980; from 1980 to 1985, the percentage expended varied minimally, but increased 6 percent during 1983 to 1985. The total increase from 1975 to 1985 was 13 percent. Assuming that the increase in the cost of cigarettes did not exceed that of inflation, it may be concluded that real household cigarette consumption increased to a greater degree from 1975 to 1985 than was indicated by the estimates of per capita consumption reported by the USDA and the National Planning Department.

The preference for tobacco in Colombia has shifted in recent decades from dark to light tobacco (Departamento Nacional de Planeación 1983); as a result, dark tobacco growing has declined also. In 1969, 94.2 percent of all tobacco produced was dark tobacco and 92.3 of cigarettes manufactured were unfiltered; in 1980, 59.2 percent of national tobacco production was light tobacco and 54 percent of manufactured cigarettes were filtered (Figure 1). By 1988, the market share for light tobacco reached 76 percent (Maxwell 1990).

Surveys

Numerous surveys are available on tobacco use in Colombia (Table 4). In 1971, the Pan American Health Organization (PAHO) conducted a survey of smoking among adults aged 15 to 74 years in eight Latin American cities including Bogotá (Joly 1977). Only the unadjusted smoking prevalence rates by age group and sex are reported for Bogotá. It is not possible to establish the actual prevalence rates by various sociodemographic variables. However, as the first survey in Colombia on smoking, it is an essential point of reference.

In 1976 the Colombian cigarette companies conducted a national market study of persons older than 14 years (Departamento Nacional de Planeación 1983). The number of persons surveyed and the methodology for this survey are unknown, but overall prevalence data from the survey are available.

In 1977 to 1980, the National Health Study in Colombia (ENS) (Rodríguez 1988), asked questions on smoking of 6,277 persons aged 15 years and older. This sample of the noninstitutional civilian population was obtained using stratification of unequal groupings; the final sampling unit was the household. Unfortunately, definitions for "smokers" and "ex-smokers" were established after the survey was completed, because the survey methodology did not provide standard definitions for these categories. The survey also did not include a category of "occasional smokers" (less than one cigarette per day); it is thus probable that the prevalences of daily smokers are overestimated. Nonetheless, the prevalences of smoking by sex, age, educational level, socioeconomic stratum, and urbanization are reported for five large regions of the country.

In 1985 a survey was conducted by researchers from the University of Antioquia in Medellín on the use of dependency-producing substances (Velázquez de Pabón 1985). The representative household sample included 2,807 persons aged 10 years and older, but excluded the very lowest socioeconomic stratum because it was considered too difficult to survey. Of the total sample, 371 were adolescents aged 10 to 15 years. The data permit reporting of prevalence of smoking by sex at any time in the year prior to the survey. For adolescents, only the prevalence for both sexes together was reported. The prevalence of smoking any time in the last year may overestimate the prevalence of daily smoking among adolescents, who still may be experimenting with cigarettes and not using tobacco on a daily basis. The data probably adequately represent the prevalence of smoking among adults.

In 1987, the University of Antioquia conducted another national study on use of dependency-producing substances (Torres 1987), among 2,800 persons aged 12 to 64 years, that was representative of the urban population of Colombia. Although "urban" is not defined in the description of the survey methodology, the investigators report data by size of city (large and intermediate) for the four largest cities of the country. Respondents were asked about the use of cigarettes, alcohol, tranquilizers, freebase cocaine, cocaine, and marijuana. This survey also defined "smoking" as having smoked at least once in the year prior to the survey.

The Latin American Center for Perinatology and Human Development (CLAP) reported the results of a 1987 survey on habits and drugs in pregnancy (PAHO 1987). This report included data on smoking prevalence among 1,480 pregnant women from two maternity centers in Colombia in the 6 months prior to their pregnancy.

In 1985, two surveys of drug use, including cigarettes, among secondary school students were conducted in Cali. The first (Climent 1986) surveyed 1,937 students from 54 private and public secondary schools, stratified by socioeconomic status. This survey determined the use of cigarettes, according to sex, in the month prior to the survey. In the second survey (Bergonzoli 1989), interviews were conducted with 512 students of public and private schools who were in their last 2 years of school. This survey's definition of "smoking" is not clear.

In 1988 and 1989 the Ministry of Education surveyed drug use among 7,513 students, aged 11 to 25 years, enrolled in basic, secondary, and vocational programs (Ministerio de Educación 1989). The sample was representative for students enrolled in these schools, which were stratified according to the type of institution (e.g., public, private, day, or night). Smoking status was reported as "never smoker," "experimental smoker" (once, occasionally, monthly), "occasional smoker" (biweekly, weekly), and "daily smoker." A total of 5,737 students (76.4 percent of the respondents) were 11 to 18 years old.

In 1991, a survey of 233 employees' smoking status was conducted in the Lorencita Villegas de Santos pediatric hospital in Bogotá. This survey asked about attitudes toward restrictive worksite smoking policies at the hospital.

Finally, Chávez (1991) surveyed 1,211 male and female physicians to investigate cardiovascular risk factors, including cigarette smoking.

Prevalence of smoking among adults

The prevalence of daily smoking among men in Bogotá in 1971 (52.4 percent) is similar to that reported in the National Health Study (ENS) for Colombia in 1979–1980 (52.2 percent). However, the ENS-derived prevalence may overestimate daily smokers because occasional smokers were included in the numerator; the 1971 Joly (PAHO) survey did not include occasional smokers in the estimates for the prevalence of daily smokers. The drug-use surveys for Medellín in 1985 and for all of Colombia in 1987 suggest that the prevalence of daily smoking among adults decreased somewhat from 1971. The 1976 tobacco-industry-sponsored marketing survey reported only a 57.6 percent prevalence of "smokers" among men (55.5 percent in urban areas and 60.9 percent in rural areas).

In the ENS, the smoking prevalence among men in cities of 100,000 or more inhabitants was estimated at 51.7 percent (compared with 52.4 percent for the entire country) and among women, 27 percent (compared with 20.2 percent for the entire country). The differences between these levels and the lower levels reported by Torres in 1987 (42.5 percent for men and 25.3 percent for women) may be due to a real decrease in the prevalence of smoking in the urban areas between 1980 and 1987 or simply to a difference in the definitions of "smoker" in the two studies. These difficulties emphasize the need to establish uniform definitions and methodologies for surveys on tobacco use in the Americas so that trends in tobacco use over time may be ascertained accurately.

In the ENS, the number of persons sampled in Bogotá permits estimated smoking prevalence in this particular location. Among men, the prevalence was 52.2 percent, similar to those reported by Joly for 1971 (Table 5). Among women, the prevalence was 26.4 percent, which is an increase in prevalence from the 6.4% reported by Joly in 1971. In 1987, Torres reported that only 35.7 percent of men and 27.4 percent of women were daily smokers in Bogotá. However, because this survey included persons aged 12 to 64 years, the prevalences would be lowered somewhat by including younger persons who have a lower prevalence of smoking than do older persons. Most disturbing is the apparent 20–percent increase in the prevalence of smoking among Bogotá women between 1971 and 1987, a pattern that has been observed to various degrees in other countries of South America.

In 1987, the prevalence of ex-smokers in Bogotá was 38.1 percent among men and 19.6 percent

Table 5. Surveys on adult tobacco use, and prevalence (percent) of current smoking by sex, Colombia, 1971 to 1987

Sponsor and year	Coverage	Ages	Definition of smoker	Prevalence			
				Men	Women	Both	N
PAHO 1971	Bogotá	15–74	≥ 100 lifetime cigs., & now smokes	52.4	20.2	34.2	1,410
ENS 1979–80	National	>14	≥ = 1 cig./day for one year	52.2	26.4	38.7	6,277
Velasquez 1985	Medellín	>15	Smoked in last year			30.0	2,432
Torres 1987	Colombia urban	15–64	Smoked in last year	42.5	25.3	33.9	2,400

among women. Thus, the differences in current smoking prevalence may be due also to men stopping smoking at greater rates than women. The dissemination of information about the health consequences of smoking is more likely to reach cities such as Bogotá before reaching rural areas; thus, quit rates (as measured by the prevalence of former smoking) likely would be higher in the cities. However, tobacco product advertising is also more pervasive in the cities, and women, who may be less cognizant of the health consequences of smoking than are men, might be affected differentially by this advertising.

Bogotá had one of the highest smoking prevalence rates in the 1971 PAHO survey, and one of the lowest rates for "heavy smoking" (as measured by the prevalence of 20 or more cigarettes smoked per day by smokers) of all eight cities surveyed. Likewise, the ENS reported a low number of cigarettes smoked per day (averages of 8.3 overall, 9.7 for men, and 6.0 for women). Of the total population, 50 percent smoked 5 or fewer cigarettes per day, and 80 percent smoked 15 or fewer cigarettes per day; the modal number of cigarettes smoked per day was 2. In the 1987 national study on urban areas (Torres 1989), 52.7 percent of men and 72 percent of women smoked 5 or fewer cigarettes per day, and only 25 percent of men and 13.6 percent of women smoked 11 or more cigarettes per day.

The ENS also reported smoking prevalence by socioeconomic stratum and educational level. An overall socioeconomic score was based on a combination of income, education, literacy, and type of housing to define four strata (low, low average, high average, and high). The age-adjusted prevalences of smoking in men were (in increasing order of socioeconomic score) 54.7 percent, 54.1 percent, 45.1 percent, and 49.1 percent. Despite a lower prevalence of smoking among men who had completed secondary school (38.3 percent) than among those who had no education (56 percent), the higher prevalence of smoking among men with a university education (54.5 percent) belies the inverse relationship between socioeconomic status and smoking noted earlier.

Among women, the age-adjusted prevalence of smoking was highest in the low and high socioeconomic and educational levels, but lower in the intermediate levels. In order of ascending socioeconomic strata, the prevalences of smoking among women were 28.9 percent, 23.9 percent, 26.1 percent, and 30.1 percent. Among women with no education, the prevalence was 32.2 percent; among those with primary school education, 23 percent; and among those with secondary school education, 28 percent. In addition, those in the high socioeconomic stratum had higher quit rates than did those in the low stratum (27.4 vs. 13.1 percent).

The ENS also asked about age at initiation of smoking. Overall, the average age of initiation was 19.8 years, with a slightly higher age for women than for men (21.2 vs. 19.1 years). The age of initiation for persons with both a higher educational attainment and higher socioeconomic status was lower than that for other educational and socioeconomic groups. The age of initiation has been declining for younger cohorts of men especially. In the cohort aged 44 to 53 years, only 61 percent of men and 42 percent of women began smoking before age 20.

Overall, in Colombia, the largest numbers of smokers are to be found in the low socioeconomic stratum because these persons have equal or higher prevalences of smoking than do high socioeconomic stratum persons and because they constitute the largest segment of the population. Hence, the estimate for the market share held by contraband cigarettes (35 to 52 percent) provided by the tobacco industry is surprisingly high, because as noted, contraband cigarettes are much more expensive.

Table 6. Surveys on smoking among adolescents, and prevalence (percent) of smoking by sex, Colombia, 1980s

Sponsor and year	Coverage	Ages	Definition of smoker	Prevalence			
				Men	Women	Both	N
Velazquez 1985	Medellín	10–15	Smoked in last year			29.6	371
Torres 1987	Colombia urban	12–15	Smoked in last year	5.3	3.8	4.6	400
Education Ministry 1988–89	Secondary students, national	11–18	Experimental	20.8	14.7	17.8	5,737
			Occasional	3.3	1.5	2.4	
			Daily	2.3	0.6	1.4	
Climent 1985	Cali students	Gr. 9–11	Smoked in last month	30.4	20.8		1,937
Bergonzoli 1985	Cali students	Gr. 10 & 11	Use/don't use				512
			Public school	6.1			
			Private school	9.5			

Prevalence of smoking among adolescents

All surveys of smoking among adolescents in Colombia have been part of drug-use surveys, and have varied in the definitions used for "smoking" (Table 6). Generally, the "smoker" in these surveys is designated as an adolescent who is experimenting with cigarettes (by use in the last year). Adult surveys in Colombia suggest that because of the relatively high smoking prevalence rates, a large majority of experimenters become addicted to nicotine. The data also suggest that more young men than young women begin to smoke during adolescence. In 1985, 29.6 percent of the adolescents in Medellín were experimenters. In 1989, only 17.8 percent of adolescent students nationally were experimenters. However, the data are rather inconsistent from city to city and nationally.

Other surveys

In the PAHO-CLAP study on habits and drugs in pregnancy, approximately 20 percent of women smoked in the 6 months prior to pregnancy (PAHO 1987). This estimate was corroborated by other researchers who reported that in 1980, 19 percent of the pregnant women in Colombia were smokers, with 150,600 children thus exposed to tobacco *in utero* each year (Chandler 1986).

In the 1991 study of the Bogotá Pediatric Hospital employees, the prevalence of smoking was 25.3 percent overall and the prevalence of ex-smoking was 25.8 percent. That these prevalences are low compared with the general population (38.4 percent) may partly reflect the comparatively young age of the group (18 to 58 years), and the reluctance of these employees to expose hospitalized children to cigarette smoke. However, it is more likely to be because many of these employees were health care professionals, in whom the knowledge of the health consequences of smoking is likely to be the highest.

In the 1991 physicians' survey (Chavez 1991), 73 percent of whom were aged 20 to 39 years, 21.3 percent overall were smokers (21.2 percent of men and 21.7 percent of women). The prevalence of smoking in the 20- to 39-year age group in the general population reported by the ENS was 62 percent among men and 30 percent among women. There appears to be no sex differential among physicians in smoking prevalence, but the prevalence of smoking is far less than that of the general population.

Other forms of tobacco use

The ENS found that only 3.1 percent of the population were pipe smokers. Along the Atlantic coast of Colombia and in the northeastern part of Antioquia, indigenous peoples still practice reverse smoking, which involves smoking with the lit end of the cigarette inside the mouth. In particular, women utilize this method to prevent dropping ashes into their laundry and onto their small children. The University of Cartagena has studied 46,902 persons through population surveys and reviewed the clinical records of patients with squamous cell carcinoma of the oral cavity (Quintero 1989). Data on reverse smoking were included in most of the case records. Based on these records, it was observed that most persons who practiced reverse smoking were rural dwellers (87 percent) and female (89.7 percent). These data do not permit an estimate of the overall prevalence of this practice, because persons in this study, and the majority of those with oral carcinoma, do not represent the general population.

In another study which screened for oral pathology in three municipalities of the Department of Bolívar on the Atlantic coast (Quintero 1984), 859 persons were examined; of these, 85 percent of men and 80 percent of women were smokers. Among male smokers, 32 (11 percent) reverse smoked, and among women, 193 (46 percent) reported reverse smoking. It appears that this custom is more common among older persons surveyed, although it is not possible to ascertain the age distribution of all respondents to this survey.

Smoking and Health

General Mortality

Significant underregistration of deaths is evident in Colombia, especially in the rural areas on the Atlantic and Pacific coasts. Because causes of death in these areas reflect rural conditions and poverty, published mortality data are more representative of the better developed areas; these areas are also more likely to suffer a greater burden of chronic disease deaths associated with smoking. The mortality pattern was dominated by cardiovascular diseases and malignancies in 1984 (PAHO 1990) (Table 7). In addition, the increase in mortality among young men due to violence has had a competitive effect as a cause of death. The greatest proportion of malignant tumors and cardiovascular

disease (e.g., cancer of the uterine cervix, hemorrhagic cerebrovascular accident, and stomach cancer) is associated with lack of access to health services (PAHO 1990).

Morbidity and Mortality Due to Lung Cancer

Since 1962, a registry of cancer incidence in Cali has been maintained according to standard registry methods. Based on these data, lung cancer incidence among men appears to have increased gradually in recent years except among the two youngest groups (Table 8). Compared with lung cancer incidence rates among males in developed countries such as Finland and the Soviet Union, rates for specific age groups are much lower in Cali (WHO 1990). For example, the lung cancer incidence rate among Finnish men aged 40 to 44 years in 1976 to 1980 was 15/100,000, while in Cali the rate for men in that age group in 1977 to 1981 was 4.8/100,000.

The population exposure to tobacco may not yet have caused a peak in lung cancer incidence in Cali, but rates as high as those reported for more developed countries may never be reached. One reason for this is the fact that Colombians smoke fewer cigarettes per day than persons in developed countries. The average number of cigarettes smoked per day by adult men in Colombia in 1983 was 5.1; in the United States in 1980, 17; and in Great Britain in 1983, 7.1. Second, when the developed countries (in particular, Great Britain) experienced peak exposure to cigarettes, most of the cigarettes smoked were unfiltered, dark tobacco

Table 7. Five leading causes of death in the general population, according to proportional mortality and rates per 100,000 population, Colombia, 1984

Cause of death	Rank order	Rate (per 100,000)	Proportional mortality (of all recorded deaths)
Heart diseases (ICD 390–429)	1	100.4	21.8
Malignant neoplasms (ICD 140–208)	2	60.3	13.1
Injuries (E800–E949, E980–E989)	3	49.9	10.8
Cerebrovascular disease (ICD 430–438)	4	38.3	8.3
Homicide (E960–E978, E990–E999)	5	33.3	7.2

Source: PAHO, 1990.

Table 8. Lung cancer incidence rates among men (per 100,000), Cali, 1962 to 1986

Ages	1962–1966	1967–1971	1972–1976	1977–1981	1982–1986
30–34	0	1.8	1.4	1.2	0
35–39	1.2	2.9	0	2.8	4.56
40–44	3	10.8	8.8	4.8	6.44
45–49	21.4	9.9	12.6	19.8	13.74
50–54	20.4	16.9	22.8	38.6	31.3
55–59	76.2	40.9	51.7	71.7	53.6
60–64	78.8	92.1	81.9	104.8	105.8
65–69	100.0	131.5	139.5	200.1	153.0
70–74	127	111.8	170	177.7	231.5

Source: WHO, Cancer incidence in five continents, Vol. I-V.

cigarettes. In Colombia, consumer preference shifted to filtered, light tobacco cigarettes at a relatively later time, during 1969 to 1987, when peak population exposure to smoking was reached. This shift will not affect the increased incidence of cardiovascular disease, but it may depress the increase in lung cancer incidence because filtered, light tobacco cigarettes may have a decreased carcinogenic potential compared with unfiltered, dark tobacco cigarettes (U.S. Department of Health and Human Services [USDHHS] 1981).

Lung cancer incidence rates are increasing for all age groups of men in Cali (Table 8), and the lung cancer mortality rates are increasing in Colombia in general (Table 9). Although the incidence rates for men only are shown for the Cali data, lung cancer mortality in Colombia for age groups 45 to 54 years and 55 to 64 years among both men and women increased overall from the period 1960 to 1964 to the period 1985 to 1987 (Figure 2); however, the mortality rates for men are much higher than for women, especially among older age groups.

This differential is due to a historically lower exposure to smoking among women, whether due to later adoption of smoking or to fewer cigarettes smoked per day. This situation is similar in Canada,

but lung cancer mortality rates are higher in Canada in the younger age groups (World Health Organization 1990). The differences between Cali, an urban area, and the national registry data, suggest that lower cigarette exposure in rural areas dampens the national incidence; in Cali, population exposure has been higher than that for the entire country and therefore, lung cancer incidence rates are higher than those reported for the entire nation.

Morbidity and Mortality Due to Other Smoking-associated Malignancies

According to registry data from the National Cancer Institute in Bogotá (Table 10), the proportion of oropharyngeal cancers declined from the late 1940s to the late 1980s. However, this decline is due to the diversion of most cases to specialty hospitals in areas where this lesion occurs more frequently because of reverse smoking (Atlantic coast and Antioquia). The proportion of lung cancer is increasing (from 0.2 percent in 1945 to 1949 to 1.7 percent in 1985 to 1989), but malignant tumors such as cancers of the uterine cervix and the stomach that may be more associated with underdevelop-

Table 9. Lung cancer mortality rates among men (per 100,000), Colombia, 1960 to 1987

Ages	1960–1964	1965–1969	1972–1974	1975–1979	1980–1984	1985–1987
35–39	0.64	1.33	1.39	1.85	1.51	1.94
40–44	6.19	2.27	4.12	2.86	4.30	4.44
45–49	4.47	6.03	6.21	7.83	9.37	9.80
50–54	8.61	10.81	13.25	13.37	19.60	20.21
55–59	16.08	16.46	19.57	24.58	32.52	39.00
60–64	27.07	32.73	34.36	37.40	49.51	61.82
65–69	30.35	45.55	45.45	55.42	65.28	82.92

Source: Unpublished data, National Cancer Institute.

Figure 2. Lung cancer mortality rates among men by age group, Colombia, 1960 to 1990

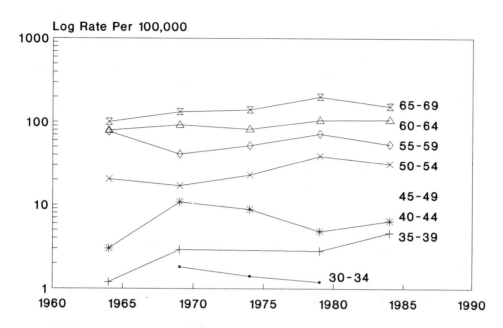

Source: Unpublished data, National Cancer Institute.

ment still occupy first and second places in percentage of diagnoses. These tumors are also associated with smoking, but dietary habits and access to screening are probably more important in the mortality outcomes than is smoking at this time in Colombia.

Oral cancer and inverse smoking in Colombia deserve special consideration. In the Department of Bolívar, of 27 persons diagnosed with squamous

cell carcinoma of the oral cavity, 18 engaged in reverse smoking (relative risk 2.9 [95 percent confidence limits 1.2–6.7]). In addition, of 377 persons with precancerous lesions, 218 practiced inverted smoking (raw relative risk 3.0 [95 percent confidence limits 2.6–3.39]) (Quintero 1984). Quintero also reviewed pathology files in the Atlantic coast departments of Córdoba from 1958 to 1981 and of Sucre from 1968 to 1981. Of 207 cases of squamous

Table 10. Malignancies diagnosed at the National Cancer Institute for three time periods, Colombia, 1945–1949, 1965–1969, 1985–1989

Site/ICD code	1945–1949		1965–1969		1985–1989	
	No.	%	No.	%	No.	%
Lung (162)	8	0.2	86	1	326	1.7
Bladder (188)	14	0.3	88	1	193	1
Oral cavity and pharynx (140–149)	296	7.2	9	0.1	49	0.3
Pancreas (157)	2	0.05	365	4.1	629	3.3
Esophagus (150)	65	1.6	260	2.9	447	2.3
Larynx (161)	50	1.2	75	0.8	220	1.2
Corpus uteri (180)	172	28.4	2,639	29.7	4,414	23
Stomach (151)	80	1.9	444	5	1,278	6.7
Other sites	2,446	59.2	4,927	55.4	11,521	60.4
All sites	4,133	100	8,893	100	19,077	100

Source: Unpublished data, National Cancer Institute.

cell carcinoma of the oral cavity in Cordoba and 122 such cases in Sucre, carcinoma of the hard and soft palate was diagnosed in 36 percent of cases in Cordoba and 46.7 percent of cases in Sucre. These proportions were comparable to those observed in India, where reverse smoking is also common among women. In other areas (i.e., Cuba, Buenos Aires, and New York City), the most frequently encountered carcinoma locations in the oral cavity were the lip and tongue, and cancers of the hard and soft palate accounted for no more than 10 percent of malignancy sites (Quintero 1986).

Quintero and Alvarez also reviewed the pathology records of the University of Antioquia for 1960 to 1986 (Quintero 1989). Of 722 cases diagnosed as squamous cell carcinoma of the oral cavity, 41.5 percent had a history of smoking and 15.6 percent practiced reverse smoking. The most common sites were tongue (31.8 percent) and palate (14.1 percent). It is clear that reverse smoking is a major cause of oropharyngeal cancer on Colombia's Atlantic coast and probably in Antioquia as well. The high temperatures of the lit end of the cigarette (900°F) and the irritative effect on mucous membranes increase exposure to the known carcinogens in cigarettes released by combustion.

Tobacco Use Prevention and Control Activities

Government Actions

Executive structure and policies

In 1982, the Bureau of Epidemiology of the Ministry of Health produced a document to encourage the Ministry's public health actions against smoking (Ministry of Health 1983). However, it was not until a 1983 workshop organized by the International Union Against Cancer (IUAC) that the National Council on Cigarettes and Health was created, the function of which was to address this public health problem (Ministry of Health 1984). The Council members are the Minister of Health (presiding), the Bureau of Medical Care of the Ministry of Health, the Director of the National Cancer Institute, the Chairman of the Colombian League Against Cancer, and a member of the press elected by consensus. The National Cancer Institute administers the Council. In 1989, a funded project entitled "Control of Smoking" was begun by the Institute. This project is designed to develop a long-term strategy to decrease the prevalence of

smoking (González 1989). In association with this project, data were to be collected in 1991 on knowledge, attitudes, and practices related to tobacco use.

Legislation

In December 1982, tobacco product advertising was restricted to after 11 p.m. (Ministerio de Comunicaciones 1982). Subsequently, the National Narcotics Council assumed responsibility for setting standards for tobacco product advertising on radio and television through a 1991 policy determination by the Ministry of Health.

Law No. 30 (31 January 1986), the "National Intoxication Statute," mandated that cigarettes or tobacco may be dispensed only to persons aged 15 and older. In addition, this decree mandated that every package of cigarettes sold in Colombia (domestic or foreign brands) must bear the warning, "Tobacco is harmful to health." The warning must occupy one-tenth of the lower end of the label.

Also in 1991, Resolution 3027, issued by the Ministry of Health, invited the civil aeronautics authority to study the prohibition of smoking on domestic airline flights. As a result of this study, smoking was prohibited on all domestic flights in Colombia (Departamento Administrativo de Aeronáutica Civil 1991). Resolution 3027 also banned smoking in all installations of the National Health System.

School-based education

The National Ministry of Education includes smoking in the Program for Prevention of Drug Addiction. A primer called "The Pleasure of Not Smoking" has been published twice by the National Council on Cigarettes and Health and the National Cancer Institute; it is distributed free of charge and is utilized in many public and private schools' curricula on behavior and health.

Public information campaigns

Since 1984, the Colombian League Against Cancer has celebrated a "nonsmoker's day" in conjunction with the American Cancer Society's "Great American Smokeout" in November of each year. In 1989, the Ministry of Health and the National Cancer Institute joined forces to celebrate the World Health Organization's World No-Tobacco Day on May 31. In 1991, a campaign entitled "Smokers, a Species on the Road of Extinction," which stresses that smoking is socially unacceptable, was launched by the National Council on Cigarettes and Health and the National Cancer Institute (Ronderos-Torres 1991).

Taxes

Cigarettes are taxed at 122 percent of the wholesale price. Of this total tax, 82 percent is for the general fund, 8 percent is for Coldeportes (sports sponsorship), and 10 percent is national value-added tax. Tobacco taxes comprised 2.9 percent of all national tax revenue in 1985 and 2.0 percent in 1988 (Ronderos-Torres 1991).

Nongovernmental Organizations

The main nongovernmental organization (NGO) active in the antismoking campaign has been the Colombian League Against Cancer, through its local chapters. Since 1990, this organization has had a National Committee for the Prevention of Smoking. In 1991, under the motto "Colombian Children and Young People Free from Smoke," this organization conducted five workshops for the education and health sectors; these workshops were sponsored by the National Cancer Institute. In addition, this NGO has been particularly visible in the public information campaigns associated with the "nonsmokers' day" and World No-Tobacco Day (Albornoz 1989).

Summary and Conclusions

The story of tobacco and health in Colombia provides several important historical lessons. First, colonial development in Colombia was largely dependent on tobacco growing. With an increase in international trade, tobacco agriculture in Colombia recently has experienced a slight resurgence. However, as a percentage of the national economy, tobacco agriculture remains small. Second, residual pockets of unusual forms of tobacco use, especially on Colombia's Atlantic coast, have created disease patterns not found elsewhere in the hemisphere. Third, a rather substantial illegal trade in foreign cigarettes is evident in Colombia. This situation is similar to the experience of other Latin American countries that had resisted the entry of multinational tobacco companies into their domestic markets. With intense advertising of illegally sold cigarettes, the domestic industries were subverted and eventually overcome by the multinationals through licensure or direct acquisition. In Colombia, the cig-

arette market has been changing steadily to the filtered light tobacco, cigarette brands sold by multinational tobacco companies. Because of increased use of cigarettes, Colombians are now experiencing increased lung cancer mortality rates and changing mortality patterns directly related to increased population exposure to cigarettes.

On the other hand, Colombia has an established scientific community, a Ministry of Health, and an NGO that are very concerned about and active in the prevention and cessation of tobacco use. A formal Government structure for the control of tobacco use is in place, and thus far, Government funds have been committed to study tobacco use and to disseminate information on the health consequences of smoking.

The information presented in this report supports the following conclusions:

1. Tobacco agriculture has been increasing in Colombia as a result of a well-integrated vertical support system and increased foreign trade in tobacco.

2. A substantial illegal trade in cigarettes is evident in Colombia, with subsequent difficulties in estimating total and per capita cigarette consumption. Per capita cigarette consumption in Colombia (estimated at 1,722 per year) is among the highest in countries of the Western Hemisphere.

3. The prevalence of smoking among men in Bogotá in 1971 was 52.4 percent, and among women, 20.2 percent. In 1987, the prevalence among men in urban areas had declined to 42.5 percent and among women it had increased to 25.3 percent. Almost 20 percent of adolescents aged 11 to 18 years had experimented with smoking in the year prior to being surveyed in 1989.

4. The incidence and mortality rates for lung cancer among both men and women are increasing, as observed in registry data on the national level and in Cali. Lung cancer mortality rates for men are substantially higher than for women, and rates for Cali are higher than for those of the nation as a whole.

5. A formal Government program to prevent and control tobacco use exists in Colombia. This specifically funded program utilizes data collection, a coalition of important Government and nongovernment agencies, and public information activities. These are essential components in the institutional approach to preventing chronic diseases associated with tobacco.

References

AGRO-ECONOMIC SERVICES AND TABACOSMOS, LTD. *The employment, tax revenue and wealth that the Tobacco Industry creates.* September 1987.

ALBORNOZ, S. Informe de Colombia. *Taller sobre Medios de Comunicación y Tabaquismo.* Caracas: June 1989.

BERGONZOLI, G., RICO, O., RAMIREZ, A., PAZ, M.I., RAMIREZ, J., RIVAS, J.C., SALINAS, A., RODRIGUEZ, O., SALAZAR, O., RINCON, N. Uso de drogas entre estudiantes de Cali, Colombia. *Bol Of Sanit Panam* 106(1):22–31, 1989.

CHANDLER, W.U. Banishing tobacco. *Worldwatch Paper,* 68, January 1986.

CHAPMAN, S., WONG, W.L. *Tobacco Control in the Third World—A Resource Atlas.* Penang, Malaysia: International Organization of Consumers Unions, 1990.

CHAVEZ, M. Factores de riesgo de enfermedad cardiovascular en la población colombiana. *Ateroma* 3(1):15–24, January 1991.

CLIMENT, C., DE ARAGON, L.V. Factores asociados con el uso de drogas en estudiantes de secundaria en Cali. Parte I. Aspectos epidemiológicos y psicométricos. *Colombia Médica* 17(2): 58–69, 1986.

CONCEJO DE BOGOTA. *Acuerdo 3 de 1983.*

DEPARTAMENTO ADMINISTRATIVO DE AERONAUTICA CIVIL. *Resolución Número 11073.* September 4, 1991.

DEPARTAMENTO ADMINISTRATIVO NACIONAL DE ESTADISTICAS. *Colombia Estadística* Vol I:183–186, 1987.

DEPARTAMENTO NACIONAL DE PLANEACION. *Definición de una política para la industria del cigarrillo.* Documento destinado al Concejo Nacional de Precios. 1970.

DEPARTAMENTO NACIONAL DE PLANEACION. La industria del tabaco en Colombia. Documento inédito, 1983.

DIRECCION DE IMPUESTOS NACIONALES. *Boletín Económico y Fiscal* No. 2, July-Sept, Bogotá, 1987.

GOMEZ, C., MAYORGA, O.A, MESTRE, C.E. *Estudio sobre la prevalencia y la incidencia de los hábitos de fumar y consumir licor en la Escuela Colombiana de Medicina.* Tesis para optar el título de Doctor en Medicina. Bogotá: Facultad de Medicina. Escuela Colombiana de Medicina. November 1988.

GONZALEZ, J., RONDEROS-TORRES, M., SALAMANCA, H. *El tabaquismo en Colombia: Un problema de salud pública. Estrategias para el control,* 1989.

HARRISON, J.P. La evolución de la comercialización del tabaco colombiano hasta 1875. En: *El siglo XIX en Colombia visto por historiadores norteamericanos.* Editorial La Carreta, p. 60, 1952.

JOLY, D.J. *Encuesta sobre las características del hábito de fumar en América Latina.* Washington, D.C.: Organización Panamericana de la Salud. Scientific Publication 337, 1977.

KALMANOVITZ, S. *La agricultura en Colombia 1950–1972. I. Evolución de la estructura agraria. II. Evolución general de la producción agrícola.* Separata del Boletín Mensual de Estadística. Departamento Administrativo Nacional de Estadísticas, May 1978.

LATIN AMERICAN CENTER FOR PERINATOLOGY AND HUMAN DEVELOPMENT (CLAP). Tabaquismo y embarazo: hay que ayudar a parar. *Salud Perinatal* 2(7):65–77, 1987.

LEAL, F. El sistema político del clientelismo. *Revista Análisis Político* No. 8, September–December 1989.

LOSADA, R., VELEZ, E. Tendencias de muertes violentas en Colombia. *Revista Coyuntura Social,* December 1989.

MAXWELL, J.C. *The Maxwell Consumer Report. International Tobacco 1988--Part One.* Richmond, Virginia: Wheat First Securities/Butcher and Singer, Inc. WFBS-5455. 1990.

MINISTERIO DE AGRICULTURA. *Anuario Estadístico del Sector Agropecuario,* 1988.

MINISTERIO DE COMUNICACIONES. *Resolución 4063 de diciembre de 1982.* Resolución reglamentaria del decreto presidencial 3040 suscrito por los Ministerios de Comunicaciones y Salud, 1982.

MINISTERIO DE EDUCACION NACIONAL. Plan Nacional de Prevención de la Drogadicción. Programa ''Promoción Juvenil y Uso Creativo del Tiempo Libre'' como Estrategia de Prevención de la Drogadicción.'' Factores asociados al consumo de sustancias psicoactivas en estudiantes de básica secundaria y media vocacional. Informe interno. Bogotá: Ministerio de Educación Nacional, 1989.

MINISTERIO DE SALUD. Tabaquismo: Un problema de salud pública. Documento interno. Bogotá: Ministerio de Salud, Dirección Epidemiología, 1983.

PAN AMERICAN HEALTH ORGANIZATION. *Health Conditions in the Americas—1990 Edition.* Washington, D.C.: Pan American Health Organization. Scientific Publication 524, 1990.

PROGRAMA DE LAS NACIONES UNIDAS PARA EL DESARROLLO. *Desarrollo Humano. Informe de 1990.* Bogotá: Tercer Mundo Editores. Programa de las Naciones Unidas Para el Desarrollo, 1990.

QUINTERO-GONZALEZ, J. Cancer y precancer en fumadores con candela hacia adentro en el Departamento de Bolívar. *Revista de Ciencia, Tecnología y Educación* 6:39-60, Universidad de Cartagena, 1984.

QUINTERO-GONZALEZ, J. Registro de carcinoma escamocelular en los departamentos de Córdoba y Sucre. *Revista de Ciencias Tecnología y Educación* 7:75-80, Universidad de Cartagena, 1986.

QUINTERO-GONZALEZ, J. *Tabaquismo en la Costa Atlántica*. Cartagena: Universidad de Cartagena. Informe. Facultad de Odontología, October 1989.

QUINTERO-GONZALEZ, J., ALVAREZ, E. Carcinoma escamocelular de cavidad oral en el departamento de Antioquia 1960-1986. Trabajo presentado para ascender en el escalafón docente de la Universidad de Cartagena. Universidad de Cartagena, Facultad de Odontología, 1989.

REPUBLICA DE COLOMBIA. *Resolución 07559 de junio de 1984*, Ministerio de Salud, 1984.

REPUBLICA DE COLOMBIA. *Resolución 4063 de diciembre de 1982*. Ministerio de Comunicaciones, 1982.

RODRIGUEZ, R. Apuntes sobre la actividad tabacalera en Colombia. Segunda edición. Mimeo. Bogotá: Instituto Nacional de Fomento Tabacalero, 1960.

RODRIGUEZ, E., RONDEROS-TORRES, M. *El hábito de fumar en Colombia. 1977-1980.* Bogotá: Organización Pa-namericana de la Salud, Ministerio de Salud, I.N.S.-I.N.C., Editorial Gente Nueva, November 1988.

TOBACCO INTERNATIONAL. Colombia: Drug cash wash, smokes smuggling linked. *Tobacco International* 191(15), April 1989a.

TOBACCO INTERNATIONAL. Colombia: Cigarette smuggling tolerated. *Tobacco International*, Latin America Issue, June 1, 1989b.

TORRES, Y., MURRELLE, L. Estudio nacional sobre alcoholismo y consumo de sustancias que producen dependencia. Mimeo. Medellín: Universidad de Antioquía, 1989.

U.S. DEPARTMENT OF HEALTH AND HUMAN SERVICES. *The Health Consequences of Smoking—The Changing Cigarette. A Report of the Surgeon General.* U.S. Department of Health and Human Services, Public Health Service, Office on Smoking and Health. DHHS Publication No. (PHS) 81-50156, January 12, 1981.

VELAZQUEZ DE PABON, E., TORRES, Y., RAMIREZ, H., SANCHEZ, M., HERNANDEZ, N.E., REBAGE, L., BUSTAMANTE, L.M. Estudio epidemiológico del uso de sustancias que producen dependencia en la población general. Mimeo. Medellín: Corporación Colombiana Contra el Alcoholismo y la Farmacodependencia. Universidad de Antioquia. Facultad de Salud Pública, Hospital Mental de Antioquia, Servicio de Farmacodependencia. Universidad Pontificia Bolivariana. Hospital Universitario San Vicente de Paul. 1985.

WORLD HEALTH ORGANIZATION. *Cancer Incidence on Five Continents.* Lyon, France: International Agency for Research in Cancer. Scientific Publication 102, 1990.

Costa Rica

General Characteristics

The Tobacco Industry
    Agriculture
    Tobacco manufacturing and production
    Marketing
    Advertising and promotional activities
    Consumption

Tobacco Use
    Surveys and limitations
    Prevalence of smoking among adults
    Prevalence of smoking among adolescents
    Other uses of tobacco
    Attitudes, knowledge, and opinions about smoking

Smoking and Health
    Mortality indicators

Tobacco Use Prevention and Control Activities
    Government action
        Executive structure and policies
        Legislation
        School-based education
        Public information campaigns
        Cessation services
        Taxes
    Action by nongovernmental agencies

Summary and Conclusions

References

General Characteristics

Costa Rica occupies 51,000 km² on the Central American Isthmus, and is bordered by Panama, Nicaragua, and both the Pacific and Atlantic Oceans. The estimated 1990 mid-year population was more than 3 million (Centro Latinoamericano de Demografía) [CELADE] 1990) (Table 1), and the age structure has changed significantly in the last 20 years due to important changes in health status. These changes include declining fertility as well as improvement in infant mortality and overall mortality. The crude mortality rate decreased from 6.6/1,000 in 1970 to 3.8/1,000 in 1988, and the infant mortality rate decreased from 61.5 to 18 per 1,000 live births over the same period (PAHO 1990). These improving health indicators have resulted from the influence exercised by democratically elected Governments to realize the goals of a national health plan implemented in 1970.

The World Bank classifies Costa Rica as a middle-income economy, with a 1988 per capita gross national product of $US1,690. However, a substantial decline in the gross domestic product with increasing external debt, impoverishment, and unemployment was experienced in the early 1980s. Costa Rica is primarily an agricultural society, on which the economy is based; exports include coffee, fruits, and formerly, tobacco.

The democratic system of government also has the objective of health for all citizens. Because Costa Rica has not had a standing army for more than 40 years, more national resources have been available for health programs and social welfare. In the last few years, almost 200,000 refugees from other Central American countries have entered Costa Rica, presenting numerous health problems such as malnutrition and high infant mortality. Again, with the Government influence demonstrated in overcoming indigenous health problems, the condition of these persons has improved (PAHO 1990). Costa Rica is positioned uniquely to manage future health problems, including those caused by widespread tobacco use.

The Tobacco Industry

Agriculture

Tobacco has been grown by indigenous people in Costa Rica for almost 1,000 years (Arce et al. 1988). In 1988, 955 ha were planted with tobacco, representing 0.24 percent of Costa Rica's total arable land. The country's tobacco farms, averaging 1.4 ha, are owned by 689 small-scale producers and are located in four main regions (Pérez Zeledón, Alajuela, Parrita, and Puriscal). Costa Rica produces flue-cured, burley, and sun-cured tobaccos.

Farmers sell their harvests to one of the three processing companies that operate in Costa Rica. Tobacco sales involve the grower, the company buyer, and a representative of the Tobacco Defense Board, which supervises the relationship between growers and the companies. The Tobacco Defense Board is a Government agency set up by a 1956 law to defend growers' rights in pricing raw tobacco. Growers are thus protected against arbitrary pricing by manufacturing companies. In 1987, growers received a total of 311,000 million colons for 1,655 MT of raw tobacco (Personal Communication, Departamento Agropecuario del Banco Central, November 18, 1991).

Costa Rica has also a system called ACIOS, whereby the Central Bank subsidizes growers with up to 70 percent of the credit needed to cover production until harvesting is completed. When the harvest is sold, the Government withholds the amount of the loan, and growers receive the net profits. This system does not permit intermediaries to control market conditions because the growers themselves deliver the harvested crops directly to manufacturing companies. The companies, working through their Tobacco Institute, also provide

Table 1. Health and economic indicators, Costa Rica, 1980s

Indicator	Year	Value
Population	1990	3,014,596
Percent < 15	1988	36.4
Percent ≥ 65	1988	4.0
Percent urban	1988	45.0
Life expectancy at birth	1985–90	
Men		72.4
Women		77.0
Total fertility rate	1988	3.2
Infant mortality rate	1988	18.0
Per 1,000 live births		
Crude mortality rate	1988	3.8
Per 1,000 persons		
Percent literate	1985	94.0
Per capita gross		
National product	1988	$US1,690
Annual percent growth		
Rate of GNP	1980–88	2.6

Sources: CELADE, 1990; World Bank, 1990.

Table 2. Production, exports, imports, and total domestic consumption, Costa Rica, 1979 to 1989

Year	Tobacco leaf (in MT)			Total domestic cigarette consumption (in billions)
	Production	Imports	Exports	
1979	2,385	274	672	2.43
1980	2,082	121	210	2.26
1981	1,608	23	41	2.34
1982	1,630	25	100	2.00
1983	1,434	35	0	2.20
1984	1,864	0	0	2.30
1985	2,306	0	0	2.40
1986	1,912	0	0	2.20
1987	1,662	17	15	2.14
1988	1,590	18	0	2.14
1989	1,571	56	0	2.08

Sources: U.S. Department of Agriculture (USDA), 1990; Maxwell, 1990.

technical assistance to growers. Growers do not otherwise receive Government agricultural assistance.

In 1980, the British-American Tobacco (BAT) subsidiary in Costa Rica launched a soil conservation program (CORENA). The company receives funding for this project from the European Economic Community and Costa Rica's Ministry of Natural Resources, Energy, and Mines. Low-interest loans are granted to farmers, and technical assistance is provided by BAT. In the first 10 years of the program, the tobacco yield per ha increased 75 percent (Barquero 1990).

Tobacco production in Costa Rica declined from 2,385 MT in 1979 to a low of 1,434 MT in 1983 (Table 2). Production increased slightly thereafter, apparently because tobacco imports increased in 1984. Costa Rican tobacco is very expensive on the international market, and as a result, nearly 100 percent of domestic production is consumed in Costa Rica.

Tobacco Manufacturing and Production

Three tobacco companies operate in Costa Rica: Republic Tobacco Co., a BAT subsidiary that is 20 percent domestically held; Tabacalera Costarricense, a Philip Morris subsidiary that is 25 percent domestically held; and Tabacalera Cachí (TAC-ASA), owned by the domestic consortium of Bejos Yamuni, which produces dark tobacco. In 1987, these companies employed 477 persons, or 0.05 percent of the country's work force (Agro-economics 1987).

Marketing

Republic Tobacco Co. holds 72.5 percent of the market share, a level that has remained stable over the last 15 years. Tabacalera Costarricense holds 27 percent, and TACASA has less than 1 percent (Maxwell 1990). Approximately 73.1 percent of cigarettes are sold in soft, 20-cigarette packs. Cigarettes are also purchased individually, especially by persons with lower income. The sale of cigarettes to persons less than 18 years old is prohibited (Executive Decree 17,967-S, 1988). The average 1990 price of a pack of cigarettes was 70.75 colons; this was equivalent to 0.45 percent of the average industrial monthly wage in Costa Rica. Therefore, if the average employed resident of Costa Rica smoked one-half pack of cigarettes per day, he or she would expend approximately 7 percent of total monthly income on cigarettes.

Advertising and Promotional Activities

In Costa Rica, advertisements for tobacco products appear throughout the mass media; however, several restrictions on advertising have been enacted by executive decree of the Government. Since 1980, cigarette advertisements have been banned from the sports and children's sections of newspapers, from sports-oriented and children's magazines, and from radio and television at hours when the majority of the audience is children. The radio and television ban is in effect throughout the day on Sundays and holidays, and before 7:00 p.m. on weekdays except during news programs. In movie theaters, no tobacco product advertising is permitted before 5:00 p.m. Other restrictions on advertising include a ban on using minors or famous personalities, such as sports figures, in print or television advertisements; models who resemble either minors or famous personalities are also banned. All advertising material must be approved by the Ministry of Health (Executive Decree No. 12,069-SPPS, 1980).

A wide variety of promotional activities is permitted and used by the tobacco companies. For example, distribution of free samples, advertising at the point of sale, posters on public transportation, coupons, concerts, and donations to sports associations are common in Costa Rica. Donations are widely publicized in the mass media. Although advertising is not allowed at sports and cultural events per se, the tobacco companies circumvent the intent of the law by setting up independent agencies that bear cigarette brand names. These agencies then sponsor events such as concerts for young people and parallel activities associated with sports events.

Consumption

Total consumption of manufactured cigarettes remained stable in Costa Rica from 1979 to 1989 (Table 2). In 1989, domestic consumption reached more than 2 billion cigarettes (USDA 1989). However, Costa Rica has one of the lowest levels of apparent per capita consumption in the Americas; fewer than 1,000 cigarettes per year for persons aged 15 years and older (Allen 1989). Total per capita consumption by all ages declined from 992 cigarettes in 1980 to 707 cigarettes in 1989 (USDA 1990; PAHO 1990).

Tobacco Use

Surveys and Limitations

Between 1984 and 1987, four national surveys asked questions about smoking in Costa Rica (Table 3). Although three of these surveys used an unspecified definition of ''smoker,'' the estimated prevalences are similar. The 1988 Gallup survey, sponsored by the American Cancer Society, used the following standard definitions ''Have you ever used 100 cigarettes in your entire life?'' If yes, ''Do you now smoke cigarettes?'' The first question establishes the category ''ever smokers'' and the second, ''current smokers.'' Former smokers are ever smokers minus current smokers (Gallup 1988). The 1986 National Household Survey utilized a national cluster sampling technique (Vargas 1989); the sampling technique for the Gallup survey is unreported. The 1984–1985 survey by Rosero-Bixby and Oberle (1987) was derived from a control group for a case-control study of cervical and breast cancer in Costa Rica. Because the control group had been age-matched to cases, the results were adjusted to the age distribution of the total female population in Costa Rica. The National Survey on Fertility and Health (Costa Rican Demographic Association 1987) interviewed women of reproductive age (15 to 49 years old).

Prevalence of Smoking among Adults

The prevalence of current smoking among men reported by all the surveys is in the mid-30 percent range (Table 3). In 1986, the prevalence of smoking among men was reported to be 34.7 percent (Vargas 1989); the national drug use survey

Table 3. Surveys on tobacco use in Costa Rica, 1980s, and prevalence (percent) of current smoking by sex

Survey sponsor/author	Year	Sample	N	Prevalence	
				Men	Women
Salud de la Mujer (Rosero-Bixby)	1984–85	Control group for cancer study among women	870		14.0
Fecundidad y Salud (Martínez-Lanza)	1986	Women 15–49 years old	3,527		12.4
Household Survey (Vargas)	1986	National	35,000	34.7	14.4
Consumo de Drogas en Costa Rica (IAFA)	1987	National, ages 14–60	2,700	32.9	10.6
Incidence of smoking in Latin America (Gallup)	1988	General population	1,213	35.0	20.0

reported a prevalence of 32.9 percent in 1987; and the Gallup survey reported a prevalence of 35 percent in 1988. Thus, it is likely that the prevalence of smoking among men in Costa Rica is slightly higher than that among men in North America and substantially lower than that among men in South American countries.

The prevalence of smoking among women is reported reliably in several different sources. The prevalence of current smoking among women on the Rosero-Bixby survey was 14.0 percent, a level similar to that (14.4 percent) reported on the 1986 National Household Survey conducted 15 months later (Vargas 1989). The prevalence of smoking among pregnant women (8.1 percent) was less than among nonpregnant women (12.7 percent); the prevalence among women who used oral contraceptives (15.5 percent) was higher than among those who did not (11.4 percent) (Rosero-Bixby and Oberle 1987). Among women of reproductive age who responded to the National Fertility and Health Survey, the estimated prevalence of current smoking was 12.4 percent (Costa Rican Demographic Association 1987). The Gallup survey, which was probably based on an urban sample, reported a higher prevalence of smoking among women aged 18 and older (20.0 percent). The Institute on Alcoholism and Drug Dependency's 1987 national survey on drug use estimated the prevalence of smoking among women at only 10.6 percent (Martínez-Lanza and Alfaro-Murillo 1987). These surveys suggest that the prevalence of smoking among women in Costa Rica is relatively low compared with most countries of South or North America, and is substantially lower than that among Costa Rican men.

The national survey on drug use reported that 73 percent of both men and women who used illegal drugs also used tobacco, while only 19 percent of those who did not use illegal drugs used tobacco (PAHO Bulletin 1990).

Relevant differences in the prevalence of smoking by occupation, education, and socioeconomic status are reported by these surveys. The working population of both men and women had a much higher prevalence of smoking than did the nonworking population (Table 4) (Martínez-Lanza 1987). The prevalence of smoking was positively correlated with level of educational attainment among women: those with progressively higher educational attainment had higher prevalences of smoking (10.3 percent for women who completed primary school, 14.1 percent for those with some secondary education, and 18.8 percent for those

who completed secondary school or had postsecondary education (Costa Rican Demographic Association 1987). Men, however, show the opposite trend. The prevalence of smoking was 43.3 percent among men who did not complete primary school, 31.6 percent for men who completed primary school, 29.3 percent for those with secondary education, and 27.2 percent for those with postsecondary education (Madrigal and Sandí 1989). The 1988 Gallup survey reported a slightly higher prevalence of smoking for those with tertiary education (29 percent) compared to those with only primary education (26 percent) (Table 5).

No significant differences in smoking prevalence rates were reported based on family income levels in the 1986 Household Survey (Vargas 1989). The prevalence of smoking was 29.9 percent for

Table 4. Prevalence (percent) of current smoking by occupation, Costa Rica, 1986 to 1987

Occupation	Prevalence (both sexes)
Unemployed	10.2
Employed	31.2
Professionals	25.9
Technical workers	42.2
Administrators	31.1
Vendors	24.8
Skilled workers and operators	35.8
Semiskilled workers and operators	35.5
Unskilled workers and operators	31.8
Personal service workers	25.7

Source: Martínez-Lanza, 1987.

Table 5. Prevalence (percent) of current and former smoking, by sex and educational attainment, Costa Rica, 1988

Category	Current smoking	Former smoking	N
Sex			
Men	35	23	609
Women	20	10	604
Educational attainment			
Primary	26	19	592
Tertiary	29	14	196

Source: Gallup, 1988.

Table 6. Prevalence (percent) of current smoking by place of residence, Costa Rica, 1986 and 1987

Place of residence	Survey on drug use 1987		Survey on fertility and health 1986
	Men	Women	Women
Metropolitan San José	37.3	16.7	19.7
Other urban areas	34.3	9.8	12.9
Rural areas	30.4	7.7	6.7

Source: Martínez-Lanza, 1987

Table 7. Prevalence (percent) of smoking among adolescents in Metropolitan San José, by sex, age, type of educational institution, and smoking by family members, Costa Rica, 1984

Category	Prevalence
Total	12.7
Sex	
Men	17.0
Women	9.6
Age	
< 15 years	9.6
15 to 20 years	14.9
Type of educational institution	
Public schools	12.5
Private schools	20.0
Family smoking status	
No family members smoke	7.3
Sibling(s) smoke	10.3
Mother smokes	13.8
Father smokes	14.5
Both parents smoke	25.5

Source: Calderón, Castro, and Montero, 1984.

persons earning less than 10,000 colons per month and 29.5 percent for persons earning 10,000 colons per month or more. For female respondents to the National Fertility Survey, however, the prevalence of smoking was higher among high-income women (18.6 percent) than among low- and middle-income women (10.1 percent) (Costa Rican Demographic Association 1987).

According to both the National Drug Use Survey and the National Fertility and Health Survey, the prevalence of smoking is higher among urban populations than among rural populations, particularly among women (Table 6). Presumably, urban women in Costa Rica are more educated and have higher educational attainment than their rural counterparts, and thus, the prevalence of smoking would be expected to be higher in urban populations.

Among male respondents to the National Drug Use Survey, the prevalence of smoking increased with age until 35 years, after which it decreased (Madrigal and Sandí 1989). Younger Costa Rican women (aged 20 to 35) in this survey had a prevalence of smoking substantially higher than older women (aged 40 to 55) (approximately 15 vs. 8 percent).

Of significance is the low number of cigarettes smoked daily among both men and women in Costa Rica (Arce et al. 1988). On both the 1986 Household Survey and the 1988 Gallup survey, most smokers smoked fewer than 10 cigarettes per day (61 percent and 53 percent of smokers, respectively). Few respondents to these surveys smoked more than 20 cigarettes per day (9 percent and 25 percent, respectively). Such low exposure will have beneficial effects on the mortality patterns for chronic diseases associated with smoking.

Prevalence of Smoking among Adolescents

Few data are available on smoking among adolescents in Costa Rica. Secondary schools in the Greater San José area were surveyed in 1984 (Calderón, Castro, and Montero 1984) (Table 7). The prevalence of smoking was higher at private schools compared with public schools (20.0 vs. 12.5 percent). This survey also reported that children from families with smokers are more likely to be smokers themselves, particularly if both parents smoke.

Other Uses of Tobacco

No data were available on the use of other forms of tobacco. Based on tobacco sales data, however, consumption of other forms of tobacco appears to be low because dark tobacco, used in cigars and perhaps hand-rolled cigarettes, accounts for less than 0.1 percent of the market (Maxwell 1990).

Attitudes, Knowledge, and Opinions about Smoking

Data on knowledge and opinions about smoking are available only for students in the San José area for 1984 (Calderón et al. 1984). No differences in knowledge about the health consequences of tobacco were reported between students in public and private schools. All students associated cigarette smoking mainly with respiratory symptoms or diseases. Only 16.6 percent associated smoking with myocardial infarctions, while 97.7 percent associated smoking with lung cancer, and 64.9 percent with bronchitis and emphysema. Based on a multipoint scale of knowledge on the health consequences of smoking, 19.4 percent of smokers and 19.3 percent of nonsmokers were classified as having a low level of knowledge; 9.7 percent of smokers and 15.8 percent of nonsmokers had a high level of knowledge.

Smoking and Health

Mortality Indicators

In Costa Rica, the number of deaths attributed to "symptoms, signs, and ill-defined conditions" (ICD 780–799) is low (2.9 percent of total deaths for men and 3.3 percent for women). Since the cause of death is reported for virtually all deaths among persons aged 15 and older, mortality data may be very reliable in assessing the disease impact of tobacco in Costa Rica.

Since 1970, the principal causes of death among adults in Costa Rica have been chronic non communicable diseases (PAHO 1990). Heart disease has been the leading cause of death, with malignant neoplasms ranking second. The mortality rate for the category "symptoms, signs, and ill-defined conditions" decreased substantially from 1980 to 1988. This decrease suggests that the assignation of cause of death has improved in the last decade. The rates for five other common causes of death were stable during these years, but ischemic heart disease and stomach cancer mortality rates may have increased slightly.

Examining both age-adjusted and age-specific rates of death for selected chronic diseases by sex for persons aged 35 years and older helps to elucidate the possible disease impact of smoking. The age-adjusted mortality rates for cardiovascular diseases (including ischemic heart disease and cerebrovascular disease) in 1983 and 1988 demonstrate a decrease in the rate among women but an increase among men (Table 8). The age-adjusted mortality rates for lip, oral cavity, and pharynx increased slightly, while trachea, bronchus, and lung

cancer mortality was essentially unchanged during this period. However, the mortality rates for cancer of the trachea, bronchi, and lungs increased among men aged 65 and older (not shown), and the mortality rate for this cancer decreased among men aged 35 to 64 years. When 5-year mortality rates are reviewed for lung cancer among men aged 45 to 64, a significant increase was observed in the age groups 45 to 54 and 55 to 64 years old between 1970 and 1974 and 1980 and 1984; after 1984, mortality rates for lung cancer decreased somewhat (Table 9). In Costa Rica, lung cancer is more frequent in urban areas, with an urban-rural ratio of 1.9 for men and 1.8 for women (Sierra et al. 1988).

These data suggest that the disease impact of smoking among women is low, and that among younger cohorts of men, the impact may be decreasing. Lung cancer is a marker for the population impact of smoking. Because smoking prevalence among Costa Rican women is quite low, and because the number of cigarettes smoked per day by both men and women is low, the mortality rates for this marker disease are low and, in younger groups, decreasing. This decrease may indicate that the economic pressures and the antismoking campaigns of the 1970s and 1980s in Costa Rica have produced some positive results. The mortality rates for cardiovascular diseases are also decreasing, further supporting this conclusion. Urban-rural differences in lung cancer mortality confirm that the exposure to tobacco of men and particularly women in urban areas is higher than that in rural areas.

Tobacco Use Prevention and Control Activities

Government Action

Executive structure and policies

The Ministry of Health has been responsible for defining policies related to tobacco use prevention and control. The Chronic Diseases Department receives support from the Department of Legal Affairs and the Department of Health Education in setting tobacco-related policies (Arce 1988). The Department of Preventive Medicine at the Caja Costarricense del Seguro Social (CCSS) implements preventive public health actions in general and, accordingly, has sponsored educational campaigns and programs to help Costa Ricans stop smoking.

Table 8. Mortality rates (per 100,000 persons) for selected diseases associated with smoking by sex and age group, Costa Rica, 1983 and 1988

| Cause of death (ICD-9 code) | Year | Age-adjusted rate | Age group-specific rates Age group | | |
			35–44	45–54	55–64
Ischemic heart disease (410–414)					
Men	1983	63.4	17.4	65.9	203.6
	1988	71.1	20.8	73.0	215.1
Women	1983	44.8	4.1	39.0	114.3
	1988	38.6	5.6	19.8	71.3
Cerebrovascular disease (430–438)					
Men	1983	27.8	3.3	26.8	69.1
	1988	30.3	6.2	24.0	76.8
Women	1983	28.0	9.9	22.0	57.1
	1988	25.1	7.0	21.9	80.2
Malignancy of the lip, oral cavity, and pharynx (140–149)					
Men	1983	1.3	0.8	—	1.8
	1988	1.8	1.4	1.0	7.7
Women	1983	0.7	—	—	1.8
	1988	0.8	—	—	1.5
Malignancy of the trachea, bronchus, and lung (162)					
Men	1983	9.1	2.5	15.9	50.9
	1988	10.2	1.4	8.3	41.5
Women	1983	3.0	—	6.1	14.3
	1988	2.9	1.4	2.1	14.9

Source: PAHO, 1986 and 1990.
Note: Age-adjusted rates are adjusted according to the age structure of the entire population of Latin America.

The Institute on Alcoholism and Drug Dependency (IAFA), a research and clinical-care institution, is a State agency under the Ministry of Health; it has

Table 9. Five-year lung cancer mortality rates among men (per 100,000), Costa Rica, 1970 to 1989

| Period | Age group | |
	45–54	55–64
1970–74	10.9	27.0
1975–79	11.2	44.6
1980–84	12.9	48.9
1985–89	10.6	44.6

Source: Dirección General de Estadística y Censos, Costa Rica, 1990.

incorporated tobacco-related issues into its research agenda, and also has sponsored smoking cessation programs. Although various Governmental and nongovernmental institutions are active in tobacco-use prevention and control in Costa Rica, no systematic national tobacco control program has been established yet. The Ministry of Health has no program on tobacco per se, but it collaborates in activities organized by nongovernmental agencies and by the CCSS.

Legislation

Most antitobacco activities have been legislative, mainly in the form of executive decrees by the Executive Branch of the Government. Although draft legislation to ban cigarette advertising repeatedly has been submitted to the Legislative Assembly, none of the bills has been passed into law.

Since 1980, all cigarette advertising and promotional activities must be approved by the Ministry of Health (Executive Decree 11,016-SPPS, 1980). Advertising is required to be objective and factual; commercials may not be broadcast during programs for children and young people, and all commercials must be approved by the Ministry of Health (Executive Decree 12,069-SPPS, 1980). A council has been established to monitor cigarette advertising; its organization was modified in 1986 (Decree 12,323-S, 1986) to include a member of the National Council on Cancer in addition to officials from the Ministry of Health.

Exposure to environmental tobacco smoke (ETS) also has been addressed by the Ministry of Health. Between 1987 and 1988, a series of decrees aimed at protecting the health of nonsmokers was issued. For example, civil servants are not allowed to smoke at work (Decree 17,398-S-J, 1987) and smoking is prohibited in cinemas and theaters (Decree 17,694-S, 1987). These decrees were later expanded (Decrees 18,216-TSS, 1988 and 18,771-S-J, 1989) to include the mandatory display of signs in visible locations, the provision of special smoking areas, and penalties for noncompliance. Smoking is also prohibited on public transportation (Decree 18,248-MOPT-S, 1988). In February 1988, it was declared that April 7 would be "Smoke-Free Day" in Costa Rica (Decree 17,969, 1988).

Packages of cigarettes manufactured in Costa Rica must bear one of the following warnings: "Smoking during pregnancy is harmful to the fetus and may provoke premature birth" or "Smoking causes lung cancer, heart disease, and emphysema" (Decree 18,780-S, 1989).

The sale of cigarettes to minors (younger than age 18 years) is prohibited (Decree 17,967-S, 1988), as is the sale of cigarettes on public transport (Decree 18,340-S-MOPT, 1988), although penalties for infringement of this ruling are not specified. Thus, as in other countries of the Americas, enforcement of laws that restrict minors' access to tobacco is probably negligible.

School-based education

During the recent revision of the primary and secondary school curricula in Costa Rica, specific segments on the effects of smoking were included. The CCSS distributes tobacco-related educational material at schools. References to smoking have been eliminated from textbooks, and content material on the health consequences of smoking has been prepared for inclusion in science textbooks. Each year, the CCSS spends approximately 1.6 million colons on school-based educational activities and public information campaigns in general.

Public information campaigns

Flyers, decals, and posters describing the harmful effects of smoking are distributed widely by the CCSS at clinics, hospitals, and to the general public. The CCSS has also produced television commercials to counter those produced by the tobacco companies, spending about 1.5 million colons each month on this activity alone. An effort also has been made by the CCSS to train journalists on health topics, including smoking.

Cessation services

The CCSS and the IAFA have offered sporadic group programs to help people stop smoking. During the initial stage of the CCSS program, 10 people were trained to lead groups. The effect of these interventions has not been evaluated.

Taxes

Five percent of Costa Rica's tax revenue is derived from the sale of tobacco products. About 75 percent of the retail sales price of a pack of 20 cigarettes is tax; 65 percent is excise tax, and 10 percent is sales tax. The sales tax is the same ad valorem tax as on other consumer goods in Costa Rica. Taxes have not been used for controlling tobacco use but rather for revenue generation.

Action by Nongovernmental Agencies

The National Anti-Tobacco Association has organized educational workshops for secondary school students. These have enjoyed support from the Ministries of Education, Health and Culture, Youth, and Sports. However, the Association does not have a guaranteed source of funding, and therefore it depends primarily on the labor of volunteers.

The Consumer Defense Committee has expanded its objectives to include the banning of all tobacco product advertising and promotion. To this end, it has lobbied for restrictive legislation, but this bill has been rejected twice in the Legislative Assembly as of 1990. The committee also has produced an antitobacco educational program on a religious radio station, and it participates in infrequent debates on tobacco-related issues.

Summary and Conclusions

In Costa Rica, tobacco is grown by small-scale farmers who are linked closely to the manufacturing industry. The Government plays an intermediary role in the sale of leaf tobacco and in the farmers' access to credit. Virtually all tobacco produced in Costa Rica is consumed internally; approximately 2.2 billion cigarettes are produced and consumed each year.

According to tobacco use surveys in the mid-1980s, the prevalence of smoking among men ranges between 32.9 and 35.0 percent and between 10.6 and 14.4 percent for women. The prevalence of smoking is higher in urban areas and among employed persons. Women with higher levels of education and income have a higher prevalence of smoking than those with less education and income. Although the prevalence of smoking among pregnant women is less than among nonpregnant women, women who use oral contraceptives have a higher smoking prevalence than those who do not. The prevalence of smoking among male adolescents was higher than among female adolescents in 1984, and the overall rate was 12.7 percent. Significantly, adolescent smoking is more common in families with smokers than in those without smokers. Among both men and women, the exposure to cigarettes is low, both in terms of prevalence and in number of cigarettes smoked per day. This exposure limitation has important implications in disease outcome as well as in the level of addiction of Costa Rican smokers. Low levels of cigarettes smoked per day may permit cessation more readily. Data are lacking that monitor public beliefs about the health consequences of smoking and on attitudes toward smoking-related policies. Data such as these can be useful in helping the Ministry of Health to advise the Government on tobacco-related policies. Data such as those reported above, especially on the use of tobacco by women, need to be communicated to the public in order to mobilize national opinions and control programs.

With regard to smoking-related diseases, the mortality rate for cardiovascular diseases has increased slightly in men but not in women. The lung cancer mortality rate increased among men aged 55 to 64 in the 1970s, but has remained stable since then. This neoplasm is more frequent in urban areas where smoking prevalence rates are higher, particularly among women. Thus, the impact of smoking on the chronic disease burden in Costa Rica is limited. Because the Government of Costa Rica has demonstrated a determination to bring good health to all of its residents, prevention of these diseases may be addressed. Cardiovascular and neoplastic diseases are the main causes of death in Costa Rica, and a substantial portion of this mortality can be prevented through the prevention and control of tobacco use.

Several health-related agencies and organizations participate in a variety of antitobacco activities in Costa Rica. At present, however, these are neither systematic nor coordinated. A series of executive decrees aimed at regulating advertising, banning smoking in public places, and requiring health warnings on cigarette packs has been executed through Ministry of Health initiatives. In addition, the sale of cigarettes to minors is prohibited. Public information campaigns and nongovernmental group activities to prevent and control smoking are evident but infrequent. Thus, an infrastructure is in place that can prevent young persons from beginning to smoke and assist adults in establishing their intention to quit.

Based on the data presented in this chapter, the following conclusions can be made:
1. Tobacco agriculture and businesses receive Government support, in particular for price supports and loans to farmers. To control tobacco use in Costa Rica, alternative crops and nontobacco agricultural activities must be embraced.
2. Despite some Government control over tobacco product advertising and promotion, there is widespread use of many different media and promotional devices to encourage young persons to smoke. Comprehensive legislation to control such advertising has been defeated repeatedly in the legislature; a complete ban on all tobacco advertising and promotion would support ongoing efforts by the Caja Costarricense del Seguro Social and Ministry of Health to prevent tobacco use by young Costa Ricans.
3. The exposure of the Costa Rican population to tobacco is relatively low by world standards, and thus the disease impact of tobacco has been limited. Prevention of chronic diseases, espe-

cially lung cancer and cardiovascular diseases caused by smoking, is possible in this setting. The most important causes of death among adult Costa Ricans are chronic and degenerative diseases. Tobacco prevention and control will need to be prioritized to overcome the future burden of these diseases.

4. The prevalence of smoking is higher among women with higher levels of education and better socioeconomic standing. As urbanization and education levels have increased, health risk behavior also seems to have increased. The positive correlation between education, income, and higher smoking rates does not appear as evident among men. Public education and information activities should address this situation.

5. Data collection and reporting on the public's tobacco use, knowledge, and attitudes are important components of the public health effort to control tobacco, and these components need to be strengthened in Costa Rica.

6. Smoking control actions have depended on Government decrees, and these may lack enforcement provisions, especially in the area of restrictions on sales to minors. These decrees will be more effective if enacted within a focused comprehensive tobacco prevention and control program that includes school-based education, public information campaigns, restrictions on tobacco advertising, and data collection and reporting.

References

ALLEN, T. Global per capita consumption of manufactured cigarettes-1987. *Chronic Diseases in Canada* 10(3):51–52, May 1989.

ARCE, R.C., ORTIZ, C., ZUÑIGA, N. *Informe sobre la situación de tabaquismo en Costa Rica, Ministerio de Salud, Costa Rica*. In PAHO, Preliminary Report on Taller Subregional para MesoAmérica, Ciudad de Guatemala, October 1988.

ASOCIACION DEMOGRAFICA COSTARRICENSE. *Encuesta Nacional de Fecundidad y Salud: Costa Rica, 1986*. San Jose, Costa Rica,1987.

BARQUERO, M. Alerta para salvar suelos. *La Nación, Suplemento Agropecuario* January 9, 1990, pp. C,1.

CALDERON, M.E., CASTRO, V.M., MONTERO, J.P. *Conocimientos, opiniones y prácticas relacionadas con el hábito de fumar*. Tésis. Facultad de Educación, Universidad de Costa Rica, 1984.

CENTRO LATINOAMERICANO DE DEMOGRAFIA.

Boletín Demográfico. Santiago: CELADE, año XXIII, No. 45, 1990.

DECRETO EJECUTIVO. No. 11016-SPPS. La Gaceta No. 3, January 4, 1980.

DECRETO EJECUTIVO. No. 12069-SPPS. La Gaceta No. 234, December 5, 1980.

DECRETO EJECUTIVO. No. 17323-S. La Gaceta No. 231, December 4, 1986.

DECRETO EJECUTIVO. No. 17393-S-J. La Gaceta No. 26, February 6, 1987.

DECRETO EJECUTIVO. No. 17694-S. La Gaceta No. 167, October 4, 1987.

DECRETO EJECUTIVO. No. 17967-S. La Gaceta No. 39, February 25, 1988.

DECRETO EJECUTIVO. No. 17969-S. La Gaceta No. 39, February 25, 1988.

DECRETO EJECUTIVO. No. 18216-TSS. La Gaceta No. 131, July 11, 1988.

DECRETO EJECUTIVO. No. 18248-MOPT-S. La Gaceta No. 139, July 21, 1988.

DECRETO EJECUTIVO. No. 18340-MOPT-S. La Gaceta No. 149, August 8, 1988.

DECRETO EJECUTIVO. No. 18771-S-J. La Gaceta No. 26, February 6, 1989.

DECRETO EJECUTIVO. No. 18780-S. La Gaceta No. 26, February 6, 1989.

MADRIGAL, J., SANDI, L.E. *Una medición estadística del hábito de fumar en Costa Rica* (en consideración para publicación), 1989.

MARTINEZ-LANZA, P., ALFARO-MURILLO, E. *Prevalencia del consumo de drogas en Costa Rica*. Instituto sobre Alcoholismo y Farmacodependencia, San José, Costa Rica, 1987.

PAN AMERICAN HEALTH ORGANIZATION. *Bulletin of PAHO*. Special Report—Epidemiologic report on the use and abuse of psychoactive substances in 16 countries of Latin America and the Caribbean. *Bulletin of PAHO* 24(1):97–143, 1990.

PAN AMERICAN HEALTH ORGANIZATION. *Health Conditions in the Americas, 1981–1984*. Washington D.C.: Pan American Health Organization, Scientific Publication No. 500, 1986.

PAN AMERICAN HEALTH ORGANIZATION. *Health Conditions in the Americas, 1990 Edition*. Washington D.C.: Pan American Health Organization, Scientific Publication No. 524, 1990.

ROSERO-BIXBY, L., OBERLE, M.W. Tabaquismo en la mujer costarricense, 1984–85. *Revista de Ciencias Sociales* (35):95–102, 1987.

SIERRA, R., PARKIN, D.M., BARRANTES, R., BIEBER, C.A., MUÑOZ-LEIVA, G., MUÑOZ-CALERO, N. *Cancer in Costa Rica*. International Agency for Research on Cancer, World Health Organization, and University of Costa Rica, IARC Technical Report No. 1, 1988.

THE MAXWELL CONSUMER REPORT. *International Tobacco 1989—Part One*. Wheat First Securities/Butcher and Singer, May 18, 1990.

UNITED STATES DEPARTMENT OF AGRICULTURE. Tobacco, Cotton and Seeds Division, Foreign Agricultural Service (unpublished tabulations), April 1990.

VARGAS, H. Prevalencia de fumado en Costa Rica. *Prevención* 2(9):1–5, March 20, 1989.

WORLD BANK, *World Development Report 1989*. New York: Oxford University Press, 1989.

WORLD BANK, *World Development Report 1990—Poverty*. New York: Oxford University Press, 1990.

Cuba

General Characteristics

The Tobacco Industry
Agriculture
Manufacturing and export
Marketing

Tobacco Use
Prevalence of smoking among adults
Prevalence of smoking among adolescents
Other tobacco consumption
Attitudes, knowledge, and opinions about smoking

Tobacco Use and Health

Tobacco Use Prevention and Control Activities
Executive structure and policies
Legislation
School-based education
Public information campaigns

Summary and Conclusions

References

General Characteristics

Cuba forms an archipelago in the Caribbean Sea at the entrance to the Gulf of Mexico. Its area of 111,000 km² is home to 10 million inhabitants—a population possessing some of the most favorable health indicators in the Americas. Between 1985 and 1988 infant mortality decreased from 16.5 to 11.9 per 1,000 live births. During the period from 1980 to 1990, total fertility declined from 4.4 to 1.83 and life expectancy at birth increased from 67 to 75 years (Table 1). Health and social services are among the most widely available in the Americas, with one physician for every 333 residents. Cuba's literacy rate is nearly 100 percent (Pan American Health Organization [PAHO] 1990).

Like other countries in the Americas, Cuba has suffered the effects of the economic crisis of the 1980s, with hard currency reserves and personal income declining in recent years. Cuban agricultural products, including tobacco, have found fewer markets as a result of the political changes experienced by the nation's chief trading partners, the former Soviet Union and the countries of Eastern Europe. Cuba traditionally has been one of the major producers and exporters of tobacco in Latin America. As one of the country's primary crops, tobacco imbues the national cultural heritage, and themes about its cultivation and use pervade Cuba's music, folklore, and other traditions (Suárez-Lugo 1988). At the same time, however,

Cuba has recognized the health consequences of the nation's high per capita consumption of tobacco and has embarked on an extensive control program that is backed strongly by its national leadership and makes use of its well-organized health system. The program includes appropriate disease surveillance and monitoring of the population's lifestyle and consumption habits.

The Tobacco Industry

Agriculture

Cuba is the second largest producer of tobacco in Latin America, after Brazil. Tobacco is one of the country's traditional crops and formerly ranked among its chief economic assets, exceeded only by sugar as a source of foreign exchange. Today tobacco production continues to be an important factor in the Cuban economy. Production has fluctuated over the years, with variations caused by adverse climatic conditions, pests, and diseases; for example, blue mold was a problem in 1980.

The cooperative and rural sectors account for 78 percent of all tobacco growing in Cuba, while 22 percent remains in the hands of the State. In 1988 a total of 56,700 ha, or the equivalent of 1.6 percent of Cuba's total agricultural land area, were planted in tobacco (Varona-Pérez 1990). Fifteen thousand persons were engaged in tobacco growing, representing 3.1 percent of all workers in the agricultural sector (Chapman 1990). Approximately 40,000 MT of dried leaf tobacco have been produced annually since 1983.

Manufacturing and Export

Tobacco manufacturing is concentrated in rural tobacco-growing areas, and is largely a manual process. There are 97 factories for processing tobacco and 6 for making cigarettes; all belong to 23 companies which together form the Unión de Empresas del Tabaco (consortium of tobacco companies). Most of the production is for domestic consumption, especially in the case of cigarettes, as opposed to other tobacco products such as cigars.

However, the overall outlook for tobacco production will depend on domestic and foreign markets, where consumption has been declining since 1985. Although the quantity of actual exports of leaf tobacco and cigarettes was lower during this last decade, the value of these exports showed an increase because of prices abroad. Cuba earns about $US90 million annually from exports, which indi-

Table 1. Health and economic indicators, Cuba, 1980–1990

Indicator	Value
Population (1990)[a]	10,608,303
Life expectancy at birth (men) (1985–90)[a]	73.48
Life expectancy at birth (women) (1985–90)[a]	77.01
Total fertility rate (1985–90)[a]	1.83
Infant mortality rate (1985–90)[a]	15.24
Literacy rate (1985)[b]	96.00%
Annual growth rate as per capita of GNP (1965–80)[b]	0.6 %
Per capita GNP (1987)[c]	N/R

Sources:

[a]Latin American Demography Center, 1990.

[b]United Nations Development Program (UNDP), 1990.

[c]This information has not been reported to any of the UN agencies nor to the World Bank. This applies to the annual growth rate of GNP per capita from 1980 on.

cates that tobacco production still constitutes a major component in the national economy.

Marketing

Since 1960, all advertising of consumer products, including tobacco, has been banned, and since 1970, cigarette packs have been imprinted with the warning FUMAR DAÑA SU SALUD [SMOKING IS HAZARDOUS TO YOUR HEALTH] (Varona-Pérez 1990). The Ministry of Agriculture has an agency responsible for analyzing the chemical composition of all brands and types of cigarettes. The tar content of unfiltered dark-tobacco cigarettes—the kind most popular in Cuba—is greater than for any other kind of cigarette, which adds to the potential hazard of smoking as a risk to health.

Tobacco is marketed in Cuba in two ways: on the rationed market, where the prices are kept low, and on the open market, where prices are high. Cigarettes are dispensed in packs of 20. Loose cigarettes have been sold only in the Province of Matanzas, and this practice was eliminated at the end of 1990. It is forbidden to sell cigarettes to minors under the age of 16, in health centers and educational institutions, and in recreational centers for children and young people.

Under the rationing program, since 1971, individuals born before January 1, 1956, have been allowed four packs of cigarettes per month at a price of 30 cents. On the open market, prices are high, and thus consumption is discouraged, principally among young people. The cigarettes cost 1.80 pesos and the tabaco negro cigarettes between 1.60 and 2.0 pesos per pack. From 1973 to 1990 the average official price increased by approximately 30 percent, which is consistent with the strategy of using price to regulate consumption. In 1989 the average monthly wage in Cuba was 188 pesos, and statistics provided by the Instituto Cubano de Investigaciones y Orientación de la Demanda Interna (Cuban Institute for Research and Guidance on Internal Demand—ICIODI) show that expenditures on cigarettes and tobacco in the last decade have ranged between 8 and 12 percent of the monthly wage (Varona-Pérez 1990).

Tobacco Use

From 1959 until 1970, cigarettes and other tobacco products were sold at low prices on a totally open market and were distributed gratis to specific sectors (e.g., sugar cane-cutters), as a result of which consumption steadily increased, peaking in 1967–1968.

The rationing of tobacco products was instituted in 1971 in order to keep prices down and guarantee quotas. This rationing, which is still being imposed, has had the effect of discouraging consumption. In August 1972, the open sale of these products was reintroduced, but at prices ranging from 1.60 to 2.00 pesos per pack for dark cigarettes, 2.40 pesos for light cigarettes, and 0.68 pesos for a cigar. At the same time the quotas were maintained. Marketing at these prices led to a substantial rise in the average price of cigarettes and cigars, amounting to yet another measure which helped to discourage consumption.

After the initial impact of the open sale of cigarettes and cigars at the higher prices, by 1985, the total per capita consumption had stabilized at approximately 2,500 to 2,800 cigarettes per year with a slightly declining trend (Table 2). Starting that year, when the campaign to discourage tobacco use got underway, consumption began to decline more sharply, falling to levels below the range just indicated.

Prevalence of Smoking among Adults

The first national survey on the prevalence of smoking was carried out by the Ministry of the Interior in 1978. In 1980, 1984, and 1988, the ICIODI—the specialized agency responsible for studying the consumption habits of the population—conducted national surveys using representative sampling techniques. In all these surveys the ''current smoker'' was defined as a person who was smoking on a daily basis at the time the survey was carried out. A common definition across surveys and the use of the same sampling frame allow for

Table 2. Cigarette consumption per capita, Cuba, 1974–1989

Period	Annual consumption per capita (15+ years)	Percent decrease
1974–1975	2,694	36.1[a]
1976–1980	2,660	1.3
1981–1985	2,620	1.5
1986–1988	2,315	11.6
1989	2,247	46.7[a]

Source: ICIODI.

[a]Estimated with reference to 1970.

reliable comparisons of prevalence in this longer period.

In 1989, a national survey conducted on the consumption of alcoholic beverages also yielded data on the prevalence of smoking. A new national survey was conducted in 1990, but its results had not been fully processed when information was requested for the present report.

In 1980, Cuba had a total of 3,192,203 smokers over the age of 17, which yields a prevalence of 52.9 percent of the population in that age group. By 1988 this prevalence had declined to 40.1 percent, and in 1989 it fell to 37.4 percent. This means that during the decade from 1980 to 1990, despite a growth in population, Cuba saw a decline of 15.5 percent in the prevalence of smoking, or an annual average decline of 1.5 percent (Table 3).

In 1988 the prevalence of smoking in the population aged 17 or over was 53.7 percent in men and 28.3 percent in women (Table 4).

Prevalence was higher in the 30–39 and 40–49 age groups, and slightly higher in rural areas than in cities (42.1 vs. 39.3 percent, respectively) (Figure 1).

Although there are no major differences in prevalence according to educational level, it can be

Table 3. Prevalence (%) of smoking among adults aged 17 and older, Cuba, 1980–1989

Year	Total population[a]	Smokers[b]	% of smokers in total population
1980	6,034,411	3,192,203	52.9
1984	6,647,307	2,805,164	42.2
1988	7,173,712	2,876,659	40.1
1989	7,529,025	2,819,318	37.4

Sources:
[a]Anuarios Estadísticos de Cuba.
[b]Encuestas Nacionales, ICIODI.

Table 4. Prevalence (%) of smoking among adults aged 17 and older, by sex, Cuba, 1988

	Males	Females
Smokers*	53.7	28.3
Nonsmokers	46.3	71.7

Source: Encuesta Nacional 1988, ICIODI.
*Includes former smokers.

Figure 1. Prevalence (%) of smoking, by place of residence, Cuba, 1978–1988

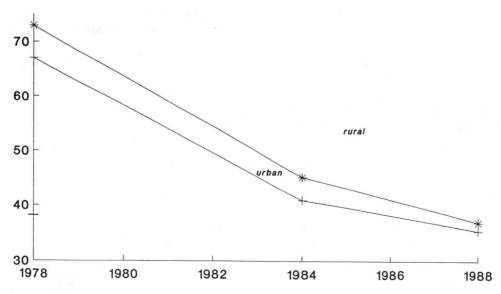

Source: ICIODI 1978, 1988a.

seen that a larger percentage of smokers is found among the population with the least amount of schooling (Table 5).

In terms of occupation, prevalence is highest among agricultural and industrial workers, with larger numbers of smokers being found in rural areas. Next in order are service workers, administrators, retirees, and administrative and clerical personnel. Prevalence is high among physicians: 3 out of every 10 are smokers (Table 6).

Prevalence is higher in the provinces where tobacco is grown: Sancti Spíritus, Cienfuegos, and Pinar del Río, and the rates among women are highest in the city of Havana. The first phenomenon corresponds to a cultural tradition and the second to greater incorporation of women into the work force.

Based on these data, it appears that both the adult prevalence and the total consumption of tobacco have shown a declining trend in recent years.

Prevalence of Smoking among Adolescents

According to a survey conducted in 1988, 95 percent of the smokers in Cuba began to smoke before the age of 30, and of these, 58.5 percent started between the ages of 13 and 16 (Varona-Pérez 1990).

Because these findings were very similar to those derived from previous surveys, the information obtained in households was compared with that elicited from adolescents interviewed outside the home setting. Thus, a national survey conducted among 1,847 students aged 13 to 17 years using a self-administered questionnaire (ICIODI

1988) revealed a prevalence of tobacco use of 5.7 percent (8.1 percent for males and 2.9 percent for females). In a 1988 household survey, the responses of adults speaking on behalf of their adolescent children indicated a prevalence of only 2.8 percent for males and 0.6 percent for females. Obviously the parents of these adolescents underestimated the extent to which their children were smoking.

Other Tobacco Consumption

Most tobacco in Cuba is consumed in the form of cigarettes. In 1988, only 8.5 percent of smokers aged 17 or over smoked cigars, 1.8 percent smoked both cigarettes and cigars, and 1 percent of the population reported that they used other types of tobacco, i.e., smoked a pipe or chewed tobacco (Varona-Pérez 1990). Cigar smoking accounts for 15.4 percent of the tobacco consumed in Cuba, and chewing tobacco accounts for only 0.5 percent.

Attitudes, Knowledge, and Opinions about Smoking

Because tobacco prevention and control activities had begun in the late 1980s, the 1988 ICIODI survey asked questions about knowledge and atti-

Table 5. Prevalence (%) of smoking among adults aged 17 or older by educational attainment, Cuba, 1988

	Smokers	Nonsmokers
Did not finish primary education	47.1	52.9
Primary school	40.5	59.5
Secondary school	39.2	60.8
Post-secondary	33.1	66.9
University	36.8	63.2

Source: Encuesta Nacional 1988, ICIODI.

Table 6. Prevalence (%) of smoking among adults aged 17 or older by occupation, Cuba, 1988

Occupation	Smokers	Nonsmokers
Agricultural and industrial worker	54.0	46.0
Service worker	49.6	50.4
Administrator	48.9	51.1
Retiree	46.0	54.0
Administrative and clerical personnel	43.7	56.3
Other professionals	36.2	63.8
Physician	33.9	66.1
Teacher	29.6	70.4
Housewife	27.2	72.8
Student	7.8	92.2

Source: Encuesta Nacional 1988, ICIODI.

tudes about smoking. Of the total population, 97 percent considered themselves "well informed" about the hazards of smoking, and smokers and nonsmokers did not differ in their response to this question. Ninety percent of respondents had received smoking-related information from television, 80 percent from the radio, and 61 percent from the print media (ICIODI 1988). The respondents were in agreement with policies that restrict smoking in public places, and almost all (98 percent) supported the newly legislated bans on smoking in enclosed spaces. At the same time, however, most of them (76 percent) also felt that the regulations were not strict enough to make an impact on smoking behavior, given the fact that there is widespread noncompliance (ICIODI 1988).

Smoking and Health

Cuba's statistics on mortality are among the most accurate in the Americas. In 1988, underreporting was estimated to be only 1.5 percent, and only 0.2 percent of all deaths were classified as "symptoms and ill-defined conditions" (PAHO 1990).

Noncommunicable diseases are the leading cause of death in Cuba in the 15 to 49 and 50 to 64 age groups. Cardiovascular diseases and cancer rank first and second, respectively, in the population aged 50 to 64. The most frequent cause of cancer death in Cuba is lung cancer (an overall age-adjusted rate of 16.2/100,000 population in 1988), with a higher rate for men (23.5/100,000) than for women (8.7/100,000) (PAHO 1990). Among the countries of the Americas, Cuba's age-adjusted mortality rate for lung cancer is surpassed only in the United States and Canada. During the period from 1980 to 1988, age-adjusted mortality for lung cancer increased slightly but not significantly.

In Cuba, the consumption of unfiltered dark tobacco cigarettes and cigars is more common than in other countries of the Americas. In light of Cuba's excessive death rates from lung cancer, Joly conducted a hospital-based study of 826 cases and controls to determine the relationship between risk for lung cancer and consumption of these types of tobacco. Odds ratios (OR) as an estimate of relative risk were calculated to determine the strength of the association between lung cancer and different forms of tobacco use. The OR were higher for dark tobacco users than for light tobacco users (OR

of 8.6 vs. 4.6 among women, and 14.3 vs. 11.2 among men). Cigar smokers had a much lower risk for lung cancer (OR = 4.0) than those who smoked only cigarettes. However, those who smoked both cigars and cigarettes had a higher OR than those who smoked only cigarettes (15.0 vs. 14.1). Based on the association found in this study, Joly also estimated that 91 percent of male lung cancer deaths and 66 percent of female lung cancer deaths could be due to smoking.

In addition to lung cancer, evidence of the disease impact of smoking in Cuba can be observed during the period 1983 to 1988 for selected cardiovascular diseases. The age-adjusted death rate for ischemic heart disease increased for both men and women until 1987 (Figure 2). However, age-adjusted mortality from cerebrovascular diseases and from cancers of the lip, oral cavity, and throat remained stable for both men and women. These diseases may have other contributing risk factors such as arterial hypertension and excess consumption of alcohol, the prevalence of which has decreased in Cuba.

Tobacco Use Prevention and Control Activities

Executive Structure and Policies

In Cuba, all activities for the prevention and control of tobacco use are carried out within a Government framework, and the Government has officially recognized that tobacco has been an important factor in the emergence of noncommunicable chronic diseases in the Cuban population (Suárez-Lugo 1988). Antismoking actions had been undertaken in the 1960s, including a ban on the advertising of tobacco products, the inclusion of a health warning on cigarette packs, and various educational activities on the part of health professionals. In 1976, the Ministry of Public Health created the National Commission on Health Promotion, with the stated objectives of reducing sedentary lifestyle, obesity, and smoking. In 1986, a national working group, Grupo de Trabajo Nacional (GTN), was established to help the antismoking campaign. A national program to reduce tobacco use was organized in 1987, and the GTN is an integral part of this program.

The GTN includes representatives from 15 different government agencies: the ministries of health, education, higher education, culture, agriculture, commerce, and transportation; institutes concerned with radio, television, sports, physical education, recreation, and aeronautics; the union of communist youth; the Organización de Pioneros José Martí (José Martí Organization of Pioneers); and the ICIODI, which acts as general coordinator. At least 100 persons participate in this group, which does not have its own budget but rather draws on resources from the participating institutions. The GTN has established units at the provincial level in an effort to regionalize its activities.

Legislation

The antismoking campaign relies primarily on public education through the mass media. Recently there has been an increase in legislative action. Early tobacco-related legislation focused on fire prevention through bans on smoking in the vicinity of flammable or explosive substances (Decree No. 41 1988). It is now also forbidden to smoke in airplanes (Resolution DJ 26/88 1988), urban public transportation, and certain other public spaces (Law No. 60 1987), as well as in education and health establishments (Rodríguez-Palacios 1988). Concern over noncompliance with these restrictions has led the GTN to redraft the existing regulations. The new version would ban smoking in meeting places, health centers, educational facilities, sport centers, public offices, and all public transportation facilities, including terminals (Varona-Pérez 1990). The bill also calls on political leaders to oversee compliance with the regulations and to impose fines on offenders. The proceeds of these fines would be turned over to the GTN to invest in the antismoking campaign.

Cuba has some restrictions on the sale of cigarettes (Varona-Pérez 1990). Cigarette sales are prohibited in health centers, schools, and other places where children and youth are found in groups. By decree, the Ministry of Commerce prohibits the sale of cigarettes to persons under the age of 16.

School-based Education

In 1989, work began on the development of an antismoking education program for children and adolescents to be implemented both in and outside the schools. The program is being assessed in terms of both its effectiveness and the feasibility of introducing it into the national education system.

Also in 1989 a process was initiated to help people give up smoking. It is being applied primarily in the community at the level of the family, which is the basic unit in the primary health care system. In addition, physicians are provided with information for helping their patients quit smoking.

Public Information Campaigns

Public information campaigns are the main component of antismoking activities in Cuba. These campaigns educate the public about the health hazards of smoking; raise the public awareness of nonsmokers' rights to breathe clean air; and encourage parents, teachers, and government officials to set an example by quitting.

Several subcampaigns are targeted at specific groups such as individuals who want to quit, household members, physicians and other influential figures such as teachers and athletes, adolescents and young people, and nonsmokers exposed to second-hand smoke. Another subcampaign emphasizes the economic effects of smoking on family income. The vehicles employed have included the mass media, posters, bumper stickers, and tee shirts bearing the message: "En vez de humo, llénese de vida" (Breathe life, not smoke!).

The first two years of the antismoking campaign have focused on education. So far, few resources have been available to help people quit. The survey mentioned earlier revealed that both smokers and nonsmokers are well informed about the health consequences of the addiction, but pharmacological aids and a few clinical programs are available only sporadically. In addition, the GTN is trying to get support from international agencies.

In 1988 Fidel Castro, the national leader, received an award from the World Health Organization on the occasion of its worldwide "No-Tobacco Day" in recognition of the Cuban Government's commitment to fight smoking and give priority to the nation's health.

Summary and Conclusions

Tobacco cultivation has played an important role in the Cuban economy and culture. Cuba has been the second largest producer and exporter of tobacco in Latin America, and per capita consumption of tobacco by Cubans is the highest in the Hemisphere. During the period 1986 to 1989 Cubans consumed 2,315 billion cigarettes a year. This excess consumption has caused lung cancer to become the leading cause of cancer mortality in Cuba, with more than 2,600 deaths from lung cancer attributable to smoking each year.

The Government and its leadership have recognized the heavy toll that smoking takes both on health and on the well-being of a struggling economy. The educational efforts that have been undertaken, and the interest shown by the State in improving the health indicators of the population, have helped to maintain a steadily declining trend in tobacco consumption which began in 1985. Despite the decline in consumption, however, the prevalence of smoking has increased among both women and young adults. In addition, Cubans continue to start smoking at an early age, although in 1988 only 5.7 percent of the adolescent population reported that they were smokers.

Legal actions are increasing under a national antismoking program, particularly smoking in public places. Physicians, who have an important role not only as opinion-makers but also as counselors to their patients who smoke, are actively involved in the antismoking campaign.

The GTN considers that it is essential to provide effective support for smokers who want to quit. Another positive aspect of the program is that it is being implemented by a multi-disciplinary and multisectoral group whose action is nationwide.

Based on the information presented in this review, the following conclusions may be drawn:

1. Tobacco production and consumption are deeply rooted in the Cuban culture, a fact that is reflected in the high prevalence of smoking. The high level of tobacco use is not so much a product of marketing as it is of strongly entrenched national custom.
2. Cuba has the third highest death rate from lung cancer in the Americas, and mortality from this form of cancer is increasing for both men and women. There are more than 2,600 lung cancer deaths attributable to smoking each year. Mortality from ischemic heart disease is also increasing. Cardiovascular and neoplastic diseases are the leading causes of death in Cuban adults.
3. The Cuban Government has recognized the need to prevent and control tobacco use among its citizens. Since 1960 there has been no advertising of tobacco products. Cuba's data systems have provided the necessary information for implementing a national tobacco prevention and control program, initiated in 1986. The effects of this program are measured by such indicators as consumption, prevalence, mortality, and the results of knowledge and attitude surveys.
4. Interventions against tobacco use have included public information using the mass media, school-based education, legislation, and a public commitment on the part of the Government's leadership to control tobacco use. Studies have shown that knowledge about the health consequences of smoking appears to be universal, but services are needed to implement cessation.
5. The prevalence of smoking declined during the 1980s by 15.5 percent. However, prevalence of smoking increased among adults aged 30 to 49 years as well as among women. Per capita cigarette and tobacco consumption fell by 46.7 percent between 1974 and 1989. However, even with these reductions, the prevalence and consumption of tobacco continue to be high in the Cuban population.

References

AGRO-ECONOMIC SERVICES LTD. AND TABACOSMOS LTD. *The employment, tax revenue and wealth that the tobacco industry creates.* 1987.

CENTRO LATINOAMERICANO DE DEMOGRAFIA. *Boletín Demográfico.* Santiago, Chile: CELADE, Año XXIII, No. 45, January 1990.

CHAPMAN, S., WONG, W.L. *Tobacco Control in the Third World—A Resource Atlas.* Penang, Malaysia: International Organization of Consumers Unions, 1990.

HEDGES, M. Trail of phony Winstons leads to Noriega, Cuba. *The Washington Times,* July 5, 1990, p. A3.

JOLY, O.G., LUBIN, J.H., CARABALLOSO, M. Dark tobacco and lung cancer in Cuba. *Journal of the National Cancer Institute* 70(6):1033–1039, June 1983.

MASIRONI, R., ROTHWELL, K. Tendences et effets du tabagisme dans le monde. *Rapp Trimest Statist Sanit Mond* 41:228–241, 1988.

PAN AMERICAN HEALTH ORGANIZATION. *Health Conditions in the Americas—1981–1984.* Washington, D.C.: Pan American Health Organization. Scientific Publication No. 500, 1986.

PAN AMERICAN HEALTH ORGANIZATION. *Health Conditions in the Americas—1990 Edition.* Washington, D.C.: Pan American Health Organization. Scientific Publication No. 524, 1990.

PAN AMERICAN HEALTH ORGANIZATION. Informe Preliminar, Taller sobre Tabaquismo y Salud, Region Mesoamérica, Ciudad de Guatemala, 11 October 1988.

RODRIGUEZ-PALACIOS, E. Estudio sobre aspectos legales del hábito de fumar. Havana, Instituto Cubano de Investigaciones y Orientación de la Demanda Interna, 1988 (mimeograph).

SUAREZ-LUGO, N. Actividades anti-tabáquicas en Cuba. Havana, 1988 (mimeograph).

UNITED NATIONS DEVELOPMENT PROGRAM. *Human Development Report 1990.* New York: Oxford University Press, 1990.

U.S. DEPARTMENT OF AGRICULTURE. Foreign Agricultural Service. Latin American and Caribbean tobacco production and consumption (unpublished tabulations), April 1990.

VARONA-PEREZ, P. Informe sobre tabaquismo, Cuba, 1990 (unpublished data).

WORLD BANK. *World Development Report 1990.* New York: Oxford University Press, 1990.

Dominican Republic

General Characteristics

The Tobacco Industry
   Agriculture
   Manufacturing and production
   Marketing, advertising, and promotion

Tobacco Use
   Consumption
   Behavioral Surveys

Smoking and Health

Tobacco Use Prevention and Control Activities
   Government policies and administrative structure
   Legislation
   Taxes
   Nongovernmental organizations

Summary and Conclusions

References

General Characteristics

The Dominican Republic is a Spanish-speaking nation occupying two-thirds of the island of Santo Domingo; it shares the island with Haiti. The estimated 1990 mid-year population was 7,170,000, and the Republic ranks third in population density among the countries of the Americas. In 1981, more than half (52 percent) of the population was urban (Pan American Health Organization [PAHO] 1988). The population of the Dominican Republic is quite young, with 37.9 percent aged less than 15 years and fewer than 3 percent 65 years or older (Table 1). The Republic experienced a significant economic depression during 1982 to 1986, with 27.2 percent unemployment in 1985, reduced social and health expenditures, and declining school enrollment. Since 1987, however, tourism and the construction industry have increased substantially and the economy has improved (PAHO 1990). Agricultural products, especially sugar, account for 21.5 percent of total exports. Of all exports, 0.1 percent is Criollo tobacco, exported primarily to Spain (PAHO 1988; Chapman 1990).

The Tobacco Industry

Agriculture

Tobacco is a major agricultural product in the Dominican Republic. According to data from the

Table 1. Health and economic indicators, Dominican Republic, 1985–1990

Indicator	Value
Population (1990)	7,169,846
% <15	37.9
% ≥65	3
Life expectancy at birth (men) (1985–90)	63.9
Life expectancy at birth (women) (1985–90)	68.1
Overall fertility (1985–90)	3.75
Infant mortality per 1,000 live births (1985–90)	65.0
Crude mortality rate per 100,000 (1985)	0.6
Illiteracy (1985)	23%
Real GNP growth rate (1980–88)	0.8%
Per capita GNP (1988)	$US720

Sources: CELADE, 1990; World Bank, 1990.

Tobacco Institute of the Dominican Republic (1988), the country had 31,000 ha of tobacco under cultivation in 1988, up from 24,000 ha in 1986 (Chapman 1990). Most tobacco agriculture is in the north part of the island. In 1987 the production of dried leaves was 21,186,500 kg; in 1988, production increased to 28,438,500 kg. Sixty-four percent of the total tobacco crop is exported as raw leaf.

In 1989 the Dominican Republic had 19,000 tobacco growers (de los Santos 1990). Of those, the Tobacco Institute provided intensive technical assistance to 900 and partial technical assistance to 10,982. The rest were controlled by small companies or operated independently (Tobacco Institute 1989a). The Tobacco Institute stated in its annual report (1989b) that the majority of tobacco growers were dissatisfied with the prices paid by the manufacturing industries and exporters that year, and some reported selling less than 50 percent of their crop. A report of the National Federation of Tobacco Producers stated that 28,000 farmers abandoned tobacco farming and moved to cities because of a decline in revenue from exports. Thus, tobacco agriculture may have reached a temporary high point in 1988 with a subsequent decline in the number of farmers and cultivated land acreage since then. Economic pressures are significant in the international tobacco market, suggesting that farmers may not be seriously committed to this particular crop.

Manufacturing and Production

Information on the production and consumption of cigarettes is provided by the Tobacco Institute (1989a, b) and other international sources (Tobacco Merchants Association 1989; Maxwell 1990). The data from all sources are virtually identical.

The State-owned Compañía Anónima Tabacalera controlled 76.9 percent of the domestic market in 1976. However, it has gradually lost market share to E. León Jiménez, a subsidiary of the Philip Morris Company. By 1989 the latter company controlled 70.7 percent of the market, while the State-owned company controlled only 29.3 percent (Maxwell 1990). Compañía Anónima Tabacalera has become a subsidiary of R. J. Reynolds, Inc. There are 13 other manufacturing companies, mainly involved in cigar production. Cigarette production increased from an estimated 3.3 billion in 1979 to 4.6 billion in 1988, 4.4 billion of which were filtered (Tobacco Merchants Association 1989) (Table 2). The production of cigars is declining. In 1983, cigar production was estimated at 80 million units, and

Table 2. Production, exports, imports (in metric tons), and per capita cigarette consumption (per person aged 15 years or older), Dominican Republic, 1979–1988

Year	Production	Exports	Imports	Per capita consumption
1979	3,353	0	0	1,284
1980	3,365	0	0	1,326
1981	3,436	0	0	1,297
1982	3,500	0	0	1,194
1983	3,600	0	0	1,180
1984	3,645	0	0	1,215
1985	3,645	0	0	1,203
1986	3,775	0	0	1,268
1987	4,576	0	0	1,396
1988	4,631	0	0	1,352

Source: Tobacco Merchants Association, 1989.

by 1988 had fallen to 53.5 million (Tobacco Merchants Association 1989). In 1984, the Dominican Republic enjoyed a $US29 million surplus trade balance in tobacco (Chapman 1990).

Marketing, Advertising, and Promotion

Marlboro cigarettes are the most popular brand sold in the Dominican Republic, with a market share that increased from 15 percent in 1978 to 51.1 percent in 1989 (Davis 1986; World Bank 1990). This increase is not surprising, given that the brand is heavily promoted throughout the country, and the environment is saturated with logos on T-shirts, street signs, bus stops, airport ticket counters, theater marquees, restaurant signs, sporting arenas, and baseball fields. A 25-foot-high air-filled Marlboro box dominates the oceanside boulevard on certain casinos in the capital city (Davis 1986).

Television advertising of cigarette products is common, especially for Marlboro.

The price of a 20-cigarette pack of the most commonly sold brand is $US0.75. However, packs of 10 cigarettes are more popular and account for 76 percent of the market (Maxwell 1990). Cigarettes are also sold individually and from vending machines (de los Santos 1990).

Tobacco Use

Consumption

Among the population aged 15 years and older, per capita cigarette consumption increased from 1,106 in 1976 to 1,361 in 1989. Ninety-four percent of the cigarettes now consumed in the Dominican Republic are filtered Virginia (blond) tobacco (Maxwell 1990). This suggests a successful market creation by the transnational tobacco companies such as that experienced in many other countries of the Americas.

Behavioral Surveys

Several surveys on tobacco use have been conducted in the Dominican Republic (Table 3). In 1985, 710 secondary school teachers in Santo Domingo were surveyed on tobacco use and knowledge about the harmful effects of tobacco. The response rate of this survey was 79 percent. Overall, 41 percent were current smokers (50.7 percent of men and 25.1 percent of women). Only 7 percent were former smokers. Most (60.5 percent) of the smokers smoked fewer than 10 cigarettes per day. "Curiosity" was the main reason given (60 percent) for initiation of smoking. Among current smokers, "custom" and "relaxation" were the most important reasons reported to continue smoking. Of the total respondents, 56.8 percent reported

Table 3. Surveys on smoking and smoking prevalence (percent) by sex, Dominican Republic, 1985–1990

| Author/Sponsor | Year | Sample | N | Prevalence | | |
				Men	Women	Both
Pimentel (1987)	1985	Teachers	710	50.7	25.1	41.5
Ferraros (1987)	1986	Secondary students	5,318			30.0
Pimentel (1991a)	1986	Physicians	580	43.0	16.9	34.5
Candelaria (1989)	1989	SESPAS employees	704	24.8	20.0	22.2
de los Santos (1990)	1990	General population	502	66.3	13.6	49.8
Vincent (1991)	1990	Households	1,388	36.0	33.1	34.9
Pimentel (1991b)	1990	Medical + dental students	754			75.2

that a ban on smoking in schools would be effective in diminishing tobacco use; 72.4 percent agreed that smoking by teachers influenced students in beginning to smoke (Pimentel et al. 1987).

In 1986, Pimentel (1991a) surveyed 580 physicians on tobacco use and respiratory symptoms. Of the total sample, 34.5 percent were current smokers (43 percent of men and 16.9 percent of women). Of smokers, 35 percent reported respiratory symptoms; only 15 percent of ex-smokers and none of the never smokers reported respiratory symptoms such as cough and dyspnea.

In 1989, 704 employees of the Ministry of Public Health and Welfare (SESPAS) who were at work on the day of the survey were asked about smoking (Candelaria and Feliz 1989). Overall, 22.2 percent (24.8 percent of men and 20.0 percent of women) were current smokers. If many of those unavailable for the survey were smokers, the prevalence of smoking may have been underestimated. Nevertheless, the prevalence of smoking among health care professionals is lower than that in the general population in most countries, and these data suggest that the Dominican Republic likely follows this pattern. However, the high rate of smoking among physicians in the Pimentel (1991a) survey was matched by the level reported among physician staff members of SESPAS (33.0 percent).

A national survey was conducted by the Ministry of Health in 1989 of 251 men and 251 women, aged 15 to 90 years (de los Santos 1990). Information on the methodology of this survey is unavailable. Among respondents aged 20 to 79 years, the prevalence of current smoking was 49.8 percent. The prevalence was 4.8 times higher among men than among women (66.3 vs. 13.6 percent). This range is similar to that reported by other Latin Caribbean countries such as Cuba.

Several surveys in Santo Domingo provide some information on smoking and health among children and adolescents. In 1986, 5,318 secondary students in Santo Domingo were surveyed as to smoking and respiratory symptoms. Of these, 30 percent were daily smokers, and of these, 41.8 percent admitted having respiratory symptoms such as coughing and nasal congestion (Ferraros et al. 1987).

Pimental (1991b) surveyed 754 medical and dental students of the Iberoamerican University. Surprisingly 75.2 percent of those students were current smokers, and 4.8 percent were former smokers. In contrast to the fewer number of cigarettes smoked per day reported by physicians, over half of the current smokers in this sample (53.4 percent) smoked more than 16 cigarettes per day.

Finally, a household survey of 1,388 persons aged 15 to 55 years and older living in Santo Domingo was performed by researchers from the University of South Florida in 1990 and 1991 (Table 4). This survey assessed knowledge about smoking as well as symptoms of morning cough and shortness of breath and respondents' educational attainment and household income. In addition, the average age at which respondents began to smoke was ascertained. Overall, the prevalence of current smoking among residents of Santo Domingo was 34.9 percent (36.0 percent among men and 33.1 percent among women). These results suggest that male and female urban residents do not differ in rates of smoking. The average age of initiation was 17.3 years. Current smokers had a lower level of educational attainment than never smokers, and there was no difference in smoking status by income. Current smokers reported significantly more morning cough and shortness of breath than never smokers, and almost all (97.4 percent) agreed smoking is dangerous to their health. However, additional questions on this survey suggested that respondents were poorly informed as to the link between smoking and specific disease entities (Vincent 1991). Only 11.3 percent had quit smoking.

Table 4. Prevalence (percent) of current, former, and never smoking among residents of Santo Domingo, Dominican Republic, 1991

Smoking status	Men		Women		Both	
	%	N	%	N	%	N
Current smoking	36.0	233	33.1	251	34.9	484
Former smoking	12.4	80	10.2	77	11.3	157
Never smoking	43.6	347	56.7	430	53.8	747
Total	100.0	647	100.0	759	100.0	1,388

Source: Vincent et al., 1991.

Smoking and Health

In 1985, 15 percent of the deaths registered in the Dominican Republic were attributed to signs, symptoms, and ill-defined conditions (ICD 780–799). Underregistration was estimated at 40.3 percent during 1980 to 1985 (PAHO 1990). This indicates a significant lack of precision in assignation of cause of death. Mortality statistics therefore should be interpreted with caution.

Among 27,844 deaths in 1985, the chief causes and greatest proportions of registered deaths were for diseases of the heart (ICD 390–492; 19.2 percent), perinatal diseases (ICD 760–769; 11.6 percent), malignant neoplasms (ICD 140–208; 7.4 percent), intestinal infections (ICD 007–009; 7.3 percent), cerebrovascular disease (ICD 430–438; 7.3 percent), and accidents (ICD E800–E949, E980–989; 7.0 percent) (PAHO 1990). Chronic diseases are the predominant cause of death in the Dominican Republic, and many of the most common causes, including perinatal conditions and fire deaths, may be associated with smoking.

In general, age-adjusted and age-specific mortality rates for cardiovascular disease and smoking-associated malignancy are higher for men than for women (Table 5). Data are available on ischemic heart disease for 1985 and 1988; based on these 2 years' data, the age-adjusted and age-specific mortality rates for this smoking-associated condition increased for men aged 35 or older. This may reflect an increase in the prevalence of cardiac risk factors among residents of the Dominican Republic in re-

cent years as well as improved reporting and death registration.

In 1984, Cruz-Tavarez (1984) reported on 64 breast-fed infants of smoking and nonsmoking mothers. Of smoking mothers, 81 percent reported inadequate quantity of breast milk, whereas 18.7 percent of nonsmoking mothers reported this problem. Health problems were more common among children of smoking mothers than those of nonsmoking mothers. These included a higher percentage in the lower three percentiles of weight at 6 months of age (44.4 vs. 11.1 percent) and a higher percentage of lung infections (31.3 vs. 6.3 percent).

In a study comparing 50 children of parents who smoked to 50 children of parents who were not smokers, Pimentel (1991b) reported that both respiratory infections (48 vs. 22 percent) and hospitalizations (26 vs. 10 percent) were more common among children of smokers compared with children of nonsmokers.

Tobacco Use Prevention and Control Activities

Government Policies and Administrative Structure

The Dominican Republic has no official policy, plan, or program for the control of tobacco use. Nevertheless, the Ministry of Public Health and Welfare has supported various related initiatives and participates in national and international ef-

Table 5. Mortality rates (per 100,000 persons) for selected tobacco-related diseases, by age and sex, Dominican Republic, 1985

Cause of death (ICD-9)	Sex	Year	Age-adjusted rate[a]	35–44	45–54	55–64
Ischemic heart disease (410–414)	men	1985	36.3	19.5	68.6	168.6
		1988	71.1	20.8	73.0	215.1
	women	1985	25.7	14.8	43.9	90.9
		1988	38.6	5.6	19.8	71.3
Cerebrovascular disease (430–438)	men	1985	31.9	10.3	57.3	124.1
	women	1985	29.7	18.3	58.4	88.5
Malignant tumor of the lip, oral cavity, and pharynx (140–149)	men	1985	1.6	0.4	3.6	6.9
	women	1985	1.0	0.7	4.0	2.4
Malignant tumor of the trachea, bronchi, and lung (162)	men	1985	4.0	1.4	7.2	25.3
	women	1985	1.1	—	2.5	6.4

Source: Pan American Health Organization, 1986 and 1990.
[a]Rates adjusted for all ages according to the population of Latin America.

forts aimed at limiting tobacco consumption, such as WHO World No-Tobacco Day. The Dominican Committee on Smoking and Health receives official support even though it acts independently of the Government and is not a functional health program (see section on Nongovernmental Organizations, below).

Legislation

The only tobacco-related legislation is a prohibition of the sale and supply of alcoholic drinks and tobacco products to minors under age 16 (Law No. 272). A bill had been submitted to the national Chamber of Deputies in 1990 to regulate and restrict the advertising of tobacco and alcohol in the mass media. In 1992, a new bill with modifications will be reconsidered by the Commission on Health of the Chamber of Deputies.

Taxes

The tax on cigarettes is equivalent to 13.4 percent of the retail price, but the structure of cigarette prices is two-tiered, with higher priced brands, such as Marlboro, taxed at a higher rate (Romero 1989). According to preliminary data from the Ministry of Finance, tobacco taxes accounted for 2.29 percent of the total Government tax revenue in 1988. However, relative earnings from tobacco decreased from 1984 to 1988 (Table 6). In 1984, tobacco products contributed 3.81 percent of revenue from taxes (Romero 1989).

Nongovernmental Organizations

In 1989, the Dominican Committee on Smoking and Health (HAFUSA) was created as a result of the First Dominican Workshop on Tobacco and Health held that year. Its honorary chairman is the

Minister of Public Health. This Committee maintains public visibility through presentations in the mass media. In addition, workshops on the effects of tobacco on health have been conducted with various organizations.

Summary and Conclusions

The Dominican Republic is typical of small agricultural countries in which tobacco growing had previously held more importance to the domestic economy. With increasing tourism and construction, tobacco agriculture declined in both volume and importance as an export crop. The multinational tobacco companies, especially Philip Morris, Inc., have succeeded in shifting both consumer tastes and national revenue from dark tobacco produced by a national monopoly to Virginia blond tobacco manufactured primarily under the cachet of the world's most widely marketed consumer product, Marlboro cigarettes. The Marlboro logo permeates Dominican society, even to the extent that cigarette advertisements pay for public street signs. It is understandable that Marlboro has increased its market share by 300 percent over the last decade.

The disease impact of tobacco is difficult to measure in the Dominican Republic. Several surveys have been performed in the country, and the data from these suggest that the prevalence of smoking among women may be increasing. Heart disease mortality rates appear to have increased from 1985 to 1988, possibly as a result of increased population exposure to tobacco, but thus far mortality rates for smoking-related malignancy are low. The high degree of underreporting and misclassification of causes of death preclude accurate analysis of smoking-attributable mortality. However, studies of the effect of smoking on breast feeding and respiratory conditions in both adults and children in the Dominican Republic provide convincing evidence of the specific negative health effects among both these groups. Given this evidence, it is surprising to find high rates of smoking among teachers and physicians and alarmingly high rates among medical and dental students.

The tobacco industry appears to be well represented through a Tobacco Institute and the National Federation of Tobacco Producers. Little organized activity for the prevention and control of tobacco use has been possible in the Dominican Republic, but resources for health and disease prevention may be increased in the near future (PAHO 1990). At this time, voluntary groups, with Minis-

Table 6. **Central Government revenue from taxes on cigarettes, in millions of $RD, Dominican Republic, 1984–1988**

Year	Tax	Percentage of tax revenue
1984	40.6	3.81
1985	51.6	3.04
1986	60.8	2.85
1987	70.1	2.46
1988	99.1	2.29

Source: Romero, 1989.

try of Health sanction, are beginning to provide the public information necessary before organized and effective tobacco control programs can be implemented.

Based on the limited data available on the Dominican Republic, the following conclusions may be drawn:

1. Approximately one-third of the general public report that they are current smokers. A lower proportion of health department employees are smokers, but over one-third of physicians are smokers. The prevalence of smoking is much higher among men than among women. Approximately 30 percent of high school students are smokers.

2. Tobacco production and consumption have declined measurably in the last decade. Tobacco provided less than 3 percent of tax revenue ($RD99.1 million) in 1988, and this proportion has decreased steadily since 1984. Tobacco farmers are abandoning tobacco because of lower international prices for Dominican exports.

3. Mortality rates for tobacco-related diseases are higher among men than among women, and for cardiac disease at least, the mortality rate has increased from 1985 to 1988. Respiratory conditions have been shown to be much more common among smokers compared with nonsmokers and among children of smokers compared with children of nonsmokers.

4. Tobacco control activities rely primarily on voluntary groups in the Dominican Republic, but the Dominican Committee on Smoking and Health was established in 1989 to focus public attention on the health effects of tobacco. Additional data, surveys, and programs are needed.

References

CANDELARIA, S., FELIZ, B.M. *Hábito de fumar en los empleados de las SESPAS.* Dirección Técnica de Sistemas, Secretaría de Estado de Salud Pública y Asistencia Social, República Dominicana, 1989.

CENTRO LATINOAMERICANO DE DEMOGRAFIA. *Boletín Demográfico.* Santiago, Chile: CELADE, vol. 13, no. 45, January 1990.

CHAPMAN, S., WONG, W.L. *Tobacco Control in the Third World—A Resource Atlas.* Penang, Malaysia: International Organization of Consumers Unions, 1990.

CRUZ-TAVAREZ, P., GARCIA, V., PIMENTEL, R.D. et al. Algunas repercusiones del tabaco sobre el niño y la producción de leche de madres fumadoras. *Archivos Dominicanos de Pediatría* 20(2): 37–40, May/August 1984.

DAVIS, R.M. Promotion of cigarettes in developing countries. *Journal of the American Medical Association* 255(8):993, 1986.

DE LOS SANTOS, T. Country Collaborator's Report, Dominican Republic. Pan American Health Organization, (unpublished), February 1990.

FERRAROS, J.M., DURAN, L.G., TOLBIO, F.A., MARTINEZ, C.L. Tabaquismo y síntomas respiratorios en la poblacion escolar. *Revista Médica Dominicana* 48:21–25, 1987.

INSTITUTO DEL TABACO. *Boletín Estadístico No. 41, 1987.* Santo Domingo: Subprograma de Planificación y Estadística, Instituto del Tabaco de República Dominicana, September 27, 1988.

INSTITUTO DEL TABACO. *Programa Tabacalero 1989–1990.* Santiago: Instituto del Tabaco de República Dominicana, September 1989a.

INSTITUTO DEL TABACO. *Memoria Anual 1989.* Santo Domingo: Instituto del Tabaco de República Dominicana, 1989b.

MAXWELL, J.C. *The Maxwell Consumer Report: International Tobacco 1989,* Part One. Richmond, Virginia: Wheat First Securities/Butcher and Singer, Inc. WFBS-5455, 18 May 1990.

PAN AMERICAN HEALTH ORGANIZATION. *Control del hábito de fumar—IV Taller Subregional: Mesoamérica,* 31 October–3 November 1988. Preliminary report, 1988.

PAN AMERICAN HEALTH ORGANIZATION. *Health Conditions in the Americas, 1990 Edition.* Washington, D.C.: Pan American Health Organization, Scientific Publication 524, 1990.

PIMENTEL, R.D., ABREU-MURENO, D.R., PENA-TORIBIO, P.I., et al. Tabaquismo en los médicos de Santo Domingo: efecto sobre la función respiratoria y actitud frente al hábito de los pacientes. *Boletín CENISMI* 1(8): 59–66, 1991a.

PIMENTEL, R.D., CUSTODIO, J., FONTANA, V., et al. Admisiones hospitalarias por infecciones bronquiales y hábitos parentales de fumar. *Boletín CENISMI* 1(4): 6–7, 1991b.

PIMENTEL, R.D., FELIZ, E., PASCUAL, Y.A., SANTOS, A.A., LEE, A.E. Opiniones en relación al tabaquismo de profesores de escuelas secundarias en Santo Domingo, República Dominicana *Revista Médica de Costa Rica* 501:165–167, 1987.

ROMERO, J. Ingresos Fisco y el ITBI. Bebidas y tabaco aportan 7.5% tributarios *Listín Diario* No. 25785 Tuesday, June 13, 1989.

TOBACCO MERCHANTS ASSOCIATION OF THE UNITED STATES. *Special Report: Production and Consumption of Tobacco Products for Selected Countries 1979-1988.* Special Report 89-3, Princeton, New Jersey, September 28, 1989.

WORLD BANK. *World Development Report 1989—Poverty.* New York: Oxford University Press, June 1989.

WORLD BANK. *World Development Report 1990.* New York: Oxford University Press, 1990.

VINCENT, A.L., BRADHAM, D.D., FISHER, S.K. A residential survey of smoking in the Dominican Republic. Unpublished manuscript dated July 21, 1991.

Ecuador

General Characteristics

Ecuador occupies 284,000 km² on the western coast of South America. The capital, Quito, at one time an important Spanish colonial center, is located in the Andes mountains. Ecuador harbors vast natural resources, especially in agriculture, but in the late 1980s experienced a severe economic crisis similar to most other Latin American nations. In 1987, a series of earthquakes damaged numerous culturally important buildings and severely disrupted services in several mountain communities. Oil, fishing, manufacturing, and forestry are important components of the gross domestic product (Pan American Health Organization [PAHO] 1990). The population is young, with approximately 40 percent younger than age 15 and only 4.2 percent older than age 65 years (World Bank 1990; Table 1). Urbanization has resulted in crowded urban centers and a gradual transculturation of the Indian and mestizo groups that reside in rural areas.

Ecuador is a tobacco-producing nation, and tobacco has been important as a domestically consumed product. Because of the young age structure of the population, chronic diseases that may be associated with tobacco use have not yet emerged as important causes of death in Ecuador. In fact, until 1984, there was no established policy for the protection and care of persons aged 65 years and older (PAHO 1990). As the population ages, the impact of tobacco-related illness may become more evident in this vulnerable population.

Table 1. Basic health and economic indicators, Ecuador, 1980s

Indicator	Year	Value
Total population	1988	10,232,000
Percent < age 15	1988	40.5
Percent ≥ age 65	1988	4.2
Percent urban	1988	55
Total fertility rate (Per 1,000 women)	1988	4.2
Literacy rate	1985	82
Life expectancy at birth	1988	66
Infant mortality rate (Per 1,000 live births)	1988	62
Crude mortality rate (Per 1,000 persons)	1988	7
GNP per capita ($US)	1988	1,120
Yearly percent change in GNP per capita	1965–88	3.1

Source: World Bank, 1990.

The Tobacco Industry

Agriculture

In 1988, Ecuador's land devoted to tobacco growing was estimated at between 1,590 and 1,968 ha (INEC 1988; Ministerio de Agricultura y Ganadería 1988), representing less than 0.1 percent of arable land. Seventy percent of tobacco farmland is in Guayas province, and the total percentage of arable land dedicated to tobacco in this province is 0.12 percent. Two large cigarette manufacturing companies produced 79.7 percent of Ecuador's leaf tobacco (3,242.1 MT) in 1988. Additional tobacco is grown specifically for use in cigars (Tobacco International 1989). Farmers appear to be dependent on these companies for advance purchase arrangements, advances of operating capital and seeds, and technical assistance (Tabea 1988). In fact, the Philip Morris Company has provided more agricultural technical assistance in Ecuador than in any other country where they have licensed or directly owned manufacturing interests (Philip Morris 1988). The financial dependence of the small- to medium-scale farmer on the tobacco company is nearly absolute.

Production of leaf tobacco has increased from an average 1,631.8 MT in the 1970s to an average 3,982 MT in the 1980s (Table 2). In these two decades, import levels of raw tobacco were approximately double those of exports so that total domestic leaf consumption increased 200 percent. However, because of a concomitant rapid population growth, per capita consumption did not increase at a comparable rate (Table 3).

Cigarette Manufacturing and Trade

Two large cigarette-manufacturing companies operate in Ecuador: Tabacalera Andina, a Philip Morris licensee that controls about 80 percent of the total market, and Fábrica de Cigarrillos El Progreso, an R. J. Reynolds licensee that controls the remainder. In 1982, four cigarette manufacturing factories owned by these two companies employed 1,060 persons, or 0.03 percent of the total Ecuadoran workforce (Samaniego 1990).

The production of cigarettes increased significantly from the middle 1970s to the middle 1980s, after which production levels were essentially unchanged through the end of the decade (USDA 1990) (Table 3). A substantial decline in total consumption may have occurred (Maxwell 1989), consonant with high inflation rates and the economic

Table 2. Production, imports, exports, and total domestic consumption of raw tobacco (in metric tons), Ecuador, 1970–1989

Year	Production	Imports	Exports	Total domestic consumption
1970	2,141	477	117	1,130
1971	790	612	70	1,475
1972	635	295	246	1,515
1973	1,713	1,144	68	2,329
1974	1,448	2,074	113	2,773
1975	1,466	1,089	157	2,345
1976	1,272	2,404	250	3,501
1977	1,805	2,967	131	4,016
1978	2,494	3,000	174	3,710
1979	2,554	2,197	373	3,370
1980	2,871	951	215	3,124
1981	3,765	620	186	3,416
1982	3,539	630	270	4,123
1983	3,300	766	216	4,242
1984	2,900	1,000	133	4,467
1985	4,062	996	424	4,172
1986	3,850	1,000	629	3,471
1987	3,850	1,000	423	3,677
1988	3,850	1,000	279	3,821
1989	3,850	900	285	3,715

Source: United States Department of Agriculture (USDA), 1990.

Table 3. Production, imports, exports, total consumption (in MT), and consumption per capita (aged 15 and older) of manufactured cigarettes, Ecuador, 1970–1989

Year	Produced	Imported	Exported	Total consumption USDA	Total consumption Maxwell	Per capita consumption
1970	1,284	473	20	1,737		525
1971	1,340	957	20	2,277		666
1972	1,327	1,424	38	2,713		769
1973	1,434	1,570	0	3,004		791
1974	1,740	1,940	0	3,680	3,570	949
1975	2,642	1,568	0	4,210	3,780	1,081
1976	3,736	0	0	3,736	3,659	928
1977	4,224	40	0	4,264	3,914	1,024
1978	3,900	36	0	3,936	3,889	914
1979	4,090	36	246	3,880	4,017	872
1980	3,932	36	256	3,712	3,740	806
1981	4,270	36	445	3,861	4,032	811
1982	4,766	36	484	4,318	4,596	876
1983	4,980	50	300	4,730	3,919	928
1984	5,000	50	300	4,750	3,983	900
1985	4,800	0	200	4,600	3,804	843
1986	4,600	0	100	4,500	3,786	798
1987	4,600	0	100	4,500	3,604	773
1988	4,600	0	100	4,500	3,076	749
1989	3,319	NA	NA	NA	3,319	535

Sources: USDA, 1990; The Maxwell Report, 1989.

crisis in the 1980s mentioned above. Importation of cigarettes is minimal, but exports became significant in the early 1980s. Nonetheless, because of raw and manufactured tobacco imports, Ecuador had an estimated negative trade balance for tobacco of $US907,000 in 1984 (Chapman 1990). In addition to legal imports, an illegal trade in cigarettes contributes an unknown quantity to total domestic consumption in Ecuador (Samaniego 1990).

Advertising and Promotion of Tobacco

In Ecuador, cigarette advertising is permitted on television after 7:30 p.m., ostensibly to limit the exposure of young persons to tobacco advertisements. However, this is an important medium for the tobacco industry. It was estimated that from 1986 to 1988, 70 percent of total cigarette advertising expenditures were for television, 21 percent were for radio, and the remaining 9 percent were split among billboards, points-of-sale, and print media (Maxwell 1989). The effect of this advertising has been measured on a 1990 Quito survey of knowledge and attitudes related to tobacco. In this survey, 90.1 percent of respondents stated they had observed television advertising, 61.9 percent had heard radio advertising, and 32.9 percent remembered seeing tobacco advertising on billboards. A smaller proportion remembered print media tobacco advertising (Ministerio de Salud Pública 1990). In countries with bans on television advertising, the greatest proportions of the tobacco advertising expenditures tend to be for radio and billboards. Philip Morris' estimated investment in advertising in Ecuador was $US1,000,000 in 1986 and 1987 (Philip Morris 1988).

An interesting advertising strategy is employed in Ecuador. Commercial "information" printed on cigarette packages, all of which are manufactured in Ecuador, is always in English (e.g., "filter cigarettes," "richly rewarding," etc.). This strategy may suggest to smokers that by smoking cigarettes they may assume a lifestyle with a higher socioeconomic status.

Tobacco Use

Per Capita Cigarette Consumption

Ecuador is among the 10 Latin American countries lowest in per capita cigarette consumption. Although the 1985 per capita consumption in Ecuador was similar to that in neighboring Peru and Bolivia, it was less than half of that for Colombia and Venezuela. Based on USDA (1990) data,

per capita consumption increased substantially in the 1970s and decreased slightly in 1986 to 1988 (Table 3). The relationship between economic capacity and the consumption of tobacco is demonstrated in this pattern, because in these years a severe economic crisis was evident in all the countries of the subregion.

Behavioral Surveys

Methodology and limitations

Numerous surveys on tobacco use are available in Ecuador. Cruz (1954) reported a tobacco-use survey performed on 535 Quito men. No information is available on the methodology used for this survey, but it may be the first such survey in Latin America.

In 1990, Confidential Report and IESOP (CEIC/IESOP) carried out a survey in Quito and Guayaquil of 600 persons aged 18 years and older. The methodology of this survey is unknown. The survey asked smokers about their age, age when they began smoking, age when they stopped, and some questions on attitudes and knowledge (Zevallos 1990).

In 1988, the Mental Health Division of the Ministry of Health and the "Our Young" Foundation (Ministerio de Salud Pública 1990) conducted a survey on the use of alcohol, tobacco, and drugs in a representative sample of the Ecuadoran population aged 10 through 65 years. The target sample of 6,800 persons was obtained by a stratified cluster sampling technique. The final sample size was 6,256, of whom 3,644 were adults (aged 20 to 65 years) and 2,612 were adolescents (aged 10 to 19 years). Among adolescents, lifetime ever use of cigarettes by sex and age was ascertained. Among adults, current smoking and ever use of cigarettes were ascertained. Current smokers were stratified into occasional smokers (seven or fewer cigarettes per day) and habitual smokers (more than seven cigarettes per day) (Aguilar 1990).

In 1990, the Ministry of Health conducted a survey of 1,805 Quito residents aged 10 years and older on smoking behavior and knowledge about smoking (Ministerio de Salud Pública 1990). In this survey, the respondent was asked if he or she consumed cigarettes regularly or occasionally, but these categories were not defined; respondents made their own judgments as to the definition.

Between 1981 and 1984 the national Comptroller General's Office conducted a survey of all 20,838 persons aged 12 to 20 years in school in 9 of

Ecuador's 20 provinces (Ministerio de Finanzas 1987). Although this survey was designed primarily to cover drug use, it also determined the prevalence of daily and occasional cigarette smoking.

The "Study on Habits and Drugs in Pregnancy" coordinated by PAHO/WHO's Latin American Center for Perinatology (CLAP 1987) in Ecuador established the prevalence of cigarette smoking among 2,009 parturient women during the 6 months before their pregnancy. Little information on the methodology for this survey is available.

Finally, in 1987 the Division of Chronic Disease Control in the Ministry of Health conducted a survey of 338 public employees at the Ministries of Health and of Education and Culture. The only information available from this survey is the prevalence of smoking at the time of the survey and the age of smoking initiation.

Prevalence of smoking among adults

In the 1954 survey, 85 percent of the male respondents smoked. It is probable that this high prevalence was observed because the only men surveyed were in the age groups in which the prevalence of smoking is highest (46 percent of the respondents were between 24 and 39 years of age). Of smokers, 38.8 percent smoked seven or more cigarettes per day, with the average daily number of cigarettes smoked at 12. By contrast, the prevalence of current cigarette smoking among men aged 18 years and older in the United States in 1955 was 59.2 percent (U.S. Department of Health and Human Services [USDHHS] 1988).

In the 1988 Ministry of Health survey of persons aged 20 to 65, 36.4 percent were current smokers, 30.8 percent were former smokers (those who did not smoke in the 30 days before the survey), and 32.8 percent had never smoked. Of smokers, 48.9 percent smoked seven or fewer cigarettes a day and the remainder smoked more than seven cigarettes a day (Ministerio de Salud Pública 1990).

The CEIC/IESOP survey found that 39.6 percent of the residents of Quito were current smokers (52 percent of men and 28 percent of women), and that the prevalence of smoking was highest among persons in the middle socioeconomic stratum (41 percent) compared to those in the upper stratum (39 percent) and those in the lower stratum (35 percent). In the second largest city of Ecuador (Guayaquil), 33.8 percent of the respondents were current smokers (48 percent among men and 20 percent

among women). In this city, the prevalences of smoking among persons in the middle and low socioeconomic strata were essentially equal (34 percent); among those in the upper socioeconomic stratum, only 25 percent were current smokers. The survey also reported that 72 and 77 percent of Quito and Guayaquil smokers, respectively, began to smoke before age 18.

Among 400 residents of Quito surveyed by Zevallos in 1991 as part of the CEIC/IESOP survey, 47 percent had smoked at some time in their lives. Among smokers, 96 percent of men and 100 percent of women believed that smoking affects their health. Almost 90 percent of smokers aged 38 to 52 expressed a desire to quit while only 59 percent of persons 18 to 27 years expressed this desire (Zevallos 1991).

In the 1990 Quito survey of behavior and attitudes among residents aged 10 years and older, the prevalence of regular smoking was 22.7 percent; of occasional smoking, 26.5 percent; and of former smoking, 18.4 percent. Unfortunately, the results for persons aged 20 and older on this survey cannot be compared to the other surveys.

Among employees of the Ministries of Health and of Education and Culture, 70 percent were current smokers. However, this population again consists of working adults, most of whom are in the age groups with the highest smoking prevalences. Of these smokers, 54 percent began to smoke before age 19 years, but none did so earlier than age 12 years.

In the CLAP study of parturient women who visited a public maternity clinic, only 6 percent of these women smoked during the 6 months prior to their pregnancy.

Based on the recent data available, the prevalence of smoking among adults in Ecuador is approximately 35 percent, and it appears that most smokers smoke fewer than seven cigarettes per day. These levels are similar to those of other countries in the Andean subregion. The decreases observed since 1954 are remarkable. Additional information on smoking by socioeconomic status from the 1988 Ministry of Health survey, which is nationally representative, will be important in understanding the relationship between smoking and variables such as education, income, urban residence, etc.

Prevalence of Smoking among Adolescents

The 1981 to 1984 survey of adolescents in the schools of nine provinces conducted by the Comptroller General's Office found that the prevalences in the different provinces varied between 41 and 75 percent for occasional smoking, between 23 and 38 percent for habitual but not daily smoking, and between 0.5 and 15 percent for daily smoking. It was reported that 20 percent of the respondents had begun to smoke before age 12.

In the 1988 Ministry of Health survey, the average lifetime prevalence of ever smoking was 45.8 percent among all adolescents. The cumulative lifetime prevalence of ever smoking is 62.7 percent at age 19, and this is nearly identical to that among adults aged 20 to 65, in whom the lifetime prevalence was 67.2 percent. Even though this analysis does not involve the same cohort, there appear to be two critical ages for experimenting with cigarettes: between 10 and 11 years and between 13 and 14 years (Figure 1). In addition, there are differences in experimentation by sex. Of males aged 10 to 19 years, an average 46.1 percent had ever smoked, but only an average 25.3 percent of females had ever smoked. Overall, 14.8 percent smoked daily; of these, 62.2 percent smoked fewer than seven cigarettes daily.

Other uses of tobacco

The single survey that gathered data on other forms of tobacco use was conducted in Quito in 1990 (Ministerio de Salud Pública 1990). It was found that 1.3 percent of the respondents smoked cigars, 0.4 percent smoked pipes, and 0.9 percent used snuff, chewing tobacco, or rolled leaf.

Knowledge and attitudes about tobacco

The CEIC/IESOP survey asked respondents if they believed that cigarettes affected health. In Quito and Guayaquil, 94 and 95.5 percent, respectively, answered in the affirmative. When stratified by smoking status, 90 and 99 percent of smokers in Quito and Guayaquil, respectively, believed that smoking affects health "a great deal"; only in Quito did some respondents (2.6 percent) answer "not at all."

The 1990 Ministry of Health survey in Quito reported that 91.8 percent of respondents believed that cigarettes damage health. Asked the source of their information on this issue, 12.7 percent named a teacher, 14.4 percent named their family, 12 percent named a physician, 11 percent named a friend, and the rest named other sources.

The CEIC/IESOP survey asked the smokers why they smoked; the most common response was "for pleasure" (61.7 percent in Guayaquil and 46.4 percent in Quito). The remainder of those surveyed in both cities divided their responses between "because" (20.3 percent in Quito and 30.5 percent in Guayaquil) and "nerves" (13 percent in Quito and 4.7 percent in Guayaquil).

In the 1990 Quito survey (Ministry of Health 1990), 7.8 percent of those surveyed answered that

Figure 1. Smoking prevalence among adolescents by age, Ecuador, 1988

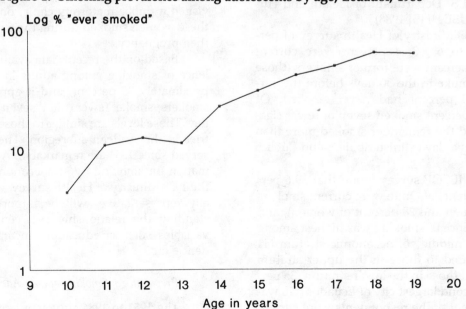

Source: Ministry of Health, 1988.

cigarettes produce benefits; when asked to specify the benefits, 82 percent responded "well-being," 8 percent responded "economic," and 10 percent responded "other." This survey also asked about attitudes toward smokers who smoke in enclosed places. Thirty-nine percent of nonsmokers responded that they "move away," 33.8 percent responded that they do not have any kind of attitude, 21.4 percent responded that they request the smoker not to smoke, and the remainder did not respond.

Smoking and Health

Morbidity

Since 1985, a cancer registry has been operative in Quito; the most recent available data from this registry are from 1988. During the 4 years of record keeping, the most frequent site for cancer incidence among men (excluding skin) was the stomach; lung cancer was the fifth most frequent site. In women, the most frequent site was the cervix, with lung cancer the fifteenth site in frequency.

The male-female ratio is 1:7 for lung cancer and 2:0 for bladder cancer.

Hospital discharge diagnoses can be used to understand the disease impact of smoking on medical care utilization. In 1987 and 1988, 13,246 discharges were due to diseases that may be associated with smoking, with a greater proportion of these diagnoses found among men (2.6 percent of total discharges). Among women, this proportion is much smaller because normal deliveries are included in the total (Table 4).

General Mortality Issues

In 1987, the estimated underregistration of deaths was approximately 30 percent (PAHO 1990). This underregistration estimate is greater in less developed parts of the country, and therefore the mortality structure for Ecuador reflects primarily the urban areas and more developed rural areas. In addition, with respect to mortality rates, underregistration may minimize certain conditions because the total population is included in the denominator.

Table 4. Hospital discharges for smoking-associated diagnoses and percentage (percent) of total by sex, Ecuador, 1987–1988

Causes	Both sexes		Men		Women	
	Discharges	%	Discharges	%	Discharges	%
Malignant tumors	1,879	0.20	1,258	0.41	621	0.10
Mouth and pharynx	145	0.02	79	0.03	66	0.01
Esophagus	204	0.02	154	0.05	50	0.01
Pancreas	374	0.04	211	0.07	163	0.03
Larynx	148	0.02	132	0.04	16	0.00
Lung	571	0.06	396	0.13	175	0.03
Bladder	244	0.03	178	0.06	66	0.01
Kidney	193	0.02	108	0.04	85	0.01
Circulatory system	9,425	0.99	5,602	1.83	3,873	0.60
Ischemic heart disease	3,491	0.36	2,244	0.73	1,247	0.19
Cerebrovascular disease	5,934	0.62	3,358	1.10	2,626	0.40
Lung disease	1,942	0.20	1,093	0.36	849	0.13
Chronic bronchitis	1,692	0.18	922	0.30	770	0.12
Emphysema	250	0.03	171	0.06	79	0.01
Total smoking-associated discharges	13,246	1.38	7,953	2.60	5,343	0.82
Total discharges *	956,595		306,418		650,177	

Source: INEC, Annual Report on Hospital Discharges, 1988.
* Includes normal deliveries.

The country's mortality structure has changed, with a reduction in total mortality from 1972 to 1987 (Table 5). There has been a substantial reduction in infectious disease mortality rates and an increase in mortality due to malignant tumors, diseases of the circulatory system, accidents, and perinatal diseases. The proportionate mortality due to malignancy more than doubled between 1972 to 1974 and 1985 to 1987. The mortality pattern in the period from 1972 to 1987 shows a trend toward causes associated with lifestyle, such as smoking and high dietary fat intake. Mosley (1990) has emphasized this shift in the mortality structure of developing countries as part of the demographic transition evident around the world. Considering that the prevalence of chronic diseases increases many years after changes in lifestyle occur, the effect of the increase in cigarette consumption described in the 1970s is understandably still not evident. It is probable that underdevelopment explains a greater proportion of deaths from diseases such as cervical cancer, gastric cancer, hypertensive disease, and hemorrhagic stroke.

Mortality Associated with Smoking

In 1984 to 1988, it was estimated that 25,933 (10 percent of total deaths) could be associated with cigarettes (Table 6). Even though the relative risks for cancers associated with smoking are higher than those for other diseases (USDHHS 1989), the proportion of these deaths among all smoking-related deaths is still low in Ecuador (1.3 percent overall). This is not surprising given the small proportion (3.8 percent) of the population aged 65 and above who are most at risk for death due to these diseases.

The specific mortality trends for lung cancer by sex among persons in two age groups (45 to 54 years and 55 to 64 years) may be considered a marker for the impact of past population exposure to cigarettes. Thus, trends in lung cancer mortality for these age groups will show the effects of smoking on successive generations of Ecuadorans. Men aged 55 to 64 years show a sustained increase in lung cancer mortality. The male-female mortality rate ratio varies inexplicably from 1968 to 1988, but

Table 5. Deaths, proportionate mortality, and age-adjusted mortality rates per 100,000 for selected causal groups, Ecuador, 1972 to 1987

	1972–1974			1978–1980			1985–1987		
	No.	%	Rate *	No.	%	Rate *	No.	%	Rate *
Infectious diseases (000–136,470–474,480–486)*	22,434	34	314.9	15,768	27.2	199.8	9,230.6	18	107.6
Malignant tumors (140–209)	2,308	3.5	41.3	3,273	5.6	43.4	4,569	8.9	48.2
Circulatory system diseases (400–404,410–414,420–429, 430–438,450–458)	5,798	8.8	101.1	6,974	12	95.6	7,980	15.6	82.6
Perinatal mortality (760–779)	2,455	3.7	31.7	3,105	5.4	42.9	3,017	5.9	43
Accidents (E810–E823, E800–E807, E825–E949)	3,487	5.3	55.2	4,650	8	60.8	4,739	9.2	49.8
Other defined causes	16,897	25.6	247.44	14,606	25.2	195.5	13,935	27.2	155.9
Symptoms and ill-defined conditions (780–796)	12,616	19.1	193.26	9,480	16.4	123.6	7,741	15.1	83.3
TOTAL	65,994	100	984.9	57,857	100	761.7	51,212	100	570.3

Source: PAHO, 1986; PAHO, 1990.
* Standardized to the 1960 Latin American population. 1972–1974 and 1978 ICD 8th Rev. 1979–1980, 1985–1987 ICD 9th Rev.

Table 6. Deaths and proportionate mortality (%) for selected diseases associated with smoking, Ecuador, 1984–1988

Related causes	Both sexes		Men		Women	
	Deaths	%	Deaths	%	Deaths	%
Malignant tumors	3,345	1.29	2,137	1.50	1,208	1.03
Mouth and pharynx	218	0.08	119	0.08	99	0.08
Esophagus	430	0.17	325	0.23	105	0.09
Pancreas	823	0.32	424	0.30	399	0.34
Larynx	165	0.06	137	0.10	28	0.02
Lung	1,279	0.49	874	0.61	405	0.35
Bladder	246	0.09	129	0.09	55	0.05
Kidney	184	0.07	129	0.09	117	0.10
Circulatory system	20,277	7.81	10,984	7.71	9,293	7.95
Ischemic heart disease	8,144	3.14	4,727	3.32	3,417	2.92
Cerebrovascular disease	12,133	4.68	6,257	4.39	5,876	5.02
Lung disease	2,311	0.89	1,353	0.95	958	0.82
Chronic bronchitis	1,837	0.71	1,013	0.71	824	0.70
Emphysema	474	0.18	340	0.24	134	0.11
Total smoking-associated deaths	25,933	9.99	14,474	10.15	11,459	9.80
Total deaths	259,508		142,550		116,958	

Source: INEC, 1988.

this variance may be due to the few cases among both men and women. The mortality rate among men is consistently almost three times that among women when 5–year grouped data are depicted. The increase in lung cancer mortality rates among men is shown clearly in these data also, but the change in lung cancer mortality rates among women is less well demonstrated. Among men and women aged 45 to 54, the mortality rate for lung cancer using 5–year grouped data shows a general increase with some periodic variability.

Tobacco Use Prevention and Control Activities

Government Activities

Policies and executive structure

Since 1986 the Division of Chronic Diseases in the Ministry of Health, through its mental health program, has had jurisdiction over tobacco-related issues. In 1988, the Ministry sponsored the National Survey of Drugs and Alcohol Prevalence (Aguilar 1990), and the Division prepared a report on smoking for the second PAHO subregional workshop in Caracas in 1986 (PAHO 1987).

On January 13, 1989, by decree of the Ministry of Health, the Interinstitutional Anti-Smoking Committee (CILA) was created. The following agencies participate in CILA: Ministries of Public Health, Education, Work, Social Welfare, Agriculture, and Industry and Trade; the Ecuadoran Institute of Social Security; SOLCA (Campaign Against Cancer Society, a semiprivate organization that conducts isolated antismoking activities); universities; churches; nongovernmental social organizations; and mass communications media. This Committee has proposed a National Anti-Smoking Campaign Plan which outlines a set of ambitious actions. These include establishing a specific organizational structure for tobacco-use prevention and control within the Ministry of Health, conducting investigations on different determinants of smoking, developing an economic policy on tobacco, developing an official institutional antitobacco educational policy, and strengthening existing tobacco-related legislation and regulations. At present, no budgetary resources have been allocated to the Ministry of Health to implement this plan; however, eight part-time staff members are working on the specific tasks. In 1989, CILA enjoyed technical assistance and financial support from PAHO.

Legislation

Article 99 of the Code of Health, issued in 1971, ordered the Ministry of Health to regulate cigarette advertising and to warn the public of the harmfulness of cigarettes (Government of Ecuador 1971). In 1973, Regulation No. 965 was implemented to support this Article; this regulation contained several provisions. First, cigarette packets must display the following warning:

"Attention: Smoking cigarettes is dangerous to your health. Ministry of Public Health of Ecuador"

Second, the same warning as well as the nicotine and tar yields of cigarettes should appear in all printed cigarette advertising. Third, the tar and nicotine yields of cigarettes manufactured in Ecuador periodically should be provided by the industry to the Ministry of Health. Fourth, direct advertising or promotion of cigarettes to children was prohibited in any form, and television advertising was prohibited before 7:30 p.m.; cigarette advertising must not be associated with sports or culture. The regulation established financial sanctions for noncompliance with these standards, but in practice the only provisions that are fulfilled are those about the warning on the packet and the restriction on television advertising. Apparently noncompliance with the other standards has not been addressed by the Ministry of Health. Information is not available about budget and personnel resources necessary for enforcement within the Ministry.

In 1987, a comprehensive tobacco-use prevention and control law was drafted for the Executive Branch of the Government. This law was vetoed because of its putative negative effect on free enterprise. In 1989, CILA prepared a new draft law, but as of 1990 it had not been discussed by the Congress of Ecuador.

School-based education

No direct instruction on smoking and health is required in the six primary-level grades in Ecuador. However, a framework for teaching this material exists in that subjects such as air pollution, environmental protection, and the importance of adequate ventilation for human health are included as a part of the natural sciences curriculum. In 1989, a pilot project named "The Program for Preventing the Use of Tobacco" was conducted in schools of the city of Portoviejo, Manabí Province, by the Ministries of Health and Education through the Interinstitutional Technical Office of Health Education (OTIDES), but the content and effectiveness of this program are not known.

Public information campaigns

The only media-based activity reported by CILA and the Ministry of Health is the World Health Organization's World No-Tobacco Day, celebrated in Ecuador each May 31st since 1989.

Taxes

The December 1989 ad valorem tax varied for different tobacco products. The rate is highest for cigarettes made with foreign or imported *tabaco rubio* (260 percent). Domestically produced filtered brands with special packaging are taxed at 240 percent, domestic filtered brands with conventional packaging at 220 percent, unfiltered domestic brands with conventional packing at 200 percent, filtered *tabaco negro* cigarettes at 70 percent, and unfiltered *tabaco negro* at 30 percent. The tax structure seems to impact the lower socioeconomic consumers least, because it is within this group that *tabaco negro* cigarettes are preferentially smoked. In fact, the Ministry of Finance observed that due to the low purchasing power of the population in 1989, consumption of unfiltered *tabaco negro* increased because of its low cost (Ministerio de Finanzas 1989). In a coherent tax policy linked to public health, these "more harmful" cigarettes should be taxed at a higher rate than *tabaco rubio* cigarettes; however, there is no such thing as a "less harmful" cigarette. The distribution of tax revenues from cigarettes in 1986 was as follows: 49.4 percent to the State Budget, 28.2 percent to FONPAR, and 22.4 percent to the National Program for Free Children's Medicine (Samaniego 1990).

Nongovernmental Activities

Medical schools, the Ecuadoran Lung Association, CEPAM (a women's organization), and several domestic pharmaceutical companies participate in public education and media activities on smoking and health. The "Our Young" Foundation, which emphasizes education against drug use, has supported behavioral research on smoking. Finally, the Seventh Day Adventist Church, as in other countries of the region, offers smoking cessation classes.

Summary and Conclusions

1. With respect to other Latin American countries, Ecuador displays intermediate smoking prevalences of approximately 36 percent among

adults and 14 percent among adolescents. Knowledge of the link between smoking and ill health is nearly universal among Quito and Guayaquil residents, but the social acceptability of smoking has not yet changed.

2. Two large transnational companies dominate an increasing domestic market for tobacco. These companies display aggressive marketing strategies, utilizing several favorable conditions: (1) advertising is permitted on television; (2) the cigarette tax policy enables market penetration into low socioeconomic strata and youth populations; and (3) there is flagrant noncompliance with and nonpunishment of infractions against existing antitobacco legislation.

3. Ecuador's nascent tobacco-use prevention and control organization (CILA) has developed ambitious plans and legislative initiatives. Due to the lack of political commitment and the scarcity of resources, the national effort has not yet been implemented. However, a structure and legislative framework for effective prevention of tobacco-related disease in a growing older population is in place.

References

AGUILAR, E. Prevalence of the improper use of alcohol, tobacco, and drugs in the Ecuadorean population. *Boletín de la OPS* 24(1):35–38, 1990.

CHAPMAN, S. WONG, W.W. *Tobacco Control in the Third World— A Resource Atlas.* Penang, Malaysia: International Organization of Consumers Unions. 1990.

CRUZ, J. Higiene mental y vicios sociales. *Archivos de Criminología y Neuropsiquiatría y Disciplinas Anexas.* 2a. época. Año II, No. 8:Oct-Dic, 1954.

DIARIO EL COMERICO. *Consumos Especiales.* Sección Economía. 5–XII. 1989.

GOVERNMENT OF ECUADOR. *Código de Salud.* Registro Oficial. DS 188–RO 158:8–11–71, 1971.

INEC. *Encuesta de superficie. Producción por muestreo de áreas.* Sistema Estadístico Agropecuario Nacional. Tomo I, p. 13, 1988.

LATIN AMERICAN CENTER FOR PERINATOLOGY AND HUMAN DEVELOPMENT (CLAP). Tabaquismo y embarazo: hay que ayudar a parar. *Salud Perinatal* 2(7):65–77, 1987.

MAXWELL, J. *The Maxwell Consumer Report: International Tobacco—Part One.* Richmond, VA: Wheat First Securities/ Butcher and Singer, 1989.

MINISTERIO DE AGRICULTURA Y GANADERIA. *Precios de los productos agropecuarios al nivel del productor.* Dependencia de Planificación, División de Estadística e Información. *Boletín* No. 14:110, 1988.

MINISTERIO DE FINANZAS. *Informe sobre el ingreso actual, cuentas especiales y transferencias del presupuesto del Estado—Año 1987.* Subsecretaría de Presupuesto, Quito, 1987.

MINISTERIO DE SALUD PUBLICA. Conocimiento y hábitos de consumo de tabaco, Quito. Informe preliminar, manuscrito inédito, Quito, 1990.

MOSLEY, W.H., JAMISON, J.T., HENDERSON, D.A. The health sector in developing countries: problems for the 1990s and beyond. *Annual Review of Public Health* 11:335–358, 1990.

PAN AMERICAN HEALTH ORGANIZATION. *Consumo de cigarrillos per cápita entre los adultos (1985).* Washington, D.C.: Pan American Health Organization, Programa de Tabaco o Salud. March 23, 1988.

PAN AMERICAN HEALTH ORGANIZATION. *Control del hábito de fumar. Segundo Taller Subregional.* Area Andina. Washington, D.C.: PAHO, 1987, p. 112.

PAN AMERICAN HEALTH ORGANIZATION. *Health Conditions in the Americas—1990 Edition.* Scientific Publication No. 524, Washington, D.C.: Pan American Health Organization, 1990.

PHILIP MORRIS INTERNATIONAL, INC. *The Activities of Philip Morris in the Third World.* Richmond, VA: Philip Morris International, Inc., April 1988.

SAMANIEGO, N. Country Collaborator's Report, unpublished data, Pan American Health Organization, 1990.

TABEA, A. *Oficio TB-105/88.* Para el Ministerio de Agricultura de Ecuador, December 28, 1988.

TOBACCO INTERNATIONAL. ASP on the move: Argentina, Ecuador now growing cigar leaf. *Tobacco International*, June 1:30, 1989.

U.S. DEPARTMENT OF AGRICULTURE. Tobacco, Cotton, and Seeds Division, Foreign Agricultural Service. No published tabulation. Washington, D.C., April 1990

U.S. DEPARTMENT OF HEALTH AND HUMAN SERVICES. *The Health Consequences of Smoking—Nicotine Addiction. A Report of the Surgeon General, 1988.* U.S. Department of Health and Human Services, Centers for Disease Control, Center for Chronic Disease Prevention and Health Promotion, Office on Smoking and Health. DHHS Publication No. (CDC) 88-8406. Rockville, MD, 1988.

U.S. DEPARTMENT OF HEALTH AND HUMAN SER-

VICES. *Reducing the Health Consequences of Smoking—25 Years of Progress. A Report of the Surgeon General, 1989.* U.S. Department of Health and Human Services. Centers for Disease Control, Center for Chronic Disease Prevention and Health Promotion, Office on Smoking and Health. DHHS Publication No. (CDC) 89–8406. Rockville, MD, 1989.

WORLD BANK. *World Development Report 1990—Poverty.* New York: Oxford University Press, 1990.

ZEVALLOS, J.C. CEIC/IESOP survey on tobacco use in Guayaquil and Quito, 1990. Unpublished data.

El Salvador

General Characteristics

The Tobacco Industry
    Agriculture
    Production, manufacturing, and total domestic consumption
    Advertising and promotion

Tobacco Use
    Per capita cigarette consumption
    Behavioral surveys

Smoking and Health

Tobacco Use Prevention and Control Activities
    Government structure and policies
    Taxation

Summary and Conclusions

References

General Characteristics

Located between Honduras, Guatemala, and Nicaragua, El Salvador occupies 21,000 km² in Central America. The native population includes Pipil and Lenca Indians, who are descended from Aztecs and speak Nahuatl or a Mayan dialect. Most of the estimated 5.1 million residents are mestizo. The population is young, with nearly 50 percent under 15 years old. The total fertility rate (4.9) is quite high (Table 1). Overall mortality declined from 10.8 per 1,000 population for the period 1980–1985 to 6.4 per 1,000 for 1985–1988. Thus, substantial future population growth can be anticipated.

El Salvador has been suffering serious social problems since the 1980s with a nearly decade-long civil war that caused "homicides and intentionally inflicted injuries" to be one of the five leading causes of death during this period (Pan American Health Organization [PAHO] 1990). The increased poverty that resulted from the war was exacerbated by a violent earthquake in the capital city, San Salvador, in 1986. The per capita gross national product ($US940 in 1988) declined 0.4 percent per year between 1965 and 1988 (PAHO 1990; World Bank 1989). More than 500,000 displaced persons are estimated to live within the borders of El Salvador, with numerous other refugees living in neighboring countries and the United States (PAHO 1990).

The Tobacco Industry

Agriculture

In 1988, 800 ha of tobacco representing 0.1 percent of arable land were planted in El Salvador (Dirección General de Estadística Agropecuaria 1989). This area is much smaller than the 2,376 ha (5 percent of arable land) planted in the 1979–1980 season (Ministerio de Planificación 1985) or the 3,000 ha in 1986 reported by Chapman and Wong (1990). During these years, tobacco production reached its highest historical level: 3,138 MT in 1980 (U.S. Department of Agriculture [USDA] 1990). A considerable decrease in production in 1980 and 1981 was accompanied by an increase in tobacco imports (from 400 MT in 1980 to 1,184 MT in 1981). Tobacco leaf production leveled off and tobacco exports decreased to 100 tons in 1983 to 1988. Most raw tobacco exported is to the United States. Both imports (mainly from Guatemala) and domes-

Table 1. Health and economic indicators, El Salvador, 1980s

Indicator	Year	Level
Population	1990	5.1 million
Life expectancy at birth (men)	(1985–1990)[a]	58.0
Life expectancy at birth (women)	(1985–1990)[a]	66.5
Total fertility rate per 1,000 women aged 15–44 years	(1985–1990)[a]	4.9
Crude mortality rate per 1,000 persons	(1985–1990)[a]	6.8
Infant mortality rate	(1985–1990)[a]	57.4
Illiteracy rate	(1985)[b]	28.0%
Real growth rate of GNP	(1980–1988)[b]	−0.4%
GNP per capita	(1988)[b]	$940

Sources: a) Centro Latinoamericano de Demografía, 1990.
b) World Bank, 1990.

tic consumption decreased during 1983 to 1988 (Table 2).

Despite this decline in production, the value added to the GNP by tobacco growing was approximately $US10.6 million (1988 value) during the period from 1980 to 1984 (1988 Ministerio de Planificación 1985).

Production, Manufacturing, and Total Domestic Consumption

Production and consumption data have been reported by the USDA (1990) and through the Maxwell Consumer Report (Maxwell 1990). Both sources indicate a recent decline in total consumption; Maxwell reports that 2.3 billion cigarettes were consumed in 1981 and only 1.4 billion in 1989. The USDA reports a decline from 2.5 billion to 1.9 billion during the same period. Total cigarettes manufactured gradually increased from approximately 2 billion cigarettes in the early 1970s to a peak of 2.5 billion in 1985. Cigarettes are sold in packages of 20 and also individually.

There are two tobacco manufacturing companies in El Salvador: Cigarrera Morazán, a subsidiary of British American Tobacco, and Tabacalera Centroamericana, a subsidiary of Philip Morris. Be-

Table 2. Production, imports, exports (in metric tons), of tobacco and total domestic consumption of cigarettes (in billions of units), El Salvador, 1978–1986

| Year | Raw tobacco (metric tons) | | | Total domestic consumption of cigarettes (billions of units) |
	Production	Imports	Exports	
1978	2,533	665	300	2.5
1979	3,183	600	200	2.5
1980	3,228	400	200	2.5
1981	2,016	1,184	356	2.5
1982	2,102	347	242	2.5
1983	1,763	657	177	2.5
1984	1,375	637	150	2.5
1985	1,256	600	130	2.3
1986	1,256	579	102	2.1
1987	1,394	300	100	1.9
1988	1,380	385	110	1.9

Sources: USDA, 1989; Maxwell, 1990.

ginning in 1979, 200 million cigarettes were imported annually in order to supply local market demands (USDA 1989). In 1989, Cigarrera Morazán had a 73.7 percent market share, down from the 87.7 percent share reported for 1984. Tabacalera Centroamericana increased its share of the domestic market during the same period (Maxwell 1990).

Advertising and Promotion

Tobacco advertising is permitted and used in all mass media. In 1988, legislation (Legislative Decree 955) restricted this advertising by prohibiting advertisement of either cigarettes or liquor during programs aimed at children on radio or television and in movie theaters. The Department of Mental Health had recommended stronger restrictions prior to the passage of this law (Urquilla-Milian 1988). Other means of promotion are also widely used and include billboards, transportation posters, tobacco industry contributions to sporting events and cultural activities, and distribution of free samples of cigarettes (Urquilla-Milian 1988).

Tobacco Use

Per Capita Cigarette Consumption

In the 1960s, annual per capita consumption of tobacco by persons aged 15 and older increased

substantially from less than 800 to almost 1,100 and then levelled off to about 1,000 cigarettes. (Figure 1). The apparent decrease in per capita consumption observed during the late 1980s is probably not so marked because a significant portion of the domestic market is now supplied via illegal trade in cigarettes. In fact, a smuggled package of cigarettes can be bought for half the price of a domestically produced package. Because it represents a loss of tax revenue, smuggling has become an issue of concern for local authorities; some control measures have been proposed (La Prensa Gráfica 1990).

In 1989, the average price per package was 5 colons ($US0.62), more than double that in 1985. Overall inflation averaged 16.8 percent per year from 1980 to 1988 (World Bank 1990); thus, the increase in price parallels that in the inflation rate. In El Salvador, the average salary for an 8-hour work day is 18 colons, or about 400 colons a month. This means that one pack of cigarettes accounts for one percent of the monthly wage, or approximately one-half the daily amount required for basic needs by an urban dweller in El Salvador (PAHO 1990).

Behavioral Surveys

Only one survey is available on tobacco use in El Salvador. In 1988, the Gallup Organization surveyed under the auspices of the American Cancer

Figure 1. Per capita cigarette consumption, El Salvador, 1964–1988 (population aged 15 and older)

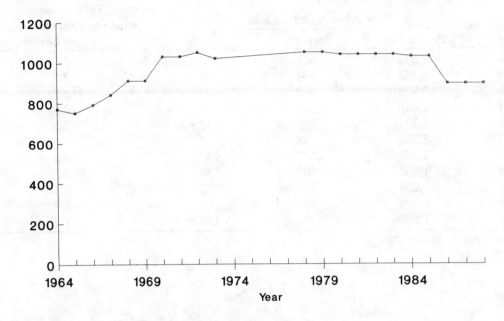

Sources: Lee, 1975 and USDA, 1990.

Society 1,300 urban residents for smoking behavior. A current smoker was defined as a person who had smoked at least 100 cigarettes during his or her lifetime (an ever smoker) and smoked at the time of the survey (Gallup 1988). Overall smoking prevalence was estimated at 25 percent, with a 38-percent prevalence among men and 12 percent among women. The highest smoking prevalence (28 percent) occurred among those aged 30 to 39. The current smoking prevalence was higher among those with higher incomes, except in the highest income stratum, which showed a lower prevalence than the national average. The prevalence of former smoking (defined as ever smokers who were not smoking at the time of the survey) was highest in this group (Table 3).

Smoking and Health

In El Salvador, only 46.5 percent of the deaths that occurred in 1983 were certified by a physician (PAHO 1986). In 1984, underreporting was estimated at 45 percent while 23 percent of all deaths reported were registered under "symptoms, signs, and morbid states" so that cause-of-death data are available on only 50 percent of the deaths in El Salvador (PAHO 1990).

Nonetheless, some indication of the effect of

Table 3. Prevalence (%) of smoking by age and family income, El Salvador, 1988

	Current smokers	Ever smokers
Total	25	8
Men	38	10
Women	12	5
Age		
18–29	24	4
30–39	28	9
40 and more	23	13
Family income monthly*		
less than 90	24	7
90–600	26	9
601–999	29	5
1,000 and more	20	10

Source: Gallup Organization Inc., 1988.
*In 1988 $US.

Table 4. Mortality rates (per 100,000 persons) for selected diseases associated with smoking, by sex and age, El Salvador, 1984

Cause of death (ICD-9 Code)	Age-adjusted rates[a]	Age group 35–44	Age group 45–54	Age group 55–64
Ischemic heart disease (410–414)				
Men	24.6	16.3	34.4	106.3
Women	14.3	7.5	25.9	47.7
Cerebrovascular disease (430–438)				
Men	20.7	8.9	24.9	80.8
Women	18.5	13.0	29.5	71.5
Malignant tumors of the lips, oral cavity, and pharynx (140–149)				
Men	0.6	2.0	0.7	3.2
Women	0.6	0.5	2.2	1.0
Malignant tumors of the trachea, bronchi, and lungs (162)				
Men	1.2	0.5	3.7	6.4
Women	0.6	0.5	0.7	2.0

Source: PAHO, 1990.

a) Rates adjusted by age to the entire population of Latin America.

smoking on the population of El Salvador can be appreciated. In 1984, the age-adjusted rate of ischemic heart disease among men was 24.6/100,000 and among women, 14.3/100,000. The mortality rate for lung cancer among men was 1.2/100,000 and 0.8/100,000 among women (Table 4). These low rates correspond with the higher smoking prevalence among men, and to a generally low population exposure to cigarettes in El Salvador.

Malignant neoplasms rank fifth as a cause of death, and cerebrovascular disease, ischemic heart disease, and bronchitis and emphysema rank sixth, seventh, and eighth, respectively. Together, these causes of death account for 14 percent of all registered causes of death (PAHO 1990).

Tobacco Use Prevention and Control Activities

Government Structure and Policies

The Department of Mental Health of the Ministry of Health and Social Welfare is responsible for smoking control activities, but has no specific budget for them. The department has made some efforts to disseminate information about smoking-related problems through conferences and sporadic television messages.

At the initiative of the Department of Mental Health, Resolution 451 was enacted in 1991. This resolution forbids smoking in the Ministry of Health buildings.

The 1988 health legislation (Código de Salud 1988) contains the above-mentioned restrictions on advertising of tobacco and alcohol to minors. In addition, the code also requires the warning "Smoking is hazardous to your health" to be printed on all packages of tobacco products, in a size specified as "not smaller than 1.5 millimeters." However, this regulation is currently under review by the Department of Mental Health. Smuggled cigarettes sold illegally would not display this warning.

Taxation

Of the total retail price of a package of 20 cigarettes, 42.5 percent is excise tax. El Salvador annually collects 98 million colons ($US20 million) in tobacco taxes. A proposal to reduce the excise tax to 35 percent of the retail price per package was considered in the Legislative Assembly in 1990. Apparently, of primary concern was the unfair competition posed by the illegal cigarette trade, primarily from Honduras, which provides cheaper cigarettes than those produced domestically. The Assembly rejected the proposal based on the fact that the

State would immediately lose 20 million colons ($US4 million) in annual taxes (La Prensa Gráfica 1990); the tax remains at 42.5 percent.

Summary and Conclusions

Tobacco as a public health problem in El Salvador has been far overshadowed by the devastation of civil war and social disruption experienced in the 1980s. Tobacco agricultural production has declined substantially, possibly as a result of the interruption of agriculture in general during this period. Although cigarette taxes generate significant revenue for the Government, the illegal trade in cigarettes has had a sufficiently negative impact on the tobacco industry to warrant efforts to decrease the tobacco taxes. In the context of national economic problems and a rising cost of living, illegal cigarette sales at cut-rate prices have permitted many smokers to maintain their tobacco use. Reported consumption data from countries such as El Salvador are systematically biased so that the apparent decline in per capita consumption since 1984 should be interpreted with caution. The level of per capita consumption is approximately one-half that reported for the United States.

The only survey of smoking behavior done in El Salvador, with unreported methodology and sampling frame, reported that more than one-third of men and over 10 percent of women are current smokers. The prevalence of ever smoking increases with income, suggesting that for urban residents, smoking is more common among men and among those with the most disposable income, a situation similar to that in most countries of the Americas. The limited mortality data available for El Salvador corroborate the much higher exposure of men compared with women and the overall lower exposure of the entire population compared with countries such as the United States and Canada where peak per capita consumption of tobacco occurred in the 1960s.

Little has been reported on nongovernmental actions against tobacco. No restrictions exist on smoking in public places or on minors' access to tobacco. There are apparently no educational activities or economic disincentives against tobacco in El Salvador. The Department of Mental Health forms the core of the minimal antitobacco program in El Salvador. Funding for such activities is scarce, and other pressing health problems have precluded the development of a comprehensive program.

Based on the information presented in this chapter, the following conclusions can be drawn:
1. El Salvador has endured a devastating 10-year civil war that has resulted in severe declines in both agricultural and industrial outputs. The tobacco sector has been no exception.
2. Reported consumption of tobacco products is distorted by a substantial illegal trade in cigarettes, primarily from Honduras. Overall smoking prevalence in certain urban areas is estimated at 25 percent.
3. The poor quality and coverage of death registration in El Salvador hinders an adequate description of mortality caused by smoking-related diseases.
4. Smoking as a public health problem has a low priority in El Salvador, which is reflected in a lack of both policies and programs against tobacco. Concern is slowly emerging through some legislative actions that mandate health warnings and restrict cigarette advertising to children.

References

CENTRO LATINOAMERICANO DE DEMOGRAFIA. *Boletín Demográfico.* CELADE, Santiago: Año XXIII, No. 45, 1990.

CHAPMAN, S., WONG, W.L. *Tobacco Control in the Third World: A Resource Atlas.* IOCU, Penang, Malaysia, 1990.

CODIGO DE SALUD. Diario Oficial 299(86):40–41, Mayo 11, 1988.

DIRECCION GENERAL DE ESTADISTICA AGROPECUARIA. *Anuario Estadístico Agropecuario.* Ministerio de Agricultura, El Salvador, 1989.

GALLUP ORGANIZATION INC. *The Incidence of Smoking in Central and South America.* Conducted for the American Cancer Society, April 1988.

LA PRENSA GRAFICA. Iniciativa de ley para bajar el impuesto al cigarrillo. Agosto 29, 1990, p. 2.

MAXWELL, J.C. JR. *The Maxwell Consumer Report: International Tobacco 1989, Part One.* Richmond, Virginia: Wheat First Securities/Butcher & Singer, Inc. WFBS-5455, May 18, 1990.

MINISTERIO DE PLANIFICACION. Indicadores Económicos y Sociales. Sección de Indicadores Económicos, Dirección General de Coordinación del Ministerio de Planificación, El Salvador, Enero-Diciembre, 1985.

MINISTERIO DE SALUD Y ASISTENCIA SOCIAL. *Salud pública en cifras, 1989*. Anuario No. 21, Unidad Estadísticas de Salud, 1991.

PAN AMERICAN HEALTH ORGANIZATION. *Health Conditions in the Americas, 1990 edition*. PAHO Scientific Publication No. 524. Washington, D.C., 1990.

UNITED STATES DEPARTMENT OF AGRICULTURE. Tobacco, Cotton, and Seeds Division, Foreign Agricultural Service, May 4, 1989 (unpublished data).

URQUILLA-MILIAN, E.A. El Salvador Country Report, in Control del Hábito de Fumar, IV Taller Subregional. Area de Mesoamérica. October 31–November 3, 1988, PAHO, unpublished manuscript.

WORLD BANK. *World Development Report 1989*. New York: Oxford University Press, 1989.

WORLD BANK. *World Development Report 1990—Poverty*. New York: Oxford University Press, 1990.

French Overseas Departments and Territories: French Guiana, Guadeloupe, Martinique and St. Pierre and Miquelon

General Characteristics

Several overseas territories and departments are included in the Republic of France. Although somewhat autonomous locally, these territories are administered centrally from Paris and are considered as parts of France that are located overseas, not colonies. A system of French law and Government services is applied, often with some local adaptations.

St. Pierre and Miquelon is a French territory located in the Gulf of St. Lawrence, just off the south coast of Newfoundland. St. Pierre and Miquelon is strategically important to the French fishing industry.

French Guiana, a large, sparsely populated department bordering on the Caribbean Sea, is located east of Guyana and Suriname. French Guiana has an area of 91,000 km², with a population density of one person per km². In 1989, the per capita gross national product (GNP) was estimated at US$3,370 (World Bank 1990). The major economic activities are shrimp processing and timber production.

Guadeloupe is composed of two main islands, Grande-Terre and Basse-Terre, which are separated by a narrow channel. However, several other smaller Caribbean islands, La Désirade, Marie-Gal-

ante, Les Saintes, St. Martin, and St. Barthélémy, are administratively part of Guadeloupe. In 1989, the per capita GNP was estimated at US$3,918 (World Bank 1990).

Martinique is located south of Guadeloupe and Dominica in the Windward Islands of the Lesser Antilles. Martinique is an island of 1,100 km², with a population density of 319 persons per km². In 1989, the per capita GNP in Martinique was US$4,075 (World Bank 1990). Martinique's major industries are tourism and oil refining; its major exports are refined petroleum products, bananas, rum, and pineapples (World Bank 1990; Encyclopedia Britannica 1990).

St. Pierre and Miquelon is the smallest of the French territories in the Americas, with a population of about 6,000 (Figure 1). French Guiana is significantly larger in geographic area than either of its sister Caribbean departments, Guadeloupe and Martinique, but the population of French Guiana is less than a third that of Guadeloupe or Martinique (approximately 90,000 vs. 338,000 vs. 330,000, respectively) (Figures 2, 3, and 4) (World Bank 1989). As shown in Figures 2 and 3, in 1985, a significant proportion of the population of Martinique and Guadeloupe was aged 10–24. This extraordinarily large cohort reflects the rapid rate of improvement in prevention of infant and childhood mortality

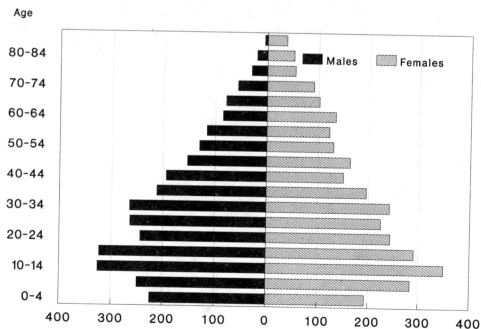

Figure 1. Population pyramid, St. Pierre and Miquelon, 1982

Source: United Nations, 1989.

Figure 2. Population pyramid, Martinique, 1985

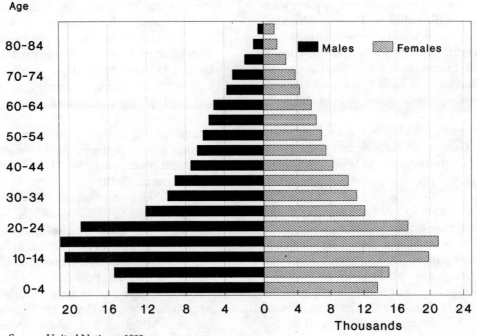

Source: United Nations, 1989.

that occurred in the 1960s (World Bank 1989). The decline in fertility since 1975 is indicated by the relatively smaller cohorts of individuals aged 0–9 (World Bank 1989). In French Guiana, although improvements have also occurred in prevention of infant and childhood mortality, by 1982 a decline in the number of births was not evident from the population pyramid (Figure 4). During the 1980s, it is likely that a large number of men aged 20 to 39 emigrated to French Guiana, creating the predominance of men in the population of those ages in 1982 (Figure 4).

In French Guiana, life expectancy at birth was estimated at 71 years in 1989. The literacy rate has been estimated at 73 percent, also in 1989 (World Bank 1990). In Guadeloupe during the 1970s and 1980s, life expectancy at birth steadily improved and the total fertility rate decreased. In 1988, life expectancy in Guadeloupe was estimated at 74 years, with 2.2 births per woman (World Bank 1989). In 1988, life expectancy at birth in Martinique was also 74 years and the total fertility rate was estimated at 2.1 births per woman (World Bank 1989). These and other social, health and demographic indicators for St. Pierre and Miquelon, Guadeloupe, Martinique and French Guiana are summarized in Table 1.

It is clear that deaths from infectious diseases among children and young people have largely been brought under control in the French Caribbean departments. With the improvements in life expectancy that took place in the 1980s, these departments can look forward to rapid increases in the proportion of the population over 45. This population will be vulnerable to a variety of chronic diseases, including smoking-related diseases.

The Tobacco Industry

Tobacco is not grown, and no tobacco products are manufactured in the four French departments in the Americas. All tobacco products are imported, mainly from the European Economic Community (EEC) (St. Pierre and Miquelon Préfecture 1989; Martinique Préfecture 1989; French Guiana Préfecture 1989).

Tobacco Use

In 1989 in St. Pierre and Miquelon, per capita tobacco consumption averaged 544 g (or 544 ciga-

Figure 3. Population pyramid, Guadeloupe, 1985

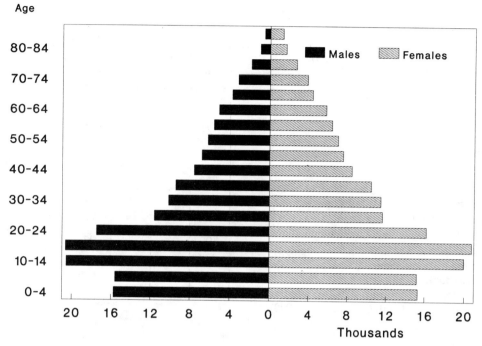

Source: United Nations, 1989.

Figure 4. Population pyramid, French Guiana, 1982

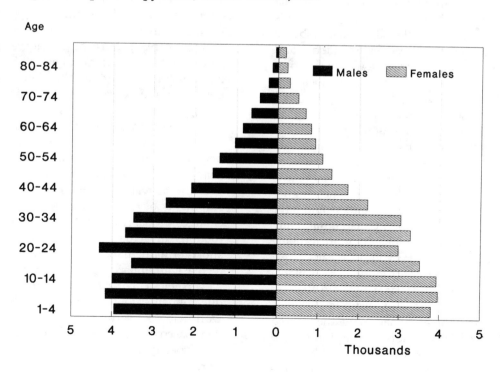

Source: United Nations, 1989.

Table 1. Selected demographic and health indicators for St. Pierre and Miquelon, Guadeloupe, Martinique, and French Guiana

	St. Pierre and Miquelon	Guadeloupe	Martinique	French Guiana
Population	6,000	320,000	330,000	110,000
Percent < 15[a]	27.0	30.7	29.8	32.6
Percent ≥ 65[a]	8.8	7.3	7.2	4.7
Total fertility rate[b]		2.2	2.1	
Crude birth rate[c]		21	18	27
Crude death rate[c]		7	7	6
Age-adjusted death rate[d]		4.2	3.3	5.6
Infant mortality rate[c]		13	11	21
Life expectancy, males[c]		70	71	68
Life expectancy, females[c]		77	77	75
Adult literacy rate (%)[c]		90	93	73

Sources: a: United Nations (1989).
b: World Bank (1989).
c: Encyclopedia Britannica (1990); World Bank (1990).
d: Pan American Health Organization (1990).

rette-equivalents) among the population aged 15 and older. In St. Pierre and Miquelon, sales of duty-free goods to visitors from neighboring Newfoundland, as well as other parts of Canada, traditionally have been an important economic activity. The sale of tobacco products is an important part of this duty-free trade. In 1989, of the 30,700 kg of tobacco products purchased duty-free in St. Pierre and Miquelon, a significant percentage was in the form of cigarettes compared with cigars and loose tobacco (22,500 vs. 300 vs. 7,900 kg, respectively). Duty-free purchases of tobacco products were almost 13 times higher than the domestic consumption of 2,400 kg (St. Pierre and Miquelon Préfecture 1989). It is probable that these duty-free tobacco products ended up in Newfoundland or other parts of Canada, where tobacco taxes are much higher than in St. Pierre and Miquelon. Some would have been legitimately imported into Canada, but many of these cigarettes and other tobacco products likely would have reached Canada by illegal means.

No data on tobacco consumption are available for Guadeloupe. However, data indicate that tobacco consumption in French Guiana in 1988 was comparable with that of Canada and the United States (2,543 cigarettes/person, among those aged 15 and older) (French Guiana Préfecture 1989; Kaiserman 1991). The Netherlands, France, and the United Kingdom were the main sources of im-

ported cigarettes for French Guiana (35, 35, and 24 percent, respectively) (French Guiana Préfecture 1989).

More complete data on trends in tobacco consumption are available for Martinique. In 1989, among those aged 15 and older, per capita consumption averaged 1,112 cigarettes (Martinique Préfecture 1989). Most of the cigarettes consumed were purchased from members of the EEC, including the United Kingdom, the Netherlands, France, Belgium, and Germany (Martinique Préfecture 1989); of the total cigarettes consumed in 1989, 40 percent were imported from the United Kingdom. Figure 5 shows long-term trends in annual adult per capita tobacco consumption in Martinique. Year-to-year fluctuations in consumption may reflect the arrival near the end of the year of large shipments of tobacco products; most likely, these changes probably do not reflect similarly large fluctuations in actual consumption. Apart from the short-term fluctuations, the data indicate an overall increase in tobacco consumption in Martinique. Nevertheless, per capita consumption in Martinique remains low compared with consumption worldwide (Kaiserman 1988). For example, per capita tobacco consumption in Canada was 2,700 cigarettes per person 15 and over in 1989 (Kaiserman 1991).

Few survey data on prevalence, attitudes, or

Figure 5. Per capita tobacco consumption in grams per person 15+, Martinique, 1956 to 1988

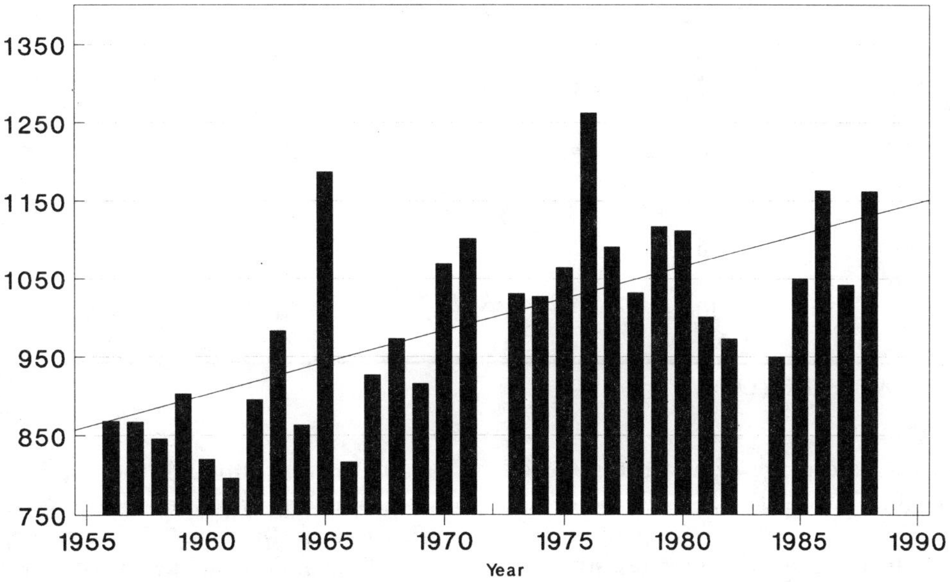

Sources: de Thoré, 1990; Martinique, 1989.

opinions on smoking are available for St. Pierre and Miquelon, or for any of the three French departments in the Caribbean.

However, in 1985–86, a survey was conducted on the health practices of individuals aged 11–13 attending school in the urban areas of French Guiana (Institute National de la Santé et de la Recherche Médicale [INSERM] 1986). Data from this survey indicated that significantly more boys than girls reported currently smoking, at least occasionally (7 vs. 2 percent, respectively).

Smoking and Health

Death registration and classification are not major problems in the Caribbean French departments. There are no indications of substantial problems of mortality under-registration, and the proportion of all deaths recorded as caused by symptoms and ill-defined conditions is lower than many other countries in the Caribbean and Central America. The proportions of all deaths due to symptoms and ill-defined conditions were 9.7 percent in Guadeloupe in 1981, 13.2 percent in French Guiana in 1984 and 11.1 percent in Martinique in 1985 (Pan American Health Organization [PAHO] 1990).

In all three Caribbean departments, chronic diseases and accidents account for all five of the leading causes of death. In Guadeloupe in 1981, the leading defined causes of death were heart disease (21.6 percent), malignant neoplasms (16.7 percent), accidents (12.7 percent), cerebrovascular disease (10.7 percent) and mental disorders (5.1 percent). In French Guiana in 1984, a similar pattern prevailed with the leading causes being heart disease (20.9 percent), accidents (14.7 percent), malignant neoplasms (12.5 percent), cerebrovascular disease (8.4 percent) and chronic liver disease and cirrhosis (6.1 percent). Chronic noncommunicable diseases were also the leading causes of death in Martinique in 1985, with the five leading defined causes of death being malignant neoplasms (22.3 percent), cerebrovascular disease (19.0 percent), heart disease (19.0 percent), accidents (7.7 percent) and diabetes mellitus (3.0 percent) (PAHO 1990).

No data are available on tobacco-related mortality for St. Pierre and Miquelon. In 1987, 25, 17, and 8 men compared with 6, 3, and 0 women died of lung cancer in Martinique, Guadeloupe, and French Guiana (INSERM 1989).

Trends since 1970 in lung cancer deaths compared with total deaths in Martinique are shown in Table 2. During 1970–87, the percentage of lung

Table 2. Total and proportionate lung cancer mortality, Martinique, 1970–87

| Year | Lung cancer deaths | | | Total deaths (Both sexes) | Percentage of deaths due to lung cancer (Both sexes) |
	Male	Female	Total		
1970	10	3	13	1953	0.67
1974	11	2	13	2296	0.57
1975	21	3	24	2190	1.10
1977	17	4	21	2155	0.97
1980	—	—	26	2109	1.23
1981	22	4	26	1873	1.39
1982	16	6	22	2070	1.06
1983	16	7	23	2034	1.13
1985	15	10	25	2140	1.17
1987	25	6	31	2007	1.54

Sources: de Thoré (1990); PAHO (1990).

cancer deaths as a percentage of all deaths more than doubled (0.7 percent vs. 1.5 percent, respectively).

Data are available from a tumor registry on the incidence of lung cancer for the entire population of Martinique. In a study of 63 incident lung cancer tumors registered in 1981–83, standardized incidence rates of lung cancer were lower than those observed in other Caribbean and American tumor registries for the same period (Table 3) (de Thoré 1990).

Tobacco Use Prevention and Control Activities

The French departments and territories located in the Americas are subject to French legislation. Regulations concerning tobacco advertising and promotion and the control of smoking in public places apply equally to the overseas territories and

Table 3. Age-standardized lung cancer incidence rates, selected tumor registries, 1980s

| Location | Incidence rates | |
	Male	Female
Martinique	11.5	1.0
Jamaica	19.8	4.0
Netherlands Antilles	30.2	3.9
Puerto Rico	16.3	5.4
Los Angeles, U.S.A. (White)	58.6	22.4
Los Angeles, U.S.A. (Black)	73.7	18.5

Source: de Thoré, 1990.

departments, although the application of tax laws varies among the territories and departments. St. Pierre and Miquelon, Martinique, Guadeloupe, and French Guiana have a "strong partial ban" on tobacco advertising (Roemer 1982). Advertising is permitted, with some restrictions, at points of sale, as well as in newspapers and magazines. Tobacco companies are prohibited from sponsoring events, except for auto racing. Passed in 1976, this ban contained loopholes that were exploited by tobacco advertisers, principally through the advertisement of matches and lighters that appear similar to cigarettes (Roemer 1986). The French National Assembly passed new legislation in 1990, effective January 1, 1993, banning all forms of tobacco advertising (Evin 1990; United Press International [UPI] 1990). This legislation will also prohibit the sale of cigarettes to minors, withdraw tobacco products from the consumer price index, and require stronger health warnings that read "seriously damages health," compared with the current warning, "abuse is dangerous." The regulation will also allow the Minister of Health to require other health warnings on the packages.

Smoking in schools, food stores, community recreation centers, elevators, and clinics and hospitals, with the exception of private rooms, is prohibited by French law. At least one-half of the seats on commercial flights must be designated as nonsmoking (Roemer 1982). However, these restrictions on smoking are not rigidly enforced. In French Guiana, for example, smoking is often observed in health care institutions (Diouf 1990). However, the new 1993 legislation bans smoking in all public places, except in the areas designated for smoking (Evin 1990; UPI 1990).

Tobacco taxation policy varies in the overseas French departments and territories from that in France. In France, approximately 75 percent of the retail price of cigarettes is tax, compared with approximately 52 percent in French Guiana (Townsend 1987, Douanes françaises, Guyane 1990). Requirements that cigarettes be sold only in licensed retail tobacconists do not apply in the overseas departments and territories. The location of retail tobacco sales is not restricted in any of the French territories in the Americas (de Thoré 1990; Diouf 1990).

Through the French Committee for Health Education, the French Government prepares a number of posters, pamphlets, and radio and television messages to encourage smoking cessation and the maintenance of a smoke-free lifestyle. Although distributed regularly to the overseas departments, these materials are used infrequently because they have not been adapted for the local population. For example, posters depicting Caucasian French models have little or no relevance in French Guiana, where the majority of the population is black (Diouf 1990). Because of the lack of financial support from central governments, local health promotion efforts to control smoking in the Caribbean departments range from minimal in Martinique (de Thoré 1990) to nonexistent in French Guiana (Diouf 1990).

Summary

The French departments and territories in the Americas are diverse in climate, ranging from sub-Arctic to tropical. Patterns of tobacco consumption are also diverse; per capita tobacco consumption in French Guiana is almost five times higher than that in St. Pierre and Miquelon. Data available for Martinique indicate a long-term trend of increased tobacco consumption from 1956 to 1988. In Martinique, the incidence of lung cancer has increased significantly during 1970–87 and has assumed greater relative importance as a cause of death. Nevertheless, lung cancer incidence for 1981–83 was the lowest recorded in the Caribbean, and one of the lowest worldwide.

Regulations prohibiting or restricting tobacco advertising and labeling and smoking in public places have been stricter than in most other Caribbean nations. However, enforcement of these laws has been erratic in metropolitan France, and may be even less effective in the overseas territories and departments, especially with respect to controlling smoking in health care institutions and public places.

Conclusions

1. High rates of tobacco consumption in French Guiana, and increasing rates of consumption in Martinique, in populations that will soon experience a rapid increase in the proportion of the population over 45 years of age presage a developing epidemic of tobacco-related death and disease.
2. New legislation, to come fully into effect on January 1, 1993, may establish comprehensive tobacco control policies and regulations in the French territories and departments as well as in France. Compliance with these actions may be problematic.
3. Monitoring of tobacco consumption in the French territories and departments could be improved by implementing regular household surveys of smoking prevalence.

References

DE THORE, J. Country Collaborator's Report, Martinique, unpublished data, PAHO, 1990.

DIOUF, M.A. Country Collaborator's Report, French Guiana, unpublished data, PAHO, 1990.

DOUANES FRANCAISES, GUYANE. Unpublished data, 1990.

ENCYCLOPEDIA BRITANNICA. *Encyclopedia Britannica World Data Annual 1990*. Encyclopedia Britannica. Chicago, 1990.

EVIN, C. Projet de loi relatif à la lutte contre le tabagisme et à la lutte contre l'alcoolisme, no. 1418. Assemblée Nationale. France, 1990.

FRENCH GUIANA PREFECTURE. Unpublished data, 1989.

INSTITUT NATIONAL DE LA SANTE ET DE LA RECHERCHE MÉDICALE. Behaviour and Health Survey of Pre-adolescents in French Guiana, unpublished data, INSERM, 1986.

INSTITUT NATIONAL DE LA SANTE ET DE LA RECHERCHE MÉDICALE. Annual Statistics of Medical Causes of Death, French Guiana, 1988, unpublished data, INSERM, 1989.

KAISERMAN, M.J., ALLEN, T.A. Global per capita consumption of manufactured cigarettes—1988. *Chronic Diseases in Canada* 11(4):56–57, July 1990.

KAISERMAN, M.J., COLLISHAW, N.E. Trends in Canadian tobacco consumption, 1980–1990. *Chronic Diseases in Canada* 12(4):50–52, July-August 1991.

MARTINIQUE PREFECTURE. Unpublished data, 1989.

PAN AMERICAN HEALTH ORGANIZATION. *Health Conditions in the Americas, 1990 Edition.* Pan American Health Organization, Pan American Sanitary Bureau, Regional Office of the World Health Organization. Scientific Publication No. 524, 1990.

ROEMER, R. *Legislative Action to Combat the World Smoking Epidemic.* World Health Organization, Geneva, 1982.

ROEMER, R. *Recent Developments in Legislation to Combat the World Smoking Epidemic.* World Health Organization, Geneva, 1986.

ST. PIERRE AND MIQUELON PRÉFECTURE. Unpublished data, 1989.

TOWNSEND, J. Price, tax and smoking in Europe. In: White, P. (ed.) *Tobacco Price and the Smoking Epidemic: Smoke-free Europe: 9.* World Health Organization Regional Office for Europe, Copenhagen, 1987.

UNITED NATIONS. *Demographic Yearbook 1988.* New York, 1989.

UNITED PRESS INTERNATIONAL. France to ban tobacco and alcohol and alcohol advertising by 1993. *United Press International Newswire.* December 13, 1990.

WORLD BANK. *The World Bank Atlas 1989.* Washington, D.C.: International Bank for Reconstruction and Development/The World Bank, November 1989.

WORLD BANK. *World Development Report 1990–Poverty.* New York: Oxford University Press, 1990.

Guatemala

General Characteristics

The Tobacco Industry
   Agriculture
   Manufacturing and production
   Marketing

Tobacco Use
   Per capita cigarette consumption
   Behavioral surveys and their limitations
   Prevalence of smoking among adults
   Prevalence of smoking among adolescents
   Other uses of tobacco and types of tobacco smoked
   Attitudes, knowledge, and opinions about smoking

Smoking and Health

Tobacco Use Prevention and Control Activities
   Government action
      Executive structure and policies
      Legislation
      School-based education and public information activities
      Taxes
   Action by nongovernmental agencies

Summary and Conclusions

References

General Characteristics

The center of the Mayan civilization in Central America during the pre-Columbian era, Guatemala still has a large native population descended from the Mayas. In 1981, 41.9 percent of the total population was Indian. Traditional cultural practices persist among these persons, and over 20 languages are spoken in addition to Spanish. Consequently, communication problems are common between Spanish-speakers and Indians, and almost half the population (45 percent) is illiterate (Table 1). Most (62 percent) of the 9 million inhabitants live in some 19,000 communities with populations of fewer than 2,000 each. These rural conditions influence the social structure, the health care delivery system, and the general health status of the country. Health and economic indicators (Table 1) reflect a high degree of poverty. The per capita gross national product (GNP) is one-twentieth that of the United States and continues to decline (0.3 percent per year). The most common causes of death in Guatemala are diarrhea, acute respiratory infections, and malnutrition (Pan American Health Organization [PAHO] 1990).

Of the total 1990 midyear population (9,197,345), 45 percent is less than 15 years old (Table 1a). The estimated total fertility rate for 1985 to 1990 is 5.8 births per childbearing-aged woman (Centro Latinoamericano de Demografía [CELADE]

Table 1. Health and economic indicators, Guatemala

Indicator	Year	Level
Population	1990	9,197,345*
Life expectancy at birth		
males	1985–1990	59.7 years*
females	1985–1990	64.4 years*
Overall fertility rate	1985–1990	5.8*
Infant mortality rate per 1,000 live births	1985–1990	58.7*
Illiteracy	1985	45%**
Real growth rate of GNP	1980–1988	−0.3%/year**
Per capita GNP $US	1988	880**

Sources: * Latin American Center for Demography (CELADE), 1990.
**World Bank, 1989.

Table 1a. Distribution of the population (percentage) by age and sex

Age	Men	Women
0–4	17.64	17.32
5–9	15.14	14.80
10–14	13.03	12.85
15–19	10.79	10.65
20–24	8.76	8.74
25–29	7.21	7.25
30–34	5.83	5.93
35–39	4.86	4.97
40–44	3.79	3.88
45–49	3.09	3.15
50–54	2.66	2.71
55–59	2.33	2.41
60–64	1.33	1.94
65–69	1.33	1.40
70–74	0.83	0.89
75–79	0.50	0.55
80 and older	0.39	0.47
Total	100.00%	100.00%
	(4,646,724)	(4,550,621)

1990). These data suggest that the population will be concentrated in younger age groups for many years. Thus, this country retains a health configuration characteristic of the less developed countries, and chronic diseases caused by tobacco have not yet emerged as major health issues.

The Tobacco Industry

Agriculture

Nine thousand ha are planted with tobacco in Guatemala. Most farms are located in the eastern and southern coastal regions of the country. Virginia and burley tobacco are grown in the east, while the crops in the south are mainly burley and aromatic or Turkish tobacco (Gremial de Fabricantes de Cigarrillos 1988). Tobacco growers rotate their fields to other crops after the seven-month tobacco-growing season.

In 1985, there were 1,190 registered tobacco growers in Guatemala. Approximately 16,500 persons were employed on a temporary or part-time basis in tobacco production, the equivalent of about 6,550 full-time workers. Tobacco provides employment for 2.2 percent of the agricultural work force in Guatemala (Agro-Economic Services and Tabacosmos 1987).

Tobacco production decreased from 7,006 MT

Table 2. Tobacco production, exports, and imports, Guatemala, 1959–1989 (in metric tons)

Year	Production	Exports	Imports
1959	1,569	0	269
1964	1,699	131	212
1969	1,890	890	371
1974	4,088	4,122	1,086
1979	7,006	4,600	800
1984	8,250	5,500	50
1989	6,537	4,801	158

Source: USDA, 1990.

in 1979 to 6,537 MT in 1989 (Table 2). Exports fluctuated minimally in response to foreign demand during this period (Mollinedo-Castillo 1988). Both production and exportation determine the quantity of tobacco available to the domestic market. Mollinedo-Castillo also reported that tobacco imports have declined as the quality of domestic tobacco has improved. The devaluation of the local currency and inflation also contributed to increased prices of imported cigarettes, thus making them inaccessible to the local population. A tobacco industry publication (Tobacco International 1989) reported that the area planted with tobacco increased in 1989, with production intended mostly for the export market (chiefly burley, which is exported to Japan, the United States, and Europe).

Manufacturing and Production

Two cigarette manufacturers operate in Guatemala, Tabacalera Centroamericana, S.A. (TACASA) and Tabacalera Nacional, S.A. (TANASA), as subsidiaries of the multinational tobacco companies Philip Morris and British American Tobacco, respectively. These manufacturers employ 1,480 persons, representing 2.0 percent of the country's industrial work force. Wages for these workers are equal to 109.4 percent of the average wage received by the entire industrial work force. Approximately 930 full-time workers are involved in the distribution of tobacco products (Agro-Economic Services and Tabacosmos, Ltd 1987).

Marketing

Most tobacco consumed in Guatemala is marketed as manufactured cigarettes, sold in packs of 20 and as individual cigarettes by street vendors. The 1990 price for a package of 20 domestic ciga-

rettes ranged from 2.25 to 4.50 quetzals ($US0.45 to $US0.90), while imported cigarettes sold for 4.5 to 6.0 quetzals ($US2.25 to $US3.00). Since the middle of 1990, packages of 10 cigarettes became available at one-half the price of 20-cigarette packs. There are no restrictions on the sale, promotion, or advertising of tobacco in Guatemala. All forms of mass media are used for advertising; other promotional activities by the tobacco companies include free tobacco samples and sponsorship of sports and cultural events.

Tobacco Use

Per Capita Cigarette Consumption

According to the 1990 Maxwell report (Table 3), per capita consumption of manufactured cigarettes declined by 61 percent between 1977 and 1988. The tobacco industry attributes this decline to a severe economic downturn within Guatemala during the 1980s and to the fact that the proportion of smokers among the growing native population is low compared with the Latino population (Tobacco International 1989).

Behavioral Surveys and Their Limitations

Guatemala City was one of the eight cities included in the 1971 PAHO study on smoking in

Table 3. Total and per capita adult cigarette consumption, Guatemala, 1976–1989

Year	Cigarettes (in billions)	Per capita consumption
1976	2.6	924.0
1977	2.7	940.0
1978	2.6	878.0
1979	2.5	856.0
1980	2.7	889.0
1981	2.2	675.0
1982	2.2	653.0
1983	2.1	603.0
1984	2.0	511.0
1985	1.9	447.0
1986	1.8	410.0
1987	2.0	430.0
1988	1.9	365.0
1989	1.9	na

Source: Maxwell, 1990.
na: not available.

Table 4. Surveys on tobacco performed in Guatemala and prevalence (percent) of current smoking by sex, 1971–1989

Survey	Year	Population surveyed	Sample size	Prevalence Men	Prevalence Women	Prevalence Both
National survey on smoking (Arango)	1989	Urban areas, ≥ 15 years old	7,372	37.8	17.7	26.8
National survey on tobacco and alcohol (DGSS)	1982	Guatemala City >10 years old	2,403	53.4	29.8	47.0
Knowledge about tobacco and its effect on health (Rojas-Espino)	1989	Employees of the Office of Public Finance	350	48.2	38.4	44.0
Smoking prevalence among students and faculty of the School of Medicine (Morales)	1987	Students and teachers of the medical school San Carlos University	170	34.0	36.0	34.4
Smoking in Latin America (Joly)	1971	Guatemala City	1,401	36.2	10.1	21.5

Latin America (Joly 1977). Since 1971, several other surveys of adult tobacco use have been completed, including another Guatemala City adult survey in 1982, a national urban adult survey in 1989, and two surveys of specific population groups (Table 4). The 1971 Guatemala City survey (Joly 1977) and the 1989 national survey of urban areas (Arango 1989) are the only population-based surveys of adult tobacco use. The National Survey on Tobacco and Alcohol targeted commercial, industrial, and educational establishments listed in a special directory. In this survey, an establishment was randomly selected from the directory, and all of the employees were interviewed on site (Dirección General de Servicios de Salud [DGSS] 1982). In addition to data on tobacco use, this survey asked if respondents felt they were well-informed as to the health issues associated with smoking. The study of faculty and students at the School of Medicine collected data not only on smoking behavior but also on knowledge, attitudes, and beliefs about tobacco and health (Morales 1987). A 1983 survey by the U.S. Centers for Disease Control (CDC) focused on women of reproductive age (15 to 44 years of age) (Anderson 1985); the results of this survey are not included in Table 4 but will be described later in this chapter.

Prevalence of Smoking among Adults

Joly (1977) reported an overall prevalence of current smoking of 21.5 percent among adults aged 15 to 74 years in Guatemala City. The overall preva-

lence of current smoking among urban adults reported on the 1989 National Survey on Smoking was 26.8 percent (Arango 1989). The 1982 survey of employed adults in Guatemala City reported a much higher overall prevalence of smoking than the other two studies (47.0 percent overall), but this difference in prevalence may be due to differences in the sampling frame rather than differences in the actual population prevalence of current smoking (DGSS 1982). The study of Treasury Department employees reported a similar prevalence of current smoking (44.0 percent overall) (Rojas-Espino 1989). These latter two surveys interviewed only persons with regular incomes, and who therefore had the ability to purchase consumer goods such as cigarettes. Morales (1987) reported an overall current smoking prevalence of 34.4 percent among students and faculty of the San Carlos University School of Medicine. This contrasts sharply with the prevalence of smoking among U.S. and Canadian physicians (less than 10 percent) reported by Pierce (1991). Further, it is remarkable that the prevalence of smoking among women in this well-educated population was similar to that among men (36 vs. 34 percent).

Between 1971 (Joly 1977) and 1989 (Arango 1989), the prevalence of current smoking among men remained relatively unchanged (from 36.1 to 37.8 percent) (Table 4). Among women, the prevalence of current smoking increased from 10.1 percent to 17.7 percent during this period. The inclusion of other Guatemalan cities in the 1989 survey may limit the comparability of these data, but it is likely that the actual 1989 prevalence in Guatemala City, especially among women, is higher than that reported for all urban areas. This is also suggested by the results of the 1982 survey of employed active persons in Guatemala City (DGSS 1982). It is likely that the prevalence of smoking among employed persons has increased substantially over the last two decades, at least in Guatemala City. It is also likely that the percentage of women who have become "economically active" increased during this period, thus facilitating smoking patterns more representative of men in previous decades.

Among men aged 20 to 24 years, 56.8 percent were current smokers in 1982 and 34.1 percent were current smokers in 1989. The prevalence of current smoking among men in middle age groups (25 to 49) was 56.4 percent in 1982 and 51.8 percent in 1989, but the prevalence among men above age 50 was approximately 30 percentage points lower than among younger men in 1982 (39.5 percent) and increased to 40.9 percent in 1989 (DGSS 1982; Arango 1989). In 1971, the prevalence of current smoking was 24.2 percent among men aged 15 to 24 years, and 45.6 percent among men aged 40 to 54. In the United States, the prevalence of smoking among men aged 65 years is substantially lower than among younger men due to increases in quitting and to differential mortality among smokers in older age groups. In poorer countries such as Guatemala, the decreased economic capabilities among older persons might also differentially affect smoking among these persons.

Joly (1977) reported that in 1971 the prevalence of smoking among women did not differ significantly by age in Guatemala City. Among women aged 25 to 39, the prevalence of current smoking was 11.9 percent; among women aged 40 to 54, 13.5 percent; and among women aged 55 to 74, 11.8 percent. In the 1982 study, however, the prevalence of current smoking among economically active women was highest (35.9 percent) in the 25 to 39 year age group compared with women aged 40 to 54 (21.3 percent) and women aged 55+ (10 percent). According to the 1989 urban survey, the highest prevalence among women (25.5 percent) was in the 25 to 34 year age group (Arango 1989).

In 1983, the nationwide CDC survey of 3,670 reproductive-aged women (15 to 44 years) reported an overall 6.6-percent prevalence of current smoking (Anderson 1985). The prevalence of current smoking was higher for older women (35 to 44 years) than for younger women (15 to 19 years) (9.8 vs. 4.4 percent). The prevalence of smoking among women with a secondary or higher level of educa-

tion was higher than for those with less educational attainment (9.4 vs. 5.2 percent). This study also reported that 4.3 percent of pregnant women were current smokers, as were 12.5 percent of women who used oral contraceptives. The prevalence of current smoking was higher among pregnant or contraceptive-using women with higher educational attainment (8.6 and 15.9 percent, respectively).

The current smoking prevalence rates for women from the 1971 (Joly 1977) and 1983 (Anderson 1985) studies are similar. However, the overall prevalence of current smoking among urban women (10.9 percent) reported by the CDC differs significantly from the results of the 1982 and 1989 surveys, which reported that the prevalence of smoking among urban women of reproductive age was 26.1 percent and 16.1 percent, respectively. The disparities are in part due to sampling differences. Another possibility is that the prevalence of smoking for women in Guatemala City was much higher than for urban women in general in 1983 and increased significantly between 1983 and 1989. However, the tobacco industry reported a drop in overall consumption between 1980 and 1988 (Maxwell 1990).

Discussion of the association between smoking and profession will be limited mainly to men because relatively few women in Guatemala are employed. According to the 1989 national urban survey (Arango 1989), agricultural laborers had the highest prevalence of current smoking (61.5 percent). The level was lowest (21.4 percent for men and 2.3 percent for women) among the native population (n=368). The prevalence among day-laborers was 56.7 percent; among skilled workers, 18.8 percent; and among public employees, 35.6 percent.

The 1982 survey reported a variable relationship between level of occupation and current smoking prevalence: 51.6 percent among technical workers, 48.8 percent among unskilled workmen, 47.4 percent among skilled workmen, and 42.9 percent among professionals.

The 1989 and the 1982 surveys reported similar prevalences for students (21.2 and 27.7 percent, respectively).

In 1982, most smokers (65.1 percent) reported smoking between one and five cigarettes per day, a low level of consumption similar to that observed in 1971, when 62.0 percent of men and 82.6 percent of women reported smoking between one and nine cigarettes per day. Approximately 25 percent of the smokers interviewed in 1971 reported that they had started smoking before age 16.

Table 5. Prevalence (percent) of ever smoking among adolescents, by age and sex, Guatemala, 1982 and 1989

Age group	Boys		Girls		Both		N	
	1982	1989	1982	1989	1982	1989	1982	1989
10–14	14.1	12.1	4.9	3.4	12.9	8.5	99	25
15–19	25.9	31.3	19.2	8.2	24.1	20.9	176	319

Sources: DGSS, 1982; Arango, 1989.

Prevalence of Smoking among Adolescents

Even though few adolescents were interviewed in the surveys summarized in Table 4, some observations can be made based on the data for 1982 and 1989 (DGSS 1982; Arango 1989) (Table 5). The prevalence of smoking among those younger than 20 years is higher among men than among women. The prevalence of smoking is significantly higher for persons in the 15 to 19 year age group compared with persons in the 10 to 14 year age group, suggesting that the onset of tobacco use occurs in the late teenage years. The populations sampled in both surveys represent economically active, employed persons. Thus, these data are not representative of the general adolescent population in Guatemala, but do describe smoking behavior among adolescents with the highest disposable incomes.

Other Uses of Tobacco and Types of Tobacco Smoked

The prevalence of pipe and cigar smoking was so low in the 1971 survey of eight Latin American cities that specific data on each city were not reported. Of all respondents, only 1 percent reported smoking a pipe and 1.6 percent reported smoking cigars.

In Guatemala City, 74.4 percent of male smokers and 83.4 percent of female smokers stated that they smoked only light tobacco, while 12.7 percent of males and 9.9 percent of females smoked only dark tobacco. Almost all smokers (89.4 percent of males and 92.8 percent of females) smoked filter cigarettes (Joly 1977). A marketing report (Maxwell 1990) indicated that the consumption of dark tobacco has decreased in Guatemala since 1976, accounting for only 2.1 percent of overall tobacco consumption in 1989.

Attitudes, Knowledge, and Opinions about Smoking

The respondents to the 1982 survey of employed persons were asked whether they considered themselves to be well-informed, somewhat informed, or uninformed as to the issue of tobacco and health. As expected, a high percentage of men and women (21.8 and 16.7 percent) with higher levels of education considered themselves to be well-informed (DGSS 1982). Among those with lower levels of educational attainment, the percentage of persons who considered themselves to be well-informed was much lower (12 and 0 percent for men and women, respectively).

In the Rojas-Espino survey (1989), Treasury Department employees were asked questions to assess their level of knowledge concerning the health risks of smoking. Those responding correctly to 16 to 20 questions were rated as well-informed, those responding correctly to 11 to 15 as average, and those with 10 or fewer correct responses were rated as having a low level of knowledge on tobacco and health. Nonsmokers rated higher than smokers, although the majority of those interviewed (64 percent of smokers and 56 percent of nonsmokers) were classified as having a low level of knowledge. These results should be interpreted with caution since they depend to a great extent on the validity of the questions asked. No description of the survey methodology or validation procedures is available.

"Level of knowledge" is a difficult concept to measure because measurement depends on the researchers' opinion of what the respondents should know and, concomitantly, on the validity of the questions. A survey of faculty and senior-year students (n=170) at the Universidad de San Carlos School of Medicine demonstrated the difficulties in assessing knowledge about tobacco (Morales-Linares 1987). The survey used a five-level scale of knowledge based on the percentage of correct responses. If 20 percent or fewer of the responses were correct, the respondent's knowledge was ranked as "none"; if 80 percent or more of the questions were answered correctly, the respondent's knowledge was ranked as "excellent." Based on survey data, 53 percent of the students and 52 percent of the teachers had a "poor" level of knowledge (between 21 percent and 40 percent of the questions answered correctly). No respondent answered more than 60 percent of the questions correctly. The sample was too small to draw any meaningful conclusions about the respondents' level of knowledge and their smoking status.

In summary, based on several small attempts to obtain information on Guatemalans' knowledge of the health risks of smoking, the level of their knowledge about the risks of smoking appears to be relatively low, especially among smokers.

Smoking and Health

The infant mortality rate in Guatemala is 59 per 1,000 live births and the life expectancy at birth is 63 years, suggesting that most deaths in Guatemala occur before age 15. An analysis of the impact of smoking on health should concentrate on the adult population aged 35 and older. However, the quality and availability of mortality data pro-

hibit analysis of the relationship between smoking and mortality. For example, 10.4 percent of deaths in 1984 were attributed to ill-defined symptoms, signs, and conditions. This designation was most common for deaths among persons younger than 5 years or older than 64 years. In addition, underreporting of mortality in 1984 was estimated by PAHO to be 18.1 percent (PAHO 1990). Thus, mortality analyses should be approached with caution.

Mortality from ischemic heart disease (IHD) increased substantially between 1981 and 1984, especially among younger men and women (Table 6). This increase may simply reflect better mortality reporting, although an upward trend in IHD mortality was observed prior to 1981. In 1974, the overall mortality rate for IHD was 5.6 per 100,000 for both sexes, and this level is 10 percent lower for men and 7 percent lower for women than levels reported in 1981. By 1984, these rates had doubled. Mortality from cerebrovascular disease and malig-

Table 6. Mortality due to selected diseases associated with smoking, according to sex and age, Guatemala, 1981 and 1984 (rates per 100,000 inhabitants)

Cause of death (ICD-9 Code)	Year	Age-adjusted rates*	Age group		
			35–44	45–54	55–64
Ischemic heart disease (410–414)					
Men	1981	9.7	6.9	21.3	35.8
	1984	21.9	14.8	31.5	73.9
Women	1981	7.1	3.8	5.2	28.8
	1984	13.9	12.4	25.2	26.9
Cerebrovascular disease (430–438)					
Men	1981	14.7	11.2	15.7	51.8
	1984	14.3	2.5	16.6	51.8
Women	1981	13.5	6.7	19.0	31.7
	1984	16.8	12.4	16.8	51.4
Malignant tumors of the lips, oral cavity, and pharynx (140–149)					
Men	1981	1.0	1.6	2.6	4.4
	1984	0.6	1.2	1.7	—
Women	1981	0.6	—	1.7	6.5
	1984	0.3	1.2	—	—
Malignant tumors of the trachea, bronchus, and lung (162)					
Men	1981	1.4	—	1.7	5.8
	1984	0.5	—	1.7	2.5
Women	1981	0.6	0.3	0.4	2.9
	1984	1.3	1.2	—	4.9

Source: Pan American Health Organization 1986 and 1990.
*Rates adjusted by age to the entire population of Latin America.

nant neoplasms remained relatively unchanged. However, the reported rates represented few events and may not present a clear picture of the trends in mortality for these diseases. From 1969 to 1984, the mortality rates for chronic bronchitis decreased from 37.7 to 8.3 per 100,000 in men and from 31 to 7.8 per 100,000 in women. These decreases may in part reflect control of infectious processes that precipitate death due to chronic bronchitis. During the same period, the mortality rate for all infectious diseases decreased from 21.8 to 6.9 per 100,000 for men and from 16.9 to 6.0 per 100,000 for women. Overall mortality has decreased over the last 20 years in Guatemala. As the chief cause of mortality, infectious disease, is controlled, the proportionate mortality due to chronic diseases will likely increase (PAHO 1988).

In Guatemala, several agencies provide health care. In general, health care is the responsibility of the Ministry of Public Health and Social Assistance, but the Guatemalan Institute of Social Security provides health care for insured workers and their families. In addition, the municipalities and the army also provide services to their constituents. As chronic diseases become more common, the health care system will undoubtedly be further overextended because of the increasing costs of health care for these diseases.

Tobacco Use Prevention and Control Activities

Government Action

Executive structure and policies

Tobacco control activities are the responsibility of the Ministry of Public Health and Social Assistance's Mental Health Department; no dedicated office covering tobacco and health has been established because of the lack of staff and budget resources. In practice, the only specific antitobacco action is guided by the National Anti-Smoking Commission. Of the 20 members serving on this voluntary coalition, 8 are Government officials, 8 are representatives of medical associations (primarily the Guatemalan Association of Physicians and Surgeons), and 4 are members of voluntary agencies (NGOs). Commission functions include public education and information, compilation of data, clinical research, governmental consultation, coordination with other agencies, and international liaison (Medina 1990).

Legislation

As of 1990, three legal measures to control smoking had been introduced in Guatemala. The first is the requirement that all cigarette packages manufactured in Guatemala display the following warning:

**"Use of this product is harmful
to your health"**

There is no requirement as to what percentage of the package's surface the warning should occupy; therefore the warning is not readable due to the small print placement, and color used. The second measure is part of the Public Transport Regulations, which bans smoking on buses. Finally, although it is more a general occupational safety measure than an intervention to reduce smoking, the Labor Health and Safety Regulation Act prohibits smoking in places where there is a danger of explosion. According to presidential directive No. 681-90 of August 3, 1990, smoking is prohibited in various places. However, there are no mechanisms for enforcement of the directive, and thus it applies mostly to government offices (Ministerio de Salud Pública y Asistencia Social 1990).

School-based education and public information activities

The National Anti-Smoking Commission is formulating a plan to introduce into the school curriculum an educational module that would cover the health effects of smoking and support prevention among young persons. Thus far, no uniform antitobacco education is provided in educational institutions. Sporadic programs related to smoking and health have appeared in the electronic and print media.

Taxes

Tobacco products accounted for 2.03 percent of the Government's total tax revenue in 1987. Although the gross amount of tax revenue has increased, the relative percentage of tobacco taxes (as part of overall taxes) has decreased since 1986 (Table 7). Taxes comprise seven percent of the average price of a pack of cigarettes in Guatemala (1989). In addition, the value added tax adds 100 percent to the price of each carton of cigarettes (10 packs of 20 cigarettes each).

Table 7. Estimated taxes collected on the sale of tobacco products and percentage of total taxes that are tobacco taxes, Guatemala, 1981–1987

Year	Tax on tobacco products	Percentage of total taxes
1981	20,587.1	3.154
1982	22,755.0	3.634
1983	24,515.4	4.279
1984	22,951.3	4.609
1985	32,539.3	4.790
1986	34,990.6	3.148
1987	47,023.6	2.034

Source: Medina, 1990.

Action by Nongovernmental Agencies

The most active NGO in tobacco and health issues is the National Anti-Smoking Commission, which originated with the Guatemalan College of Physicians and Surgeons. In addition, a Youth Subcommission of the National Anti-Smoking Commission organized the First Youth Congress on Smoking in 1990. The objectives for this congress were to provide incentives, instruction, and training to encourage the young people of Guatemala to be smoke-free (Medina 1990). During a 1–day session, discussions and presentations were conducted with various youth groups, educators, and youth leaders on issues related to smoking and health.

Summary and Conclusions

Tobacco agriculture in Guatemala is based on small-scale farmers who usually rotate their crops for part of the year. Thus, they are not totally dependent on tobacco for their survival. Overall, the tobacco agricultural and manufacturing sectors employ only 2.0 percent of the country's total work force. Tobacco production has expanded over the past 5 years, although this expansion apparently has been directed to the export market. Domestic consumption has fallen during this period as the buying power of Guatemalans decreased.

The domestic market is divided equally between a Philip Morris subsidiary and the British American Tobacco subsidiary. Both companies promote their products throughout the media and use a variety of advertising strategies. There are no legal restrictions on advertising and promotion of tobacco products in Guatemala.

Several surveys have been carried out in Guatemala to assess the prevalence of smoking. They differ greatly in methodology, most notably in the sampling frames. A 1971 PAHO survey of Guatemala City residents reported that the prevalence of current smoking was 36.2 percent among men and 10.1 percent among women. A 1989 survey covering all urban areas reported a similar prevalence (37.8 percent) among men and an increased prevalence (17.7 percent) among women. These data suggest that the percentage of urban women who are smokers has increased but the prevalence of smoking among urban men has remained relatively stable in the the last two decades. A nationally representative CDC survey of reproductive-aged (15 to 44 years) women reported a current smoking prevalence of 6.6 percent overall and 10.9 percent for urban areas. In this survey, it was found that women who used oral contraceptives had a higher prevalence of current smoking than those who did not.

Minimal data on knowledge, attitudes, and practices regarding smoking in Guatemala are available from several surveys. The level of knowledge about the health consequences of tobacco use reported in these surveys was in general somewhat low, but it is difficult to generalize the results of these surveys to the entire population.

The mortality data in Guatemala suggest that the impact of smoking on diseases such as lung cancer, cardiovascular disease, and chronic obstructive pulmonary disease has not yet become evident. Although the mortality rate for ischemic heart disease increased between 1981 and 1984, the mortality rates for respiratory disease and lung cancer remained relatively low.

Legislation to control tobacco advertising and the access to tobacco by minors is essentially nonexistent. Government involvement in tobacco prevention and control is limited to participation in the National Anti-Smoking Commission. This coalition depends on the voluntary efforts of its membership; it receives the most substantive support from nongovernmental organizations. It is, however, one of the few functional national coalitions against tobacco in Central or South America. This coalition could eventually provide the structure for an effective tobacco control campaign. It has already begun to provide leadership in the area of school education.

Based on the data presented above, the following conclusions can be drawn:

1. Tobacco growing and cigarette manufacturing are not of major economic importance to Guatemala in terms of employment and tax revenue. These activities employ 2.0 percent of the work force and contribute 2.03 percent of the nation's tax revenue.

2. Per capita consumption of tobacco in Guatemala declined more than 50 percent between 1981 and 1989.

3. The prevalence of current smoking changed very little among urban men between 1971 and 1989 but appears to have increased among urban women during this period.

4. Guatemalan women with a higher level of education have a higher prevalence of smoking than those with less education. Women who use oral contraceptives have a higher prevalence of current smoking than those who do not.

5. The effects of smoking on health have not been analyzed sufficiently in Guatemala. It is difficult to interpret mortality statistics because of ongoing problems with data quality and the low number of adult deaths.

6. The Government's involvement in controlling smoking is quite limited, and legislative actions are uncommon except for a presidential directive which limits smoking in public places. However, a voluntary national coalition against smoking includes Government representatives and may serve as the nucleus for an effective tobacco prevention and control program if resources become available.

References

AGRO-ECONOMIC SERVICES LTD, and TABACOS-MOS LTD. *The employment, tax revenue and wealth that the tobacco industry creates.* September 1987.

ANDERSON, J.E. Smoking during pregnancy and while using oral contraceptives. Presented at the International Conference on Smoking and Reproductive Health, San Francisco, October 1985.

ARANGO, L. Encuesta nacional de tabaquismo. Comisión Nacional de Lucha contra el Tabaco (resultados no publicados), 1989.

CENTRO LATINOAMERICANO DE DEMOGRAFIA. *Boletín Demográfico.* CELADE, Santiago: año XXIII, No. 45, 1990.

DIRECCION GENERAL DE SERVICIOS DE SALUD.

Encuesta sobre alcohol y tabaco, División de Programación; Departamento de Estadística; Dirección General de Servicios de Salud (publicación interna), 1982.

GREMIAL DE FABRICANTES DE CIGARRILLOS. *El Tabaco: su importante aporte al desarrollo socio-económico de Guatemala,* 1988.

JOLY, D.J. *Encuesta sobre las características del hábito de fumar en América Latina.* Organización Panamericana de la Salud, Publicación Científica No. 337, Washington, D.C., 1977.

MAXWELL, J. *The Maxwell Consumer Report,* International Tobacco 1989, part one, May 1990.

MEDINA, R.L. Country collaborator's report, Guatemala. Unpublished data, Pan American Health Organization, 1990.

MINISTERIO DE SALUD PUBLICA. Acuerdo Gubernamental No. 681-90, August 3, 1990.

MOLLINEDO-CASTILLO, E.V., ESCOBAR de JUAREZ de MINERVA, B.L., LEAL-LOPEZ, M.L., CASTILLO-RIVERA, A.F. *Cultivo de Tabaco.* Tesis, Facultad de Ciencias Ecoómicas, Universidad de San Carlos, Guatemala, 1988, pp. 52–102.

MORALES-LINARES, J.C. *Tabaquismo: determinación de la prevalencia y el grado de información sobre tabaquismo en estudiantes y docentes de la facultad de Ciencias Médicas de la Universidad de San Carlos.* Tesis. Facultad de Ciencias Médicas, Universidad de San Carlos, Guatemala, 1987.

PAN AMERICAN HEALTH ORGANIZATION. *Las condiciones de salud en las Américas 1981–1984.* Publicación Científica No. 500, Organización Panamericana de la Salud, Washington, D.C., 1986.

PAN AMERICAN HEALTH ORGANIZATION. *Evolución de la mortalidad en las Américas (1968–1987):* Guatemala, 1988, pp. 404–419.

PAN AMERICAN HEALTH ORGANIZATION. *Las condiciones de salud en las Américas.* Scientific Publication No. 524, Organización Panamericana de la Salud, Washington, D.C., 1990.

PIERCE, J.P. Progress and problems in international public health efforts to reduce tobacco usage. *Annual Review of Public Health* 12:383–400, 1991.

ROJAS-ESPINO, N.J. *Conocimiento sobre tabaquismo y daños a las salud.* Tesis. Facultad de Ciencias Médicas, Universidad de San Carlos, Guatemala, 1989.

TOBACCO INTERNATIONAL. *Guatemala: economy up; cigarette sales to follow.* June 1, 1989.

WORLD BANK. *World Development Report 1989.* New York: Oxford University Press, 1989

Guyana

General Characteristics

Although located on the north central coast of the South American mainland, Guyana is considered a Caribbean nation. Covering a total land area of 215,000 km², Guyana is divided into 10 regions. More than 80 percent of the population lives on the coastal plains that comprise 5 percent of the land area; the remainder live in rural communities in the highlands and savannahs of the interior. In 1986, the population was estimated at 756,072. According to the United Nations Economic Commission for Latin America and the Caribbean (ECLAC), 28 percent of the total population resides in five urban areas: Georgetown, New Amsterdam, Linden, Corriverton, and Rose Hall (ECLAC 1987). Formerly a British colony, Guyana is now a cooperative republic within the Commonwealth (Pan American Health Organization [PAHO] 1990).

The decline in the prices of sugar and bauxite, Guyana's two main exports, during the late 1970s led to a steady decline in the economy (PAHO, 1990). In 1989, the per capita gross domestic product (GDP) was $US207, less than 50 percent that of 1988 ($US476) (ECLAC 1990). The largest contributors to the GDP are agriculture, mining, and manufacturing, which account for more than 50 percent of the GDP and employ 45 percent of the labor force.

Since 1980, changes in economic conditions have prompted increased emigration at an average rate of 8,500 persons per year or more than 1 percent of the population for the period 1986 to 1989 (Statistical Bureau 1988). These emigrants have been mainly young professionals and skilled persons: 65 percent of emigrants were aged 15 to 34 years and the male:female ratio was 1:1.2. This, together with a birth rate that decreased from 33.7 per 1,000 population in 1970 to 23.8 per 1,000 population in 1986, has resulted in a population growth rate that has declined steadily from 3.25 percent per year in 1960 to 0.78 percent per year in 1986 (PAHO 1990).

Comparison of the age distribution of the 1980 population with the results of the 1986 GUYREDEM survey and mid-year estimates for 1990 shows a still young but slowly aging population (PAHO 1990, ECLAC 1987). Persons less than 15 years old comprised 33 percent of the 1990 population, compared with 37 percent in 1986 and 40 percent in 1980. There was a corresponding increase in the proportion of the population in the 25 to 44 year age group, from 21 percent in 1980 to 25 percent in 1985 and 29 percent in 1990, that represents a growing reservoir for later development of chronic diseases, including those related to tobacco use.

All demographic data must be interpreted very cautiously. The size and terrain of the country militate against the routine collection of accurate vital events data, a situation exacerbated by the lack of physical and manpower resources.

The Ministry of Health is responsible for improving and protecting the health of the Guyanese population. This is done through 4 regional hospitals, 5 specialized hospitals, 20 district hospitals, 159 health centers, and 15 health posts. In addition, 7 private hospitals and 16 dispensaries are owned by the sugar corporations (PAHO 1990).

For the 83 percent of the population living along Guyana's coastal area, health care is fairly accessible. Care to the 10 percent of the population living in the hinterlands is provided by mobile services and community health workers, usually nurse-midwives and medics. The promotion of primary health care has been the goal of the health authorities. Therefore, access to care may be illustrated better by the number of preventive health care workers relative to the population: per 10,000 population, there are 9.8 nurses, 5.1 midwives, and 1.6 medics (PAHO, 1990). This severe shortage of human resources in the public sector has resulted from emigration.

There has been a gradual deterioration of the health status of the people of Guyana (Table 1). The crude death rate has increased from 7.1 in 1979 to 7.98 in 1986. During the same period, infant mortality increased from 33.5 to 49.0 per 1,000 live births (PAHO, 1986 and 1990).

The Tobacco Industry

Agriculture

In 1989, 385 ha of land, or 0.23 percent of the total cropland, was under tobacco cultivation; 200 ha of this land was individual farm holdings while the remaining 185 are owned or leased by the Demerara Tobacco Company (Demtoco). Of the total labor force of 270,000, 400 individuals (0.15 percent) are employed in the tobacco industry, including 100 of the 25,000 total farmers (0.4 percent) (Ministry of Health 1990).

Demtoco plans to improve tobacco production by increasing the acreage under cultivation, by means of a provisional lease of 1,250 ha of farm-

Table 1. Basic health and demographic indicators, Guyana, 1979 and 1986

Indicator	1979	1986
Crude birth rate (per 1,000 population)	27.2	23.8
Total fertility rate (per woman)	3.8	2.8
Crude death rate (per 1,000 population)	7.1	7.98
Infant mortality rate (per 1,000 live births)	33.5	49.0
Life expectancy at birth		
(male)	NA	65.8
(female)	NA	70.9

Sources: PAHO, 1986; PAHO, 1990.
NA   Not available.

land. This lease supplements a 1984 grant of 809 ha from the Government of Guyana (Demtoco, 1988). Financial support in the form of lines of credit, release of foreign exchange, and relaxation of import restrictions for acquisition of machinery and supplies is provided through Government authority. However, foreign exchange is in very short supply in Guyana, a nation heavily in debt.

The only tobacco company in Guyana has 30 percent local ownership and 70 percent ownership by the multinational British American Tobacco Company Limited. Tobacco farmers are retained by the firm, supplied with tools and materials at cost (including wood for curing), and paid a set price based on the grade of tobacco produced (Guyana Chronicle 1988). The company provides its farmers with medical, educational, and transportation support services. In some cases, farmers are allowed to homestead.

Manufacturing, Marketing, and Taxation

Demtoco manufactures and packages filter-tip, king-sized, Bristol cigarettes, the only legal brand on the market. It is estimated that at least 50 percent of the domestic market is supplied by some 14 foreign brands, imported illegally from Brazil and Suriname. These brands, including Topten, Ronhill, Buckingham, and Champion, are not subject to consumption tax because of their illegal source, and they are therefore sold at a lower price than the Bristol cigarettes (GUY$13 vs. GUY$20). The result has been a substantial decrease in the sale of Bristol cigarettes, from 478,000,000 in 1988 to 265,700,000 in 1989, despite claims that smokers prefer Bristol (Guyana Chronicle 1989). The decline in overall national economic activity also may have decreased purchases of cigarettes.

The tobacco industry does not contribute significantly to either the manufacturing or agricultural sectors of the economy, accounting for less than 2 percent of the GDP. In an effort to reduce the dependence on foreign exchange for importation of tobacco, Demtoco has been increasing local production. In 1989, 150,000 kg, or one-third of the tobacco needed for cigarette manufacture, was grown locally. The tobacco industry does not generate foreign exchange, and difficulty in obtaining foreign exchange for purchase of new equipment and parts for maintenance has hampered expansion plans. However, the company has embarked on a diversification program to grow fruit and vegetables for local and overseas markets. These measures would improve the efficiency of land utilization during out-of-crop periods, as well as help to generate foreign exchange (Demtoco 1988).

Tobacco Use

There have been no surveys on tobacco use in Guyana. Cigarette production was used initially to estimate per capita cigarette consumption; however, the drastic decline in production reported for 1989 could be explained only by the influx of foreign brands on the market (Guyana Chronicle 1989) (Figure 1). Given that in 1980, Demtoco's production of 550,000,000 cigarettes represented 75 percent of the market, consumption at that time may be estimated at 1,100 cigarettes per adult aged 15 and older. If the 1989 production of 265,700,000 cigarettes represented 50 percent of the domestic market, then consumption per adult (1,050) has not changed significantly. The legitimate cigarette market was $US6.1 million in 1989 while the illegal supply was estimated at an additional $US3 million (Ministry of Health 1990).

Smoking and Health

Because of the remoteness of some communities, reporting of vital events, especially deaths, may be delayed by months or even years. Further, the person attending and/or reporting the death may not be medically qualified. This situation raises doubts about the completeness of the data and about the accuracy of the reported cause of death. The fact that the category "signs, symptoms

Figure 1. Cigarette production, in millions of cigarettes, Guyana, 1980–1989

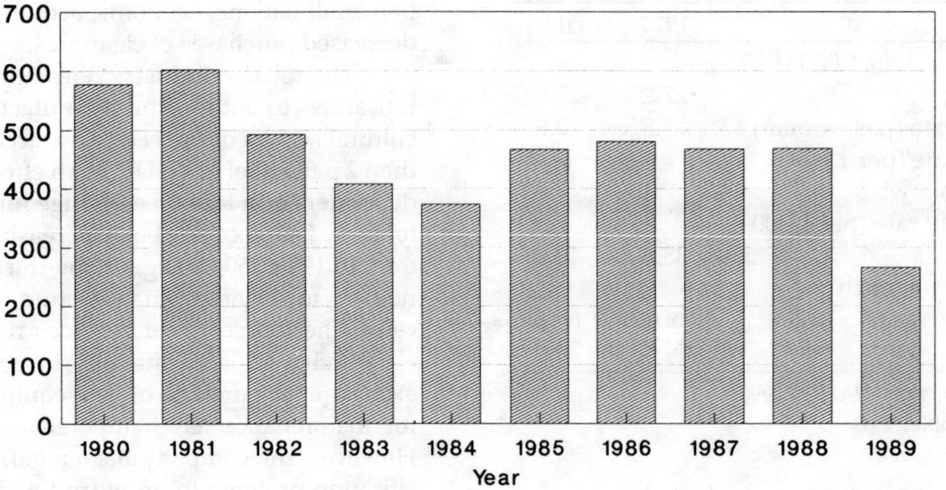

Source: Guyana Statistical Bureau

and ill-defined conditions'' was the third leading cause of death in Guyana, accounting for one-tenth of all deaths, endorses this concern (PAHO 1990). The last year for which mortality data by cause are available is 1984. At that time persons trained in coding cause of death were on the staff of the Ministry of Health.

If ''signs, symptoms and ill-defined conditions'' are excluded, the pattern of mortality has changed little during the past 7 years (Table 2). Figure 2 demonstrates the similarity of proportionate mortality due to diseases that may be caused by smoking. The apparent increase in proportionate mortality from diabetes and other causes may be an artifact of the relatively poorer quality of the 1979

data, when benign neoplasms reputedly caused as many (and sometimes more) deaths than malignant ones.

In 1984, of an estimated total 6,000 deaths, 28 were attributed to chronic obstructive pulmonary disease (COPD) and 14 to lung cancer. The numbers and rates of these and other tobacco-related diseases are much lower than prevailing rates in Canada and the United States (Table 3). A long history of lower smoking prevalence, younger age structure, and problems of mortality reporting in Guyana could all contribute to these lower rates of smoking-related disease. This may change, however, as the large cohorts of young adults under age 35 mature into middle age. If there are substantial

Table 2. Five leading causes of death, Guyana, 1979 and 1984

Causes of death	1979		1984	
	Rank	% of total*	Rank	% of total*
Signs, symptoms and ill-defined conditions		13.2		10.8
Deaths from defined causes		100.0		100.0
Diseases of the heart (398–429)	1	16.4	1	20.5
Cerebrovascular diseases (430–438)	2	14.0	2	13.7
Accidents (E800–E949, E980–E989)	3	2.7	3	7.5
Malignant neoplasms (140–208)	5	1.0	4	6.6
Nutritional deficiencies	not ranked		5	5.8

Sources: PAHO, 1986; PAHO, 1990.

*Percent by cause based on total number of deaths from defined causes.

Figure 2. Proportional mortality by age and sex, Guyana, 1979 and 1984 (selected causes)

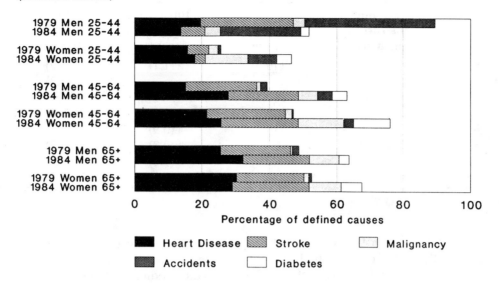

Sources: PAHO, 1986; PAHO, 1990.

proportions of smokers in these cohorts, increases in rates of smoking-related diseases can be expected.

The Caribbean Epidemiology Center (CAREC) has suggested that there is a difference in the effects of cigarette smoking among people of the Caribbean subregion due to dietary and genetic factors (CAREC 1977).

In a study during the 1970s of patients with chronic expectoration (the frequency of which

ranged up to 14 percent, depending on sex, age, location, and ethnic group), it was noted that the majority of cigarette smokers manifested little more than a life-long tendency to cough and phlegm (Miller and Ashcroft 1971; Miller 1974). The few patients who do develop COPD are of similar age and as susceptible to hypoxia and right heart failure as COPD patients in industrialized countries.

With the exception of cerebrovascular disease in the 45 to 54 year age group, there is a substantially higher proportion of deaths due to tobacco-related diseases among males than females aged 35 to 65 years or older (Table 4). Mention is made of occasional cases of fatal lipoid pneumonia with cor pulmonale, due to smoking tobacco flavored with mineral oil in Guyana.

Tobacco Use Prevention and Control Activities

Guyana has no departments or special programs for tobacco use prevention and control; smoking appears not to be considered a priority health problem. No official or legislative controls or restrictions exist with respect to the use of tobacco or its promotion.

The levy of a 100 percent consumption tax on the sale of cigarettes has probably contributed to a curtailing of sales of Bristol cigarettes (Stabroek News 1989; Guyana Chronicle 1988), although this was not the purpose of the levy. The cigarette tax revenue of $US300,000 in 1989 represented 35 per-

Table 3. Crude death rates per 100,000 population for selected tobacco-related diseases, Guyana, Canada, USA, last available year

Cause	Guyana (1984)	Canada (1988)	USA (1987)
Bronchitis, emphysema, and asthma (490–493)	5.2	8.9	9.2
Other respiratory diseases (010–012, 480–487)	19.6	26.0	29.1
Cancer of the lung (162)	1.6	50.2	53.4
Cancer of the respiratory tract (140–149)	0.3	5.3	4.5
Malignant neoplasms of other sites (rest of 140–208)	27.7	139.1	145.0

Source: PAHO, 1990.

Table 4. Numbers of deaths and proportionate mortality of tobacco-related diseases by age and sex, Guyana, 1984

Age	Sex	Chronic obstructive lung disease	Lung cancer	Tobacco-related cancers	Coronary heart disease	Cerebro-vascular disease
35–44	Male	—	1 (0.5)	2 (1.1)	15 (8.2)	18 (9.8)
	Female	—	—	—	5 (5.3)	4 (4.2)
45–54	Male	—	1 (0.4)	—	38 (13.8)	42 (15.3)
	Female	—	1 (0.6)	1 (0.6)	9 (5.1)	39 (22.0)
55–64	Male	3 (0.7)	3 (0.7)	4 (0.9)	52 (11.8)	104 (23.7)
	Female	4 (1.2)	—	1 (0.3)	14 (4.2)	58 (17.2)
65+	Male	15 (2.4)	6 (1.0)	6 (1.0)	81 (12.9)	155 (24.8)
	Female	6 (0.9)	2 (0.3)	1 (0.2)	36 (5.6)	150 (23.4)

Source: Unpublished data, Ministry of Health 1990.

cent of all consumption taxes in Guyana in that year (Ministry of Health 1990). However, both the primary purpose and the secondary effect of the levy may be defeated by the illegal trade in cigarettes.

No restrictions on tobacco advertising have been established, and cigarette advertisements appear on radio, in newspapers, on billboards, and on posters. There is also indirect advertisement through sponsorship of sporting and cultural events and an active projection of Demtoco's benevolent corporate image. For example, Demtoco donated $US1,500 to the New Amsterdam Hospital for rehabilitation. The company also sponsors scholarships for deserving high school students.

No legal restrictions exist concerning tobacco use or sales, and health warnings are found only on the illegally imported brands. No restrictions prohibit smoking in health facilities, on public transport, at worksites, or in restaurants. In movie theaters, smoking is permitted only in lobbies. Although students are not permitted to smoke in school, teachers may smoke (Ministry of Health 1990).

Any antismoking campaigns and other tobacco control activities usually are instigated by international health organizations, although executed by the Health Education Unit of the Ministry of Health. These campaigns include the ''Great American Smokeout'' of the American Lung Association and ''World No-Tobacco Day'' of the World Health Organization. These focus each year on the ill effects of smoking on health, particularly among pregnant women and unborn children. Unfortunately all of the information used in these campaigns relates to developed countries. A program has been organized by the National Coordinating Council for Drug Education to contribute teaching material to the school curriculum. Tobacco prevention education is included in the material being developed by the Council (Ministry of Health 1990).

Lack of information on the prevalence of tobacco use and its ill-health effects, combined with a national perception that smoking is not a priority health problem, serves to create an environment that is not conducive to the introduction of tobacco control interventions. However, since there are active campaigns against alcohol and drug abuse, it may be possible to use these as vehicles for the promotion of nonsmoking. Additionally, enforcement of the levy on foreign brands may reduce consumption (Ministry of Health 1990).

Summary

The Guyanese economy experienced a substantial decline during the 1980s, with implications in all sectors. Many of the country's skilled persons, including health workers, have emigrated. Shortage of foreign exchange has hindered acquisition of drugs and maintenance of medical equipment, thereby making curative medicine more difficult and expensive. In such an economic climate, disease prevention is particularly important, especially for tobacco-related diseases.

The economic changes have also affected the industrial and agricultural sectors, including the tobacco industry. The turnover of farmers and an inability to maintain existing machinery or procure new equipment have severely hampered the viability of the industry. The promise of development of self sufficiency in tobacco has not been realized. The tobacco industry imposes a net drain on

Guyana's scarce foreign exchange reserves, both for tobacco leaf and tobacco manufacturing machinery.

Another negative aspect of the tobacco industry is the use of wood for curing. Although Demtoco has initiated a reforestation project, it is not known what the effect will be of the time lag between destruction and regrowth.

Despite the shortage of money in the economy, personal expenditure on tobacco is staggering. One pack of cigarettes represents a half-day's wage. Total national expenditure is equivalent to half a million man-months. Estimated per capita consumption of cigarettes did not decrease between 1980 and 1989.

A possible argument in favor of tobacco growing may be the generation of employment, but even this argument is spurious because less than 0.15 percent of the labor force is employed in the industry.

When the economic drain caused by tobacco production and consumption is considered together with an unknown expenditure in tobacco-related health costs, $US5 million in foreign exchange to generate the local equivalent of $US3 million in revenue, and potential environmental damage due to deforestation, there arises a grave disparity between negative and positive outcomes of tobacco use. However, until the actual consumption can be determined and until there is more reliable data to indicate otherwise, the common perception that tobacco-related disease is not a current priority health problem is understandable. Continuing effectiveness in discouraging tobacco consumption now will prevent the development of a future epidemic of tobacco-related diseases.

Conclusions

1. Although the public health burden of smoking is difficult to estimate, several health indicators including crude mortality and infant mortality rates show a worsening of health status since 1979. Preventing smoking-related diseases is particularly important under such conditions.
2. A negative balance of trade for the tobacco industry is reported for Guyana. Hard currency is thus exported to maintain smoking among Guyanese.
3. An extensive illegal trade in cigarettes facilitates sustained per capita consumption of cigarettes at low prices in Guyana.

4. International health organizations and the National Coordinating Council for Drug Education provide some antismoking interventions in Guyana.

References

CARIBBEAN COMMISSION. Population Census of the Commonwealth Caribbean—Guyana, Volumes 1 and 2. 1980–1981.

CARIBBEAN EPIDEMIOLOGY CENTER. Cigarette smoking and chronic obstructive lung disease in the Caribbean. *CAREC Surveillance Report* 3(6):1–3, June 1977.

DEMERARA TOBACCO COMPANY LIMITED. 1988 Annual Reports & Accounts. 1988.

GUYANA CHRONICLE. Demtoco effects $302,000 (US) savings annually. 1988.

GUYANA CHRONICLE. Lowering of tax could keep 'Kings' on the market—Demtoco. 1989.

GUYANA STATISTICAL BUREAU. *Quarterly Statistical Abstract*. 1988.

MILLER, G.J. Cigarette smoking and irreversible airways obstruction in the West Indies. *Thorax* 29(5):495–504, September 1974.

MILLER, G.J., ASHCROFT, M.T. A community survey of respiratory disease among East Indian and African adults in Guyana. *Thorax* 26(3):331–338, May 1971.

MINISTRY OF HEALTH. Country Collaborator's Report, Guyana, unpublished data, PAHO, 1990.

PAN AMERICAN HEALTH ORGANIZATION. *Health Conditions in the Americas, 1981–1984*. Pan American Health Organization, Pan American Sanitary Bureau. Scientific Publication No. 500, 1986.

PAN AMERICAN HEALTH ORGANIZATION. *Health Conditions in the Americas, 1990 Edition*. Pan American Health Organization, Pan American Sanitary Bureau, Scientific Publication No. 524, 1990.

STABROEK NEWS. Consumption tax kills cigarette sales 1989.

UNITED NATIONS ECONOMIC COMMISSION FOR LATIN AMERICA AND THE CARIBBEAN. Preliminary Results and Tables from GUYREDEM. 1987.

UNITED NATIONS ECONOMIC COMMISSION FOR LATIN AMERICA AND THE CARIBBEAN. Selected Statistical Indicators of the Caribbean Countries, Vol. 2. 1990.

Haiti

General Characteristics

Haiti, a French- and Creole-speaking country, shares the island of Hispaniola with its eastern neighbor, the Dominican Republic. Agricultural activity is important in Haiti, accounting for 32 percent of the gross national product (GNP) in 1989 (Encyclopedia Britannica 1990). In 1989, the per capita GNP was US$356, the lowest in the Western Hemisphere (Encyclopedia Britannica 1990). The Haitian per capita GNP declined by 2.1 percent per year from 1980 to 1988 (World Bank 1989). Only 38 percent of the population between 6 and 24 years of age attends school and 63 percent of the population is illiterate (Pan American Health Organization [PAHO] 1990).

The estimated 1990 mid-year population of Haiti was 6.3 million. Life expectancy at birth has improved since 1970, when it was at 48 years (World Bank 1989). Even so, in 1989, life expectancy at birth was 55 years for men and 56 years for women, among the lowest in the Caribbean sub-region (World Bank 1990). In 1985, 40.1 percent of the population was under 15 years of age and 3.8 percent was 65 and older (PAHO 1990). Haiti has a young population; more than half the population is under 20 years of age.

The Haitian population is characteristic of countries with high birth rates and high death rates. Although the total fertility rate declined from 5.9 births per woman in 1970 to 4.7 in 1988 (World Bank 1989), 20 percent of all children die before their fifth birthday (PAHO 1990). The crude birth rate was estimated at 35.4 per 1,000 during 1980 to 1985, while the infant mortality rate was estimated at 128 per 1,000 live births for the same period (PAHO 1990). Crude birth and fertility rates have not started to decline in Haiti, in contrast to what has been observed in all the countries of the Caribbean and in most developing countries. In fact, during the last 10 years the average number of children per woman has increased from 5.5 to 6.5.

Infectious diseases are the main causes of morbidity and mortality. Diarrhea and respiratory infections account for 50 percent of all deaths among children under 5 years of age (PAHO 1990). Among adults, malaria is a serious problem, but recent epidemiologic data do not permit an estimate of the exact magnitude. AIDS is also widespread in Haiti; 3,086 cases were registered between 1981 and 1990, and women now account for 40 percent of all Haitian AIDS cases (PAHO 1990). The seroprevalence of HIV among the sexually active urban population is 5 to 10 percent.

The current health priorities in Haiti involve controlling infectious and communicable diseases through improving nutritional deficiencies and providing clean drinking water supplies and proper sewage disposal facilities (PAHO 1990). Faced with serious health problems posed by infectious and communicable diseases, Haitians have not assigned any priority to controlling tobacco use.

The Tobacco Industry

It is difficult to estimate how much tobacco is consumed in Haiti. United States Department of Agriculture (USDA) estimates for Haiti of tobacco dry weight production, imports of unmanufactured tobacco leaf, and total domestic consumption of unmanufactured tobacco are provided in Table 1 (USDA 1990). However, the accuracy of these data is questionable. It is unlikely that domestic production did not decline from 1983 to 1989, or that imports more than doubled from 500 MT in 1985 to 1,200 MT in 1986, only to fall to 700 MT in 1987. Nonetheless, it is probably safe to conclude that somewhat less than half of the tobacco consumed in Haiti is grown there, with the remainder being imported. No tobacco is exported.

Tobacco Use

The USDA also has provided estimates of trends in cigarette consumption in Haiti (USDA 1990). Estimated annual cigarette consumption per

Table 1. Production, imports, and total domestic consumption of unmanufactured tobacco, Haiti, 1979–1989 (MT)

Year	Production	Imports	Total domestic consumption
1979	431	635	1066
1980	527	635	1162
1981	374	635	1009
1982	570	555	1125
1983	680	500	1180
1984	680	700	1380
1985	680	500	1180
1986	680	1200	1880
1987	680	700	1380
1988	680	1000	1680
1989	680	1000	1680

Source: USDA (1990).

Figure 1. Cigarette consumption per adult 15+, Haiti, 1979 to 1989

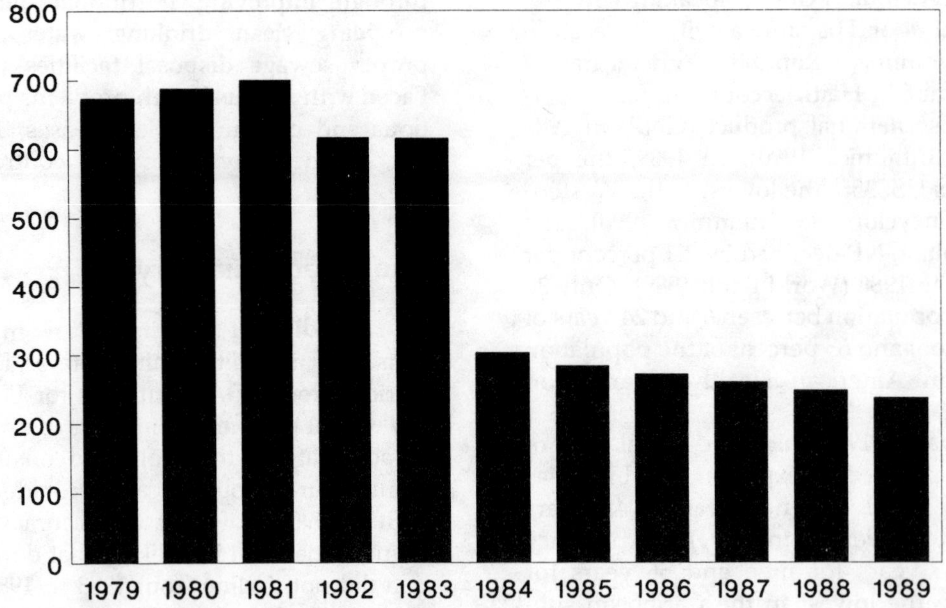

Source: USDA, 1990.

person 15 years of age and older has been derived from these data (Figure 1). These data suggest that tobacco consumption dropped suddenly in 1984, and declined slowly thereafter. However, further examination of the tobacco consumption data suggests not that consumption declined markedly, but that the data are inaccurate.

Table 2 provides figures for both domestic production and imports of cigarettes for the period 1977 to 1989, with comparisons of data from both the USDA and the Haitian Institute of Statistics and Information (USDA 1990; Institut Haïtien de Statistique et d'Informatique (IHSI) 1980, 1981, 1982a, 1982b). Unfortunately, the official data are not available for the years since 1982, but IHSI data for the period 1977 to 1982 do not appear to vary widely from that reported by the USDA. However, it is implausible that imports dropped so precipitously in 1984, with no compensatory increase in domestic production, as the USDA figures imply. A likely explanation is that during the political and civil unrest that occurred in Haiti from 1984 to 1989, official control of cigarette imports was lost and cigarettes were smuggled into Haiti while other imports simply went unreported. Under these circumstances, it is likely that cigarette consumption has remained in the range of 600 to 700 cigarettes

per capita per year for persons 15 years of age and older, as was reported in the period 1979 to 1983. No further information is available on tobacco consumption or smoking prevalence in Haiti.

Summary

Like tobacco sales data, Haitian mortality data are also questionable. No age- or cause-specific mortality data for Haiti have been published. Similarly, no morbidity data are available for smoking-related diseases. The priorities of the Ministry of Health mirror the health problems that face the nation. The priorities being addressed are: diarrheal diseases, diseases preventable by vaccination, tuberculosis, protection of women and children, family planning, malnutrition, malaria, and AIDS (PAHO 1990). This list does not include tobacco, and no organized programs or interventions exist to address the problem of tobacco use. Infant mortality and childhood mortality have been and remain the major public health problems in Haiti. Relatively few persons survive long enough to suffer the tobacco-related diseases that usually develop only after age 45.

Data collection remains problematic in many sectors in Haiti. There are problems in many areas

Table 2. Production and imports of cigarettes as reported from various sources (millions of cigarettes), Haiti, 1977 to 1989

Year	Production		Imports	
	USDA	IHSI	USDA	IHSI
1977	785	815	1000	583
1978	864	958	1000	627
1979	950	1004	1000	1351
1980	1050	1094	1000	
1981	1125	1062	1000	
1982	900	921	1000	
1983	925		1000	
1984	940		19	
1985	887	957*	13	
1986	870		30	
1987	870		30	
1988	870		30	
1989	870		30	

Sources: USDA (1990).
　　　　Institut Haïtien de Statistique et d'Informatique (1980, 1981, 1982a, 1982b).
*Encyclopedia Britannica (1990).

of collection of social, economic, demographic, and health data. Despite these problems, it is known that tobacco products are consumed in Haiti, and have been present there for a long time. Even with this rudimentary knowledge, it is possible to assert that the solutions to current public health problems in Haiti contain the seeds of the next. As progress continues in conquering childhood and infant mortality and in bringing infectious and communicable diseases under control, more people will survive into middle age. They then will be at risk for many chronic diseases that are the most common causes of death elsewhere in the Caribbean and in North America. Inattention to tobacco use by young people in Haiti during the 1990s dictates that many of them will be at high risk of death from a tobacco-related cause when they reach their fifties and sixties. The greater the success in conquering mortality from infectious and communicable diseases and the resultant larger number of people surviving to older ages, the greater will be the eventual death toll from tobacco-related diseases in middle age.

Effective programs of prevention of tobacco use, particularly among young people, could prevent the development in Haiti of an epidemic of tobacco use on the scale currently being experienced in Europe, Canada and the United States. However, the clear and present health problems in Haiti are many and the resources are few. In these circumstances, the implementation of elaborate, comprehensive programs to discourage tobacco use is probably not indicated. Simple, effective legislative and economic activities may be the most important interventions at this time in Haiti.

Recognizing such problems, a WHO expert committee in 1983 proposed a series of recommendations for comprehensive tobacco control programs to be carried out in developing countries (WHO 1983). Many of these recommendations are relevant to Haiti and merit further study for their application in that country. Notable among them is the need to take effective action now to prevent future problems and a call for prohibitions on tobacco advertising and promotion, as well as on the sale of tobacco products to children. These recommendations also call for the development of carefully planned and adequately funded educational programs and the integration of smoking and health action campaigns into the national primary health care system.

Even before these recommendations are undertaken, however, a first priority would be to re-establish full administrative control of the tobacco trade. If manufacturing and importing of tobacco products were controlled well enough to minimize smuggling and to ensure that tobacco taxes were collected on virtually all the cigarettes sold in Haiti, many purposes would be served. Trends in tobacco consumption could be monitored properly, permitting confidence to be restored in the statistics on Haitian tobacco consumption. Such action would serve to reduce smuggling and other unlawful activities and very probably would reduce tobacco consumption, because the price of all cigarettes would include tobacco taxes and therefore be higher. Moreover, the collection of tobacco taxes would provide much-needed State revenues for carrying out public health actions to address the nation's priority health problems and provide a basis from which to implement the recommendations made by the WHO Expert Committee (WHO 1983).

Conclusions

1. The priority health problems being addressed by Haiti do not include tobacco, and no organized programs or interventions exist to address the problem of tobacco use. Infant mortality and childhood mortality have been and remain the major public health problems in Haiti. Relatively

few persons survive long enough to develop the tobacco-related diseases that usually occur after age 45.

2. Tobacco consumption data for Haiti, particularly import data, are incomplete and of questionable quality. However, it is estimated that the current annual rate of cigarette consumption is at least in the range of 600 to 700 cigarettes per person 15 years of age and older.

3. As a first priority for tobacco control in Haiti, action should be undertaken to ensure that State taxes are collected on all cigarettes sold, whether imported or manufactured locally. Complete statistics should be published on the volume and monetary value of both imported and locally manufactured cigarettes.

References

ENCYCLOPEDIA BRITANNICA. *Encyclopedia Britannica World Data Annual 1990*. Encyclopedia Britannica. Chicago, 1990.

INSTITUT HAITIEN DE STATISTIQUE ET D'INFORMATIQUE. *Bulletin trimestriel de statistique*. No. 120, 4th quarter, 1980.

INSTITUT HAITIEN DE STATISTIQUE ET D'INFORMATIQUE. *Bulletin trimestriel de statistique*. No. 124, 4th quarter, 1981.

INSTITUT HAITIEN DE STATISTIQUE ET D'INFORMATIQUE. *Bulletin trimestriel de statistique*. Nos. 127 and 128, 3rd and 4th quarters, 1982a.

INSTITUT HAITIEN DE STATISTIQUE ET D'INFORMATIQUE. *Bulletin trimestriel de statistique: Supplement annuel*. No. XII, 1980, 1981, 1982b.

PAN AMERICAN HEALTH ORGANIZATION. *Health Conditions in the Americas, 1990 Edition*. Pan American Health Organization, Pan American Sanitary Bureau, Regional Office of the World Health Organization. Scientific Publication No. 524, 1990.

UNITED NATIONS. *Demographic Yearbook 1988*. New York, 1989.

UNITED STATES DEPARTMENT OF AGRICULTURE. Tobacco Cotton and Seeds Division, Foreign Agricultural Service. Unpublished data, April 1990.

WORLD BANK. *The World Bank Atlas 1989*. Washington, D.C.: International Bank for Reconstruction and Development/The World Bank, November 1989.

WORLD BANK. *World Development Report 1990—Poverty*. New York: Oxford University Press. 1990.

WORLD HEALTH ORGANIZATION. *Smoking Control Strategies in Developing Countries: Report of a WHO Expert Committee*. World Health Organization. Technical Report Series Number 695. Geneva, 1983.

Honduras

General Characteristics

The Tobacco Industry
  Agriculture
  Manufacturing and production
  Tobacco trade and sales
  Advertising and promotion

Tobacco Use
  Per capita cigarette consumption
  Behavioral surveys
  Prevalence of smoking among adults
  Attitudes and beliefs about worksite smoking
  Prevalence of smoking among adolescents

Smoking and Health

Tobacco Use Prevention and Control Activities
  Executive structure and policies
  Education
  Public information activities
  Action by nongovernmental agencies
  Smoking cessation activities

Summary and Conclusions

References

General Characteristics

Honduras is a subtropical country occupying 112,088 km² on the Central American isthmus. The estimated 1990 midyear population was 4,758,800 (Table 1) (Banco Central de Honduras, 1988); the annual population growth rate reported for the period 1980 to 1988 was 3 percent (Pan American Health Organization [PAHO] 1990). According to 1988 population projections, 45.9 percent of the population is younger than 15 years old; 51.1 percent is 15 to 64 years old; and only 3.0 percent is 65 or older. Over half (58 percent in 1988) the population lives in rural areas (PAHO 1990). Overall mortality, infant mortality, and total fertility decreased between 1983 and 1988. Like many other nations of the Americas, Honduras experienced a severe economic crisis that began in 1981 and worsened between 1985 and 1988. This crisis was manifested in a major devaluation of the lempira, severe inflation, and increased national debt (from $US3.4 billion in 1986 to $US4.5 billion in 1990) (Secretaría de Hacienda y Crédito Público 1991). Productive activity drastically declined during this period, with increased unemployment and inflation. Because of regional instability, Honduras has an estimated 40,000 refugees along its borders with El Salvador, Guatemala, and Nicaragua. Spanish is the national language, with several Indian dialects spoken throughout the country as well as English on the Atlantic coast.

The Tobacco Industry

Agriculture

According to Government sources, land planted with tobacco increased from 6,258 ha in 1987 to 8,511 ha in 1990 (Banco Central de Honduras 1991), or the equivalent of approximately 0.5 percent of the country's total arable land. In 1989, 4,600 MT (dry weight) of tobacco were produced on this land; 43 percent was burley, 27 percent cigar leaf, 29 percent flue-cured, and one percent oriental tobacco (U.S. Department of Agriculture [USDA] 1990b). Tobacco production declined by almost 50 percent in the last 10 years (Table 2). This decline can be attributed in part to an epidemic of blue mold that began in 1980 and affected mainly cigar leaf, which is produced for export. The Government has been striving to control this epidemic since 1987 (Tobacco International 1989).

Table 1. Health and economic indicators, Honduras, 1980s and 1990s

Indicator	Year	Level
Population	1990***	4,758,800
Life expectancy at birth, males	1965–1970	48.2
	1985–1990*	62.0
Life expectancy at birth, females	1965–1970	52.7
	1985–1990*	66.1
Total fertility rate	1985–1990*	5.6
Infant mortality rate	1965–1970	123.7
	1985–1990*	68.4
Crude mortality rate	1988	8.0
Population growth (percent/year)	1980–1988*	3
Percent illiterate	1985	41.0
Real growth rate of GDP (percent/year)	1980–1988**	1.0
Per capita GNP	1987**	$US850

Sources: *Latin American Center for Demography, 1990.
**World Bank, 1989; World Bank, 1990.
***Banco Central de Honduras, 1991.

Manufacturing and Production

Tabacalera Hondureña, S.A. (TAHSA) is a subsidiary of the British American Tobacco Company and operates 15 small plants in Honduras. It holds 98 percent of the domestic market share and produces 2.3 billion units yearly for 13 different brands. Philip Morris recently entered the Honduran cigarette market with a new company, CIGARSA, which imports three cigarette brands from Guatemala. To protect the domestic industry, the Government subsequently placed quotas on cigarette imports (Tobacco International 1989).

Tobacco Trade and Sales

Nearly half of all leaf tobacco grown is exported each year (Table 2). TAHSA produces primarily manufactured cigarettes using domestic tobacco, and in 1988 only 26 million of the 2.3 billion cigarettes manufactured in Honduras were exported (USDA 1990). According to Government sources, export revenues for tobacco increased from $US3.9 million in 1988 to $US9.6 million in 1990 (Secretaría de Hacienda y Crédito Público 1991). Total Government revenue from cigarettes increased from $US34.8 million in 1986 to $US57.5 million in 1990.

Table 2. Production, imports, exports of tobacco, and total domestic consumption of cigarettes, Honduras, 1978–1990

Year	Raw tobacco (metric tons)			Total domestic consumption of cigarettes (billions of units)
	Production	Imports	Exports	
1978	7,046	680	4,522	2.3
1979	9,496	319	4,489	2.5
1980	6,723	520	2,938	2.1
1981	6,530	700	2,800	2.1
1982	6,095	600	2,800	2.3
1983	5,099	200	1,600	2.3
1984	5,049	500	1,600	2.3
1985	5,139	500	1,800	2.3
1986	3,982	212	1,498	2.3
1987	3,963	212	1,260	2.3
1988	3,804	50	1,124	2.3
1989	3,775	50	1,800	2.5
1990	4,600	50	2,520	2.5

Sources: USDA, 1990; Tabacalera Hondureña, S.A., 1990.

Domestically, cigarettes are sold in packs of 20 at a price ranging between 1 and 2 lempiras ($US0.23 to 0.46) (Banco Central de Honduras 1991); cigarettes are also sold individually by street vendors.

Advertising and Promotion

Cigarette advertisements appear in all the mass media. However, commercials on television are now prohibited during the daytime. Nevertheless, an estimated 60.8 hours of airtime per program per year are devoted to cigarette advertisements despite increasing costs for these advertisements (Almandares 1991). Newspaper advertisements appear mostly in the sports sections, with an average of 288 advertisements appearing per year in the nation's four largest newspapers (Pon 1989).

The National Constitution states that censorship laws may be passed in the interest of protecting ethical and cultural values; it specifically stipulates that advertising of alcoholic beverages and tobacco products will be regulated by law (Constitución de la República de Honduras 1988). Responsibility for this area has been assigned to the Honduran Institute for the Prevention of Alcoholism and Drug Dependency (Decree 136-89 1989). More restrictive legislation currently is being considered for advertising and promotional activities.

Tobacco Use

Per Capita Cigarette Consumption

According to USDA data (USDA 1990a), total tobacco consumption in Honduras has remained stable over the last 10 years at approximately 2.3 billion cigarettes per year (Table 2). However, because of an increase in the population, the yearly per capita consumption of tobacco for persons aged 15 years and older has decreased from an estimated 1,346 in 1979 to 807 in 1988 (Table 3). The tobacco industry has observed that sales have been concentrated primarily in the lower-cost and lower-quality brands (Tobacco International 1989). It is apparent that declining consumption was linked to a declining economy in the 1980s.

Table 3. Estimated yearly per capita consumption of manufactured cigarettes, adults aged 15 and older, Honduras, 1979–1990

Year	Adult per capita cigarette consumption
1979	1,346
1981	1,066
1985	995
1988	807

Source: USDA, 1990a.

Table 4. Surveys on smoking and prevalence (percent) of current smoking by sex, Honduras, 1980

Survey	Year	Sample	Sample size	Prevalence (%) of smoking Men	Women	Both
Flores de Kunkar (1986)	1986	Students waiting to begin university	694	29.0	4.1	17
Survey of Family Health (Ministerio de Salud Pública 1987)	1987	Women aged 15 to 44 (national)	10,142	—	6.0	—
Ministerio de Salud Pública (1987)	1987	Ministry of Public Health employees	293	21.5		
Gallup (1988)	1988	Urban population	1,200	36.0	11.0	24.0
Hernández-González (1989)	1989	Rural and urban areas, aged 15–30 years	1,000 (urban) 1,000 (rural)	76.0 56.6	14.5 1.3	55.7 36.2
Amaya-Alemán (1990)	1989	Valle and Choluteca secondary students	1,491	77.2	22.9	64.6

Behavioral Surveys

Several surveys on the prevalence of smoking have been carried out in Honduras; each has covered a specific sector of the population (Table 4). The first survey, done in 1986, involved a group of young adults, aged 15 to 26 years, who were waiting to begin their university studies (Flores de Kunkar 1986). A 1987 survey on epidemiology and family health investigated smoking by women of reproductive age (15 to 44 years) (Ministerio de Salud Pública 1987b). The third survey was carried out in urban areas and focused on the population aged 18 and older (Gallup, Inc. 1988); the definition of "smoker" in this survey differed from the earlier two. In the Gallup survey, "ever smokers" were those respondents who had smoked at least 100 cigarettes in their lifetimes, and "current smokers" were still smoking at the time of the survey. For the other surveys, "smokers" included even occasional smokers, whether or not they had smoked 100 cigarettes in their lifetimes.

Fourth, employees of the Ministry of Public Health were surveyed in 1987 regarding their smoking behavior as well as their attitudes toward workplace tobacco smoke exposure and restrictions on smoking in the workplace. This survey was designed to evaluate a change in policy in Ministry of Public Health workplaces (Ministerio de Salud Pública 1987a). Finally, two doctoral theses by candidates at the Faculty of Medical Sciences in Tegucigalpa reported the results of comparative tobacco-use surveys among residents of rural and urban areas (Hernández-González 1989) and among secondary students (Amaya-Alemán 1990).

Prevalence of Smoking among Adults

The 1988 Gallup survey reported that the overall prevalence of current smoking was 24.0 percent, with 36 percent among men and 11 percent among women; 16 percent smoked in the 18 to 24 year age group, a level slightly higher than that reported for persons aged 15 to 30 years in Flores de Kunkar's study of university entrants (17 percent overall, 29.0 percent among men, and 4.1 percent among women). The survey of women aged 15 to 44 (Ministerio de Salud Pública 1987b) reported a prevalence of regular smoking among these women that was somewhat higher than among women aged 15 to 30 in the Flores de Kunkar (1986) study (6.0 vs. 3.9 percent). Overall, the prevalence of smoking among Ministry of Public Health employees was 21.5 percent; the highest prevalence rates were reported for porters and drivers (31.6 percent) and technical employees (24.3 percent) and the lowest rates for university graduates (22.5 percent) and secretaries (12.3 percent) (Ministerio de Salud Pública 1987a).

In the Gallup survey, the prevalence of smoking was higher among the population with secondary or postsecondary education (26 percent) than for those with less education (22 percent). However, the prevalence of former smoking was also higher among those with higher levels of educational attainment: 36 percent among those with primary education, 40 percent among those with secondary education, and 45 percent among those with postsecondary education (Gallup 1988).

The Ministry of Public Health reported several sociodemographic differences for women of reproductive age. Among women in the metropolitan Tegucigalpa area, 8.0 percent were current smokers, while the prevalence rate among women living in rural areas was only 5.0 percent. The prevalence of smoking among employed women was higher than among unemployed women (9.0 vs. 4.8 percent), and the prevalence of smoking among women with the highest level of education (university or higher) was higher (12.0 percent) than among those with primary education (4.7 percent), secondary education (5.6 percent), or no education (9.7 percent). Women who used oral contraceptives had a higher prevalence of smoking than women who did not (8.3 vs. 5.8 percent). Almost all smokers (96.2 percent) reported smoking fewer than 21 cigarettes per day; 86.8 percent smoked fewer than 11 cigarettes per day (Ministerio de Salud Pública 1987b). The data suggest that the smoking prevalence among women in Honduras is quite low, but that women with the most education, the highest income potential, and the most urbanization are at the highest risk for smoking. In addition, because of the higher prevalence of smoking among women who use oral contraceptives, the risk of cardiovascular complications associated with oral contraceptives might increase among these women (U.S. Department of Health and Human Services 1980).

Attitudes and Beliefs about Worksite Smoking

The 1987 survey of Ministry of Public Health employees was designed to determine support for a planned policy that would restrict smoking in health department facilities. Overall, 77.4 percent were bothered by environmental tobacco smoke (ETS) in the workplace; 90.4 percent desired that there would be no smoking in the workplace; and 69.8 percent favored an actual regulation of smoking at the worksite. Of the 293 respondents, 71.4 percent reported that they were exposed to ETS in their individual worksites (Ministerio de Salud Pública 1987a).

Prevalence of Smoking among Adolescents

The Flores de Kunkar study (1986) reported that the prevalence of smoking among men and women under age 20 was 5.2 percent and 1.3 per-

cent, respectively. Most of the total sample (n=694, aged 15 to 30 years) reported that the age of initiation of smoking was between 15 and 18 years. Among this educated, pre-university group of students, only 50 percent knew that smoking was associated with lung cancer and other diseases (Flores de Kunkar 1986).

Among persons aged 15 to 30 in Catacomas (an urban area) and Olandro (a rural area), the prevalence of smoking was higher in the urban area, and much higher among men than among women (Table 4). Among secondary students in Valle and Choluteca, the prevalence of ever smoking among young men (77.2 percent) and young women (22.9 percent) was extraordinarily high (Table 4).

Smoking and Health

It is difficult to assess the impact of smoking on the health of Hondurans because of the small number of deaths reported for smoking-related diseases and because of problems associated with mortality reporting in Honduras. In 1983, only 11 percent of deaths were certified by a physician (PAHO 1986). In 1981, 35 percent of all deaths were attributed to symptoms, signs, and ill-defined conditions; the proportion was somewhat lower (25 percent) for the 35 to 64 year age group (PAHO 1990). The trends in the age-adjusted mortality rates for ischemic heart disease and cerebrovascular disease show no change between 1971 and 1981 (Table 5), despite the substantial drop in the percentage of deaths categorized "symptoms, signs, and ill-defined conditions" (PAHO 1986, 1990). These data suggest that the prevalence of smoking and other cardiovascular disease risk factors did not increase among the population in that decade.

Stomach cancer is the most common cause of recorded cancer death among men in Honduras

Table 5. **Age- and sex-adjusted mortality rates (per 100,000 persons) for selected cardiovascular diseases associated with smoking, 1971 and 1981**

Cause of death (ICD-9 Code)	Year	
	1971	1981
Ischemic heart disease (410–414)	6.2	4.5
Cerebrovascular disease (430–438)	17.7	17.1

Source: PAHO, 1986 and 1990.

Table 6. Age-adjusted mortality rates (per 100,000 persons) for selected diseases associated with smoking, by age and sex, Honduras, 1981

Cause of death (ICD-9 Code)	Age-adjusted mortality rate	Age group		
		35–44	45–54	55–64
Ischemic heart disease (410–414)				
Men	5.4	1.3	10.5	20.7
Women	3.6	1.3	3.5	15.0
Cerebrovascular disease (430–438)				
Men	17.4	6.9	15.8	40.0
Women	16.8	13.2	15.8	43.5
Malignancies of the lip, oral cavity, and pharynx (140–149)				
Men	0.2	—	0.9	—
Women	0.2	1.3	—	—
Malignancies of the trachea, bronchi, and lungs (162)				
Men	0.5	—	—	1.4
Women	0.2	0.6	0.9	1.4

Source: PAHO, 1990.

(19.4 percent of all cancer deaths), and cervical cancer is the chief cause of recorded cancer death among women (54.6 percent of all recorded cancer deaths). These cancers are both associated with smoking as well as with other risk factors. Lung cancer, the chief cause of which is smoking, was the seventh-ranked cause of recorded cancer death (2.4 percent of all cancer deaths) among men and was not among the top 12 causes of recorded cancer death among women (PAHO 1990). In Honduras, the very low number of cigarettes smoked per day explains in part the pattern and low levels of lung cancer mortality.

Among persons aged 55 to 64 years, the age-adjusted mortality rate for ischemic heart disease for men was somewhat higher than for women, but the cerebrovascular mortality rate for women in this age group was slightly higher than for men (Table 6). The age-adjusted mortality rates for oropharyngeal cancers and lung cancer are quite similar for both men and women.

Tobacco Use Prevention and Control Activities

Executive Structure and Policies

The Honduran Institute for the Prevention of Alcoholism and Drug Dependency, established in 1988, coordinates antismoking activities. The Institute has a staff of five part-time employees. Since its inception, the Institute has focused its efforts on promoting legislation and providing coordination between Government and nongovernmental agencies.

The Institute has submitted draft legislation to the Congress that would ban smoking in public and private schools, in cinemas and theaters, on public transportation, in the workplace, and at sports facilities. This draft legislation also calls for a mandatory warning on cigarette packages indicating the health risks of smoking, a ban on tobacco sales to minors, and a ban on the sale of single cigarettes. The bill also establishes penalties and fines, which would be used to finance the Institute's programs. Although this comprehensive legislative package has not yet been passed, a regulation was passed in 1987 that banned smoking in cinemas during the showing of movies for children and ordered the placement of "NO SMOKING" signs in these facilities.

In February 1991, the Department of Communications, Public Works, and Transportation decreed that smoking would not be permitted in transportation vehicles carrying eight or fewer passengers (Secretaría de Estado en el Despacho de Communicaciones, Obras Públicas, y Transporte 1991).

No other legislative actions have been enacted to control or prevent tobacco use in Honduras, and there are no regulations on tar and nicotine levels for tobacco products.

Education

Information on smoking is not included in the official school curriculum at any level. The Institute, however, gives occasional lectures on drug dependency (including smoking) at schools.

Public Information Activities

Although no formal, widespread activities in public information are reported, the topic of smoking is nevertheless addressed by radio, television, and print media reports on scientific issues, especially during the period surrounding World No-Tobacco Day (May 31). The National Smoking Control Commission (CONACTA) supports a radio program on tobacco and health, broadcast by the National College of Medicine. Honduras is a member of the Latin American Coordinating Committee on Smoking Control, sponsored by the American Cancer Society and PAHO.

Action by Nongovernmental Agencies

CONACTA was established in September 1988. Its resources are derived from the Honduran Cancer Society, direct solicitations, and local tobacco control committees which exist in different areas of the country. The commission organizes national and local workshops on treatment and prevention of smoking that are presented to community organizations, unions, student groups, religious groups, and the general public. The committee also coordinates activities for World No-Tobacco Day each year, and in 1991 sponsored a demonstration by 20,000 persons in conjunction with this event. CONACTA helped develop a national plan for tobacco control. In addition, CONACTA staged a campaign to donate fruit trees to communities dependent on tobacco growing as part of a crop substitution program. The Commission sponsored a national survey on tobacco use in October 1991 and has developed a training program or antitobacco education that will affect more than 10,000 young persons (Almendares 1991).

Smoking Cessation Activities

The Seventh Day Adventist Church offers to the general public a 5-day program to quit smoking. In addition, the Ministry of Public Health and the Honduran Cancer Society occasionally address smoking cessation as part of their regular community activities (Almendares 1991).

Summary and Conclusions

Honduras is a very poor country with a low and falling level of domestic tobacco consumption. Tobacco exports may have some economic significance to a small sector of the population, but consumer purchasing capabilities for most Hondurans preclude the widespread use of manufactured cigarettes. The Government has been actively involved in developing tobacco agriculture and in protecting the domestic industry from foreign cigarette imports. Advertising and promotional activities for tobacco products are extensive, but these advertisements must be submitted for Government approval to ensure that ethical and cultural values are not undermined. Tobacco product advertising is now prohibited prior to 7:00 p.m. on radio and television.

The prevalence of smoking among the adult urban population in Honduras is 11 percent for women and 36 percent for men (Gallup 1988). It is important to note the higher prevalence rates of smoking among women with greater incomes and educational attainment compared to women with lesser incomes and educational attainment. The prevalence of smoking among urban women is higher than that among rural women. The prevalence of smoking among young persons (aged 15 to 30) waiting to begin their university studies was 29.0 percent among males and 4.1 percent among females. However, among residents of two different communities, a comparison of rural and urban persons' tobacco use reported that the current smoking prevalence in both communities was extraordinarily high (55.7 and 36.2 percent, respectively) in 1989. Even more disturbing is a recent report of the ever-smoking prevalence among secondary students (77.2 percent among men and 22.9 percent among women).

The impact of tobacco on mortality and morbidity in Honduras is difficult to quantify due to problems with mortality reporting and due to the fact that diseases associated with smoking, such as lung and oropharyngeal cancers, are still rare causes of death. In addition, the proportion of the population aged 65 and older, in whom these diseases have a greater impact, is very small (3.0 percent in 1990). Thus, it is difficult to predict the future effects of smoking among Hondurans.

Actions to prevent and control the use of tobacco in Honduras are growing, and an administrative structure within the Government, the Honduran Institute for the Prevention of Alcoholism and Drug Dependency, has been assigned responsibility for coordinating the country's antismoking program. To this end, the Institute has proposed legislation to control smoking in public places and to increase restrictions on tobacco advertising. Recently, the National Smoking Control Commission (CONACTA) has organized workshops and informational activities on tobacco and health in the media and for smokers in particular. Several nongovernmental organizations have provided support for the official antismoking program. These include the Seventh Day Adventist Church, which offers cessation programs in Honduras as it does in most countries of the Americas; the Honduran Cancer Society, which also offers support for cessation; and the National Smoking Control Commission.

Based on the data presented in this report, the following conclusions can be drawn:

1. Although the percentage of agricultural and industrial workers involved in tobacco production is small in Honduras, tobacco is economically important as an agricultural export. The Government supports efforts to enhance production and protect the local industry.

2. According to the limited research available on smoking behavior in Honduras, estimated prevalence is relatively low, particularly among women. Educated, urban, employed women have a higher prevalence of current smoking than those with less education, higher unemployment, and a rural lifestyle. The consumption of tobacco appears closely linked to economic capability in Honduras, and knowledge of the health consequences of smoking among Hondurans may be quite limited.

3. The recently established National Smoking Control Commission provides a framework for coordinated antitobacco activities. The Commission has proposed more restrictive legislation on the advertising of tobacco products, on smoking in public, and on access to tobacco by minors. It has also supported public information and media activities against smoking. Nongovernmental organizations help support the national campaign through collaborative efforts, cessation programs, and World No-Tobacco Day activities.

4. In Honduras, the consequences of smoking are not as yet reflected in mortality figures, which in part is due to the low coverage of death registration and lack of diagnostic precision, but also to the fact that most deaths in the country occur before age 15.

References

ALMENDARES, J. Country collaborator's report, Honduras. Pan American Health Organization, unpublished data, 1991.

AMAYA-ALEMAN, D.D., AGUILAR-REYES, M.G., CARRASCO-NUNEZ, E.A. *Prevalencia de alcoholismo y tabaquismo en estudiantes de educación secundaria de Valle y Choluteco*. Previa Opción al Título de Doctor en Medicina y Cirugía. Tegucigalpa, Honduras, 1990.

BANCO CENTRAL DE HONDURAS. *Honduras en Cifras 1988–1990*. Departamento de Estudios Económicos. Tegucigalpa, M.D.C., Honduras, C.A., June 1991.

CENTRO LATINOAMERICANO DE DEMOGRAFIA. *Boletín Demográfico*. CELADE, Santiago, 23(45), 1990.

CONSTITUCION DE LA REPUBLICA DE HONDURAS. *Congreso Nacional de Honduras, Edición Conmemorativa, 1988.*

DECRETO No. 136–89. *La Gaceta*, año CXIII, No. 25959, Tegucigalpa, Honduras, 14 October 1989.

FLORES DE KUNKAR, A., ALMENDARES, J. Estudio de tabaquismo en población de pre-ingreso universitario. Dirección de Investigación Científica, Universidad Nacional Autónoma de Honduras (datos no publicados), 1986.

GALLUP ORGANIZATION INC. *The incidence of smoking in Central and Latin America*. Conducted for the American Cancer Society, April 1988.

HERNANDEZ-GONZALEZ, S.Y., GALDEMA-SANTA CRUZ, G.E. *Estudio comparativo sobre la prevalencia del tabaquismo en personas de 15 a 30 años*. Area urbana y rural, Catacomas, Olancho. Tesis. Previa Opción al Título de Médico y Cirujano. Tegucigalpa, Honduras, 1989.

MINISTERIO DE SALUD PUBLICA. *Encuesta para conocer la actitud del personal de salud frente al fumado en ambientes de trabajo*. Ministerio de Salud Pública, Tegucigalpa, January 1987a.

MINISTERIO DE SALUD PUBLICA. *Encuesta nacional de epidemiología y salud familiar*. Tegucigalpa, 1987b.

PAN AMERICAN HEALTH ORGANIZATION. *Health Conditions in the Americas, 1981–1984*. Washington, D.C. PAHO Scientific Publication No. 500, 1986.

PAN AMERICAN HEALTH ORGANIZATION. *Health Conditions in the Americas, 1990 edition.* Washington, D.C. PAHO Scientific Publication No. 524, 1990.

PON, A.M., ARAGON, A., HERNANDEZ, V., ESPAÑA, R., ALMENDARES, J. *Propaganda y publicidad del fumado en Honduras.* Trabajo presentado en VII Semana Científica de la Universidad Nacional Autónoma de Honduras, Ciudad Universitaria "José Trinidad Reyes," Tegucigalpa, Honduras, October 1989.

SECRETARIA DE ESTADO EN EL DESPACHO DE COMUNICACIONES, OBRAS PUBLICAS, Y TRANSPORTE. *Acuerdo presidencial No. 00345.* 22 February 1991.

SECRETARIA DE HACIENDA Y CREDITO PUBLICO. *Memoria 1990.* Presentada al Soberano Congreso Nacional de Tegucigalpa, M.D.C., January 1991.

TABACALERA HONDURENA, S.A. *Reporte Annual 1990.*

TOBACCO INTERNATIONAL. Latin America Issue, June 1, 1989, pp. 5-6.

U.S. DEPARTMENT OF AGRICULTURE. Tobacco, Cotton, and Seeds Division, Foreign Agricultural Service, 1990a.

U.S. DEPARTMENT OF AGRICULTURE. *World Tobacco Situation.* U.S. Department of Agriculture, Foreign Agricultural Service, Circular Series, FT 5-90, May 1990b.

U.S. DEPARTMENT OF HEALTH AND HUMAN SERVICES. *The Health Consequences of Smoking for Women—A Report of the Surgeon General.* U.S. Department of Health and Human Services, Public Health Service, Office of the Assistant Secretary for Health, Office on Smoking and Health, 1980.

WORLD BANK. *World Development Report 1989.* New York: Oxford University Press, 1989.

WORLD BANK. *World Development Report 1990—Poverty.* New York: Oxford University Press, 1990.

Jamaica

General Characteristics

The Tobacco Industry
   Agriculture
   Manufacturing
   Marketing

Tobacco Use
   Consumption data
   Survey data

Smoking and Health
   Data sources and quality
   Mortality
   The Kingston and St. Andrew Tumour Registry

Tobacco Use Prevention and Control Activities
   The National Council on Drug Abuse
   Taxation
   Legislative controls and policies
   National health organizations
   Summary of tobacco prevention and control activities

Summary

Conclusions

References

General Characteristics

Jamaica, with a population of 2.4 million, is the most populous English-speaking country in the Caribbean. Tourism and bauxite production are the major economic activities in Jamaica. In 1988, the per capita gross national product (GNP) was US$1,080. From 1980 to 1988, the rate of economic growth, measured in change in per capita GNP, dropped an average of 2.1 percent per year (World Bank 1989).

The population of Jamaica shows the effects of a 20-year decline in the total fertility rate: since 1970, the number of individuals in the 0 to 4, 5 to 9, 10 to 14, and 15 to 19 age groups has remained approximately the same. In 1985, an estimated 36.7 percent of the population was under 15 years, while those 65 years of age and over accounted for only 6.1 percent of the population (Pan American Health Organization [PAHO] 1990).

During 1980 to 1988, average life expectancy at birth increased from 67 to 74 years. The total fertility rate continued to decline during 1970 to 1988, from 5.4 to 2.8 live births per woman (World Bank 1989). In 1987, the crude birth rate in Jamaica was 21.9 births per 1,000 population (PAHO 1990). Jamaica experienced comparatively low rates of childhood mortality during the 1970s and 1980s. In 1984, the infant mortality rate (i.e., among children less than 1 year old) was 16.5 per 1,000 in Jamaica compared with 56.6 per 1,000 in the Dominican Republic in 1985 (PAHO 1990). In 1984, crude and age-adjusted mortality rates per 1,000 population were 6.0 and 4.5, respectively, in Jamaica.

The population and vital statistics presented above indicate that Jamaica recently has experienced an epidemiologic transition from a country of high birth and death rates to one where death rates are now very low and birth rates continue to decrease toward population replacement levels. Because much of this change occurred during the 1980s, a large proportion of the population is under 15 years of age. As this cohort enters adulthood in future decades, individuals will become susceptible to chronic diseases, including tobacco-related diseases such as cancer, heart disease, and chronic obstructive lung diseases.

The Tobacco Industry

Agriculture

Until 1987, the State had legislative authority to regulate and control tobacco growing in Jamaica (Statutes of Jamaica 1967) through a seven-member Tobacco Control Authority reporting to the Minister of Agriculture. However, in 1987, the appointments of members of the Tobacco Control Authority expired and the organization ceased activities. The Government no longer has any authority over the tobacco industry.

In 1988, the 354 tobacco farmers accounted for 0.14 percent of the total number of farmers in Jamaica (Agricultural Products of Jamaica, Ltd. 1990). For 1988, the entire Jamaican tobacco crop was grown on 584 ha, or less than 0.05 percent of all agricultural land in the country.

In the 1980s, as the previously expanding cigar industry began to decline, growers of cigar tobacco gradually shifted their production to vegetable and fruit crops because it was in their best economic interest (Agricultural Products of Jamaica, Ltd. 1990). However, because there is a strong demand for cigarettes in Jamaica and because growing tobacco for cigarettes is very lucrative relative to other crops, it is unlikely that other crops will be substituted for cigarette tobacco (PAHO 1988).

Jamaica is essentially self-sufficient in tobacco growing; although some tobacco leaf is imported, an approximately equal amount is exported. Trends in tobacco leaf production, imports, exports, and consumption for 1979 through 1989 are illustrated in Figure 1 (United States Department of Agriculture [USDA] 1990).

Manufacturing

The Carreras Group Limited with its majority shareholder and controlling parent company, Rothman's International, virtually controls the Jamaican cigarette market. Two smaller private cigar manufacturing concerns also currently operate in Jamaica. When a company engages in growing, manufacturing, wholesaling, and retailing a single commodity, it is said to be vertically integrated. Conversely, horizontally integrated companies are those involved in a single aspect, such as manufacturing, of several commodities. Carreras enjoys a high degree of vertical integration in the local tobacco industry based on ownership of numerous subsidiary companies, including two farming and leaf-processing companies, three companies that produce printing and packaging materials for the tobacco industry, a tobacco manufacturing company, the Cigarette Company of Jamaica, and a tobacco research and development firm. However, Carreras also has diversified horizontally into a

Figure 1. Tobacco leaf production, exports, imports, and total domestic consumption (metric tons) Jamaica, 1979–1989

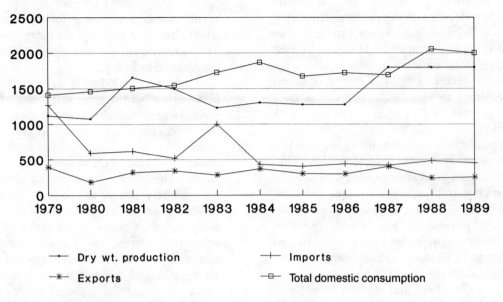

Source: USDA, 1990.

non-tobacco sector through another subsidiary, the Jamaica Biscuit Company (Carreras Group [Jamaica] Ltd. 1989).

It has been argued that such vertical integration has helped stabilize cigarette tobacco agriculture in Jamaica. This economic stability, rare in other sectors of Jamaican agriculture, militates against any eventual policy of tobacco crop substitution.

One large cigarette factory and four smaller factories that manufacture cigars are located in Jamaica. In 1988 and 1989, these factories employed 285 people accounting for 0.03 percent of the total labor force (Jamaican Ministry of Labour 1989).

Marketing

The major brands of cigarettes in Jamaica are Craven "A," Matterhorn, Benson & Hedges, Rothman's, and Dunhill. In 1989, Craven "A" held a 77-percent share of the total Jamaican cigarette market (Maxwell 1990). No cigarettes are imported into Jamaica, and there is no evidence of illegal trade in tobacco products (Barnaby 1990).

Cigarettes are sold in packs of 20 and range in price from J$8 to J$10 (US$1.46 to US$1.83) (Statistical Institute of Jamaica 1990). With weekly wages for employed persons averaging J$485.95, the

average Jamaican worker would need to work 44 minutes to earn the average price of J$9 for one pack of 20 domestically produced cigarettes (Statistical Institute of Jamaica 1990).

Tobacco Use

Consumption Data

Of total tobacco consumed in Jamaica, 97 percent is in the form of domestically produced cigarettes with the remainder in the form of cigars. Of total Jamaican cigarette production, approximately 3 percent is exported, mainly to other Caribbean countries. No cigarettes are imported (Statistical Institute of Jamaica 1987, 1989).

Per capita cigarette consumption data are available from the Maxwell Report (1990) and the Statistical Institute of Jamaica (1987, 1989). For 1979 to 1985, cigarette consumption reported by Maxwell averaged 3.5 percent per year lower than that reported by the Government source; for 1986 to 1988, cigarette consumption reported by Maxwell averaged 0.64 percent per year higher than that reported by the Statistical Institute of Jamaica. However, reported trends in consumption of cigarettes per adult are similar for the two sources. Calculations based on population projections by the Statistical Institute of Jamaica (1987, 1989) and these data show that although there was a slight downward trend in annual per capita cigarette consumption among persons aged 15 years and older from 1979 to 1986, dropping 25 percent to a low of 760, cigarette consumption per adult subsequently increased 14.7 percent to approximately 872 in 1989 (Figure 2).

Survey Data

In 1987, the Medical Association of Jamaica (MAJ) commissioned a survey of smoking prevalence among Jamaicans aged 10 years and older. Estimates of smoking prevalence by age and sex, based on the results of this survey, are presented in Table 1. However, only 1,000 persons were sampled and the stratification was reported to have been inadequate (PAHO 1988). Although survey methodology was reported to be weak and the prevalence rates are reported in non-standard age groups, data from this study are the only available estimates of current smoking prevalence for Jamaica. Survey results indicated that of those surveyed, a greater percentage of men than women reported smoking (25.1 vs. 5.9 percent, respectively). Smoking prevalence among Jamaicans in the 32- to 41-year-old age group in 1987 was comparable with that observed in 1989 among Canadians

aged 35 to 44 (32.4 vs. 35.4 percent, respectively); however, smoking prevalence among Jamaicans aged 16 to 21 years was 7.9 percent compared with 25.2 percent among Canadians aged 15 to 19 years (PAHO 1988; Stephens 1991).

A 1987 Jamaica Household Survey, sponsored by the National Council on Drug Abuse (1987a), collected data on lifetime prevalence of cigarette use and cigarette use within the last 30 days by selected age groups and demographic characteristics (Table 2).

Table 1. Percentage of current smokers in the Jamaican population ten years of age and older, by age and sex, Jamaica, 1987

Age groups	Percentage of smokers		
	Both sexes	Males	Females
10–15	2.3	3.2	1.3
16–21	7.9	14.1	1.8
22–31	18.8	34.3	3.9
32–41	32.4	49.2	16.3
42–51	25.1	42.6	8.2
51+	16.1	24.6	8.6
Total	15.3	25.1	5.9

Source: PAHO, 1988.

Figure 2. Cigarette consumption (in thousands) per adult 15+, Jamaica, 1979 to 1989

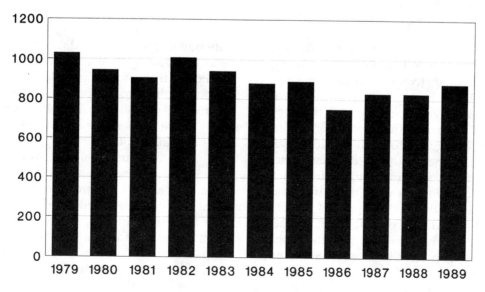

Sources: 1. Statistical Institute of Jamaica, Prod. Stat. '87.
2. Maxwell, 1990.

Table 2. Percentage of Jamaicans who ever smoked cigarettes, by selected demographic characteristics, 1987

Demographic characteristics	Age groups				
	< 20	20–29	30–39	40+	Total
Sex					
Male	19.7	49.1	69.7	68.3	51.4
Female	3.0	12.7	22.1	21.6	14.8
Education					
No formal	4.0	17.1	12.2	46.4	7.7
6th form or less	24.0	37.1	48.0	44.4	41.2
High school	20.4	23.4	44.0	47.7	28.7
Some college/graduate	*	11.5	37.2	23.1	21.1
Employment					
Unemployed	9.0	24.3	37.2	32.0	20.2
Unskilled	26.3	42.0	48.5	52.4	47.4
Semi-skilled	29.2	32.6	50.4	54.3	42.8
Skilled	*	16.4	37.2	37.0	29.9
Religion					
None	26.9	51.2	66.6	70.4	53.4
Anglican/R. Catholic	14.7	27.4	51.6	47.8	36.6
Baptist/Methodist/Church of God	7.7	24.9	39.2	41.9	28.4
Rastafarian	*	68.3	81.3	83.0	74.3
Pentecostal/J. Witness/7th Day Adventist	7.2	22.6	35.3	33.1	23.9
Other	8.7	26.8	28.9	38.9	25.9
Church Attendance					
More than 1/week	4.9	12.9	23.6	26.0	17.0
More than 1/month	5.0	18.1	35.5	41.3	24.6
Less than 1/month	12.0	25.0	43.6	52.3	33.0
None in past year	17.4	42.2	57.5	55.9	44.9

Source: National Council on Drug Abuse, 1987a.

* Fewer than 10 respondents in category

The 1987 Jamaica Household Survey indicated that tobacco may serve as a gateway drug among the Jamaican population (National Council on Drug Abuse 1987a). Of smokers of both "ganja" (marijuana) and cigarettes, 76 percent reported that they began smoking cigarettes first and later added ganja to their smoking repertoire; 21 percent began smoking both substances at about the same time; and 3 percent began smoking ganja before they began smoking cigarettes. Among those who had smoked cigarettes in the last 30 days, 2.4 percent reported that they had used cocaine at some time. Among those who had not smoked cigarettes in the last 30 days, only 0.1 percent reported having used cocaine at least once.

Another 1987 survey reported on lifetime use and use in the last 30 days of both tobacco and alcohol among adolescents aged 11 to 21 years and attending school (National Council on Drug Abuse 1987b) (Table 3). Similar surveys in Canada have indicated that smoking prevalence is higher among dropouts than among those who continue to attend school (Flay 1990). Thus, the 1987 Jamaican survey may have underestimated smoking prevalence among adolescents.

In a 1979 survey of adolescents aged 14 to 20 years attending school in the districts of Kingston and St. Andrew, 21 percent of boys and 13.5 percent of girls reported continued tobacco use (Barnaby 1979). In 1987, among adolescents aged 11 to 21 years attending school, use of tobacco in the last 30 days was reported at 7.3 and 3.1 percent for boys and girls, respectively (National Council on Drug Abuse 1987b). The data from these two studies indicate that prevalence of smoking among Jamaican schoolchildren declined somewhat from

Table 3. Percentage of secondary students who used tobacco in the past month and those who ever used tobacco, Jamaica, 1987

	Past month	Ever
All students	**5.1**	**29.1**
Sex		
Male	7.3	39.8
Female	3.1	19.4
Age		
13–14	3.8	43.6
15–16	4.7	25.0
17–18	6.0	27.5
19–21	3.7	50.0
Grade		
9	4.5	25.3
11	6.0	32.8
13	6.5	50.0
Region		
Metropolitan	8.1	90.0
Coastal urban	3.1	25.8
Inland urban	3.7	25.5
Rural	4.8	21.2
Tourism	4.3	32.7

Source: National Council on Drug Abuse, 1987b.

1979 to 1987. However, additional studies are needed to substantiate these findings.

In both the 1979 and 1987 surveys, students cited curiosity (62 and 41 percent, respectively) and peer group pressure (15 and 34 percent, respectively) most frequently as reasons for starting to smoke (Barnaby 1979; Jamaican Ministry of Health and National Council on Drug Abuse 1987b).

Smoking and Health

Data Sources and Quality

Chronic diseases account for most of the defined causes of death in Jamaica. Of the total number of deaths reported in 1984, 23.1 percent were attributed to coronary heart disease, 17.3 percent to malignant neoplasms, 16.3 percent to cerebrovascular diseases, 5.9 percent to diabetes mellitus, and 4.4 percent to intestinal infections (PAHO 1990). The first three of these chronic diseases together accounted for 56.7 percent of all defined causes of death. Mortality data in Jamaica may not be completely reliable. Of the total number of deaths reported in Jamaica in 1984, symptoms and ill-defined conditions accounted for 12.7 per-

cent, compared with 2.5 percent in Trinidad and Tobago in 1986. Moreover, under-registration of deaths is still problematic in Jamaica (PAHO 1990).

Mortality

The 1989 U.S. Surgeon General's Report identified smoking as causally related to a number of diseases, including coronary heart disease; cerebrovascular disease; chronic obstructive lung disease; lung cancer; and cancers of the lip, oral cavity, pharynx, larynx, esophagus, pancreas, bladder, and kidney (United States Department of Health and Human Services [USDHHS] 1989). Tables 4 and 5 present the number of smoking-related deaths and age-specific death rates, respectively, for these causes of death reported among persons in Jamaica aged 35 and older in 1984.

Lung cancer mortality was 4.8 times greater among Jamaican men aged 55 to 64 than among women in the same age group. The large gender differential observed in mortality rates for smoking-related diseases in Jamaica may be due to the fact that the prevalence of smoking among Jamaican females is much lower than among Jamaican males. As indicated in Table 1, Jamaican males were 3.5 times more likely than females to have ever smoked (Jamaican Ministry of Health and National Council on Drug Abuse 1987a).

In 1984, the lung cancer mortality among Jamaican males aged 55 to 64 was approximately one-third that of Canadian males in the same year and approximately one-third that of U.S. males in 1983 (46.3 vs. 141.5 vs. 145.4 per 100,000 persons, respectively); however, this rate is more than 20 percent greater than in Trinidad and Tobago in 1986 (35.9 per 100,000 persons) (PAHO 1986, 1990).

Maternal smoking increases the risk of perinatal mortality by 24 to 144 percent depending on birthweight (Malloy 1988). Because many perinatal deaths are not reported in Jamaica, it is impossible to assess accurately the impact of maternal smoking during pregnancy on Jamaican children. For example, in the rural parish of Clarendon in 1984, of the total number of perinatal deaths, 98 percent of stillbirths and 34 percent of all infant deaths were not reported (Jamaican Ministry of Health 1989b). Thus, national surveys to identify smoking prevalence among pregnant women and more consistent perinatal death registration are necessary to assess reliably smoking-related perinatal mortality in Jamaica.

Table 4. Number of deaths from selected smoking-related causes among persons 35 years of age and over, Jamaica, 1984

Age	Ischemic heart disease	Cerebrovascular disease	Chronic obstructive lung disease	Lung cancer	Cancers of the lip, oral cavity, pharynx, larynx, esophagus, pancreas, bladder, and kidney
35–44					
Men	6	28	4	9	0
Women	7	11	5	3	0
45–54					
Men	18	47	18	23	10
Women	22	44	11	6	6
55–64					
Men	71	107	31	46	40
Women	54	134	9	11	12
65–74					
Men	132	280	35	52	45
Women	102	246	18	15	26
75+					
Men	172	368	59	40	54
Women	198	645	35	10	22

Source: Jamaican Ministry of Health 1989a.

Table 5. Mortality rates per 100,000 from selected smoking-related causes among persons 35 years of age and over, Jamaica, 1984

Age	Ischemic heart disease	Cerebrovascular disease	Chronic obstructive lung disease	Lung cancer	Cancers of the lip, oral cavity, pharynx, larynx, esophagus, pancreas, bladder, and kidney
35–44					
Men	8.0	37.4	5.3	12.0	0
Women	8.2	12.8	5.8	3.5	0
45–54					
Men	28.1	73.4	28.1	35.9	15.6
Women	30.2	60.4	15.1	8.2	8.2
55–64					
Men	124.3	187.4	54.3	80.6	70.1
Women	81.9	203.3	13.7	16.7	18.2
65–74					
Men	319.6	678.0	84.7	125.9	109.0
Women	211.2	509.3	37.3	31.1	53.8
75+					
Men	792.6	1695.9	271.9	184.3	248.9
Women	668.9	2179.1	118.2	33.8	74.3

Source: Jamaican Ministry of Health 1989a.

The Kingston and St. Andrew Tumour Registry

In selected geographic areas around the world, all new malignant tumors are reported to a central registry for that area. Usually, tumor registration areas cover areas smaller than an entire nation. One of the few tumor registries in the Caribbean region is located in the urban districts of Kingston and St. Andrew in Jamaica. Since 1958, data from this registry have been used to assess trends in incidence for cancers discovered among residents of the major urban area of Jamaica. Among women, incidence rates for cancers at sites known to be associated with smoking are low and stable or declining (Table 6). These data most likely again reflect historic and continuing low prevalence of lifetime smoking among Jamaican females (Tables 1 and 2). Similarly among men, the incidence rates for smoking-related cancers are also low and stable or declining, with the notable exception of lung cancer.

Incidence rates for lung cancer are five times higher among men than women in Kingston and St. Andrew (21.1 vs. 3.9 per 100,000, respectively). It is encouraging to note that the lung cancer rates for Jamaican males rank in the lowest quintile of

Table 6. Age-standardized incidence rates for smoking-related tumors, Kingston and St. Andrew districts, Jamaica, 1967 to 1987

Tumor site (ICD-9 code)	Rank among 80 tumor registries worldwide 1967–72	Incidence rates per 100,000 Period of registration			
		1967–72	1973–77	1978–82	1983–87
Lip (140)					
Men	66	0.3	1.0	0.5	0.0
Women	38	0.2	0.4	0.3	0.1
Tongue (141)					
Men	15	2.7	1.9	0.7	2.4
Women	30	0.6	1.0	0.4	1.0
Oral cavity (143–45)					
Men	21	3.2	0.8	3.0	1.7
Women	22	1.2	1.4	0.4	0.4
Pharynx (146–49)					
Men	3.5	3.5	2.5		
Women		0.9	1.3	0.8	
Esophagus (150)					
Men	12	9.1	7.1	5.8	4.4
Women	5	4.7	3.0	3.2	2.3
Pancreas (157)					
Men	67	4.0	2.3	3.5	3.7
Women	70	2.5	3.2	2.3	2.1
Larynx (161)					
Men	56	3.7	4.6	5.3	3.7
Women	53	0.4	0.4	0.4	0.3
Lung (162)					
Men	66	21.2	19.8	19.1	21.1
Women	63	5.0	4.0	3.2	3.9
Bladder (188)					
Men	54	8.6	8.5	6.4	4.4
Women	39	3.2	3.9	2.0	1.7
Other urinary organs (189)					
Men	65	2.5	2.9	2.2	2.0
Women	72	1.1	.0	0.6	2.0

Sources: Segi 1977.
Jamaica Cancer Registry 1989.

incidence rates reported in 80 international cancer registries (Segi 1977). Moreover, the male lung cancer incidence rate among residents of Kingston and St. Andrew has remained stable since 1967 (Table 6).

All smoking-related tumor sites, except the lung, are also associated with major risk factors other than smoking, such as alcohol abuse. Changes in patterns of exposure to these other risk factors may explain observed declines in cancer incidence at other sites such as the oral cavity and esophagus. Nonetheless, smoking is the single most important risk factor for lung cancer (USDHHS 1989) and past smoking patterns among men in Jamaica (Tables 1 and 2) undoubtedly have contributed to the higher incidence of lung cancer observed in the Registry data. The 1989 U.S. Surgeon General's Report estimated that of the total lung cancer deaths in the United States, 90 percent among men and 79 percent among women were attributable to smoking in 1985 (USDHHS 1989).

Tobacco Use Prevention and Control Activities

The National Council on Drug Abuse

The National Council on Drug Abuse, funded by the Jamaican Ministry of Health, conducts health education activities and provides technical information to promote Government and interagency coordination in prevention and control of substance abuse. The prevention and control of tobacco use forms an integral part of the Council's functions. The Council has a full-time, salaried staff of seven individuals.

Taxation

Tobacco taxes imposed and collected in Jamaica are an important source of Government revenue. Of the retail price of cigarettes, 42 percent is allocated to the Government in the form of an excise tax. In 1989, the Government collected J$262 million in cigarette excise taxes, accounting for approximately 18 percent of all excise taxes collected and approximately 4 percent of all Government revenues (Jamaica Customs and Excise Department 1990). Cigarette taxes in Jamaica are higher than in some other Caribbean countries such as St. Lucia and Dominica (18 and 35 percent, respectively). However, taxes on cigarettes are relatively low as a percentage of total price in Jamaica when compared

to the situation in Canada and the United Kingdom (42 vs. 67 and 75 percent, respectively).

Legislative Controls and Policies

Currently, no legislation restricts tobacco advertising. However, Carreras has withdrawn voluntarily from advertising its tobacco products on television. Of Carreras' 1989 total advertising expenditures, 25 percent was targeted to radio, 30 percent to billboards, 10 percent to point of sale, and 4 percent to print media advertising (Maxwell 1990). Carreras also sponsors sporting and cultural events, most notably the annual awards for Sportsman and Sportswoman of the Year (Barnaby 1990).

The Medical Association of Jamaica and the Ministry of Health were instrumental in persuading Carreras Ltd. to print a health warning on all cigarette packages sold in Jamaica. However, tar and nicotine information is not required on cigarette packages. Each cigarette pack bears the following health warning:

CHIEF MEDICAL OFFICER'S WARNING: Cigarettes can be dangerous to your health.

Currently, no laws restrict smoking in public places and workplaces in Jamaica. However, voluntary restrictions and local regulation of smoking in enclosed locations are widespread. Some public places, workplaces, and modes of transit offer limited protection from involuntary exposure to tobacco smoke (Barnaby 1990; PAHO 1988).

National Health Organizations

The Medical Association of Jamaica, the Jamaican Heart Foundation, and the Jamaica Cancer Society have been particularly active in undertaking tobacco control activities (Barnaby 1990; PAHO 1988). In conjunction with the Ministry of Health and the National Council on Drug Abuse, these and other major health and service organizations periodically sponsor antismoking promotional and educational activities. Antismoking education has been incorporated into the health education curricula of primary and secondary schools. At least six Jamaican life insurance companies offer lower premiums to nonsmokers than to smokers.

Smoking cessation programs are offered by the Seventh Day Adventist Church and by several private practitioners in Jamaica. However, no studies have been conducted to assess the effectiveness of these various smoking cessation programs (Barnaby 1990).

Summary of Tobacco Prevention and Control Activities

Tobacco use prevention and control activities in Jamaica are addressed most vigorously by the Medical Association of Jamaica. The National Council on Drug Abuse, a coalition of Government and nongovernment representatives, has prioritized illicit drugs, and their legislative subcommittee is planning additional tobacco-related interventions. The Ministry of Health has demonstrated a financial commitment to these efforts through the Council, and thus institutional support for tobacco control may have additional potential for development. It is important to note the leadership also demonstrated by the Jamaican Heart Foundation and Cancer Society. Professional and voluntary organization activities have been critical in the development of effective educational campaigns to control tobacco use.

Summary

Like many other countries in the English-speaking Caribbean, Jamaica has a single dominant tobacco producer that is controlled by one of the large transnational tobacco companies. Despite relatively low taxes as a percentage of the price, Jamaican cigarettes are relatively expensive when compared with those in many other Caribbean countries. The tobacco industry is highly vertically integrated into tobacco agriculture and promotional activities in Jamaica, and there are few restrictions on tobacco advertising. Jamaica is one of the few Caribbean countries to require a warning on packages of cigarettes manufactured.

Per capita cigarette consumption declined from 1979 to 1986 and then increased from 1986 to 1989. The initial decline in consumption may have been linked to declining economic conditions in Jamaica during this period. Reasons for the more recent increase in per capita consumption are unclear. Additional data on promotional activities by the tobacco industry as well as on tobacco prevention and control activities would be helpful in understanding these trends.

Recent survey data suggest a favorable trend in the uptake of tobacco use. The percentages of both men and women aged 20 to 29 who ever smoked are considerably lower than those observed for older cohorts. Lifetime prevalence of smoking is highest among persons aged 32 to 51 and lowest among persons aged 10 to 21. Among Jamaican adolescent schoolchildren, 30-day smoking prevalence is less than 10 percent. If young persons continue to demonstrate such modest levels of uptake of tobacco use, favorable changes in the chronic disease burden in Jamaica may be anticipated.

Accurate assessment of tobacco use among both adults and youth is essential to evaluate the overall tobacco and health situation. Improved reporting and analyses of chronic disease mortality will assist public health workers and policy makers in evaluating both the disease burden caused by smoking and the beneficial effects of tobacco use prevention and control campaigns. Improvements in data collection systems are essential for future planning of tobacco control in Jamaica.

National health organizations offer coordinated, active antismoking promotional and educational programs in Jamaica. Antismoking education has been integrated into public school curricula. Evaluation studies of these activities would help to strengthen the programs and to support the development of programs for high-risk groups such as pregnant women and young persons.

Conclusions

1. In 1989, Jamaicans smoked, on average, 872 cigarettes per person aged 15 years and older. This is less than one-third the level of the highest rates of adult per capita cigarette consumption in the world, which are observed in Cuba and some countries of southern and eastern Europe.

2. Only 8 percent of Jamaicans aged 16 to 21 smoke cigarettes. If over 90 percent of Jamaican teenagers continue to maintain their nonsmoking status, lung cancer incidence rates are expected to remain stable for several more years and then slowly to decline among both men and women.

3. Even though cause of death reporting is somewhat incomplete in Jamaica, recent data (1984) suggest a significant mortality burden for chronic diseases that are causally linked to tobacco use. These include: coronary heart disease (23.1 percent of total mortality), malignant neoplasms (17.3 percent of total mortality), and cerebrovascular diseases (16.3 percent of total mortality).

4. An infrastructure to support tobacco use prevention and control exists in Jamaica and is linked to drug abuse prevention activities. Voluntary and health professional organizations provide leadership in efforts to inform the public about the health consequences of tobacco.

References

AGRICULTURAL PRODUCTS OF JAMAICA, LTD. Unpublished data, 1990.

BARNABY, L. *Drug Use and Adolescence*. Jamaican Ministry of Health, Community Mental Health Services, 1979.

BARNABY, L. Country Collaborator's Report, Jamaica. Pan American Health Organization, unpublished data, 1990.

CARRERAS GROUP (JAMAICA) LTD. *Annual Report*. 1989.

JAMAICA CANCER REGISTRY. University of the West Indies, Department of Pathology, Kingston, Jamaica. Unpublished data, 1989.

JAMAICA CUSTOMS AND EXCISE DEPARTMENT. Unpublished data, 1990.

JAMAICAN MINISTRY OF HEALTH. *Death by Cause, Age and Sex, Kingston, Jamaica, 1984*.

JAMAICAN MINISTRY OF HEALTH. Health Information Unit, unpublished data, 1989a.

JAMAICAN MINISTRY OF HEALTH. Health Information Unit, unpublished data, 1989b.

JAMAICAN MINISTRY OF LABOUR. *Factory Inspectorate*, Kingston, Jamaica, 1989.

KAISERMAN, M.J., ALLEN, T.A. Global per capita consumption of manufactured cigarettes—1988. *Chronic Diseases in Canada* 11(4):56–57, July 1990.

MALLOY, M.H., KLEINMAN, J.C., LAND, G.H., SCHRAMM, W.F. The association of maternal smoking with age and cause of infant death. *American Journal of Epidemiology* 128(1):46–55, July 1988.

MAXWELL, J.C. JR. *The Maxwell Consumer Report. International Tobacco 1989*, Part Three. Richmond, Virginia:Wheat First Securities/Butcher & Singer, Inc. WFBS-5685, October 30, 1990.

NATIONAL COUNCIL ON DRUG ABUSE. *Drug Use in Jamaican Households*, 1987a.

NATIONAL COUNCIL ON DRUG ABUSE. *Drug Use in Jamaican Students at Post-primary Level*, 1987b.

PAN AMERICAN HEALTH ORGANIZATION. *Health Conditions in the Americas, 1981–1984*, Volume I. Pan American Health Organization, Pan American Sanitary Bureau, Regional Office of the World Health Organization. Scientific Publication No. 500, 1986.

PAN AMERICAN HEALTH ORGANIZATION. *Smoking Control: Third Subregional Workshop, Caribbean Area, Kingston, Jamaica, 1987*. Pan American Health Organization, Pan American Sanitary Bureau, Regional Office of the World Health Organization. Technical Paper No. 20, 1988.

PAN AMERICAN HEALTH ORGANIZATION. *Health Conditions in the Americas, 1990 Edition*. Pan American Health Organization, Pan American Sanitary Bureau, Regional Office of the World Health Organization. Scientific Publication No. 524, 1990.

SEGI, M. *Cancer Incidence in Five Continents, Volume III: 1976*. International Agency for Research on Cancer. IARC Scientific Publication No. 15, 1977.

STATISTICAL INSTITUTE OF JAMAICA. *Production Statistics 1987*. Kingston, Jamaica, 1987.

STATISTICAL INSTITUTE OF JAMAICA. *Statistical Review 1989*. Kingston, Jamaica, 1989.

STATISTICAL INSTITUTE OF JAMAICA. *Weekly Estimates of Average Earnings Per Week of All Employees in Large Establishments, 1986–89*. In press, 1990.

STATUTES OF JAMAICA. *The Tobacco Industry Regulation Act*. No. 24, December 4, 1967.

STEPHENS, T. Smoking in Canada—1989. Unpublished manuscript prepared for the Tobacco Programs Unit, Health Promotion Directorate, Health and Welfare, Ottawa, Canada, 1991.

U. S. DEPARTMENT OF AGRICULTURE. Unpublished data, Tobacco Cotton and Seeds Division, Foreign Agricultural Service, April 1990.

U.S. DEPARTMENT OF HEALTH AND HUMAN SERVICES. *Reducing the Health Consequences of Smoking: 25 Years of Progress. A Report of the Surgeon General*. U.S. Department of Health and Human Services, Public Health Service, Centers for Disease Control, Center for Chronic Disease Prevention and Health Promotion, Office on Smoking and Health. DHHS Publication No. (CDC) 89–8411, 1989.

WORLD BANK. *The World Bank Atlas 1989*. Washington, D.C.: International Bank for Reconstruction and Development/The World Bank, November 1989.

Mexico

General Characteristics

The Tobacco Industry
   Agriculture
   Manufacturing
   Cigarette sales and trade
   Advertising and promotion

Tobacco Use
   Per capita cigarette consumption
   Behavioral surveys on tobacco use
   Prevalence of smoking among adults
   Prevalence of smoking among adolescents
   Other uses of tobacco
   Attitudes, knowledge, and opinions about smoking

Smoking and Health

Tobacco Use Prevention and Control Activities
   Government action
      Executive structure and policies
      Legislation
      Taxes
   School education
   Public information activities and cessation programs
   Nongovernmental action

Summary

Conclusions

References

General Characteristics

Mexico occupies 1,958,000 km² south of the United States. For better or worse, numerous cultural influences cross the border from its northern neighbor including those related to tobacco use, marketing, and promotion. Although Mexico enjoyed an economic boom based on oil production in the early 1980s, the standard of living for most of the population has deteriorated since then (Pan American Health Organization [PAHO] 1990). Agricultural activity also declined, but tobacco production apparently was not as affected by the general economic situation (Tobacco Merchants Association of the U.S. 1989). As of 1987, Mexico had the fourth highest total tobacco growing acreage in Latin America, after Brazil, Cuba, and Argentina (Chapman 1990). Mexico produces approximately 1.0 percent of the world's tobacco crop (Food and Agriculture Organization [FAO] 1990).

Included in the economic decline has been health services. Diarrhea and respiratory infections are still leading causes of death, but chronic diseases have begun to affect mortality patterns. The infant mortality rate is still quite high at 46/1,000 live births, but this rate is nearly one-half the level (82/1,000 live births) in 1965 (Table 1).

Mexico is one of the most populous nation of Latin America and the Caribbean, with an estimated 1988 mid-year population of 83.7 million (World Bank 1990). The growth rate of the population from 1980 to 1988 was 2.2 percent per year, and the age structure (38.6 percent less than 15 years old) and total fertility rate (3.58/1,000 women) indicate that Mexico will have a young and growing population for several decades. This fact has not been lost on the tobacco industry in Mexico, which has recognized the importance of marketing tobacco to young persons (Weingarten 1987). However, health indicators in general have improved for Mexicans. Fertility for women of child-bearing age has declined from 6.76/1,000 in 1986 to 3.58/1,000 in 1990, and the population less than age 15 has declined from 43 percent in 1980. Thus, future health policy in Mexico must address chronic diseases of adults; many of these will be caused by smoking among the 9 million adult smokers (aged 15 years and older) estimated in Mexico in 1988.

The Tobacco Industry

Agriculture

In the 1930s, only 15,000 ha of tobacco were farmed, but this land area increased to 54,000 ha in 1964. Since then, tobacco production and ha planted with tobacco decreased to levels similar to those prior to 1937 (Tabamex 1988). In 1989, an estimated 33,029 ha of tobacco were planted in Mexico, 43 percent of which is of the Burley variety (U.S. Department of Agriculture [USDA] 1990b). Tobacco production declined from a record high (due to extraordinarily favorable agricultural conditions) of 94,000 MT in 1980 to a projected 32,680 MT in 1990 (Table 2). The FAO projects that production will

Table 1. Health and economic indicators, Mexico, 1980s

Indicator	Year	Value
Population	1988	83,700,000
Percent <15 years old	1988	38.6
Percent urban	1988	71.0
Life expectancy at birth		
Men	1985–90	65.7
Women	1985–90	72.3
Total fertility rate per 1,000 women	1985–90	3.58
Infant mortality rate per 1,000 live births	1988	46.0
Crude mortality rate per 1,000 persons	1988	6.0
Percent literate	1985	10.0
Per capita gross national product	1988	$1,760
Average annual percent growth rate of GNP	1980–88	0.7

Sources: CELADE, 1990; World Bank, 1990.

Table 2. Raw tobacco production, exports, and total domestic consumption (in metric tons) and land area planted in tobacco (in ha), Mexico, 1979–1990

Year	Area planted in tobacco*	Production**	Exports**	Total domestic consumption**
1979	46,000	72,000	11,000	51,600
1980	42,000	94,000	18,000	53,300
1981	36,000	58,000	12,000	53,100
1982	40,000	67,000	37,000	53,000
1983	37,000	53,000	11,000	49,700
1984	31,000	41,000	13,000	49,200
1985	39,000	48,000	9,000	55,100
1986	46,128	69,303	11,135	47,000
1987	47,443	47,667	8,050	51,300
1988	44,895	66,643	15,588	47,100
1989	33,029	53,350	11,065	51,300
1990	22,860	32,680	10,400	—

Sources: Secretaría de Agricultura y Recursos Hidráulicos, México, 1979–1985; USDA, 1990a; consumption data from Maxwell, 1990.
* Hectares
** Metric Tons

increase due to a 3-percent increase in domestic demand. This increase in demand is largely due to the projected increase in the size of the adult Mexican population (FAO 1990).

Currently, 18,025 farmers grow tobacco in Mexico. Approximately 85 percent of tobacco is produced in the western state of Nayarit, and most of the remaining tobacco production is in the southern states of Veracruz, Chiapas, and Oxaca (Labrandero 1990). According to tobacco industry sources, 351,000 persons are employed at least part-time in tobacco agriculture, the equivalent of 117,000 full-time jobs (Agroeconomic Services Ltd., and Tabacosmos Ltd. 1987). However, this represents only 2.2 percent of Mexico's agricultural labor force (Chapman 1990).

Tobacco exports fluctuated widely in the past, but have remained relatively stable since 1983, representing 0.2 percent of the total national exports (Agroeconomic Services Ltd. and Tabacosmos Ltd. 1987; Tabamex 1987) (Table 2). Little tobacco had been imported into Mexico because no import licenses could be obtained until local growers sold all of their produce. Nonetheless, recent free-market policies have permitted regulatory changes, and imports have increased substantially from 0.5 MT in 1983 to 3,000 MT in 1989; estimates for 1990 indicate that tobacco imports will approach 6,600 MT

(USDA 1990b; Agroeconomic Services Ltd. and Tabacosmos Ltd. 1987).

Manufacturing

Since 1972, Tabacos Mexicanos (Tabamex), a company with 52-percent Government ownership, has been the only buyer of tobacco leaf in Mexico. The company also owns curing and processing plants. Tobacco growers, through the Confederación Nacional de Campesinos, own 24 percent of Tabamex, while cigarette manufacturing companies also own 24 percent. Tabamex purchases tobacco at prices established before the planting season. Thus, growers have had little incentive to increase production.

Until 1987, Tabamex's annual earnings averaged $US10,000,000. In the 1987–1988 season, however, floods destroyed 40 percent of the Nayarit tobacco crop (Weingarten 1987). Due to additional national economic problems, the Government froze prices on most basic products, including cigarettes, to control inflation. Subsequent restructuring of the Mexican economy permitted the sale, to private concerns, of the Government's share of Tabamex. The Government then created the Comité Nacional de Tabaco, which is responsible for setting tobacco prices. Tobacco producers, cigarette manufacturers, and the Government are represented on the committee (USDA 1990b).

In 1989 three cigarette manufacturing companies operated in Mexico: La Moderna, a subsidiary of British-American Tobacco; Cigarros La Tabacalera Mexicana (CIGATAM), a subsidiary of Philip Morris; and La Libertad, owned primarily by Mexican interests. Together, these companies produced an estimated 51.3 billion cigarettes in 1989. Throughout the 1980s, cigarette production fluctuated very little, from 47 to 55 billion units (USDA 1990).

According to a 1988 Tabamex report, the contribution of the tobacco manufacturing industry to the overall national economy is minimal, estimated at 0.31 percent (14,390,000 million 1980 pesos) of the gross domestic product (GDP). This level has remained stable over time (Instituto Nacional de Estadística, Geografía e Informática 1989). According to tobacco industry sources, tobacco manufacturing provided jobs for 5,163 persons in 1988, or 0.2 percent of all jobs in the formal economy (Agroeconomics Ltd. and Tabacosmos Ltd. 1987).

Cigarette sales and trade

Cigarettes are sold in packages of 20 and 14 units, and also singly. The 1988 price ranged from 170 to 1,550 pesos per package ($US0.05–0.52) (Labrandero 1990). In 1989, the average price for a package of domestic cigarettes was $US0.40; if an average worker consumed 20 cigarettes per day, this expense would be equivalent to 6 percent of the average household income (Chapman 1990). Convenience stores sell 80.4 percent of cigarettes sold in Mexico, while 11.3 percent is sold in tobacco shops, and 8.3 percent in other locations (Maxwell 1990).

La Moderna now controls 59.1 percent of the domestic cigarette market, down from 70.7 percent in 1979. Tabacalera Mexicana's market share increased from 28.2 percent in 1979 to 40.9 percent in 1989. This company produces the world's most widely marketed consumer product, Marlboro cigarettes. In Mexico, Marlboro promotions have been extensive, including exclusive rights to sponsor television coverage of the national football championships (Chapman 1990). La Libertad has less than 0.1 percent of the total market (Maxwell 1990).

Mexico does not import cigarettes because stiff tariffs make foreign brands noncompetitive. However, the country has considered exporting domestically produced cigarettes to China, Afghanistan, Iran, and African nations. It is expected that if manufacturers do not increase cigarette exports, they will attempt to increase domestic consumption. Recently, cigars manufactured by Tabamex were exported to the United States in considerable quantity (Weingarten 1987).

Advertising and promotion

Cigarette advertising is permitted and used in all mass media. However, prior authorization of the content of these ads is required from the Secretaría de la Gobernación. By law, cigarette ads must not associate smoking with sports, civic, or religious activities, and persons younger than age 25 are not to appear in these commercials (Secretaría de Salud 1986).

In 1988, 48 percent of total cigarette advertising expenditures was for television, 20 percent for radio, and 19 percent for outdoor billboards (Maxwell 1990). Television advertising has decreased since 1982, when 88.8 percent of total tobacco advertising expenditures (1,815 million pesos) were for television. This sum purchased 5,956 commercials in 1 year. By 1988, the number of commercials decreased to 5,492 with a total value of 128,938 million pesos, but tobacco product advertising increased in other media such as radio and billboards. A 1990 study conducted by the Instituto Nacional del Consumidor reported that in 1987, advertising accounted for 7.63 percent of the total television air time; 1.74 percent of the total air time (and 22.8 percent of all advertising time) was cigarette advertising (Chan-Escalante 1990).

Tobacco Use

Per Capita Cigarette Consumption

In 1923, the adult (age 15 years and older) per capita cigarette consumption was a modest 900 cigarettes per year. Per capita consumption increased substantially in the mid-1930s and then fluctuated between 1,360 and 1,750 units per year (Lee 1975; Maxwell 1990). Apparent per capita consumption decreased from 1,617 in 1987 to a projected 990 in 1989 (based on 51.3 billion cigarettes consumed and a population aged 15 and older numbering 52 million in 1989) (Figure 1). This dramatic decline in consumption is due in part to increasing cigarette prices, decreased consumer buying power, and antismoking activity in Mexico. Part of the decline is artifactual, however, because different data sources were used in estimating per capita con-

Figure 1. Per capita consumption of cigarettes, Mexico, 1923–89 (cigarettes per person age 15 or older)

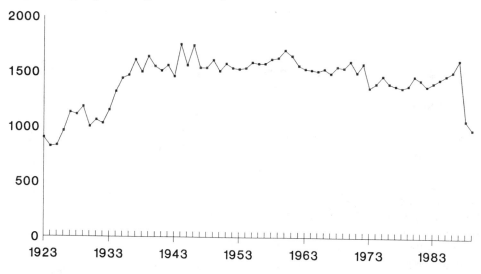

Sources: Lee 1975; The Maxwell Consumer Report 1990.

sumption between 1987 and 1989. Nonetheless, recent per capita consumption estimates by Maxwell and the FAO confirm that tobacco consumption in Mexico is declining.

In 1988, 77.6 percent of all cigarettes consumed were filtered and made of tabaco rubio, and 22.4 percent of cigarettes were unfiltered and made of tabaco negro (Maxwell 1990).

Behavioral Surveys on Tobacco Use

In 1971, PAHO sponsored an eight-city survey on smoking in Latin America, including Mexico City (Joly 1977). Since then several other surveys on smoking have been conducted in various parts of the country and among different population groups (Table 3). Nationally representative surveys were conducted in 1986 and in 1988. In 1986, the Secretaría de Salud directed the Encuesta Nacional de Salud (ENSA) (Secretaría de Salud 1988a). In 1988, the same institution carried out the Encuesta Nacional de Adicciones (ENA) (Secretaría de Salud 1990). In 1988, the American Cancer Society commissioned the Gallup Organization to perform a survey on smoking among Mexico City residents aged 18 years and older (Gallup 1988). Little infor-

Table 3. Surveys on tobacco use and prevalence (percent) of current (daily) smoking by sex, Mexico, 1971–1988

Author/Sponsor	Year	Sample	N	Prevalence of current smoking		
				Men	Women	Both
Joly (PAHO)	1971	Mexico City Age 15–74	1,574	43.6	16.0	28.7
National Health Survey (ENSA), Secretaría de Salud	1986	National Age ≥ 12	14,528	27.4	8.4	17.4
National Survey on Addictions, (ENA), Secretaría de Salud	1988	Urban residents Age 12–65	12,581	43.1	20.0	25.8
Gallup (American Cancer Society)	1988	Mexico City Age ≥ 18	2,600	37.0	17.0	

mation on the sampling methodology for this survey is available.

ENSA 1986 used a household cluster sampling technique. After the household was selected, an individual was identified to respond about himself or herself and all other members of the household. This proxy technique may lead to underreporting of smoking prevalence if the respondent is not aware of household members' smoking status. ENA 1988 used the same sampling frame as ENSA 1986, but sampled only urban areas. The respondent only was surveyed about his or her own tobacco and drug use (Secretaría de Salud 1988a and 1990). Thus, underreporting of tobacco use is unlikely in this survey. The definition of smoker in the 1971 PAHO study (Joly 1977) is different from that used in ENSA 1986 and ENA 1988. The 1971 PAHO survey and the 1988 Gallup survey used the U.S. definition by which an individual is defined as a smoker when he or she has smoked at least 100 cigarettes in his or her lifetime and smokes at the time of the survey. ENSA and ENA defined a smoker as an individual who currently smokes every day. Both the sampling methodology and the definition of "smoker" affect the reported prevalence from these various surveys.

Prevalence of Smoking among Adults

The national adult prevalence of daily smoking reported by ENSA 1986 is lower than that reported among urban respondents by ENA 1988 (17.4 vs. 25.8 percent), suggesting that the prevalence of smoking among urban residents is higher than in the general population (Table 4). However, both surveys report a south-north gradient in current smoking prevalence, with lower prevalence in the south and higher prevalence in the north (Tapia-Conyer 1989a and 1989b).

Among both men and women, the prevalence of smoking was highest in Mexico City in 1988. It is interesting that the lowest prevalence of daily smoking among urban men is reported for the northwest region (28.4 percent), where the prevalence among women (16.6 percent) is one of the highest prevalences among women in all urban areas.

Because the 1971 PAHO survey and 1986 and 1988 surveys provide data on Mexico City, some general comparisons may be made for these time periods. The overall prevalence of current smoking among Mexico City residents reported by the 1971 survey was 28.7 percent. In 1988, the prevalence of daily smoking was 25.8 percent overall. The ENSA

Table 4. Prevalence of current daily smoking by sex and geographic area, Mexico, 1988

Region	Prevalence of current daily smoking	
	Men	Women
Noroccidental	28.4	16.6
Nororiental	38.1	15.5
Centro Norte	38.9	14.2
Distrito Federal	43.1	20.8
Centro	38.5	13.9
Centro Sur	33.7	10.7
Sur	37.2	25.1
Mexico total	38.3	14.4

Source: Secretaría de Salud, 1990.

1986 overall prevalence was only 17.4 percent, but the sample may have been quite different from ENA 1988 in that persons living in Mexico City's surrounding countryside might have been included, thus lowering the overall prevalence of smoking because of the more rural and impoverished nature of these households. By sex, little change in the prevalence of smoking among men occurred between 1971 (43.6 percent) and the ENA 1988 (43.1 percent). Among women, however, the prevalence of smoking increased from 16 percent in 1971 to 20 percent in 1988. The prevalence of smoking reported on the Gallup survey for men (37 percent) and women (17 percent) was somewhat lower than that reported by ENA 1988 (Table 3).

The 1986 Household survey permits stratification by age and region. The highest prevalence among younger respondents (less than 40 years old) was in Mexico City, while the highest prevalence among those older than 40 years was in the northwest region. The prevalence of daily smoking among the 30- to 39-year age group is the highest for all age groups in each region of the country.

The Gallup survey reported that the prevalence of smoking among persons of "upper social class" was higher than among persons of "low social class" (34 vs. 27 percent), but no definition for these categories is available (Gallup 1988).

Analyses of both ENSA 1986 and ENA 1988 data show that approximately two-thirds of smokers in Mexico smoked fewer than 10 cigarettes per day (Tapia-Conyer et al. 1989a; PAHO 1990).

The 1988 survey ascertained exposure to environmental tobacco smoke (ETS) for nonsmokers aged 12 to 65 who lived with smokers. Between

Table 5. Prevalence (percent) of exposure to environmental tobacco smoke (passive smoking) among nonsmokers by region, 1988

Region	Prevalence (%) of passive smoking
Noroccidental	28.2
Nororiental	31.1
Centro Norte	31.3
Distrito Federal	32.7
Centro	35.0
Centro Sur	29.2
Sur	25.1
Mexico total	31.5

Source: Secretaría de Salud, 1990.

25.1 and 35 percent of nonsmokers in this age group living in urban areas are exposed to ETS in their homes (Table 5). However, if children less than age 12 and adults older than age 65 were included, the rate of ETS exposure would be much higher.

Smoking among health personnel affects the development of antismoking policies. Two surveys on tobacco use among physicians in Mexico City have been performed. In 1983, the prevalence of daily smoking was 33 percent among 495 physicians working in university hospitals (Puente-Silva 1985). More recently, a 1989 telephone survey of Mexico City physicians reported that 22.8 percent were current smokers (Meneses 1989). This prevalence is higher than that reported in ENSA 1986 (16.7 percent) for Mexico City, but lower than that (31 percent) reported in ENA 1988 and in the 1983 survey mentioned above. The average age of smoking initiation reported in the 1989 physicians' survey was 17.7 years, and of current smokers, 51.9 percent had ever made a serious attempt to quit smoking.

In a survey conducted among the personnel of the Instituto Nacional de Enfermedades Respiratorias, only 55 percent of the sample responded. Among these respondents the prevalence of current smoking was 27.7 percent (41.3 percent among men and 18.4 percent among women) (Gutiérrez de Velasco 1988). If the results can be generalized to the rest of the Institute, employees of this respiratory disease hospital have a higher prevalence of smoking than do physicians in Mexico City and a prevalence similar to that reported by ENA 1988 for the general public in Mexico City.

Prevalence of Smoking among Adolescents

In 1988, 9,967 secondary school students were surveyed for the National Study on the Use of Drugs in the Student Population (Medina-Mora 1990). Nationally, 42.2 percent had tried cigarettes at least once, 19.5 percent had smoked at least once in the last 30 days, and 6 percent smoked on a daily basis. However, this level of experimentation is lower than that reported in a 1980 study conducted among 3,408 secondary students in Mexico City and suburban areas (46.9 percent) and among 4,049 Mexico City students surveyed in 1978 (53.2 percent) (Castro-Sariñana 1982).

Finally, 88,735 first-year students of the Universidad Nacional Autónoma de Mexico, UNAM (National Autonomous University of Mexico) were surveyed on tobacco use in 1988. Among these high socioeconomic status adolescents, 9.3 percent had smoked daily for the last 12 months. Among these smokers, 76.6 percent said that they smoked "for pleasure," 18.2 percent to "relieve stress," and 16.7 percent to "imitate others" (peer pressure) (Dirección General de Servicios Médicos 1988).

Other Uses of Tobacco

No survey data are available regarding other forms of tobacco consumed in Mexico besides manufactured cigarettes. However, Mexico produces 16.2 million cigars each year. Of this total, only 5.8 million are consumed domestically, and the rest are exported (Tobacco Merchants Association of the U.S. 1989).

Attitudes, Knowledge, and Opinions about Smoking

Data were collected on knowledge about the harmful effects of smoking on health for the 1988 ENA (Secretaría de Salud 1990). Over 90 percent of those surveyed in all regions of the country responded correctly to the questions about knowledge. However, 30 percent of respondents affirmed that smoking helps a person to relax and to relieve stress, 46.5 percent thought that smoking is a form of entertainment, and 65.2 percent considered tobacco smoking to be less harmful to health than illicit drugs. However, 95.1 percent of respondents also "requested more information about smoking."

The 1989 Mexico City physicians' survey asked about their knowledge of specific health effects of smoking, about counseling their patients to quit, and about their attitudes toward restricting smoking in medical or public settings. More than 90 percent of all physicians, regardless of smoking status, believed that smoking causes emphysema, lung cancer, chronic bronchitis, mouth and throat cancer, and heart disease. However, approximately 15 percent also believed that smoking causes diabetes and kidney stones (for which there are no published associations). Among current smokers, 36.4 percent stated that they counseled all their patients to quit smoking, but 51.3 percent of nonsmoking physicians counseled all their patients to quit smoking. Approximately three-quarters of physicians felt that smoking should be restricted in medical facilities, whereas approximately 90 percent felt that smoking should be restricted in restaurants (Meneses 1989).

Smoking and Health

There were 400,079 deaths in Mexico in 1986, with 15.5 percent estimated underreporting. Signs and ill-defined conditions (ICD 780–799) represented 3.1 percent of deaths among men and 4.0 percent among women for that year (PAHO 1986,

1990). The age-adjusted mortality rate for ill-defined conditions decreased from 1981 to 1986 (Figure 2). Thus, recent mortality data for Mexico permit a reasonably accurate estimate of the impact of smoking on the population.

Of the five leading causes of death in Mexico in 1986, heart diseases (ICD 390–429) ranked first (n=50,739) and malignant neoplasms (ICD 140–208) ranked second (n=35,930). Many of these deaths may be smoking-associated. Trend analyses for selected smoking-associated deaths may reveal patterns related to changing exposure to cigarette smoking in Mexico.

Age-adjusted mortality rates for four disease categories known to be causally related to smoking were analyzed for 1982 and 1986 (unpublished tabulations, PAHO 1990) (Table 6). Lung cancer (ICD 162) is the most frequent cause of cancer death in Mexico (11.9 percent of all cancer deaths). In 1986, 4,412 deaths were due to lung cancer (PAHO 1990), and according to U.S. attributable risk estimates (U.S. Department of Health and Human Services [USDHHS] 1989), 87 percent (n=3,838) of these deaths may be attributed to smoking. The age-adjusted lung cancer mortality rate for men was more than twice that for women in 1986, but the rates

Table 6. Age-adjusted mortality rates (per 100,000 persons) for selected smoking-related conditions and age-specific mortality rates by sex for persons aged 35–64, Mexico, 1982 and 1986

Cause of death	Sex	Year	Age-adjusted rate*	Age-specific rates		
				35–44	45–54	55–64
Ischemic heart disease	Male	1982	30.9	17.8	55.8	148.7
(ICD 410–414)	Male	1986	31.5	16.5	52.8	144.7
	Female	1982	17.7	7.3	19.3	65.0
	Female	1986	18.7	6.2	19.7	60.4
Cerebrovascular disease	Male	1982	22.8	10.7	32.5	84.6
(ICD 430–438)	Male	1986	22.2	8.8	27.2	75.7
	Female	1982	22.0	12.7	31.8	71.3
	Female	1986	21.8	9.1	26.9	64.8
Malignancy of lip, oral cavity,	Male	1982	0.9	0.4	1.7	5.7
and pharynx (ICD 140–149)	Male	1986	1.0	0.3	1.4	6.3
	Female	1982	0.4	0.3	1.4	6.3
	Female	1986	0.4	0.5	0.8	1.6
Malignancy of trachea, bronchus,	Male	1982	7.3	2.4	13.1	44.9
and lung (ICD 162)	Male	1986	8.4	2.3	13.1	48.0
	Female	1982	2.7	1.5	5.2	15.4
	Female	1986	3.4	1.9	6.2	18.6

Source: PAHO, 1986 and 1990.

* Rates adjusted for all ages to the total population of Latin America.

increased for both sexes from 1982 to 1986. The observed increase in rate is more apparent for men aged 55 to 64 years, but for women, the increase is more apparent for both those aged 45 to 54 years and 55 to 64 years (Table 6). The age-adjusted mortality rate for lung cancer among men now ranks in the upper half of countries in the Americas for which there are reliable data (PAHO 1990). Based on these data, it appears that the impact of smoking, evidenced by the increasing lung cancer mortality rate, is increasing in Mexico, and that the impact on women as yet is lower than on men.

Malignant tumors of the lip, oral cavity, and pharynx (ICD 140–149), which are strongly associated with smoking, are very infrequent in Mexico; the age-adjusted mortality rates for both men and women were unchanged from 1982 to 1986.

Because the exposure to tobacco in terms of prevalence and number of cigarettes smoked per day is relatively low in Mexico, national mortality rates may not reflect the disease impact of smoking in the most heavily exposed populations, i.e., those living in Mexico City. Additional analyses of mortality patterns among these populations would undoubtedly show a greater impact of smoking than do those performed on the national population.

Tobacco Use Prevention and Control Activities

Government Action

Executive structure and policies

The Ley General de Salud, issued in 1983, called for a Government program to combat drug addiction, including tobacco use (Secretaría de Salud 1983). Within this general framework, the Government created the Consejo Nacional Contra las Adicciones, presided over by the Secretary of Health, in 1986. The Programa Contra el Tabaquismo was also created as a collaborative effort of the Health Secretariat, the National Council Against Addictions, and the National Institute of Respiratory Diseases (Secretaría de Salud 1986). Prior to this public health effort, antismoking activities were limited to cessation programs concentrated in Mexico City university hospitals (Puente-Silva 1986). By their nature, these programs had a curative rather than a preventive approach.

The Programa Contra el Tabaquismo has four objectives: to develop antitobacco education for schools and the general public; to improve the di-

agnosis, treatment, and rehabilitation for smoking-related conditions; to strengthen the legal framework for smoking control; and to improve scientific research on tobacco and health. A series of strategies, lines of action, and concrete activities was designed to achieve these objectives. Four technical committees, including representatives of several institutions, are responsible for the implementation of the program (Secretaría de Salud 1986).

The first year of the national antitobacco program highlighted school-based and public education activities (Rubio et al. 1990). In addition, 12 scientific research projects were sponsored. Of these, eight were biomedical, three addressed psychosocial issues, and one analyzed the economics of tobacco product television advertising (Chan-Escalante 1989). In 1989, the Taller Intersectorial de Derecho Sanitario Mexicano discussed the problem of smoking and made several legislative proposals.

Legislation

The Mexican constitution guarantees the right to good health. The Ley General de Salud acknowledged that smoking is harmful to health through several components of the law. First, it included provisions for the National Antismoking Program to conduct research and education. It also required on tobacco packages a warning which reads: ''This product may be harmful to your health.'' In addition, the sale of tobacco products to minors is prohibited and product advertising is regulated. With respect to tobacco products, commercial messages may only provide information about the quality of the product and about manufacturing techniques. Tobacco neither can be presented as a symbol of good health nor can it be associated with positive social values. The law forbids the participation of children or adolescents in tobacco advertisements and forbids targeting these ads to them as consumers. In 1987, the law was amended so that the above restriction applied to persons younger than 25 years and that the message, ''Smoking **is** harmful to your health,'' is included in all audio or visual advertisements for tobacco (Secretaría de Salud 1987). Other warnings that mention specific smoking-related risks were also included. The law mandates that nicotine and tar yields for cigarettes be provided to consumers, and that cigarettes are insect- and pesticide-free (Secretaría de Salud 1988b).

Although these restrictions on advertising are a clear statement of the Government's commitment to prevent tobacco use by young persons, the substantial funds devoted to tobacco promotion in Mexico by the multinational tobacco companies may overwhelm these control efforts. In addition to the Marlboro sponsorship of national football championships, tobacco sponsorships include international motor racing, horse racing, the Acapulco International Film Festival, and rock concerts (Chapman 1990).

In 1990, a Federal decree issued by the Minister of Health banned smoking from classrooms, auditoria, health facilities, gas stations, public transportation, Government offices serving the public, and movie theaters. Enclosed food service facilities are required to have nonsmoking areas. The regulations accompanying this decree provide for enforcement through surveillance, inspections, notifications, and sanctions for violators (Asamblea de Representantes del Distrito Federal 88–91, 1990). The extent to which the clean indoor air legislation is enforced is unknown.

Taxes

In 1985, the Government collected 107,305 million pesos in tobacco-related taxes. This represented 1.7 percent of total Government revenue and an increase from 1.1 percent of total revenue ($US 305,100,000) in 1983 (Chapman 1990).

School Education

The National Antismoking Program proposed the inclusion of information on the health consequences of smoking in primary school textbooks to the Secretaría de Educación Pública. It has also produced booklets and other educational materials that are used by the school system, parents' associations, and Children's Brigades (Dirección de Educación Para la Salud 1987). It is reported that three universities have expanded teaching on smoking and health in medicine, psychology, and social work curricula (Labrandero 1990).

Public Information Activities and Cessation Programs

Antismoking messages have been disseminated by the National Antismoking Program through both printed and electronic mass media. The Program has participated routinely in the World Health Organization sponsored World No-Tobacco Day.

Although public information activities have focused on preventing smoking, cessation pro-

grams are available. Cessation clinics are offered by several hospitals in Mexico City and other states.

Nongovernmental Action

In 1985, the nongovernmental Comité Mexicano para el Estudio y Control del Tabaquismo (COMECTA) was created. COMECTA promotes intersectoral collaboration and employs five persons full time in tobacco control activities, and produces radio and television public educational programs (Chapman 1990).

Summary

Because of a variety of climatic and economic changes, tobacco production has decreased in Mexico since 1980. The partially Government-owned tobacco intermediary organization has been sold to private concerns, and pricing policies for growers are now set by the National Tobacco Committee, in which growers participate. The Government of Mexico is now faced with a familiar two-pronged dilemma: maintaining an ongoing commitment to support small farmers who benefit from cash crops such as tobacco while simultaneously forging a commitment to control the emerging chronic diseases caused by tobacco use among their citizens. A newfound interest in exporting tobacco parallels that same interest found in the United States, where tobacco farmers have benefited from recent hard-edged trade policies that support U.S. tobacco sales abroad.

Advertising and promotion of tobacco products are permitted and used in all forms and through all mass media. Tobacco sponsorship of sports, cultural events, and youth-oriented events is widespread, despite legislative restrictions designed to decrease advertising targeted toward youth. Television is the primary medium for tobacco advertising. Tobacco advertisements and cigarette packages display unequivocal warnings stating that tobacco is harmful to human health.

Per capita cigarette consumption has decreased recently after a steady increase that began in the 1930s. However, projections have been made by the FAO for increased total consumption due to an increase in the size of the adult population. Although the prevalence of smoking among men has not decreased since 1971, at least in Mexico City, the prevalence among women has increased substantially. Interestingly, survey data show the existence of a south-north gradient in prevalence, with the highest prevalence in the north. Whether this results from a greater cultural and economic influence because of the closer proximity of the United States to these regions is not known. In addition to this gradient, survey data show a similar effect of urbanization on tobacco prevalence. The prevalence of smoking is higher in urban centers than in rural areas for both men and women.

Surveys of physicians and hospital employees suggest that the prevalence of smoking among these well-educated persons is similar to or higher than the prevalence of smoking among the general public. These professionals clearly understand the health consequences of smoking, but they have not yet adopted the nonsmoking norm. In developed nations, the nonsmoking norm was embraced by physicians prior to diffusion into the general public. Thus, widespread changes in public behavior provoked by changes in public beliefs and knowledge about smoking do not appear imminent in Mexico. The decline in per capita consumption of cigarettes is primarily a result of decreased consumer buying power, and this pattern is similar to that of the middle-income nations in the rest of Latin America.

The disease impact of smoking is already evident in Mexico. Cancer of the trachea, bronchus, and lung is the most common type of cancer death, and each year, nearly 4,000 lung cancer deaths may be attributed to cigarette smoking among Mexicans. The true disease burden is likely much larger given the fact that cardiovascular diseases are the most common cause of death in Mexico overall. The age-specific mortality rate for lung cancer, a marker of the population exposure to tobacco, is increasing among both men and women aged 55 and older, and is increasing at a faster rate among women than among men for younger Mexicans.

The Ley General de Salud created one of the few Government-sponsored antismoking programs in the Americas. Among the achievements of the program are school-based and public education campaigns and the introduction of new legislation aimed at restricting smoking in public places. Research on smoking and health has been limited primarily to biomedical subjects, but the National Program is positioned uniquely to support policy-related and economic research geared toward fostering widespread behavioral change and social norms. The Government program may also benefit from a centralized nongovernmental National Committee for the Study and Control of Smoking (COMECTA), which can act as a coalition to unify public support for tobacco prevention and control through public information activities and coordination of various other nongovernmental groups.

Conclusions

1. The disease burden of tobacco use is emerging among Mexicans, as evidenced by the increasing age-specific rates for lung cancer among both men and women aged 55 years and older. Nearly 4,000 lung cancer deaths and an undetermined number of cardiovascular disease deaths are caused each year by smoking in Mexico.

2. The prevalence of smoking among men in Mexico City has remained stable since 1971, but that among women has increased. Approximately 9,000,000 adult Mexicans were daily smokers in 1988.

3. The prevalence of smoking is higher in the north and in urban areas of Mexico than in the south or in rural areas. The prevalence of smoking among Mexican physicians is similar to that of the general public, suggesting that the nonsmoking norm has not yet been embraced by those who are the best informed about the health consequences of smoking.

4. Tobacco advertising and promotion are widespread, despite legislative controls on content and coverage of these advertisements. Sports, cultural, and youth-oriented events are vigorously sponsored by the tobacco industry.

5. A substantial Government commitment to tobacco control is evident in the establishment, by law, of a National Antismoking Program. The program develops school-based and public educational campaigns, research on smoking and health, and legislative actions to combat tobacco use. Nongovernmental programs, most notably COMECTA, are active in changing norms on smoking among Mexicans.

References

AGROECONOMIC SERVICES LTD. and TABACOSMOS LTD. *The Employment, Tax Revenue and Wealth that the Tobacco Industry Creates: an Economic Study.* Agroeconomic Services Ltd. and Tabacosmos Ltd., September 1987.

ASAMBLEA DE REPRESENTANTES DEL DISTRITO FEDERAL 88–91. Reglamento para la Protección de los no fumadores en el Distrito Federal. *Diario Oficial* 6 August 1990.

CASTRO-SARINANA, M.E., MAYA, M.A., AGUILAR,

M.A. Consumo de sustancias tóxicas y tabaco entre la población estudiantil de 14 a 18 años. *Salud Pública de México* 24(5):565–574, Sept.–Oct. 1982.

CENTRO LATINOAMERICANO DE DEMOGRAFIA. CELADE. *Boletín Demográfico* 23(45), Santiago, 1990.

CHAN-ESCALANTE, J. El gasto publicitario en la televisión de la ciudad de México para la promoción del consumo de tabaco. In: Rubio, H., Labrandero, M., Selman, M., Martínez-Rossier, J., Perez-Neria, J., Yañez, R.M., et al. Avances del Programa contra el Tabaquismo. *Revista del Instituto Nacional de Enfermedades Respiratorias (supl.)* 2(3):1–45, February 1990.

CHAPMAN, S., WONG, W.L. *Tobacco Control in the Third World—a Resource Atlas.* Penang, Malaysia: International Organization of Consumers Unions, 1990.

DIRECCION DE EDUCACION PARA LA SALUD. La prevención de las adicciones-farmacodependencia, problemas relacionados con el abuso del alcohol y tabaquismo. *Unidad Educativa para el Cuidado de la Salud. No. 15.* Subsecretaría de Servicios de Salud, Secretaría de Salud, México, 1987.

DIRECCION GENERAL DE SERVICIOS MEDICOS. Exámen médico para alumnos de primer ingreso 1988. Dirección General de Servicios Médicos, Universidad Nacional Autónoma de México, (Unpublished data), 1988.

FOOD AND AGRICULTURE ORGANIZATION OF THE UNITED NATIONS. Tobacco: supply, demand, and trade projections, 1995 and 2000. *FAO Economic and Social Development Paper 86.* Rome: FAO, 1990.

GALLUP ORGANIZATION. The Incidence of Smoking in Central and Latin America. Conducted for: The American Cancer Society. Princeton, New Jersey: The Gallup Organization, Inc., April 1988.

GUTIERREZ DE VELASCO, C., YANEZ-CLAVEL, R.M. Encuesta para conocer el hábito tabáquico de los trabajadores del Instituto Nacional de Enfermedades Respiratorias. Instituto Nacional de Enfermedades Respiratorias, México, 1988.

INSTITUTO NACIONAL DE ESTADISTICA, GEOGRAFIA E INFORMATICA. Encuesta industrial anual 1989 México, 1989.

JOLY, D.J. *El hábito de fumar en América Latina.* Washington, D.C.: Pan American Health Organization, Scientific Publication 337, 1977.

LABRANDERO, M. Country collaborator's report, Mexico. (Unpublished data). Pan American Health Organization, 1990.

LEE, P.N. *Tobacco Consumption in Various Countries.* Research paper 6, 4th edition. London: Tobacco Research Council, 1975.

MAXWELL, J.P. International Tobacco—Part One 1989. Richmond, Virginia: The Maxwell Consumer Report, 18 May 1990.

MEDINA-MORA, M.E., DE LA FUENTE, R. Estudio nacional sobre uso de drogas en la población estudiantil de la República Mexicana. In: Rubio, H., Labrandero, M., Selman, M., Martinez-Rossier, J., Perez-Neria, J., Yañez, R.M., et al. Avances del Programa contra el Tabaquismo. *Revista del Instituto Nacional de Enfermedades Respiratorias (supl.)* 2(3):1–45, February 1990.

MENESES, F., STETLER, H., PIERCE, J. A telephone survey of smoking among practicing physicians in Mexico City, unpublished data, 1989.

PAN AMERICAN HEALTH ORGANIZATION. *Health Conditions in the Americas, 1981–1984.* Washington, D.C.: PAHO, Scientific Publication 500, 1986.

PAN AMERICAN HEALTH ORGANIZATION. *Health Conditions in the Americas.* Washington, D.C.: PAHO, Scientific Publication 524, 1990.

PUENTE-SILVA, F.G. Resultados sobre el hábito de fumar en tres muestras (población suburbana/rural, personal médico de siete centros hospitalarios y personal de Petróleos Mexicanos), implicaciones y consideraciones. *Salud Mental* 8(3):60–65, September 1985.

PUENTE-SILVA, F.G. Tabaquismo en México. *Boletín de la Oficina Sanitaria Panamericana* 10(3):234–246, September 1986.

RUBIO, H., LABRANDERO, M., SELMAN, M., MARTINEZ-ROSSIER, J., PEREZ-NERIA, J., YANEZ, R.M., et al. Avances del Programa contra el Tabaquismo. *Revista del Instituto Nacional de Enfermedades Respiratorias (supl.)* 2(3):1–45, February 1990.

SECRETARIA DE SALUD. *Ley General de Salud.* Dirección General de Asuntos Jurídicos, Secretaría de Salud, México, 1983.

SECRETARIA DE SALUD. Decreto por el que se reforma y adiciona la Ley General de Salud. *Diario Oficial de la Federación.* 27 May 1987, pp. 7–13.

SECRETARIA DE SALUD. *Encuesta nacional de salud.* Secretaría de Salud, Subsecretaría de Servicios de Salud, Dirección General de Epidemiología, Sistema Nacional de Encuestas de Salud, México, 1988.

SECRETARIA DE SALUD. Reglamento de la Ley General de Salud en materia de control sanitario de actividades, establecimientos, productos y servicios. *Diario Oficial de la Federación.* 18 January 1988b.

SECRETARIA DE SALUD. *Encuesta nacional de adicciones.* Secretaría de Salud, Subsecretaría de Servicios de Salud, Dirección General de Epidemiología, Sistema Nacional de Encuestas de Salud, México, 1990.

SECRETARIA DE SALUD. *Programa contra el Tabaquismo.* Secretaría de Salud, Consejo Nacional contra las Adicciones, Instituto Nacional de Enfermedades Respiratorias, Organización Panamericana de la Salud, México, 1986.

TABAMEX. *Historia y Cultura del Tabaco en México.* México: Secretaría de Agricultura y Recursos Hidráulicos, 1988.

TAPIA-CONYER, R., LAZCANO-RAMIREZ, F., MEDINA-MORA, M.E., SOLACHE, G., LEON, G., OTERO, B.R., et al. Situación epidemiológica del tabaquismo en México: una comparación entre la Encuesta Nacional de Salud y la Encuesta Nacional de Adicciones (unpublished paper), 1989a.

TAPIA-CONYER, R., LAZCANO-RAMIREZ, F., REVUELTA-HERRERA, M., SEPULVEDA-AMOR, J. El consumo de tabaco en México: resultados de la Encuesta Nacional de Salud. *Boletín Mensual de Epidemiología* 4(3):33–39, March 1989b.

TOBACCO MERCHANTS ASSOCIATION OF THE U.S. Production and consumption of tobacco products for selected countries 1979–1988. *Special Report.* 89-3, September 28, 1989.

U.S. DEPARTMENT OF AGRICULTURE. Tobacco Production, Exports and Imports 1979–1989. Unpublished tabulations. U.S. Department of Agriculture; Tobacco, Cotton, and Seeds Division; Foreign Agricultural Service, 1990a.

U.S. DEPARTMENT OF AGRICULTURE. *World Tobacco Situation.* U.S. Department of Agriculture, Foreign Agricultural Service, August 1990b.

WEINGARTEN, S. Tobacco grows into Mexico's hot moneymaker. *The Atlanta Journal and Constitution,* July 3, 1987, p. 11.

WORLD BANK, *World Development Report 1990—Poverty.* New York: Oxford University Press, 1990.

Nicaragua

General Characteristics

Nicaragua is situated on the Central American isthmus between Costa Rica to the south and Honduras and El Salvador to the north. The country has been torn by civil war for much of the past decade, leading to a severe economic recession (Pan American Health Organization [PAHO] 1990). The war has clearly affected health status, especially evidenced by the limited mortality data available for parts of Nicaragua. For young adults in this country, external causes of death, e.g., homicide and other violent actions, were the causes of death most frequently reported.

The estimated 1990 mid-year population in Nicaragua was 3,870,000, 46 percent of which was younger than 15 years old. With a total fertility rate of 5.5, one of the highest in Latin America, the age structure of the population will continue to be concentrated in younger age groups for the foreseeable future. Only 59 percent of the population is urban (World Bank 1990). It should be noted that no census has been conducted since 1971 in Nicaragua.

The infant mortality rate was 61.6 per 1,000 live births during 1985 to 1990, and life expectancy at birth was 62.0 years for men and 64.6 years for women (Table 1). These figures are similar to those reported for the neighboring Central American countries of Honduras, El Salvador, and Guatemala (CELADE 1990).

Table 1. Health and economic indicators, Nicaragua, 1980s and 1990

Indicator	Year	Value
Population	1990	3,870,180
Percent < age 15	1988	46.1
Percent ≥ age 65	1988	2.9
Percent urban	1988	59
Life expectancy at birth	1985–1990	
Men		62.0
Women		64.6
Total fertility rate	1985–1990	5.5
Infant mortality rate	1985–1990	61.6
Per 1,000 live births		
Crude mortality rate	1988	41
Per capita gross national product ($US)	1987	830
Percent change in GNP Per year	1980–1988	−4.7

Sources: World Bank, 1989, 1990; CELADE, 1990.

In 1987, the per capita gross national product (GNP) of Nicaragua was one of the lowest in the Americas: $US830 (Table 1). During 1980 to 1988, the per capita GNP in fact decreased 4.7 percent per year. Inflation has been as high as 1,500 percent in 1985. In 1988, some economic and social stabilization began to emerge, but the course of the economy under this new political situation has yet to be determined (PAHO 1990).

The current health situation of Nicaragua is a product of the economic problems in the late 1980s, as well as generally poor living conditions for the majority of Nicaraguans. Despite the establishment of a National Health System in 1981, accessibility to health care is still limited. Since 1988, additional efforts to extend coverage have included the establishment of new health care facilities and several prevention programs. However, until 1991, the long state of war and economic disruption greatly limited resources available for health. Currently, 4.7 percent of the GNP is spent on health care each year.

The Tobacco Industry

Agriculture

In 1987, an estimated 2,000 ha were planted with tobacco (Chapman 1990). Tobacco is mainly grown in northern Nicaragua, but there are also plantations on the islands of Omotepe and Moyogalpa in Lake Managua. Approximately 50 of the 204 Nicaraguan tobacco growers farm lands were given to them by the Government. TANIC (Tabacalera Nicaraguense), the Nicaraguan subsidiary of British-American Tobacco Company, SA, (BAT), is vertically integrated into the entire tobacco agro-industry. It acts as a guarantor for farmers' loans from the Bank of Nicaragua and provides technical support to farmers from the planting phase through the sale of raw leaf. The Government does not fix raw leaf prices nor does it mediate in domestic or international raw tobacco sales. Quality control and price-setting are solely the responsibility of TANIC.

In contrast to tobacco farmers, those who farm other crops have no loan guarantees, no guaranteed purchasers for their crops, and no Government incentives to grow basic foodstuffs or other products for domestic consumption (Robles 1991). Thus, despite the war, production and exports of Nicaraguan tobacco did not decrease during the pe-

Table 2. Production, imports, exports, and total domestic consumption of leaf tobacco (in metric tons), Nicaragua, 1978–1989

Year	Production	Imports	Exports	Total domestic consumption
1978	2,981	93	1,106	1,200
1979	2,745	0	1,400	1,200
1980	4,192	0	423	1,400
1981	3,691	43	657	1,600
1982	2,783	0	570	2,170
1983	3,900	566	773	3,035
1984	4,550	444	1,068	3,600
1985	4,550	740	501	4,000
1986	4,550	409	142	4,350
1987	4,550	335	209	4,325
1988	4,550	400	160	4,200
1989	4,550	400	160	4,200

Source: USDA, 1990.

riod 1978–89 (Table 2). Moreover, tobacco production increased to 4,550 MT in 1984 and has since stayed at that level.

Tobacco Manufacturing and Marketing

TANIC is the only cigarette manufacturing company operating in Nicaragua. It produces several different cigarette brands, of which the most popular are Windsor, Belmont, Belmont Menthol, and Alas (Cardosa 1991). Because cigarette advertising has been prohibited since 1979, the major promotional strategy used by TANIC is an effective distribution system with wide availability of cigarettes throughout the country. Cigarettes are commonly sold by the single unit in Nicaragua. In addition, cigars are manufactured in the north, but these have lost economic importance as domestic consumption of cigars has declined (Robles 1991). Nicaraguan tobacco is well regarded abroad. Thus exports increased from 570 MT in 1982 to 1,068 MT in 1984 and remained at that level through 1988 but has decreased since then (Table 2) (U.S. Department of Agriculture [USDA] 1990).

Tobacco Use

Per Capita Cigarette Consumption

Total and per capita domestic cigarette consumption increased over the past 15 years. Total consumption increased from 1,648 MT in 1973 to 2,400 MT in 1988 (Table 2). The apparent per capita consumption for persons aged 15 and older increased from 1,878 cigarettes in 1973 to 2,400 in 1983, remaining at that level through 1986 (USDA 1990) (per capita consumption was 1,140 cigarettes in 1965) (Figure 1). A TANIC company spokesman attributed the increase in per capita consumption to a much better availability of cigarettes compared with other basic goods. However, since 1988, increased availability of consumer products and a higher cost of living have been evident (Robles 1991). Adult per capita cigarette consumption has decreased sharply since 1988 due to economic pressures and was 1,400 in 1990, even lower than the 1973 figure.

Behavioral Surveys and Limitations

Only two surveys that address tobacco use have been carried out in Nicaragua. The first was part of the Nicaragua-Sweden Cooperative Program on Occupational Health Research (Quintero 1989) that surveyed workers from Region II in northern Nicaragua. The sample included 402 men and 118 women who were either rural agricultural workers or urban industrial workers. The mean age of respondents was 33 years for men and 25 years for women.

The second survey was conducted on high school students in Managua in 1988 (Moncada-Rodríguez 1988). A sample of 510 students was drawn from a total of 20,739 students enrolled in high school in the capital. Of the 507 respondents, 47 were younger than 15 years old, 130 were aged 15 to 16, 191 were aged 17 to 18, and 139 were older than 18 years.

The data from these two surveys apply only to adolescents and young adults; therefore, it is not possible to generalize the results to the entire Nicaraguan population. In addition, the definition of "smoker" was not provided for either survey. In the adolescent survey, occasional and regular smokers were not differentiated, and therefore the prevalences reported may be overestimates of the true behavior of Managua adolescents.

Prevalence of Smoking among Young Working Adults

In the workers' survey, the reported prevalence of smoking was 43.5 percent overall, with a much higher prevalence among men than among women (51 vs. 16 percent) (Table 3) (Quintero 1989). The prevalence of smoking was higher for

Figure 1. Cigarette consumption (per adult 15 and over) Nicaragua, 1978–1986

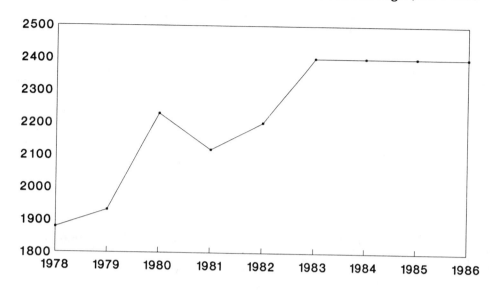

Source: USDA, 1990.

both men and women older than age 25 years than for those younger than 25 years. The prevalence rate among men was quite high compared to reported rates from other Central American countries (for example, in Guatemala City, 38 percent among men and 18 percent among women; in Honduras urban areas, 36 percent among men and 11 percent among women; in El Salvador, 38 percent among men and 12 percent among women). The higher rate in Nicaragua is in part attributable to the younger age of the sample and to their ability to afford cigarettes. In many other countries of the Americas, a determinant of higher smoking prevalence appears to be economic capability, and it is more

likely that younger working adults would have sufficient income to permit them to purchase cigarettes.

Prevalence of Smoking among Adolescents

The prevalence of smoking among Managua high school students was 48.7 percent: 39.8 among males and 52.2 among females (Table 4). This figure includes all experimenters, occasional smokers, and regular smokers. The smoking prevalence among adolescent females is much higher than among young adult workers in Region II, suggesting that young women are initiating smoking more readily than did older cohorts of women. In addi-

Table 3. Prevalence (percent) cigarette smoking among rural and urban workers in Region II, by sex and age group, Nicaragua, 1989

Category	Men			Women		
	<25 yrs (n=63)	≥25 yrs (n=339)	Total (n=402)	<25 yrs (n=27)	≥25 yrs (n=91)	Total (n=118)
Smokers (%)	46	53	51	4	20	16
Ex-smokers (%)	—	6	5	—	4	3
Nonsmokers (%)	54	42	44	96	76	81
Mean age	20	35	33	20	33	26

Source: Quintero, 1989.

Table 4. Prevalence (percent) of cigarette smoking among adolescents, by sex, age group, and smoking status of friends, Managua, 1988

Category	Smoker	Ex-smoker	Never smoked	N
Sex				
Females	52.2	6.8	35.3	232
Males	39.8	4.6	55.5	236
Age group				
<15	19.1	2.1	78.7	47
15–16	42.3	5.3	52.3	130
17–18	49.2	5.2	45.5	191
over 18	64.0	2.8	33.0	139
Friends' smoking status				
None	19.3	1.6	79.0	62
Some	47.4	2.5	50.0	358
All	78.6	1.6	19.6	61

Source: Moncada-Rodríguez, 1988.

tion, the prevalence of smoking among adults and adolescents in Managua may be higher as a result of the urban setting, particularly for women. The prevalence of smoking among adolescents increases with age, reaching a high of 64 percent for those more than 18 years old; this level is almost 50 percent higher than the prevalence among Region II workers, suggesting an urban-rural difference in cigarette use similar to that of other countries of the Americas.

In addition, the prevalence of smoking is higher among those who have friends who smoke (Table 4). The prevalence of smoking among those who report that all of their friends are smokers is 78.6 percent, and only 19.3 percent among those who report that none of their friends are smokers. Although the question may have been ambiguous, these differences are large enough to suggest the possibility of peer pressure in the initiation of smoking among Managua high school students.

Most (90.3 percent) of the 217 smokers smoked fewer than 10 cigarettes per day. The proportion of smokers who began to smoke before age 15 was 37.6 percent; 40.4 percent began at ages 15 to 17, and 22.0 percent began after age 17.

Smoking and Health

National mortality data for Nicaragua are incomplete and are not published by international agencies. Therefore, in order to begin to assess the disease impact of several smoking-related diseases, mortality data for Managua only (Region III) were used to calculate rates for selected smoking-related diseases by sex for persons aged 15 to 34, 35 to 49, and 50 and older (Table 5). Because Managua is the capital city, under-registration of deaths should be minimal. In addition, in Region III, deaths attributed to signs, symptoms and ill-defined causes account for only 4.1 percent of all registered deaths. Mortality data were supplied by the Ministry of Health, and population data were provided by the Nicaraguan Institute of Statistics and CELADE. Although no census has been carried out in Nicaragua since 1971, population data were estimated using data from the 1989 electoral registration records.

External causes of death (such as homicide, violent death, and war) were the most important causes of death in the age groups 15 to 34 and 35 to 49 in Managua. Among persons aged 50 years and older, myocardial infarction was the leading cause of death (age group-specific mortality rate 169.8 per 100,000 persons), and external causes were the second leading cause (88.9 per 100,000) (Table 5). Stomach cancer was the leading cause of cancer death for persons aged 50 years and older, and the mortality rate for infectious diseases was lower than that for external causes as well as chronic diseases (lung cancer, stomach cancer, chronic lung disease, and myocardial infarction). The relative impact of chronic diseases may increase, given the reduction of armed struggle in Nicaragua.

Table 5. Mortality rates (per 100,000 persons) by age group for selected causes of death by age, Region III, Managua, Nicaragua, 1989

Cause of death (ICD-9 code)	Age group in years		
	15–34	35–49	50 and older
All causes	106.6	226.8	1,692.0
Intestinal infections (ICD-9 001-009)	1.3	4.0	18.5
Malignant tumor of stomach (ICD-9 151)	1.1	2.4	49.7
Malignant tumor of trachea, bronchi, and lungs (ICD-9 162)	0	1.6	21.9
Myocardial infarction (ICD-9 410)	2.1	11.1	169.8
Bronchitis, emphysema, and asthma (ICD-9 490–493)	0.5	3.2	23.1
External causes of injury and poisoning (ICD-9 E800–E819)	56.9	45.2	88.9
Percent of diagnoses = symptoms, signs, and ill-defined conditions (ICD-9 780-799)	2.2	1.7	7.2

Source: Unpublished data, Ministry of Health, Population Directorate, Nicaraguan Institute of Statistics (INEC), Population Estimates and Projections 1950–2025, INEC-CELADE, 1991.

Mortality rates for several chronic diseases related to smoking show that heart disease has emerged as the most frequently reported cause of death in Managua for persons aged 50 and older. Trend data are not available, but it is clear from the limited data available that Nicaragua will display mortality patterns similar to those of other Central American countries as the pall of violence is lifted and life expectancy is extended. Cardiovascular diseases will lead the list of chronic disease mortality rates among older adults for the foreseeable future, but as the large population of Nicaraguans that smokes ages, diseases such as lung cancer and chronic obstructive pulmonary disease will become more important. In addition, it appears that young women, who will soon be reaching child-bearing age, have initiated smoking in large numbers, at least in Managua. The impact on infant mortality and fetal loss may be substantial in the near future. In the United States, as much as 10 percent of infant mortality is attributable to smoking by pregnant women and mothers (Malloy 1988).

Tobacco Use Prevention and Control Activities

The Department of Chronic Diseases of the Ministry of Health has responsibility for the prevention of tobacco-related diseases in Nicaragua. The only substantive intervention against tobacco in Nicaragua thus far is the 1979 ban on tobacco product advertising. Other health problems have dominated the attention of the Ministry, but an awareness of the need for tobacco prevention programs and basic legislative policies that might inhibit tobacco consumption has been expressed (Robles 1991).

Summary and Conclusions

Economic and social disruption has taken a severe toll on the population of Nicaragua, evidenced by a decline in the per capita GNP, a persistently high infant mortality rate, and increased impoverishment of many citizens. It is impressive in the face of this discouraging situation that tobacco production increased during 1978 to 1988, and that the prevalence of smoking among young employed persons and adolescents is among the highest of all the Central American countries. Despite the lack of tobacco product advertising, the distribution of cigarettes was efficient enough to maintain access to this consumer product, even when other goods were in short supply in the 1980s. Vertical integration of the tobacco industry has supported sustained tobacco production and consumption. Revenue data from taxes are unavailable, but it is not likely that the Nicaraguan government is profiting greatly from tobacco consumption given that the sole manufacturing company is not owned or operated by the government but by a multinational tobacco conglomerate.

As Nicaragua looks to the problems of the future, it is certain that tobacco-related disease will emerge as a major health concern. As data systems are refined to permit analyses of mortality patterns, chronic disease deaths among older adults will increase in importance within these patterns. As Nicaragua regains control over basic health services and data collection systems, controlling tobacco use among the population should be included in health planning.

Based on the data reported above, the following conclusions can be drawn:

1. Tobacco production and consumption have been maintained at relatively high levels in Nicaragua despite the deterioration of services and availability of other consumer goods due to widespread social and economic disruption.
2. More than 50 percent of employed men in parts of Nicaragua are current smokers, but only 6.4 percent of employed women are smokers. However, among Managua adolescents, more than 50 percent of females are either occasional or daily smokers. These prevalence rates are among the highest of the Central American countries. Patterns of tobacco use should be monitored among all Nicaraguans in the future.
3. Few tobacco control activities are as yet evident in Nicaragua, and a long-standing ban on tobacco product advertising is counterbalanced by the effective cigarette distribution system of the multinational tobacco subsidiary in Nicaragua.

References

CARDOSA, A. Country Collaborator's Report. Unpublished data, PAHO, 1991.

CENTRO LATINOAMERICANO DE DEMOGRAFIA. *Boletín Demográfico.* CELADE, Santiago, Year XXIII, No. 45, 1990.

CHAPMAN, S., WONG, W.L. *Tobacco Control in the Third World—A Resource Atlas.* Penang, Malaysia: International Organization of Consumers Unions, 1990.

MALLOY, M.H., KLEINMAN, J.C., LAND, G.H., SCHRAMM, W.F. The association of maternal smoking with age and cause of infant death. *American Journal of Epidemiology* 128(1):46–55, 1988.

MONCADA-RODRIGUEZ, N., ESPINAL-BOTTEL, O., GUTIERREZ-SERRANO, R. *Hábito de fumar en estudiantes de secundaria,* Managua, Setiembre 1988. VII Jornada Universitaria de Desarrollo Científico. Universidad Nacional Autónoma de Nicaragua, Recinto Universitario "Rubén Darío," Facultad de Ciencias Médicas, Managua, Nicaragua, 1988.

PAN AMERICAN HEALTH ORGANIZATION. *Health Conditions in the Americas.* Washington D.C.: Pan American Health Organization. Scientific Publication No. 524, 1990.

QUINTERO, C., ANDERSSON, K., MCCONNELL, R., HOGSTEDT, C., *Valores de referencia para función pulmonar en trabajadores nicaragüenses.* Universidad Nacional Autónoma de Nicaragua, Swedish Board of Occupational Safety and Health, Department of Occupational Medicine, Orebro, 1989.

ROBLES, S. Consultancy Report, Managua, February 5–8, 1991. Washington, D.C.: Pan American Health Organization, 1991.

U.S. DEPARTMENT OF AGRICULTURE. Tobacco production, imports, exports, and consumption, Latin America and the Caribbean, unpublished tabulations. U.S. Department of Agriculture, Tobacco, Cotton, and Seeds Division, Foreign Agricultural Service, Washington, D.C., 1990.

WORLD BANK. *World Development Report 1989.* New York: Oxford University Press, 1989.

WORLD BANK. *World Development Report 1990—Poverty.* New York: Oxford University Press, 1990.

Organization of Eastern Caribbean States: Antigua and Barbuda, Dominica, Grenada, St. Kitts and Nevis, Saint Lucia, and St. Vincent and the Grenadines

General Characteristics

The Tobacco Industry
    Tobacco taxation and government revenues

Tobacco Use

Smoking and Health

Tobacco Use Prevention and Control Activities
    Antigua and Barbuda
    Dominica
    Grenada
    St. Kitts and Nevis
    Saint Lucia
    St. Vincent and the Grenadines

Summary

Conclusions

References

General Characteristics

This chapter will review tobacco use in the six small English-speaking island nations of the Organization of Eastern Caribbean States (OECS)—Antigua and Barbuda, Dominica, Grenada, St. Kitts and Nevis, Saint Lucia, and St. Vincent and the Grenadines. All were once British colonies, and all have become independent since 1945; each has a population of fewer than 300,000 (Figures 1, 2, 3, 4, 5). However, St. Kitts and Nevis constitute a federal state within the British Commonwealth. Anguilla and Montserrat are also members of the OECS, but they are not included in this chapter. The OECS was established in June 1981 under the Treaty of Basseterre to strengthen regionalization of the Eastern Caribbean. The objectives of the OECS are to promote unity and cooperation among members in defense of their sovereignty, territorial integrity, and independence (OECS in Perspective 1987). The Eastern Caribbean dollar ($EC) is the common currency for all the members.

Most Government revenues for these states are derived from tourism and agriculture. St. Vincent and the Grenadines produces approximately half of the world's supply of arrowroot in addition to tobacco used for cigarette manufacture. Bananas and grapefruit are the principal economic products of Dominica. Although both tourism and agriculture are major economic activities in Saint Lucia, agriculture accounted for 73 percent of all export earnings in 1986 (United Nations 1988).

Antigua, Barbuda, and the uninhabited island of Redonda occupy 440 km² east of the Leeward Islands and north of Guadeloupe, and constitute a unitary state. Dominica, an island of 750 km² in the Eastern Caribbean between Guadeloupe and Martinique, gained its independence from Britain in 1978. Grenada occupies 344 km² at the southern end of the Windward Islands. St. Kitts and Nevis are located in the Leeward Islands east of the U.S. Virgin Islands, and occupy 360 km². Saint Lucia is an island of 616 km², located south of Martinique in the Eastern Caribbean. St. Vincent and the Grenadines consists of a chain of islands in the southeastern Windward Islands of the Caribbean; an independent nation since 1979, these islands encompass 389 km² (Encyclopedia Britannica 1990).

Population pyramids have been constructed from the most recent population data available for five of the six countries (no recent population data are available for Antigua and Barbuda) (Figures 1,

Figure 1. Population pyramid, Grenada, 1981

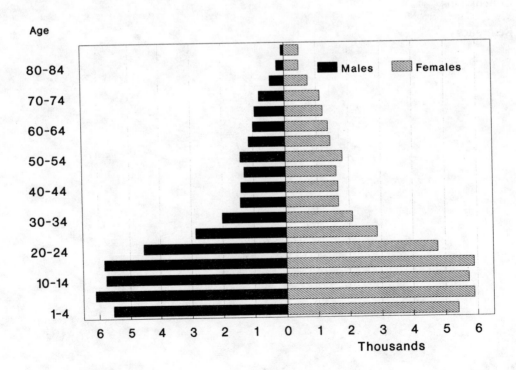

Source: United Nations, 1988.

Figure 2. Population pyramid, Dominica, 1981

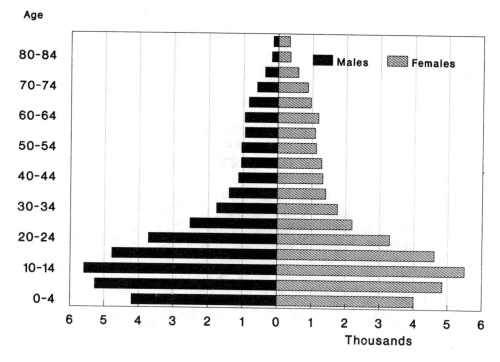

Source: United Nations, 1988.

Figure 3. Population pyramid, Saint Lucia, 1990

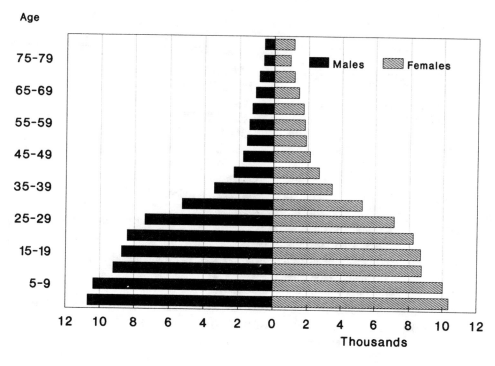

Source: ECLAC, 1990.

Figure 4. Population pyramid, St. Vincent and the Grenadines, 1990

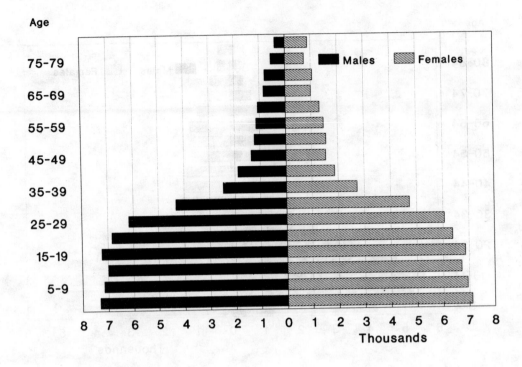

Source: ECLAC, 1990.

Figure 5. Population pyramid, St. Kitts and Nevis, 1990

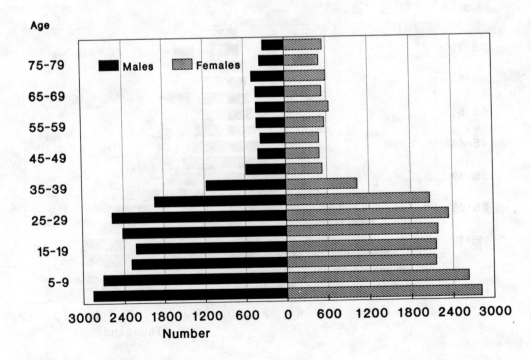

Source: ECLAC, 1990.

2, 3, 4, 5). The five countries for which recent population data are available have similar population structures, characterized by small cohorts aged 40 and older and large cohorts under age 20.

In 1988, life expectancy at birth ranged from 64 years in St. Kitts and Nevis to 73 years in Dominica for men. For women, life expectancy ranged from 70 years in St. Kitts and Nevis to 78 years in Dominica. The 1988 per capita gross national product (GNP) for these nations ranged from US$1,100 in St. Vincent and the Grenadines to US$2,800 in Antigua and Barbuda (World Bank 1989). In none of the countries are the infectious diseases of childhood any longer a major cause of death (Pan American Health Organization [PAHO] 1990). Instead, chronic diseases are emerging as the leading causes of death, indicating that behavioral risk factors such as tobacco use are of immediate concern to these relatively healthy populations (Table 1).

The Tobacco Industry

In the OECS, tobacco is grown only in St. Vincent and the Grenadines, but tobacco products are manufactured in all nations except Antigua and Barbuda and St. Kitts and Nevis. In 1988, 56 MT of tobacco were grown by nine farmers on 31 ha in St. Vincent and the Grenadines. Almost all of this tobacco was grown under contract to the West Indian Tobacco Company, and was exported for manufacture and consumption in Trinidad and Tobago (Browne 1990).

Virtually all tobacco consumed in the OECS is in the form of manufactured cigarettes (Pigott 1990, Browne 1990, Gittens 1990, Hendrickson 1990). Tobacco consumed in Antigua and Barbuda is imported mainly from the United States, the United Kingdom, and Canada. Eight importers supply 38 retailers with approximately 21 brands of cigarettes and 3 other types of tobacco products. Benson & Hedges, 555, Marlboro, Kool, and du Maurier are the most popular cigarette brands (Pigott 1990).

In Dominica, the James Garraway tobacco manufacturing company produces the most popular cigarette brand, Hillsborough, which held an 84-percent market share in 1989. Three imported brands (Benson & Hedges, 555 State Express, and Kool) accounted for the rest (Fortune 1990).

The privately held Caribbean Tobacco Com-

Table 1. Health and economic indicators for independent countries of the Organization of Eastern Caribbean States, latest available data

Indicator	Antigua and Barbuda	Dominica	Grenada	St. Kitts and Nevis	Saint Lucia	St. Vincent and the Grenadines
Area (km^2)[c]	440	750	344	360	620	340
Population, 1988[b]	78,726	81,000	102,000	43,000	145,000	122,000
Population <15 (%)[a]	—	40	39	34	44	44
Population >65 (%)[a]	—	7	7	9	6	6
Ann. pop. growth, 1980–88 (%)[b]	1.4	1.3	1.9	−0.3	2.0	1.4
GNP per capita, 1988 (US$)[b]	2,800	1,650	1,370	2,770	1,540	1,100
Ann. GNP/capita growth rate, 1980–88 (%)[b]	4.0	3.1	3.5	4.9	2.3	4.3
Total fertility rate[b]	1.9	3.0	3.2	2.7	3.4	2.7
Crude birth rate[c]	14	26	37	24	34	27
Crude death rate[c]	5	5	7	10	5	6
Age-adjusted death rate[d]	—	3.8	—	—	5.3	5.2
Infant mortality rate[c]	20	14	30	41	18	26
Life expectancy, Males[c]	70	73	69	64	68	69
Life expectancy, Females[c]	73	78	74	70	73	74
Literacy rate (%)[c]	90	95	85	90	90	85

Sources: a: United Nations, 1990.
          b: World Bank, 1989.
          c: Encyclopedia Britannica, 1990; World Bank, 1990.
          d: PAHO, 1990.

pany, Ltd. operates one factory and employed 21 people in 1989 in Grenada (Gittens 1990). From 1984 to 1988, Grenada annually imported an average of 21,701 kg of unmanufactured tobacco and 4,508 kg of cigarettes (Gittens 1990). Annual domestic production of cigarettes varied between 19.6 million and 24.5 million cigarettes during the decade 1979 to 1988. All cigarettes produced and imported were consumed locally. Locally produced cigarettes have an average level of 20 mg tar and 2.4 mg nicotine (Bhola 1989). Phoenix and Dunhill are the most popular brands.

St. Kitts and Nevis import for domestic consumption cigarettes from the United Kingdom and Barbados. The most popular brands sold are 555 (50-percent market share) and Marlboro Lite (40-percent market share) (Gittens 1990).

In Saint Lucia, the independent cigarette manufacturing firm N.Y. Daher Cigarette Company employs 32 persons and holds 78 percent of the domestic market. Diamond, a plain-end cigarette, is the leading brand in the country. A variety of imported brands account for the remaining market share (Louisy 1990).

Two tobacco manufacturing companies operate in St. Vincent and the Grenadines: the West Indian Tobacco Company, which exports processed tobacco leaf to Trinidad and Tobago, and the St. Vincent Manufacturing Company, which manufactures cigarettes from imported tobacco leaf for domestic consumption. In 1988, 22 MT of tobacco leaf were imported into St. Vincent and the Grenadines. The most popular brand, Empire, is produced locally and accounted for 69 percent of total tobacco sales in 1988. The imported brand, 555 State Express, accounted for 19 percent of total sales (Browne 1990).

Tobacco Taxation and Government Revenues

The tourist destinations of the Caribbean are well-known for duty-free shopping, including cigarettes and other tobacco products; however, taxes are levied on cigarettes produced and consumed domestically in all the countries. Cigarette package prices are high relative to average wages in most countries of the OECS. Cigarettes are made more affordable through the use of 10–cigarette packs. To better understand the economic impact of tobacco on these countries, including Government dependence on cigarette taxes, total revenues per pack and as a percentage of total Government revenue were calculated. In addition, the time an average wage earner must work to earn enough to purchase a package of cigarettes was estimated (Table 2).

In Antigua and Barbuda, the total Government revenue collected from manufactured and unmanufactured tobacco increased from EC$56,950 in 1986 to EC$190,347 in 1987. This increase may not

Table 2. Cigarette taxes, per pack, as a percentage of pack price, as Government revenue and as a percentage of Government revenue, in $EC. Organization of Eastern Caribbean States, most recent year available

Country	Average price per pack in EC$	% of price = tax	Total Government cigarette tax revenue (year)	% of Government revenue = cigarette tax	Minutes needed to earn price of cigarette pack
Antigua and Barbuda	*$3.30–$3.80		$190,347 (1987)		30 minutes
Dominica	*$2.00–$4.00	23 ($.70)		1.4	40 minutes
Grenada	*$2.15 local *$5.20 imported	55			50 minutes
St. Kitts and Nevis	**$2.00–3.50				48 minutes
Saint Lucia	**$1.25 local **$2.00 imported	10	$840,000 (1988)	0.5	100 minutes
St. Vincent and the Grenadines	*$2.00 local *$4.50 imported	41 ($1.60)		1	50 minutes

Source: Unpublished data (Louisy 1990, Pigott 1990, Fortune 1990, Browne 1990, Gittens 1990, Hendrickson 1990).
1 $US = 2.7 $EC
* 20 cigarettes per pack
**10 cigarettes per pack

reflect accurately the increase in tobacco consumption in this nation because up to 50 percent of cigarettes sold in Antigua and Barbuda are contraband (Pigott 1990). In addition, substantial sales of cigarettes to tourists occur in the two duty-free shopping complexes in Antigua and Barbuda. Prices in these shops are about EC$3.51 (US$1.30) per pack of 20. The annual average sales figure for 1989 in one of the tourist shops was approximately EC$19,572. However, sales vary according to the tourist season (Pigott 1990).

An estimated EC$1.2 million illegal trade in cigarettes is also reported annually in Grenada (Gittens 1990). The national tax on cigarettes is the highest in the OECS, consisting of 30 percent value added tax (VAT) on the retail price and a 25 percent surcharge per pack.

The apparent contribution of tobacco taxes to the total Government revenue in the OECS is minimal: range from 0.5 percent in Saint Lucia to 1.4 percent in Dominica. However, the diversion of individual consumer resources by tobacco purchases is substantial: in most of the countries, a worker who consumes one pack of cigarettes per day will spend almost 1 hour per day to satisfy his or her addiction to nicotine. The effect of this diversion on the economy of these small nations is unknown.

Tobacco Use

Data on per capita cigarette consumption are sparse for the OECS countries. With few exceptions, both reported domestic consumption and population data are insufficient to produce reliable estimates in each locale for the entire 10-year period from 1979 to 1989. However, some general trends may be discerned using data reported by individual Governments and estimated yearly populations reported by the Pan American Health Organization (1990).

In Antigua and Barbuda, yearly adult per capita cigarette consumption during 1979 to 1989 cannot be calculated because population estimates for persons 15 years or older are not available. However, based on data supplied by Government sources, the number of imported cigarettes available to residents apparently decreased by more than 70 percent from approximately 106,000,000 units in 1984 to 30,000,000 units in 1987. For 1987, the apparent total per capita cigarette consumption was 389 for all 77,093 persons populating this nation, down from 1,412 in 1984 for the estimated population of 75,067 (PAHO 1990; Pigott 1990).

This apparent dramatic decline in consumption is likely to be an artifact. An increase in illegal trade, coupled with inaccurate import data, contributes to the difficulties in estimating true per capita consumption.

The data for Dominica appear to be more reliable. For persons aged 15 and older in Dominica, per capita cigarette consumption decreased linearly from 892 in 1979 to 657 in 1989, at an average annual rate of 3 percent. The total decline in consumption was 26 percent in these 10 years (Fortune 1990). This change in consumption seems reasonable and may reflect a real change in tobacco use among the residents of Dominica (Figure 6).

In Grenada, apparent per capita cigarette consumption among persons aged 15 years and older changed very little from 1984 to 1988, from approximately 450 to 495 cigarettes per year. Data are not available earlier than 1984, and the extent of illegal trade in cigarettes is unknown.

In Saint Lucia, adult annual per capita cigarette consumption apparently decreased from 1,208 in 1979 to 737 in 1983. However, adult consumption subsequently increased to 830 cigarettes per year by 1988 (Figure 7); even so, this level was 31 percent lower than that for 1979 (Louisy 1990). In the 1982 Household Budget Survey performed by the Government Statistical Department (PAHO 1988), 25 percent of households consumed 9.5 packs of locally made Diamond cigarettes per month and 10 percent of households consumed 1.8 packs of imported "555" cigarettes per month. In an unpublished survey of 48 professionals, 23 percent were "smokers," 43 percent were "nonsmokers," and 29 percent had "unknown" tobacco-use behavior.

Cigarette consumption per person aged 15 and older in St. Vincent and the Grenadines declined overall from 1979 to 1989 (Figure 8). Although adult per capita cigarette consumption declined from 651 in 1982 to 417 in 1986, adult consumption increased to 477 by 1989. The total number of cigarettes smoked in St. Vincent and the Grenadines declined steadily from 36.5 million in 1979 to 24.7 million in 1986. However, by 1986 to 1988, the number of cigarettes consumed by adults in this nation had increased to 29.6 million (Browne 1990).

No data are available on the per capita cigarette consumption in St. Kitts and Nevis.

In small countries such as these, population-based surveys of health risk behaviors would provide better data and better understanding of tobacco use among residents. Illegal trade in ciga-

Figure 6. Adult per capita cigarette consumption (age 15+), Dominica, 1979–1989

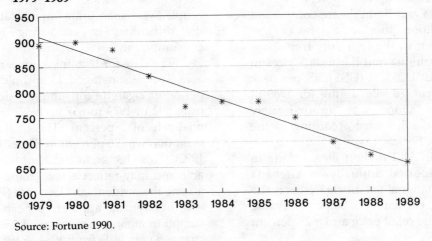

Source: Fortune 1990.

Figure 7. Adult per capita cigarette consumption (age 15+), in thousands, Saint Lucia, 1979–1989

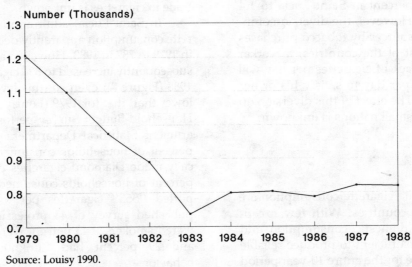

Source: Louisy 1990.

Figure 8. Adult per capita cigarette consumption (age 15+), St. Vincent and the Grenadines, 1979–89

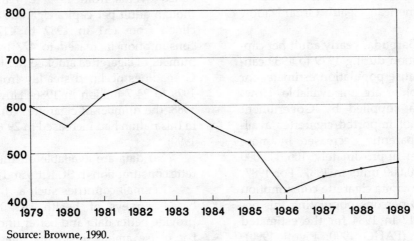

Source: Browne, 1990.

rettes, large sales of tobacco to tourists, and difficulties in collecting data on both consumption and population contribute to the problems in estimating tobacco use among residents of OECS countries. Unfortunately, there have been no household surveys to determine the prevalence of smoking in any of the countries reviewed here. The data available suggest that the residents of most OECS countries have a very low level of tobacco consumption. The apparently consistent data for Dominica suggest that tobacco consumption is declining. Available data for Saint Lucia, St. Vincent and the Grenadines, and Antigua and Barbuda also suggest that tobacco consumption is declining overall in the Eastern Caribbean. Undocumented reports by health department officials suggest that the overall climate in the OECS countries is one of decreasing tobacco use.

Smoking and Health

Mortality data are insufficient to analyze trends in the smoking-related diseases such as lung cancer, coronary heart disease, cerebrovascular disease, chronic obstructive lung disease, and cancers of the lip, oral cavity, pharynx, larynx, esophagus, and kidney for Antigua and Barbuda, Grenada, St. Kitts and Nevis, Saint Lucia, and St. Vincent and the Grenadines. Few deaths are recorded for these diseases in Antigua and Barbuda or Grenada.

It should be reasonable, however, to attribute almost all lung cancer deaths to cigarette smoking; data from U.S. studies suggest that 87 percent of lung cancer mortality is caused by smoking (U.S. Department of Health and Human Services 1989). Thus, considering only lung cancer (although this diagnosis is far from certain where diagnostic facilities are scarce) may help illuminate the current impact of smoking in the small nations of the OECS. There were 729 deaths from all causes in Antigua in 1988 and Barbuda and Grenada in 1984 collectively. Of these, 9 deaths (approximately 1 percent) were recorded as lung cancer (Pigott 1990; PAHO 1990). Of 481 deaths from all causes in St. Kitts and Nevis in 1984, 3 were due to lung cancer (PAHO 1990). Of 885 deaths recorded in Saint Lucia in 1985, only 5 were caused by lung cancer (PAHO 1990). In 1988, five lung cancer deaths were reported for St. Vincent and the Grenadines (Browne 1990). The Pan American Health Organization estimated the lung cancer mortality rate at 1.9 per 100,000 for 1983 in St. Vincent and the Grenadines, but this estimate is based on only two lung cancer deaths (PAHO 1986).

Another approach to understanding mortality patterns in small countries is to pool the number of deaths for several years and to calculate both mortality rates and proportional mortality for selected smoking-related causes of death. Pooled mortality data are available for Dominica for 1984 through 1988: there were 35 reported lung cancer deaths (30 for men and 5 for women, respectively). Of 1,908 total deaths for this period, 371 (17.9 percent) were due to coronary heart disease, cerebrovascular disease, chronic obstructive lung disease, lung cancer, and other smoking-related cancers (Table 3; Fortune 1990). With the exception of cerebrovascular disease, the data suggest that the mortality rates for smoking-related diseases are substantially higher for men than for women. This difference then suggests that the prevalence of risk factors for these diseases (in particular smoking) is higher for men than for women. The data must be interpreted with caution because of the small number of recorded deaths on the island. By comparison, lung cancer mortality rates in Dominica are much lower than those for Canada and the United States (Table 4).

Tobacco Use Prevention and Control Activities

None of the islands in the OECS has a formal Government program or policy on tobacco-use prevention and control. Nor are there sustained school-based or public education programs against smoking. Legislative actions against tobacco are essentially nonexistent in the OECS. There are no restrictions on tobacco advertising in these countries, and tobacco products are frequently advertised on radio and television and in newspapers and magazines. In addition to print media advertising, free samples and giveaways of promotional items have been reported (Fortune 1990). The local cigarette company in Grenada spends approximately EC$10,000 per year sponsoring various sports including basketball, football, table tennis, and body building. The company also sponsors Carnival bands and donates money to churches and schools (PAHO 1988; Bhola 1989). There are no laws requiring tobacco companies to publish tar and nicotine levels on cigarette packs and no regulations requiring health warnings on cigarette packages. Cigarettes imported from Canada and the United States display a health warning only if required by law in the respective destination countries. There are no restrictions on the retail sale of tobacco products to minors in any of the countries of the OECS.

Table 3. Number of deaths from selected smoking-related causes among persons 35 years of age and over, Dominica, 1984–1988

Age	Coronary heart disease	Cerebrovascular disease	Chronic obstructive lung disease	Lung cancer	Cancers of the lip, oral cavity, pharynx, larynx, esophagus, pancreas, bladder, and kidney
35–64					
Men	13	13	8	12	7
Women	7	19	6	3	5
65 and over					
Men	24	55	22	18	9
Women	28	80	15	4	6

Source: Fortune, 1990.

With regard to tobacco control efforts, many of the OECS countries have access to U.S. cable television programming, and thus, exposure to tobacco advertising on television is uncommon. Some U.S. anti-smoking messages are available to the television audiences. Most nations report ad hoc public awareness programs in response to the World Health Organization's (WHO) World No-Tobacco Day each May 31. It is reported that most of the schools in OECS countries prohibit smoking by students, but it is also reported that these restrictions are often ignored.

Drug abuse has recently become an area of concern for OECS countries. The Caribbean Community (CARICOM), of which all six OECS countries are full members, mandated the implementation of the Regional Program for Drug Abuse Abatement and Control at its Heads of Government meeting in 1987. This program focuses on the reduction of illicit drug abuse, but alcohol, tobacco, and prescribed drugs are included in the mandate. The interventions call for youth education and training of teachers. Other components include treatment and rehabilitation, data collection and epidemiology, and law enforcement. In order to implement this mandate, the CARICOM Secretariat, based in Guyana, recommended the formation of a National Drug Abuse Council in each country. These Councils should be multisectoral in order to address the broad issues of drug abuse (including tobacco) in these countries. Many of the OECS countries are still in the process of setting up these committees, and it is too early to evaluate their effectiveness (CARICOM 1990).

Table 4. Rates of death per 100,000 from selected smoking-related causes among persons 35 years of age and over, Dominica, 1984 to 1988

Age	Coronary heart disease	Cerebrovascular disease	Chronic obstructive lung disease	Lung cancer	Cancers of the lip, oral cavity, pharynx, larynx, esophagus, pancreas, bladder, and kidney
35–64					
Men	39.4	39.4	24.2	27.2	21.2
Women	17.0	46.2	14.6	4.9	12.2
65 and over					
Men	227.5	521.3	208.5	170.6	85.3
Women	193.8	553.6	103.8	27.7	41.5

Source: Fortune, 1990.

Antigua and Barbuda

In 1988 and 1989, the Health Education Unit and the Ministry of Home Affairs of Antigua and Barbuda organized for World No-Tobacco Day a public awareness program consisting of posters placed in buildings across the islands and several newspaper articles. The Ministry of Home Affairs now also works closely with the Ministry of Education to provide in primary and secondary schools health education on substance abuse including tobacco (Pigott 1990). Several church groups have established community discussions on tobacco cessation. The Seventh Day Adventist Church in Antigua and Barbuda actively has promoted a lifestyle which condemns smoking. The Church sponsors lectures, demonstrations, and exhibitions at health fairs. The Church also distributes information to young adults on the health effects of smoking. Five of the seven insurance companies in Antigua and Barbuda have recognized the risks associated with tobacco consumption and offer discounts on life insurance policies to nonsmokers. One company, which did not offer discounts, excluded smokers from certain types of coverage (Pigott 1990).

Dominica

Although there are no laws restricting smoking indoors, administrative bans on smoking apply in most Dominican health care facilities, buses, and schools. Smoking is prohibited on all LIAT aircraft of 19 seats or fewer. The central Government increases national taxes on cigarettes at least once per year, not to depress tobacco use but to increase revenues. The Drug Abuse Task Force occasionally publishes news articles concerning tobacco use. Some churches sponsor smoking cessation programs (Fortune 1990).

Grenada

Voluntary restrictions on smoking are common in public places including workplaces, health facilities, buses, Government buildings, theaters, cinemas, and restaurants. The Ministry of Education has prohibited children from smoking in school for many years, but no prevention education is undertaken in the schools. Efforts have been made to raise public awareness through the WHO No-Tobacco Day by featuring the Minister of Health and Chief Medical Officer on radio programs (Gittens 1990).

St. Kitts and Nevis

No education or smoking prevention programs have been initiated by the Government or by nongovernmental organizations in St. Kitts and Nevis. Pall Mall cigarettes is the only brand carrying a warning on its packet. The warning states "Smoking causes lung cancer, heart disease and may complicate pregnancy." A Drug Abuse Prevention Program stressing antismoking messages has been introduced to children in Grades 5 and 6. No treatment programs are available in St. Kitts and Nevis (Hendrickson 1990)

Saint Lucia

In Saint Lucia, a license is required for retail sales of tobacco. There are no laws restricting smoking indoors, but voluntary restrictions limit smoking in supermarkets, gas stations, hospitals, schools, and on some scheduled commercial flights. Approximately half of the life insurance companies on Saint Lucia have recognized the benefits of a smoke-free lifestyle and offer insurance to nonsmokers at much lower rates. The Seventh Day Adventist schools include anti-smoking messages as part of their regular curriculum, and the church sponsored a cessation program in 1987. The local cancer society counsels against tobacco use and distributes stickers and desk-cards (PAHO 1988; Louisy 1990).

St. Vincent and the Grenadines

Although no laws restrict smoking indoors, administrative bans on smoking apply in schools. No sustained anti-tobacco education and information programs have been implemented by nongovernmental organizations. However, the Ministry of Health and Environment frequently produces promotional and educational materials in an effort to discourage tobacco use (Browne 1990).

Summary

Few data or organizational resources are available to describe or intervene against tobacco use in OECS countries. However, voluntary efforts and anecdotal reports suggest that public sentiment supports a nonsmoking norm. After an organizational base for tobacco control is established, periodic household surveys of smoking and other health risk behaviors would be more helpful in building a database on tobacco control than would data on tobacco consumption. From these surveys, target groups could be determined for subsequent intervention strategies that might include legislation and smoking cessation, health promotion, and education programs.

Sustained health promotion activities adopting a holistic approach to healthy lifestyles and positive well-being should be implemented in the OECS to minimize the future impact of chronic diseases on their populations. The National Drug Abuse Councils seem to be a good forum in which to establish multisectoral approaches to tobacco and other drugs if sufficient human and financial resources can be assigned.

Conclusions

1. Per capita cigarette consumption in most countries of the Organization of Eastern Caribbean States (OECS) is low and declining. A consistent downward trend is less evident in Saint Lucia and St. Vincent and the Grenadines. No data on health risk behavior are available for any of the OECS countries.
2. While reliable mortality data are sparse, it also appears that mortality from lung cancer, and possibly other smoking-related causes, is very low in these six countries. This situation presents an opportunity for true primary prevention of an epidemic of tobacco-related diseases.
3. Restrictions on smoking in schools, hospitals, and other public places are minimal in OECS countries, relying primarily on voluntary efforts. No systematic school-based or public education campaigns are reported for these countries.
4. The price of cigarettes is relatively low in Antigua and Barbuda, Grenada, St. Kitts and Nevis, and Saint Lucia. Cigarette tax increases, in addition to increasing Government revenue, would serve to deter further tobacco consumption.

References

BHOLA, R. Country Collaborator's Report, Grenada. Unpublished data, PAHO, 1989.

BROWNE, C.F. Country Collaborator's Report, St. Vincent and the Grenadines, Unpublished data, PAHO, 1990.

CARICOM. Caribbean Development and Cooperation Committee (CDCC), Port-of-Spain, Trinidad. Publication No. LC/CAR/G.293, March 19, 1990.

ECONOMIC COMMISSION FOR LATIN AMERICA AND THE CARIBBEAN. Unpublished tabulations. Port-of-Spain, Trinidad, 1990.

ENCYCLOPEDIA BRITANNICA. *Encyclopedia Britannica World Data Annual 1990*. Encyclopedia Britannica. Chicago, 1990.

FORTUNE, R. Country Collaborator's Report, Dominica, Unpublished data, PAHO, 1990.

GITTENS, A. Country Collaborator's Report, Grenada, Unpublished data, PAHO, 1990.

HENDRICKSON, V. Country Collaborator's Report, St. Kitts and Nevis. Unpublished data, PAHO, 1990.

LOUISY, D. Country Collaborator's Report, Saint Lucia. Unpublished data, PAHO, 1990.

OECS In Perspective (Brochure) 1987.

PAN AMERICAN HEALTH ORGANIZATION. *Health Conditions in the Americas, 1981–1984, Volume I*. Pan American Health Organization, Washington, D.C., Scientific Publication No. 500, 1986.

PAN AMERICAN HEALTH ORGANIZATION. *Health Conditions in the Americas, 1990 Edition, Volume I*. Pan American Health Organization, Washington, D.C., Scientific Publication No. 524, 1990.

PAN AMERICAN HEALTH ORGANIZATION. *Smoking Control—Third Subregional Workshop, Caribbean Area.* Kingston, Jamaica, 8–11 December 1987. Technical Paper No. 20, Pan American Health Organization, Washington, D.C., 1988.

PIGOTT, S. Country Collaborator's Report, Antigua and Barbuda. Unpublished data, PAHO, 1990.

UNITED NATIONS. *Demographic Yearbook 1988.* New York, 1989.

UNITED NATIONS. *Caribbean Countries: Agricultural Statistics, Volume VII.* Economic Commission for Latin America and the Caribbean. Scientific Publication No. LC/CAR/G.272, 1988.

UNITED NATIONS. *Selected Statistical Indicators of Caribbean Countries, Volume II, 1990.* Economic Commission for Latin America and the Caribbean. Subregional Headquarters for the OECS, 1990.

WORLD BANK. *The World Bank Atlas 1989.* Washington, D.C.: International Bank for Reconstruction and Development/The World Bank, November 1989.

WORLD BANK. *World Development Report 1990—Poverty.* New York: Oxford University Press. 1990.

Panama

General Characteristics

The Tobacco Industry
    Agriculture
    Manufacturing
    Trade
    Advertising and promotion

Tobacco Use
    Behavioral surveys of tobacco use
        Available surveys and their limitations
        Prevalence of smoking among adults
        Prevalence of smoking among adolescents
        Other uses of tobacco
        Attitudes, knowledge, and opinions about smoking

Smoking and Health

Tobacco Use Prevention and Control Activities
    Government activities
        Executive structure and policies
        Legislation
        Taxes
        Education
    Action by nongovernmental agencies

Summary

Conclusions

References

General Characteristics

Panama occupies 77,381 km² at the southern end of the Central American isthmus. Based on trade and commerce, the principal economic activities of Panama reflect the importance of the Panama Canal and the banking system, which was until recently one of the most important of the hemisphere. The majority of the Panamanian population is concentrated in younger age groups. In 1990, of the total population of 2.4 million, 35 percent were younger than age 15. The total fertility rate is estimated at 3.14 (Centro Latinoamericano de Demografia [CELADE] 1990). As health conditions improved during the two decades since 1970, the infant mortality rate declined from 51.6/1,000 live births in 1970 to 22.7/1,000 in 1990, and life expectancy from birth increased from 64.3 years in 1970 to 72.1 years in 1990 (Table 1). Thus, chronic diseases associated with tobacco are expected to become more prevalent as the Panamanian population ages and as infant and childhood mortality continue to decrease.

These changes in health status reflect generally improved economic capacity and living conditions. In 1988, the per capita gross national product (GNP) was estimated at $US2,120, ranking sixth in the Americas. The real annual growth rate of GNP from 1980 to 1988 was 2.2 percent (World Bank 1990). As the standard of living improved over the last decade, Panamanians may have acquired consumption and behavioral patterns, including increased rates of cigarette smoking, that are similar to more developed countries.

The Government allocates 5 percent of the GNP to health programs. However, because of the recent political crisis in Panama, these funds may be diverted to stimulate economic development. In the 1980s, the Caja del Seguro Social extended its coverage to include health care. Of the total population, 64.5 percent were covered by this program in 1987 (Pan American Health Organization [PAHO] 1990). It is anticipated that a greater proportion of these resources will be needed to apply to costly treatments for chronic diseases such as lung cancer, cardiovascular disease, and chronic lung disease as these diseases become more prevalent in an aging population. However, recent changes in economic and political conditions may severely limit the resources available for health care and preventive services.

The Tobacco Industry

Agriculture

Tobacco has been grown in Panama for centuries. In 1988, the Statistics and Census Directorate published a report on cigarette production and its socioeconomic effects in Panama for the years 1980 to 1987 (León and Alain 1988). Data from that report and from additional sources of the Ministry of Agriculture (Dirección de Estadística y Censo 1989) and the U.S. Department of Agriculture (USDA) (1990) suggest that decreasing domestic and worldwide demand has led to decreased production during the decade of the 1980s (Table 2). The land allocated for tobacco production decreased from 1,037 ha in 1980 to 800 ha in 1989, or approximately 0.2 to 0.3 percent of Panama's total arable land (Dirección de Estadística y Censo 1989). Total tobacco production peaked in 1979 at 1,508 MT and declined to 1,148 MT in 1982. During 1982 to 1989, tobacco production remained relatively stable, with 1,172 MT produced in 1989. Imports have had only minor variations since 1980. Tobacco exports have remained at approximately 400 MT per year since 1982.

In 1988, Panama's tobacco was grown by 740 farmers, mostly on small farms in the northern province of Chiriquí. Many varieties of tobacco are

Table 1. Health and economic indicators, Panama

Indicator	Year	Level
Population	1990	2,400,000
Percentage < age 15	1990	35
Percentage urban	1988	54
Life expectancy at birth (males)	1965–1970	63.1
	1985–1990	70.2
Life expectancy at birth (females)	1965–1970	65.5
	1985–1990	74.1
Total fertility rate per 1,000	1985–1990	3.14
Crude birth rate per 1,000 women	1988	26.0
Crude mortality rate per 1,000	1988	5.0
Infant mortality rate per 1,000 live births	1965–1970	51.6
	1985–1990	22.7
Percent illiterate	1985	12.0
Real growth rate of GNP (percent/year)	1980–1988	2.2
Per capita GNP	1988	$US2,120

Sources: CELADE, 1990. World Bank, 1990.
Note: GNP = Gross national product.

Table 2. Tobacco leaf production and imports; cigarettes manufactured and per capita cigarette consumption in Panama, 1960–88

Year	Domestic leaf production (unmanufactured) (MT)	Imports (MT)	Total manufactured cigarettes produced (milllions)	Total cigarettes imported (millions)	Yearly cigarette consumption per capita age ≥ 15 yrs
1960	541	133	658	17	1,080
1965	1,078	213	826	15	1,172
1970	716	269	1,011	8	1,228
1975	801	175	1,045	0	1,074
1980	1,397	228	1,100	5	1,036
1981	1,254	348	1,200	1	1,086
1982	1,148	91	1,100	31	968
1983	1,416	238	1,100	30	882
1984	1,037	265	1,100	30	883
1985	1,209	109	1,125	30	875
1986	1,240	94	1,150	30	894
1987	1,172	133	1,150	30	842
1988	1,172	133	1,150	30	794

Source: USDA, 1990.
Note: MT = metric tons.

grown by these farmers; of the total cropland, 460 ha was burley tobacco, followed by 160 ha of creole-type, 110 ha of Virginia, 20 ha of Sumatra, 10 ha of Copán, and 40 ha of other varieties (León and Alain 1988). Growers sell approximately 95 percent of their crop to the three cigarette manufacturing companies operating in Panama.

Manufacturing

Two of the three tobacco-manufacturing companies in Panama are now under control of the major transnational corporations. Tabacalera Nacional, S.A., is controlled by Philip Morris while Tabacalera Istmeña is a subsidiary of British-American Tobacco. Panamá Cigar has both domestic and foreign backing and produces mainly dark tobacco for cigars (Chong 1990).

In 1987, 410 people were employed directly by the tobacco-manufacturing industry, earning average yearly wages of 966 balboas ($US966) (León and Alain 1988). Just as tobacco agricultural production declined, tobacco manufacture and trade also decreased in the last decade. In 1980, tobacco manufacturing represented 3.6 percent of total Panamanian industrial activity; by 1987, the proportion had dropped to 2.7 percent. The aggregate economic value of the tobacco industry declined from 6.6 million balboas ($US6.6 million) in 1980 to 5.2 million balboas ($US5.2 million) in 1987. This de-

cline was attributed to decreased consumption associated with an active campaign against drugs and tobacco, as well as to an increase in the illegal trade in tobacco products from the former Canal Zone (León and Alain 1988).

Trade

USDA data indicate that all domestically manufactured cigarettes are consumed by Panamanian residents. In 1988, 1,150 million cigarettes were manufactured, 30 million cigarettes were imported, and the resulting total domestic consumption was 1,180 million units (USDA 1990). However, because the extent of the illegal trade in cigarettes is not known, these figures may substantially underreport total consumption.

The tobacco industry receives no preferential treatment such as price supports or development projects from the Government, but it does benefit from customs protection that applies to all domestically produced goods. In 1986, for example, the tobacco industry saved 83,385 balboas ($US83,385) in import duty exemptions for raw and manufactured tobacco (Chong 1990). Maximum tobacco prices are set through resolutions of the Oficina de Regulación de Precios (Decreto de Gabinete No. 60, 1969). These may serve to support tobacco sales through price controls, but illegal trade in tobacco may subvert the intent of these controls.

Advertising and Promotion

Tobacco advertising is prolific on television and radio and in magazines and newspapers. Cigarette brand names are used in promotion of sports and cultural events, both through direct advertising and by sponsorship. Food stores, refreshment stands, national highways, public transport vehicles, and sports stadia display cigarette advertisements (Chong 1990).

A framework for control of tobacco advertising in Panama is in place, and several regulatory actions have been taken against tobacco advertising. A 1970 Ministry of Health decree requires that all cigarette advertisements include the warning "Caution: Smoking is harmful to your health" (Ministry of Health 1970). In 1978, a Commission on Advertising was established under the Ministry of Health. According to the Sanitary Code, any advertising that may exploit the public or that may advertise products harmful to health is prohibited. The Commission's function is to approve advertising contents for cigarettes, alcoholic beverages, drugs, beauty products, and foods, and to ensure that advertising is factual and that advertisements do not show individuals consuming tobacco or liquor (Ministry of Health 1990). In 1985, the Ministry of Government and Justice issued a resolution ordering advertising agencies to submit technical reports explaining the contents of advertisements, either prior to public display or within the first 2 days of distribution. These reports are filed for information purposes only.

Thus, both the Health and Government and Justice Ministries review information on tobacco product advertising, but regulatory activities on advertising are minimal. Even though human imagery in this advertising is limited, tobacco advertisements in Panama rely on saturation of the environment with cigarette brand logos. For example, in a recent promotional television announcement for a boxing match between Roberto Durán and Sugar Ray Leonard (held in the United States), Roberto Durán, a Panamanian, displayed a tee shirt bearing the Viceroy logo and flashed a "V" sign just as the Viceroy logo covered the screen; Viceroy is the leading cigarette brand in Panama (Chong 1990).

Tobacco Use

During 1980 to 1988, apparent per capita cigarette consumption decreased in Panama (Table 2); it is not known how much of this decrease was offset by the illegal trade in cigarettes described above, but survey data confirm this general trend. A comparison between 1972 and 1983 surveys on family living conditions in Panama City and Colón indicates a decrease in the proportion of overall household spending on cigarettes, although the exact percentage is not available (León and Alain 1988). This study also showed that families with higher incomes spent proportionally more on cigarettes than did those at lower income levels. These findings were also confirmed by a survey performed for the Adult Health Department of the Ministry of Health in 1989 (Chong 1990).

Tar and nicotine levels for brands produced by Tabacalera Nacional and Tabacalera Istmeña are reported as part of company quality control data (Tabacalera Nacional, S.A. 1989). Tar and nicotine levels for the five leading cigarette brands sold in Panama varied minimally, from 13.04 to 15.73 mg of tar per cigarette and from 0.90 to 1.19 mg of nicotine per cigarette. Brands advertised as "light" had lower levels: 10.94 mg of tar and 0.77 mg of nicotine per cigarette. When brands sold in both the United States and Panama (Viceroy, Marlboro, Kool, and Lucky Strike) were compared using tar and nicotine levels reported by the U.S. Federal Trade Commission, the U.S.-manufactured brands had slightly higher levels of these components (U.S. Federal Trade Commission 1988) (Table 3).

Packs of 10 cigarettes are the most popular size sold in Panama because of the lower selling price, but 20-cigarette packs are also available throughout the country (Chong 1990).

About 28 percent of the tobacco consumed in

Table 3. Tar and nicotine yields in mg per cigarette for the five top-selling brands of cigarettes in Panama, with comparison to U.S. manufactured brands of the same name, 1988

Brand	Tar		Nicotine	
	Panama	U.S.	Panama	U.S.
Viceroy	14.87	15	1.19	1.00
Marlboro	15.05	17	0.98	1.10
Kool	13.21	16	1.05	1.10
Mentolados	14.40		0.93	
Lucky Strike	14.28	17	1.05	0.90

Sources: Tabacalera Nacional, 1989; U.S. Federal Trade Commission, 1988.

Panama is in the form of loose tobacco for cigarettes made by hand, 0.9 percent is consumed as cigars, and 0.1 percent is loose tobacco for pipes. Consumption of smokeless tobacco is nonexistent (Chong 1990).

Behavioral Surveys of Tobacco Use

Available surveys and their limitations

Several surveys carried out in Panama over the past 10 years collected data on cigarette smoking prevalence among adults and adolescents (Table 4). Only one survey was nationally representative (National Association Against Cancer 1983); the others focused on specific population groups. None of the survey results have been published; the data presented here were derived from raw data sources (Chong 1990). The 1982 survey of medical students (Carrasco 1982) suggests future directions the medical profession may take in tobacco control.

The surveys differed in their definitions of "smoker." Three of them (Carrasco 1982, National Association Against Cancer 1986 and 1989) defined a smoker as a "person who currently smokes

daily." The others include in the category of "smoker" occasional smokers who may not smoke every day (Table 4). The population groups studied also differ substantially, ranging from high school and medical students to Ministry of Health staff and retired persons. Consequently, direct comparisons between the surveys are difficult.

Prevalence of smoking among adults

The 1983 National Association Against Cancer survey reported an overall prevalence of current smoking at 38 percent (56.1 percent among men and 20.0 percent among women) (Table 4). The prevalence of smoking among men was highest (64 percent) for those aged 20 to 30 years, with the rates decreasing somewhat as age increases. Of men aged 50 and older, 46 percent were current smokers. No major age differences were observed with regard to current smoking prevalence among women. Persons with higher incomes and a higher level of education tended to have a higher frequency of smoking. These data are consistent with the 1983 survey of household expenditures mentioned above in which the proportion of household income devoted to purchasing cigarettes was

Table 4. Surveys on smoking and prevalence (percent) of current cigarette smoking among men and women in Panama, 1982–89

Survey	Year	Population sampled	Sample size	Definition of "smoker"	Prevalence of current smoking		
					Male	Female	Total
Medical students survey (Carrasco)	1982	Faculty of Medicine students	230	Currently smokes daily			18.7
Study of smoking among adults (National Association Against Cancer)	1983	Population aged 18 and older residing in Panama	1,631	Has smoked continuously or occasionally over the last 6 months and currently smokes	56.1	20.0	38.0
Smoking and health (National Association Against Cancer)	1984	Secondary school students aged 11 to 18	11,385	Has smoked at least once a week over the last 3 months	10.1	3.9	7.0
Smoking control (National Association Against Cancer)	1986	Ministry of Health employees	411	Currently smokes daily	28.3	10.3	18.0
Smoking among retirees (Ministry of Health)	1989	Aged 55 and older who collect pensions at the Ministry of Health	100	Currently smokes daily	48.0	13.0	33.0

Source: Chong, 1990.

higher in upper-income households compared with lower-income households. However, the prevalence of smoking was higher in rural than in urban areas (44 vs. 34 percent). This relationship differs from that in other countries of Central America. However, approximately 28 percent of tobacco consumed in rural areas is loose tobacco for hand-rolled cigarettes. In addition, the sampling process in rural areas may have facilitated over-reporting of tobacco use in those areas. Among male smokers, 61 percent reported smoking one to 12 cigarettes daily and only 1.3 percent smoked more than 40 cigarettes a day. Among women, 82 percent of the smokers reported smoking from one to 12 cigarettes a day and 3.6 percent smoked more than 40 cigarettes daily (National Association Against Cancer 1983).

In the 1989 survey by the Department of Adult Health (Ministry of Health 1989a), the prevalence of current smoking among 58 men aged 55 years and older was 48 percent; this level is similar to the 46-percent level reported for men aged 50 years and older in the 1983 national survey. Among women surveyed, the 1983 survey reported that 24 percent of those aged 55 years and older were current smokers (National Association Against Cancer 1983), while only 13 percent of the 42 women surveyed in 1989 were current smokers. This decline among women may not be real because of selection bias (i.e., pensioners only were surveyed in 1989) and a small sample size.

The 1982 survey of medical students reported that 18.7 percent of 230 students were current smokers and 9.6 percent were former smokers. This distribution indicates that those future health professionals had barely begun to heed information about the health risks of smoking (Carrasco 1982).

Detailed data from the 1986 survey of Ministry of Health employees are not available. However, the overall prevalence of current smoking among the entire sample of 411 persons was 18 percent (26.8 percent among men and 10.0 percent among women); 7 percent reported that they were ex-smokers (National Association Against Cancer 1986). In 1990, another survey of all Ministry of Health employees reported that 12 percent were current smokers (Chong 1990). Theses prevalences are substantially lower than the reported 1983 national prevalence; in most countries of the Americas, health professionals can be expected to have a lower prevalence of smoking than the general population. The extent to which response bias affected the surveys' estimates is unknown.

Prevalence of smoking among adolescents

Although several small surveys on tobacco use among children and adolescents have been done in Panama (Chong 1990), the data from these surveys were not available for this report. However, the National Association Against Cancer and the Ministry of Education of Panama have performed one the largest and most representative surveys of youth in the Americas. In 1984, 11,385 urban and rural secondary students at public and private schools were interviewed (National Association Against Cancer 1984). The sample represented 9.3 percent of all secondary school enrollment and included students aged 11 to 18 years. Overall, smoking prevalence (defined as "weekly smoker") was 7 percent (10.1 percent among males and 3.9 percent among females). No data were reported on daily or experimental smokers or on the number of cigarettes smoked per day.

Other uses of tobacco

Survey data for persons aged 55 years and older collecting pensions from the Ministry of Health (Ministry of Health 1989a) indicated that 4 to 7 percent smoked cigars. Pipe smoking and tobacco chewing were not reported in this survey. In the coastal provinces of Colón, Darién, and Bocas del Toro, inverted smoking, in which the cigarette's burning end is held inside the mouth, is still practiced by Antillean Indian descendants (Chong 1990).

Attitudes, knowledge, and opinions about smoking

A series of small surveys on attitudes toward smoking was carried out in 1989 by the Adult Health Department of the Ministry of Health in several schools in Coclé province. Because the same questions were asked in all of the surveys, it is possible to compare their results (total n=969). The percentage of students who reported that they were current smokers is very low in all of these surveys (Table 5), and in several cases, the percentage of students refusing to answer questions about their behavior was quite high (up to 24 percent). However, responses to the question "If someone is smoking near you. . ." were more complete: the majority of respondents answered that it bothered them. Of students at the Escuela de Artes y Oficios, 41 percent said that it bothered them "but they understood." The lowest percentage of students

Table 5. Responses to the question: "If someone smokes near you," and prevalence (percent) of current smoking in various student population groups, Panama, 1989 (percentages)

Responses	Primary school	Secondary school (Public)	Secondary school (Private)	Escuela de Artes y Oficios	Night school	University
It doesn't matter to them	20.6	25.0	22.0	23.6	28.3	12.7
Bothers them but they understand	9.5	22.4	14.0	41.0	17.4	26.1
Bothers them	42.9	39.5	43.8	20.8	39.1	35.9
Oppose	3.2	0.0	7.8	3.4	2.2	9.9
Are indifferent	0.0	3.9	7.5	0.6	0.0	7.7
Think it's a bad idea	17.5	6.6	3.4	9.0	10.9	7.7
Think it's a good idea	1.6	0.0	0.6	1.1	0.0	0.0
No reply	4.8	2.6	0.9	0.6	2.2	0.0
Number surveyed	63	76	464	178	46	142
Age range (at last birthday)	5–14	8–34	8–19	8–34	20–44	20–54
Percentage of smokers	0.0*	1.3	6.0	4.5	4.0	4.0

Source: Ministry of Health, 1989b.

*24% of the respondents did not indicate whether or not they smoked.

who were not bothered by smoking (12.7 percent) was found among university students and the highest percentage (28.3 percent) was found among night school students. Very few students (0 to 1.6 percent of respondents) replied that they thought smoking was a "good idea." The responses to these surveys suggest that the vast majority of students are nonsmokers, and that most are bothered by others' smoking but display a high level of tolerance and acceptance (Ministerio de Salud 1989b).

Knowledge and attitudes about smoking were explored in greater detail in the 1984 national survey of students (National Association Against Cancer and the Ministry of Education 1984). A total of 2,157 students aged 12 to 17 who identified themselves as smokers were asked true/false questions on tobacco and health. More than half the respondents answered correctly these questions on knowledge of tobacco and health consequences. Of those older than 17, 49.3 percent answered most questions on tobacco and health correctly. When asked whether cigarette smoke was harmful to persons other than the smoker and whether smoking by pregnant women can affect the fetus, approximately 77 percent of the students replied in the affirmative. However, when asked more specific questions, such as whether nicotine causes blood vessels to constrict, the majority said they did not know (60 percent for the nicotine question).

A second part of the questionnaire was de-signed to produce a 5-level attitude scale. The responses were collapsed into two strata: those with a predominately negative attitude (dislike smoking and smokers), and those with a predominately positive attitude (do not care about smoking or are smokers themselves). Of the students in the 12 to 17 age group, 74.3 percent had a negative attitude towards smoking. Of those older than 17, only 66 percent had a predominately negative attitude, perhaps reflecting that it is at about this age that the initiation of smoking occurs in Panama. It is interesting to note that 86 percent responded that they did not feel that they had to smoke even when they are with friends who smoke, and 85 percent said that teachers should not be allowed to smoke at school. Opinions on banning cigarette advertising were divided: 40 percent agreed that cigarette advertising should be banned and 56 percent did not agree. Only 6 percent of students aged 12 to 17 were allowed to smoke by their parents; this level corresponds to the reported overall prevalence of smoking in this age group (7 percent).

These data suggest that Panamanian students were reasonably well-informed on the health consequences of smoking in 1984, but that smoking by others was tolerable.

Smoking and Health

In 1978, an estimated 75 percent of deaths in Panama were certified by a physician, and 11 percent of deaths were classified as due to "symptoms and ill-defined conditions" (ICD 780-799). This proportion declined to 8.3 percent in 1981 to 1987 (PAHO 1990), indicating a gradual improvement in the quality of mortality data in Panama. Deaths attributed to ill-defined conditions were more frequent among the elderly and among women. However, because estimated underregistration in Panama is still 23.1 percent of all deaths (PAHO 1986, 1990), mortality statistics should be interpreted with caution.

Table 6 presents age-adjusted and age-specific mortality rates for several smoking-related diseases in 1984 and 1987. Myocardial infarction and other ischemic heart (IHD) disease are grouped as IHD. The IHD mortality rates for men and women in the 45–54-year age group increased from 1984 to 1987 (50.0 to 64.3 per 100,000 among men and 9.9 to 18.4 per 100,000 among women). The IHD mortality rate for women aged 35 to 44 years more than doubled

in the 3 years; however, in this age group few deaths were reported, and therefore the calculated rate is questionable. The increased IHD rate in the 45–54-year age group could be attributed in part to improved diagnoses; this explanation is reinforced by the decline in the proportion of deaths in Panama classified as ill-defined. In addition, IHD mortality could have increased among women due to increased smoking and increased usage of oral contraceptives, as has been seen in other Latin American countries (Rosero-Bixby and Oberle 1987; Anderson 1985). However, from 1984 to 1987, the age-adjusted mortality rate for IHD increased slightly for men but not for women. The age-adjusted mortality rates for cerebrovascular disease increased for both men and women during this period (Table 6).

From 1981 to 1987, the age-adjusted mortality rates for lung cancer and stomach cancer remained stable at relatively low levels. The mortality rate

Table 6. Mortality rates (per 100,000 inhabitants) for selected smoking-related diseases, by sex and age, Panama, 1984 and 1987

Cause of death (ICD-9)	Year	Rate*	Age groups 35–44	45–54	55–64
Ischemic heart disease (410–414)					
Men	1984	43.5	15.7	50.0	179.2
	1987	44.3	12.6	64.3	137.7
Women	1984	34.2	2.9	9.9	111.8
	1987	33.9	7.0	18.4	84.6
Cerebrovascular disease (430–438)					
Men	1984	24.8	6.5	24.3	73.6
	1987	33.1	8.4	30.3	114.1
Women	1984	28.3	8.8	36.6	82.4
	1987	31.4	7.9	27.6	88.3
Malignant neoplasm of lips, oral cavity, and pharynx (140–149)					
Men	1984	1.3	0.9	1.4	3.8
	1987	2.3	1.7	3.8	7.2
Women	1984	1.2	—	1.4	7.8
	1987	1.2	0.9	2.6	7.5
Malignant neoplasm of the trachea, bronchi, and lungs (162)					
Men	1984	8.0	4.6	18.9	34.0
	1987	8.0	4.2	13.9	50.7
Women	1984	2.5	5.9	5.6	7.8
	1987	3.1	2.6	5.3	26.3

Source: PAHO, 1990.
*Rates adjusted for all ages, based on overall population in Latin America.

among persons aged 55 to 64 for cancer of the trachea, bronchi, and lungs (ICD 162) increased from 1984 to 1987 from 34.0 to 50.7 per 100,000 in men and from 7.8 to 26.3 per 100,000 in women (Table 6). This increase may reflect the historical exposure of the population to cigarette smoking. However, mortality reporting and diagnostic accuracy have improved during this period. In addition, mortality rates may be unstable due to the low number of cases in this particular age group (e.g., 28 among men and 14 among women in 1987). To increase the stability of the mortality rate estimate, 3 years' data (1985 to 1987) for the 55–64-year age group were collapsed to calculate male and female mortality rates: 53.6 per 100,000 for men and 24.0 per 100,000 for women; these rates are comparable to those reported in Table 6. Thus, the increase in mortality rates for smoking-related diseases, particularly myocardial infarction and lung cancer, is probably real. The change was more substantial for women. The health consequences of smoking among Panamanians are becoming evident in this relatively healthy country. Opportunities for preventing many chronic disease deaths lie in addressing tobacco use and other behavioral risk factors.

Tobacco Use Prevention and Control Activities

Government Activities

Executive structure and policies

The Ministry of Health's Adult Health Department is responsible for smoking prevention and control activities. In May 1990, a public education and information program developed by the Department was aimed specifically at preventing smoking among adolescents and encouraging adults to quit smoking (Ministry of Health 1990). The program does not have its own budget; rather, it establishes guidelines and identifies regional and local activities. Public health activities by the local health departments include tobacco issues as part of their adult health programs.

In 1989, a national commission was established by Resolution of the Ministry of Health to study the problem of smoking in Panama. The commission is an interdisciplinary group of professionals whose role is to report on progress in tobacco control and on the impact of different smoking prevention programs (Ministerio de Salud 1989c).

Legislation

The first smoking-related regulations issued in Panama appeared in 1970, with restrictions on advertising described above (Ministry of Health 1970). Subsequently, in 1978, a presidential resolution created under the Ministry of Health the Commission on Advertising, whose function is to verify the accuracy of advertisements for cigarettes, liquor, and other consumer products, and to ensure that the advertisements do not show anyone consuming cigarettes or liquor. In 1991, by Resolution of the Ministry of Health, smoking was prohibited in health facilities and vehicles of the health secretariat.

A presidential decree established National No-Smoking Day in 1987 (Executive Decree 76, 1987), and in 1989 a law was passed banning smoking in offices that are open to the public (Official Gazette 1989). This law states that "smoking is harmful to individual and public health" and instructs the Ministry of Education, the Caja del Seguro Social, the Ministry of Health, and the media to participate in ongoing educational campaigns on the health impact of tobacco. It also ordered that tobacco product packaging must bear the warning "smoking is harmful to your health." Sanctions were established for individuals who smoke in offices open to the public, but not for institutions or industries that fail to observe the other two components of the law.

In 1981, a mayoral decree was made in Panama City (Office of the Mayor 1981) prohibiting smoking in churches, theaters, cinemas, and on public transport. In 1990, the 1981 decree was expanded by the Office of the Mayor (1990). The new decree orders owners and managers of restaurants and cafeterias to provide separate areas for smokers and nonsmokers; it does not stipulate how large each area must be, but penalties are set for owners and clients who do not comply.

There are no restrictions on the sale of cigarettes to minors or on tar and nicotine yields for cigarettes manufactured in Panama (Chong 1990).

Taxes

Taxes compose 60 percent of the retail price of a pack of cigarettes in Panama. Tobacco-related economic activities (production and sales) generated 2 percent of the overall national tax revenue in 1988. However, revenue from tobacco taxes has fluctuated substantially over the past 10 years, from 9 million balboas ($US9 million) in 1979 to just over

13 million in 1983, gradually returning to approximately 9 million in 1988. This revenue is not earmarked in any way for health programs, but is deposited in the National Treasury.

Education

The Ministry of Education is required by law to include information on the health impact of smoking in the school curriculum (Official Gazette 1989). Specifically, this topic is included in science courses during the first year of secondary school. The students participate actively by preparing antismoking papers and murals in schools, especially during Science Week.

The community-based tobacco-use-prevention program previously mentioned aims to educate and inform the public at the local level. In addition, radio and television stations periodically broadcast presentations and panel discussions on smoking. Posters, flyers, and educational brochures are distributed by the national program at various health institutions and schools. These activities are supplemented by staff training seminars.

Action by Nongovernmental Agencies

Several nongovernmental organizations provide support in tobacco control efforts. These organizations include the Organización Panameña Antituberculosa (OPAT), which distributes an antismoking poster, and the Seventh Day Adventist Church, which conducts 5-day smoking cessation classes for the public. The Civic Support Committee for No-Smoking Day (COCIA) and the National Association Against Cancer (ANCEC) have been involved actively in tobacco control for several years. Both of these organizations offer cessation programs, and their members frequently publish articles in the media on the problem of smoking. These organizations are also actively involved in lobbying for antismoking policies and legislation. ANCEC has carried out several surveys of the prevalence of smoking in Panama (see Table 4).

Most insurance companies in Panama offer a 10- to 25-percent discount on life insurance premiums for nonsmokers. However, one company offers this option to men but not to women (Chong 1990).

Summary

Tobacco leaf production and cigarette manufacturing in Panama have declined to a stable level since around 1982. The decline reported by central data sources for per capita consumption is uncertain, largely because of the unknown level of illegal trade in cigarettes. Nevertheless, tobacco remains somewhat important to the Panamanian economy. The three tobacco companies functioning in Panama create 2.7 percent of the nation's total industrial activity. However, the economic burden of smoking-related diseases and disability has not been calculated. The mortality burden of sentinel diseases such as lung cancer and cardiovascular disease has begun to increase, and thus, the economic "benefit" of this industry must be reconsidered. The future impact of these diseases is likely to be substantial. Given the scarce resources for health in Panama, the economic burden on the health care system created by smoking-related disease will be disastrous.

Panama has a rather unique set of laws applying to tobacco product advertising. The use of cigarette logos is pervasive throughout sporting, cultural, transportation, and other segments of society. However, the Ministry of Health has been charged with ensuring that advertising claims for tobacco and alcohol are factual. This may restrict advertisers from promoting "safe" cigarettes or in implying improved social and athletic performance through the use of the products. As a result, brand logos appear to saturate Panamanian society. Tobacco advertisements and packages must include a warning on health risks. Advertisements must not show models consuming alcohol or tobacco, and appeals to young people are supposed to be avoided.

Tobacco consumption has declined over the last 10 years and currently accounts for a lower percentage of basic family consumption than it did in 1980. Approximately 28 percent of tobacco is consumed as loose tobacco in cigarettes made by hand, possibly in response to high cigarette prices in Panama. The tar and nicotine levels of Panamanian-made cigarettes are very similar to levels reported by the U.S. Federal Trade Commission for like-branded U.S. cigarettes.

In 1983, the overall prevalence of smoking in Panama was estimated at 38 percent (56 percent for men and 20 percent for women). More recent data covering the entire country are not available. In contrast to other Central American countries, the prevalence of smoking in Panama is higher in rural areas than in the cities. Among adolescents aged 11 to 18, the prevalence of weekly smoking was 7 percent in 1984.

The 1989 survey data from several different

schools in Coclé province show that most respondents were well-informed as to the health consequences of smoking, and most showed a negative attitude towards smoking. If students in the rest of the country have similar attitudes and understanding of the health risks of smoking, the mandated school education on tobacco may have had a positive effect. Careful evaluation of this program has not been undertaken, nor is the extent to which this education actually is implemented certain.

The Ministry of Health's Adult Health Department has been assigned responsibility for activities to control smoking. However, it has few resources available for this task, since this is only one of its many programs. Efforts have been made to identify the extent of the problem through national and target group surveys and to promote educational intervention. Panama has a national commission in which other health sector agencies participate. Although this commission is an official Government agency, it does not have a separate budget.

Many legislative restrictions on smoking in public places have been enacted in Panama City, and several of these extend to the rest of the country. The degree to which compliance with the restrictions is enforced is unknown, but it is clear that governmental and particularly nongovernmental groups have gained visibility for a non-smoking norm.

Conclusions

1. Tobacco agriculture, production of manufactured cigarettes, and reported per capita consumption of cigarettes have been relatively stable in Panama since 1982. A substantial illegal trade in cigarettes is evident.
2. The burden of tobacco-related disease is increasing in Panama. Cardiovascular and lung cancer mortality rates recently have increased among both men and women, with a substantially greater increase among women. This suggests that the exposure of Panamanian women to tobacco has increased in recent decades.
3. Tobacco accounts for 2.7 percent of economic activity in Panama, but the economic costs of tobacco-attributable disease have not been determined.
4. Modest legislative actions against tobacco use have been taken in Panama, including censorship of tobacco advertising content, the addition of warning labels to cigarette packages and advertising, and local clean-indoor-air policies. Cigarette brand logos saturate the Panamanian environment, and advertising of tobacco products is pervasive in radio, television, sports, cultural activities, and outdoor venues.
5. An existing infrastructure to control tobacco in Panama includes a designated Government agency, an active National Association Against Cancer, and a recently named national coalition of health professionals. National data on adult and youth tobacco use have been collected in Panama, and data on knowledge and attitudes toward tobacco among youth have been reported.

References

ANDERSON, J.E. *Smoking during pregnancy and while using oral contraceptives*. Data from seven surveys in western hemisphere populations. Paper presented at The International Conference on Smoking and Reproductive Health, San Francisco, California, October 15–17, 1985.

CARRASCO, I. Hábito de fumar en estudiantes de la Facultad de Medicina, Panama (unpublished data), 1982.

CENTRO LATINOAMERICANO DE DEMOGRAFIA. *Boletín Demográfico*. CELADE, Santiago: año XXIII, No. 45, 1990.

CHONG, N. Country collaborator's report, Panama. Pan American Health Organization (unpublished data), 1990.

DIRECCION DE ESTADISTICA Y CENSO. Superficie sembrada y cosecha de tabaco y caña de azúcar: Año agrícola 1987–88, Estadística Panamá. *Boletín* 6:1–5, 1989.

LEON, M.A., ALAIN, A. La producción cigarrillera en Panamá y sus efectos socioeconómicos: Años 1980–87. Dirección de Estadística y Censo, Panamá, 1988.

MINISTERIO DE SALUD. Ministerial Decree No. 56, March 17, 1970.

MINISTERIO DE SALUD. Hábito del tabaco en jubilados y pensionados, Ministry of Health, Adult Health Department (unpublished data), 1989a.

MINISTERIO DE SALUD. El hábito de fumar en los estudiantes, Ministry of Health, Adult Health Department (unpublished data), 1989b.

MINISTERIO DE SALUD. Ministerial Resolution No. 31561, November 8, 1989c.

MINISTERIO DE SALUD. Programa de prevención del tabaquismo, Ministry of Health, Adult Health Department. Internal document, 1990.

NATIONAL ASSOCIATION AGAINST CANCER. Control del hábito de fumar, personal del Ministerio de Salud (unpublished data), 1986.

NATIONAL ASSOCIATION AGAINST CANCER. Investigación sobre el hábito de fumar: adultos de la República de Panamá (unpublished data), 1983.

NATIONAL ASSOCIATION AGAINST CANCER, MINISTRY OF EDUCATION. El hábito de fumar y la salud (unpublished data), 1984.

OFFICIAL GAZETTE. Año LXXXV, No 21,326, Panama City, Panamá, July 3, 1989.

OFFICE OF THE MAYOR. Decree No. 17, Panama City, Panama, April 22, 1981.

OFFICE OF THE MAYOR. Decree No. 291, Panama City, Panama, March 8, 1990,

PAN AMERICAN HEALTH ORGANIZATION. *Health Conditions in the Americas, 1981–1984*. Washington DC: Pan American Health Organization, Scientific Publication No. 500. 1986.

PAN AMERICAN HEALTH ORGANIZATION. *Health Conditions in the Americas, 1990 edition*. Washington DC: Pan American Health Organization, Scientific Publication No. 524. 1990.

REPUBLIC OF PANAMA. Executive Decree No. 76, March 18, 1987.

ROSERO-BIXBY, L., OBERLE, M.W. Tabaquismo en la mujer costarricense, 1984–85. *Revista Ciencias Sociales* 35:95–102, 1987.

TABACALERA NACIONAL S.A. Departamento de Control de Calidad, *Niveles de tar y nicotina en marcas de Tabacal y Tisa*, August 1989.

U.S. DEPARTMENT OF AGRICULTURE. Tobacco, Cotton, and Seeds Division, Foreign Agricultural Service (unpublished data), 1990.

WORLD BANK. *World Development Report, 1989*. New York: Oxford University Press, 1989.

WORLD BANK. *World Development Report, 1990—Poverty*. New York: Oxford University Press, 1990.

Paraguay

General Characteristics

The Tobacco Industry
    Agriculture
    Manufacturing, production, and trade
    Advertising and marketing
    Taxes and expenditures for cigarettes

Tobacco Use
    Consumption data
    Behavioral surveys
        Prevalence of smoking among adults
        Prevalence of smoking among adolescents

Smoking and Health
    Mortality indicators

Tobacco Use Prevention and Control Activities
    Government action
    Action by nongovernmental agencies

Summary

Conclusions

References

General Characteristics

Paraguay is the eleventh largest country in the Americas, occupying a landlocked 406,756 km² in South America. With the 1990 mid-year population estimated at 4.3 million, the republic ranks nineteenth in the Americas in population (World Bank 1989; World Bank 1990).

Approximately 60 percent of the 1990 population was 15 years or younger. Slow aging of the population is evident; by the year 2000, an estimated 62 percent of the population will be 15 years or older. Thus, chronic diseases associated with tobacco are likely to become more apparent when a larger proportion of Paraguayans reaches the ages at which these diseases occur. Life expectancy at birth increased from 62.6 years in 1950 to 66.4 years in 1987. Infant mortality declined from 73.4 to 41.0 per 1,000 live births during this period. Approximately 54 percent of the population lives in rural areas (Pan American Health Organization [PAHO] 1990; Centro Latinoamericano Demográfico [CELADE] 1990) (Table 1).

Based on per capita yearly income, the World Bank classifies Paraguay in the lower middle level of the world economic community (World Bank 1990). Per capita gross domestic product (GDP) grew at a rate of 3.4 percent per year between 1965 and 1987 (World Bank 1989), and in 1988 reached $US1,180 (World Bank 1990). Inflation averaged 22 percent per year between 1980 and 1988. The per capita foreign debt ($US510 in 1987 [World Bank 1989]) is equivalent to approximately one-half of the per capita gross national product (GNP) (PAHO 1990), but this rate is one of the smallest relative debts in Latin America (PAHO 1990). National revenue derives primarily from agriculture: in 1986, agriculture (including tobacco) accounted for 27.2 percent of the country's GDP (World Bank 1989).

The country is administratively divided into 19 Departments, through which the health care system is regionalized. The Ministry of Health provides guidance and direction to health care, but there is a growing private sector providing health services. In 1987, 35 percent of hospitalizations were in Ministry hospitals, 27.4 percent were in private institutions, 13.4 percent were in university hospitals, and 6.6 percent were in military facilities (PAHO 1990).

The Tobacco Industry

Agriculture

Data on tobacco production are reported by the U.S. Department of Agriculture (USDA), the Ministry of Industry and Commerce of the Government of Paraguay, the Tobacco Merchants Association of the United States (TMA), and the United Nations Food and Agriculture Organization (FAO). Reported data on production between 1959 and 1989 vary considerably from year to year, with the different sources reporting somewhat contradictory figures. According to the USDA, it appears that dry weight production peaked in 1975 at 34,830 MT and dropped 82 percent to 6,271 MT in 1989 (Table 2). However, alternative industry reports show markedly higher production (25,000 MT) for 1985 than did the USDA (6,222 MT). The Ministry of Industry and Commerce reported peak production in 1985 of 24,867 MT, with a decline to 4,500 MT in 1989 (Chaparro 1990b).

According to FAO, Paraguay was the ninth largest tobacco-producing country in the hemisphere during 1984 to 1986. In this period, a yearly average of 18,700 MT was produced, but this quantity represented a 30–percent decline from average yearly production (26,600 MT) 10 years earlier. In 1984 to 1986, Paraguay produced less than 0.7 percent (by dry weight) of the total hemispheric tobacco crop and about 0.3 percent of the entire global crop (FAO 1990). Production is projected to decline to 14,200 MT by the year 2000. Thus, a clear downward trend in tobacco production is evident

Table 1. Health and economic indicators, Paraguay, 1980s

Area (km²)	406,756
Population (1990)	4,277,000
Population <15 years (%) (1990)	59.6
Total fertility rate per 1,000 (1988)	4.5
Crude mortality rate per 1,000 (1988)	6.0
Life expectancy at birth	
Men	65.2
Women	69.5
Infant mortality per 1,000 live births (1988)	41.0
Percent urban population (1988)	46.0
Per capita gross national product (1988)	$US1,180
Annual rate of inflation (1980–1988)	22.1

Sources: CELADE, 1990; World Bank, 1990; Encyclopedia Britannica, 1990.

in Paraguay, indicating that both foreign and domestic markets for this agricultural product are changing. However, according to a tobacco industry correspondent, this trend completely reversed in 1990, showing a rather remarkable 50-percent increase over the production recorded in 1988 (Misdorp 1990). This claim cannot be substantiated with existing data. However, the newly installed Government has emphasized an expansion of agricultural development for export, including private investment in the agricultural sector (PAHO 1990). Thus, tobacco agricultural products appear to be an important component in Paraguay's current agricultural and economic development strategy.

In 1990, 5,000 farmers were reported to be involved in agricultural production (Chaparro 1990b). Tobacco production is concentrated in four Departments: San Pedro, Kanindeyu, Caguazu, and Caazapa. Information published in the Annual Report of the Ministry of Agriculture and Livestock indicates that agricultural land used to grow air-cured dark tobacco increased from 1,225 ha in the 1988–1989 season to 2,600 ha the following year. Only 85 ha are devoted to burley tobacco. Based on these data, 0.065 percent of Paraguay's total arable land is used for tobacco. The reported increase in land used for tobacco is unlikely, given the need for substantial investments in seedlings, equipment, personnel, and supplies necessary to support such dramatic growth, especially when both exported tobacco and domestic consumption appear to be decreasing (Table 2). Production is almost entirely from small family holdings averaging 1 to 1.5 ha (Misdorp 1990); these farms produce primarily *tabaco negro*. No crop substitution program for replacing tobacco is reported (Chaparro 1990b); in fact, farmers were offered better prices for tobacco in 1990 than for alternative crops such as cotton and beans (Misdorp 1990).

Exporters have been encouraging producers to switch to a variety of tobacco with a wider leaf and greater productivity (up to 3,500 kg/ha). All three sources of production data indicate that exports of unmanufactured tobacco showed a downward trend similar to that for production. For example, according to the USDA (1990), exports decreased from 12,483 MT in 1979 to 6,200 MT in 1989 (Table 2).

The Government has provided support for the tobacco industry through the National Tobacco Program (Programa Nacional del Tabaco—PRONATA), which was established under Executive Decree No. 26055/67 in 1967 and is aimed at increasing and enhancing national production (Chaparro 1990b). PRONATA is managed by representatives of the domestic tobacco industry and banks. It plays a role in tobacco policy, support for technical assistance, distribution of seeds, and financial support. For example, in 1985, the Banco Nacional de Fomento (National Development Bank) approved a loan of G$236 million ($US1 = 1,200 guaranis) to La Vencedora, the largest Paraguayan tobacco manufacturer, and a loan of $G150 million in 1988 to Tabacalera Boquerón, S.A. (Chaparro 1990b).

Manufacturing, Production, and Trade

Cigarette production data are available from the USDA, the TMA, and the General Accounting

Table 2. Tobacco production, exportation, importation, and total domestic consumption, in metric tons, Paraguay, 1979–1989

Year	Production	Exports	Imports	Total domestic consumption
1979	20,910	12,483	0	2,300
1980	13,600	14,858	7	1,900
1981	8,700	8,994	0	1,800
1982	10,200	8,656	383	1,600
1983	15,300	12,379	1,302	2,250
1984	17,000	11,685	603	3,050
1985	6,222	6,122	1,582	2,740
1986	4,931	5,089	387	2,800
1987	10,200	8,194	1,450	2,750
1988	6,271	6,321	400	2,650
1989	6,271	6,200	900	2,450

Source: USDA, 1990.

Table 3. Production, exportation, importation, and total consumption of manufactured cigarettes (millions), Paraguay, 1978–1988

Year	Production	Export	Import	Consumption
1978	800	0	1,788	1,788
1979	808	0	2,540	2,542
1980	648	0	1,911	2,559
1981	756	0	1,212	1,968
1982	1,800	0	200	2,000
1983	1,950	0	50	2,000
1984	1,950	0	60	2,010
1985	2,100	0	50	2,150
1986	2,500	0	40	2,540
1987	2,650	0	30	2,680
1988	2,730	0	25	2,755

Source: U.S. Department of Agriculture, 1990.

Office of the Government of Paraguay. According to the TMA (1989), cigarette production increased from an estimated 345 million cigarettes in 1969 to 800 million cigarettes in 1978, growing at 10.9 percent per year (Table 3). Between 1979 and 1988, yearly cigarette production increased almost three-fold from 808 million to 2.73 billion; unfiltered cigarettes accounted for approximately 46 percent of all cigarettes manufactured in Paraguay in 1988 (TMA 1989). In contrast, filtered, low-tar cigarettes are more commonly produced in more mature tobacco markets such as the United States, where 94 percent of the total cigarettes sold in 1988 were filtered (U.S. Federal Trade Commission [FTC] 1988). The U.S. market for filtered cigarettes has developed in large part due to the widespread information about the health consequences of tobacco use and the linkage of increased health risks to high-tar, unfiltered cigarettes (U.S. Department of Health and Human Services [USDHHS] 1989). The 46–percent market share of unfiltered cigarettes produced in Paraguay is similar to that of unfiltered cigarettes in the United States around 1958, when information about the adverse health consequences of tobacco use was just emerging (FTC 1988; USDHHS 1989). In Latin American countries with higher socioeconomic status, such as Argentina and Chile, almost 100 percent of cigarettes produced in 1988 were filtered (TMA 1989).

Data on imports of tobacco products are available from the USDA (1990) and from the Customs Department. With increased total consumption of manufactured cigarettes (FAO 1990; USDA 1990; TMA 1989), it may be expected that both raw tobacco and manufactured cigarette imports have increased. In 1980, 7 MT of imported raw tobacco were reported by the USDA; this level increased to

383 MT in 1982 and peaked at 1,580 MT in 1985. In 1989, 900 MT were imported. Reported imported manufactured cigarettes peaked at 2,542 million in 1979 and then declined substantially to only 25 million in 1988 according to the USDA. However, the Customs Department reported that 1,028 millon cigarettes were imported in 1988 (Chaparro 1990b). The reasons for inconsistencies in these data are not clear, but a significant illegal market for tobacco products appears to exist in Paraguay (Misdorp 1990).

Three companies manufacture cigarettes in Paraguay, one produces cigars, and two are involved in tobacco-leaf packing. According to Government sources, the industry employs about 650 people, or 0.22 percent of the country's industrial labor force (Chaparro 1990b).

La Vencedora, a private company, is the largest manufacturer of cigarettes in Paraguay, with 60 to 70 percent of the market share. Next in order of importance with 30 percent of market share is SABA Imports, a subsidiary of Brown & Williams Tobacco Co. Tabacalera Boquerón, another private company, has 2 to 3 percent of the market share.

The illegal trade in tobacco with the neighboring countries of Argentina and Brazil may be equivalent to more than half the quantity of all registered exchanged goods. Tobacco products play a dominant role in such illegal trade from Paraguay (Tobacco Journal International 1990). Reliable data are not available on the volume of illegally traded tobacco, but it has been estimated that about 60 percent of imported cigarettes are re-exported to neighboring countries as contraband. This illegal market may escape taxation on several levels, including import, export, and excise taxes, both in Paraguay and in the neighboring countries. The average price of a package of 20 domestic cigarettes in Paraguay was $US0.25 in 1989. Based on an average monthly industrial wage of $US160.00, a worker smoking 10 cigarettes per day would devote 2.3 percent of his monthly income to tobacco.

Advertising and Marketing

Legal restrictions on tobacco advertising and promotions in Paraguay were enacted by decree in 1989, but they reportedly are not observed (Chaparro 1990b). Advertising of tobacco products and alcohol on television is banned before 7:00 p.m. according to Decree 4012 dated December 12, 1989. However, because of a clause permitting tobacco and alcohol advertising if referring to foreign events or residents, tobacco product advertising circumvents the restrictions intended by the law. Thematic association of advertising with youth and sports is prohibited, and the use of messages "aimed at influencing behavior" is prohibited. Advertisements can only mention the quality and origin of the products (Public Law 836 [1980], paragraphs #202 and 203). Although permitted, on-screen advertising at movie theaters is relatively uncommon. Promotional activities have not been used in political campaigns, on public transportation, or at cultural events. However, posters are placed on traffic and street signs and at bus shelters (Chaparro 1990b).

Information on expenditures for tobacco advertising and promotion is available only for La Vencedora, S.A., the largest cigarette manufacturer. In 1989, $G20 million per month ($US17,000) was spent on tobacco advertising. Overall, 19.2 percent of total advertising expenditures ($G36,632 million) were for alcohol and tobacco. Of this sum, half was spent on television and radio advertising. In 1989, La Vencedora offered prizes of $US800 in drawings in which participants sent in empty Clayton cigarette packs, the main product of La Vencedora, with their names written on them (Chaparro 1990b).

Taxes and Expenditures for Cigarettes

Overall, taxes account for 10 percent of the average sales price of cigarettes (Chaparro 1990b), a rate far lower than that for many other countries in the Americas. However, some brands of dark tobacco cigarettes are taxed at a higher rate (35 percent of the sales price). Because of the negative price elasticity of demand for cigarettes in Paraguay, this higher tax may serve to promote the use of lower-tar, lower-risk cigarettes. Recently cigarettes and alcohol were placed in a special category for import taxes. Because these goods are ostensibly for the tourist market, the tax rate was set at a rather low 7 percent. On approximately 1.6 billion cigarettes imported in 1990, $US5.8 million in tax revenue was collected (Ultima Hora 1990).

Tax revenues from tobacco have increased substantially in the mid-1980s. In 1984, cigarette tax revenues were $G1,281.7 million ($US5.34 million), and in 1989, the total was $G5,222 million ($US4.35 million). Imported cigarettes generate more than half the total Government tobacco tax revenue, despite prices that are almost double those of locally produced cigarettes (Misdorp 1990). In 1989, imported cigarettes accounted for approximately $G3,313,528,000 ($US2,720,466).

Tobacco Use

Consumption Data

Domestic consumption data are available from the USDA, from the TMA for 1983 to 1986, from the FAO for 1974 to 1976 and 1984 to 1986, and from the General Accounting Office of the Government of Paraguay (Chaparro 1990b) (Table 2). Because of the illegal trade in both imported and domestically manufactured cigarettes described above, production, export, and import estimates from standard central data sources may be particularly unreliable when used to estimate domestic per capita consumption in Paraguay.

Most tobacco consumed in Paraguay is in the form of manufactured cigarettes. Cigars account for 2 percent of the tobacco consumed. Snuff and chewing tobacco account for 5 to 10 percent and are used mainly by rural inhabitants, many of whom smoke cigarettes as well. Approximately 3 percent of the domestically produced *tabaco negro* is used for hand-rolled cigarettes (Chaparro 1990b). Thirty percent of all cigarettes sold in Paraguay are reported by industry correspondents to be *tabaco negro* (Misdorp 1990). Of particular concern is the report of increasing sales of single cigarettes, especially to the "younger generation" (Misdorp 1990). Marketing this more affordable form of cigarettes is effective in its appeal to those with little disposable income.

Total consumption of cigarettes increased from 2,000 million to 2,340 million between 1983 and 1986, according to the TMA (1989). According to USDA, total consumption was 1,788 million cigarettes in 1978 and increased to 2,559 million in 1980;

a decline to 1,968 million in 1981 was followed by a steady increase to 2,755 million in 1988. Finally, Ministry of Agriculture data (Riquelme 1989) show that total consumption declined from 19,977 MT in 1984 to 1,500 MT in 1989.

Using USDA consumption data and population data from the World Bank (1990), estimated domestic per capita cigarette consumption for persons aged 15 and older decreased from 1,428 in 1979 to a low of 950 in 1984. Since 1984, yearly per capita cigarette consumption has increased by an average of 5 percent per year, to 1,143 in 1988. A 1988 World Health Organization (WHO) report based on USDA data reported apparent per capita consumption of cigarettes by adults at 960 in 1970 and 1,000 in 1985, indicating a 4–percent increase for the 15–year period (Chapman 1990).

Thus, the yearly per capita consumption pattern in Paraguay demonstrates a decline during the mid-1980s with a recent moderate increase in consumption. These data should be considered in the context of the illegal tobacco trade: consumption actually may have declined if this illegal trade increased substantially in recent years. Negative economic pressures may have depressed the domestic market for manufactured cigarettes in the mid-1980s, but more recent economic stability (PAHO 1990) may have led to increased consumption. The association between better economic conditions and increased consumption of tobacco in Paraguay is more characteristic of countries in the World Bank's lower income group than of those with higher economic development such as the United States, Canada, and Brazil. In these nations, tobacco use is increasingly more representative of persons in lower socioeconomic groups (USDHHS 1989; Costa E Silva 1990). The *tabaco negro* market in Paraguay (30 percent of the total

market) is gradually being replaced by *tabaco rubio*, a trend characteristic of more developed countries. Unfiltered cigarettes are still consumed by more than 50 percent of Paraguayans. Thus, it appears that the cigarette market in Paraguay has not yet been influenced to the same extent as in the United States by widespread knowledge about the health consequences of tobacco. Some researchers have advocated that low-tar, filtered cigarettes should be marketed to countries such as Paraguay to reduce immediately the risk of lung cancer. Risks for chronic obstructive pulmonary disease and cardiovascular disease probably would not be affected by this intervention, and thus, health education is still the most important component of public health efforts to decrease exposure to tobacco in developing nations.

Behavioral Surveys

In 1990, national data on tobacco use were collected as part of the National Health Survey by the Instituto de Investigaciones en Ciencias de la Salud (1990). Data are also available on the prevalence of smoking for several small population groups (Table 4).

Prevalence of smoking among adults

Smoking data for the National Health Survey were available only for the entire sample (0 to 65 years and older). Thus, these data do not represent adult smoking prevalence. Among all males surveyed, 24.1 percent were smokers; among all females, 5.5 percent were smokers. Most (71 percent) smoked filtered cigarettes, but almost 20 percent of men smoked cigars. Of cigarette smokers, over half (54.3 percent) smoked fewer than 10 cigarettes per

Table 4. Surveys on the prevalence of smoking, Paraguay, 1980s

| Author/Sponsor | Date | Sample area | N | Age group | Prevalence (%) | | |
					Men	Women	Total
Instituto de Investigaciones en Ciencias de la Salud	1990	National	8,287	0–65+	24.1	5.5	14.8
Martínez	1989	Santiago Medical students	394	16–36	17.7	14.4	16.5
Chaparro	1989	National Physicians	837	20–80	35.2	23.9	31.7
Estigarribia	1988	Asunción physicians teaching hospital	375		25.1	24.3	24.8

Source: Chaparro, 1990a.

day. Of cigar smokers, 71 percent smoked fewer than 5 cigars per day. Additional analyses of these data will be important in understanding tobacco use in Paraguay (Instituto de Investigaciones en Ciencias de la Salud 1990).

Studies from other nations show a very low (10 percent) prevalence of current smoking among physicians, who are ostensibly most knowledgeable about the health consequences of smoking (Pierce 1991). Physicians may in fact be considered a sentinel group for changes in tobacco use among the population as a whole, although it is not known whether this supposition holds true for medical students. Several surveys of physicians and medical students have been performed in Paraguay (Table 4).

In 1989, 394 medical students aged 16 to 36 years (54.7 percent of all 720 medical students in Paraguay) were surveyed using personal interviews to assess their prevalence of smoking (Martínez 1989). Overall, 16.5 percent of medical students were classified as ''current smokers.'' The prevalence of current smoking among male students was only slightly higher than that among female students (17.7 vs. 14.4 percent). Among smokers, 70.8 percent smoked 10 or fewer cigarettes per day; 15.2 percent smoked 11 to 20 cigarettes per day; and only 9.2 percent smoked more than 20 cigarettes per day.

In a nationwide study of 837 physicians conducted in 1988 and 1989 (Chaparro 1990a), 31.7 percent were current smokers and 22 percent were ex-smokers (Table 5). Current smoking prevalence was higher among men than among women (35.2 vs.

23.9 percent). The prevalence of current smoking was inversely associated with age, being highest (42.9 percent) among the youngest age group (20 to 24 years) and lowest (6.7 percent) among the oldest age group (65 to 80 years). In this survey, 50.4 percent of smokers smoked fewer than 15 cigarettes per day; 31.6 percent smoked 15 to 24 cigarettes per day; and only 13.9 percent smoked 25 or more cigarettes per day. Almost all physician smokers (92.1 percent) used filtered, *tabaco rubio* cigarettes.

In a 1988 personal interview survey of 375 physicians and medical students from the Catholic teaching hospital in Asunción (Estigarribia 1989), the prevalence of smoking was somewhat lower than reported in the Chaparro survey: 24.8 percent overall, 25.1 percent among men, and 24.3 percent among women. Of smokers, 59.3 percent smoked fewer than 10 cigarettes per day.

Prevalence of smoking among adolescents

No data are available on tobacco use among Paraguayan adolescents. However, in the Chaparro study (1990a), 10.5 percent of physicians reported their age of initiation as 11 to 14 years; 47 percent began between 15 and 19 years of age; and 38.3 percent did not begin smoking until at least age 20 years. In the 1990 Household Survey, 87 percent of smokers reported beginning before age 20. Thus, the onset of regular tobacco use in Paraguay is probably an adolescent phenomenon, as seen in other countries (USDHHS 1989; Pierce 1991).

No other data are available on the use of other forms of tobacco in Paraguay or on attitudes and opinions about tobacco. In the 1989 physicians' survey (Chaparro 1990a), only 30.4 percent considered smoking to be ''an undesirable behavior.'' Clearly, the high prevalence of smoking among physicians and their relatively weak condemnation of tobacco use indicate that the public opinions of tobacco use in Paraguay are not strongly negative.

Smoking and Health

Mortality Indicators

It is difficult to quantify the impact of smoking-related diseases because of significant underreporting of mortality in general in Paraguay. For example, in 1988 the expected number of deaths was 28,000, but only 13,511 deaths were actually reported; of these only 7,268 were certified by a physician (PAHO 1990). Not all areas of Paraguay are represented in the mortality reporting system.

Table 5. Prevalence (percent) of current and former smoking among physicians, Paraguay, 1989

Category	N	Current smokers (%)	Ex-smokers (%)
Total	837	31.7	22.0
Sex			
Men	205	35.2	24.2
Women	255	23.5	16.9
Age group			
20–24	7	42.9	28.6
25–34	307	33.8	17.3
35–44	308	32.8	21.4
45–55	130	33.8	23.1
56–64	58	20.7	39.7
65–80	15	6.7	40.0

Source: Chaparro, 1990a.

Figure 1. Proportionate mortality of reported deaths among men aged 35 and older, Paraguay, 1988

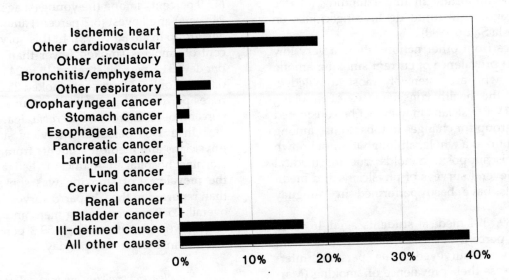

Source: PAHO 1990.

In 1988, 8,571 deaths among persons aged 35 years and older were certified. In this age category, approximately 15 percent of all causes are "Symptoms and Ill-defined Conditions" (ICD 780–799), the second largest of the major groups of causes. Significant under- or misreporting of cause of death is suggested when percentages of deaths categorized as "ill defined" exceed 10 percent (PAHO 1990).

Smoking may have contributed to several of the most commonly reported causes of death among men aged 35 and older in Paraguay in 1988 (Figure 1). The most common cause of death was "other cardiovascular diseases" and among these ischemic heart disease the leading cause. Respiratory disease (4 percent) and lung cancer (2 percent) were the fourth and fifth most common causes of death, respectively. Each of these may be related to tobacco use. Because lung cancer mortality is so low, it is likely that exposure to tobacco among Paraguayans is not yet as important. However, the large proportion of cardiac deaths among Paraguayans suggests that smoking as well as other cardiac risk factors may be influencing the mortality patterns already.

Additional data from the Paraguayan National Tumor Registry help in defining the disease impact of tobacco on health in Paraguay. This registry, though not nationally representative, collects data on incident cases of cancer by site, age, and

sex. Between 1975 to 1977 and 1988 to 1989, the age-adjusted incidence of lung cancer among men doubled from 7.9 per 100,000 to 18.1 per 100,000. Part of this increase is due to improved registration and diagnosis, but a substantial proportion of the increased male lung cancer incidence rate is due to cumulative population exposure to cigarettes.

Tobacco Use Prevention and Control Activities

Government Action

Recently, the Minister of Health prohibited smoking in clinics, offices, and waiting rooms under the jurisdiction of the Ministry of Health and Social Welfare (Ministerio de Salud Pública y Bienestar Social 1990a). This resolution also called on the Department of Health Education to initiate public education campaigns using intersectoral collaboration. The Government does not provide formal smoking cessation programs (Chaparro 1990b).

Considerable progress has been made regarding health warnings in tobacco product advertising and on cigarette packages (Table 6). As a result of Ministerial Resolution No. 428 of November 22, 1990, warnings must appear on both imported and domestically made cigarette packages. The warning reads: **"Smoking is Harmful to Health."** Ministerial Resolution No. 246 of May 27, 1991, mandated that the warning must appear on tobacco

Table 6. Tobacco-related policies in Paraguay

- Asunción Municipal Law No. 15,381 (February 11, 1984): bans smoking in public places, such as cinemas and theaters.
- Asunción Municipal Law on Transportation No. 298 (August 1971): bans smoking in urban passenger vehicles.
- National Decree No. 4012 (December 12, 1989): prohibits advertising of tobacco and alcoholic beverages before 9:00 p.m. Prohibits encouraging, through advertising, the use of these products. Advertisements may only mention the quality and origin of the products.
- Ministerial Resolution No. 428 (November 23, 1990): mandates health warning "Smoking is harmful to health" on cigarette packages.
- Ministerial Resolution No. 206 (January 23, 1990): prohibits smoking in clinics, offices, and waiting rooms under the jurisdiction of the Ministry of Health and Social Welfare. Calls on Department of Health Education to initiate a public information campaign.
- Ministerial Resolution No. 246 (May 27, 1991): Mandated health warning on imported cigarettes, in advertisements in all periodicals and newspapers, and on television advertisements for tobacco.

product advertisements in magazines and newspapers as well as outdoor advertising. In addition, a minimum of 3 seconds must be devoted to a legible health warning displayed during television commercials. Compliance with this Resolution is reported to be complete despite the fact that two television channels in Paraguay are owned by tobacco companies. National legislation has been enacted that restricts tobacco and alcohol advertising before 7:00 p.m. on television, but there is little compliance with this legislation. This legislation also mandates that only the quality and origin of the products may be indicated in the advertisements. Local legislation in Asunción, the capital city, bans smoking in cinemas, theaters, and urban public transportation vehicles (Table 6). However, it is reported that most of these legislative measures have not been implemented or enforced (Chaparro 1990b).

The schools do not systematically teach about the health consequences of tobacco use, although it is reported that some discussion of the harmful effects of smoking is carried out in the fourth, fifth, and sixth grades. The Paraguayan Anti-Smoking Association has named school education as one of its most important objectives (Latin American Coordinating Committee 1990b).

Action by Nongovernmental Agencies

Action against smoking in Paraguay has been taken primarily by nongovernmental organizations. Two private hospitals (Baptist and Adventist) have restricted smoking in their facilities (Latin American Coordinating Committee 1990). The Paraguayan Anti-Smoking League (Liga Paraguaya

Contra el Tabaquismo) has recommended restrictions on smoking in all hospitals. The Association of Young Paraguayans against Drug Abuse (Asociación de Jóvenes Paraguayos Contra el Abuso de Drogas—JOPACAD) requested in 1989 that the Ministry of Health pass restrictive legislation on tobacco use by minors (Chaparro 1990b). The Paraguayan Tuberculosis and Pneumonology Society (Sociedad Paraguaya de Tisiología y Neumología) recently published a public information booklet, "En Defensa de la Salud Popular: Campaña Nacional Contra el Tabaquismo," on the risks of smoking. With the cooperation of domestic pharmaceutical companies, 3,000 copies of this pamphlet were distributed to physicians (Latin American Coordinating Committee 1990). Several radio stations and newspapers have disseminated information about the health consequences of tobacco. Business relationships with tobacco manufacturing companies have prevented other news organizations from disseminating such information (specifically, television channels). The PRE-VER Association and the Providence Foundation have been involved in campaigns against drug abuse, including tobacco (Chaparro 1990b).

Summary

Paraguay has extensive investment in tobacco production and trade, and special treatment is given to tobacco exports. In association with economic instability in the 1980s, declines in per capita cigarette consumption have been observed. The prevalence of smoking among males of all ages is almost five times that among females of all ages, but national data on adult smoking prevalence are not available. The majority of smokers smoke fewer than 10 cigarettes per day. Data from the Paraguayan Tumor Registry indicate a doubling in the lung cancer incidence rate for men between the 1970s and 1980s.

Progress against smoking has begun in Paraguay, a country dependent to a large extent on the tobacco industry. Specifically, health warnings are now required for cigarette packages as well as tobacco product advertising. The Ministry of Health and Social Welfare has demonstrated leadership by prohibiting smoking in enclosed areas under Ministerial jurisdiction. Thus, the social transformation to an environment less supportive of smoking may have begun in Paraguay.

Conclusions

1. Paraguay is a country in pursuit of economic development and social, economic, and political stability. It produces, exports, and imports raw tobacco; manufactured cigarettes are also imported. The per capita consumption of cigarettes appears to have declined in the last decade, although data on consumption may be unreliable because of the significant illegal trade with neighboring countries in cigarettes.
2. Epidemiologic data on tobacco use and its disease impact are limited. Tumor registry data show that lung cancer incidence among men doubled in those areas covered by the registry from 1975 to 1989. Data on physicians' smoking behavior suggest that population prevalence rates are high compared with those in more developed nations. The prevalence of smoking among males is almost five times that among females (all ages), based on a national household survey.
3. Cigarette excise taxes are relatively low, but this source of income represents a substantial portion of total Government revenues. No specific Government policy or program exists to control tobacco use. Nongovernmental agencies play a leading role in tobacco control and education activities in Paraguay.
4. Recent actions by the Ministry of Health and Social Welfare have been successful in implementing health warnings on cigarette packages and tobacco product advertising.

References

CABRERA, V., GALDONA, C.M. *Actitud hacia el tabaquismo. 1989.* Asunción, 1989.

CASTRO, V.C.A. Personal communication from "Despacho Contaduría General." 1989.

CENTRO LATINOAMERICANO DE DEMOGRAFIA. *Boletín Demográfico.* No. 45. Santiago, Chile, January 1990.

CHAPARRO ABENTE, G. *Incidencia del tabaquismo en el gremio médico 1988–1989.* Typescript, 1990a.

CHAPARRO ABENTE, G. Country Collaborator's Report, Paraguay. Unpublished data, Pan American Health Organization, 1990b.

CHAPMAN, S., WONG, L.W. *Tobacco Control in the Third World—A Resource Atlas.* Penang, Malaysia: International Organization of Consumers Unions, 1990.

COSTA E. SILVA, V.L. Tabaguismo—um problema de saúde pública no Brasil. *Jornal Brasileiro de Medicina* 59(2):14–24, Agosto 1990.

ENCYCLOPEDIA BRITANNICA. *1989 Yearbook.* Chicago: Encyclopedia Britannica, 1990.

ESTIGARRIBIA, L.C. *Prevalencia del tabaquismo entre los médicos del Hospital de Clínicas. 1988.* Typescript, 1989.

FOOD AND AGRICULTURE ORGANIZATION OF THE UNITED NATIONS. *Tobacco: Supply, Demand and Trade Projections, 1995 and 2000.* Rome: 1990.

INSTITUTO DE INVESTIGACIONES EN CIENCIAS DE LA SALUD. Memorias—Paraguay: Encuesta Nacional de Salud 1990–EFACIM, 1990.

LATIN AMERICAN COORDINATING COMMITTEE ON SMOKING CONTROL. *Report of Sixth Annual Meeting, January 25–27, 1990.* American Cancer Society, Atlanta, Georgia, 1990.

MARTINEZ, G. *El hábito de fumar en los estudiantes de medicina-Universidad de Asunción.* Typescript, 1989.

MINISTERIO DE SALUD PUBLICA Y BIENESTAR SOCIAL. *Resolución S.G. No. 206,* January 23, 1990a.

MINISTERIO DE SALUD PUBLICA Y BIENESTAR SOCIAL. *Resolución S.G. No. 428,* Asunción, November 22, 1990b.

MINISTERIO DE SALUD PUBLICA Y BIENESTAR SOCIAL. *Resolución S.G. No. 246,* Asunción, May 27, 1991.

MISDORP, S. Paraguay report. *Tobacco International* 36, June 1, 1990.

PAN AMERICAN HEALTH ORGANIZATION. *Health Conditions in the Americas.* Scientific Publication No. 524. Washington, D.C.: Pan American Health Organization, 1990.

PIERCE, J.P. Progress and problems in international public health efforts to reduce tobacco usage. *Annual Review of Public Health* 12:383–400, 1991.

RIQUELME, P. Personal communication, Paraguayan Ministry of Industry and Commerce. Asunción, 1989.

TOBACCO MERCHANTS ASSOCIATION OF THE UNITED STATES, INC. Production and consumption of tobacco products for selected countries 1974–1988. *Special Report 89-3*, September 28, 1989.

ULTIMA HORA. *Establecer 7% de tributo para importación especial.* Martes 16 de enero de 1990.

U.S. DEPARTMENT OF AGRICULTURE. Tobacco, Cotton, and Seeds Division, Foreign Agricultural Service. Unpublished tabulations, Washington, D.C., April 1990.

U.S. DEPARTMENT OF HEALTH AND HUMAN SERVICES. *Reducing the Health Consequences of Smoking: 25 Years of Progress. A Report of the Surgeon General.* U.S. Department of Health and Human Services, Public Health Service, Centers for Disease Control, Center for Chronic Disease Prevention and Health Promotion, Office on Smoking and Health. DHHS publication No. (CDC) 89–8411, January 1989.

U.S. FEDERAL TRADE COMMISSION. *Tar, nicotine and carbon monoxide of the smoke of 272 varieties of domestic cigarettes.* Washington, D.C. 1988.

WORLD BANK. *World Development Report 1989.* New York: Oxford University Press, 1989.

WORLD BANK. *World Development Report 1990––Poverty.* New York: Oxford University Press, 1990.

Peru

General Characteristics

The Tobacco Industry
    Agriculture
    Production and trade
    Tobacco advertising and promotion

Tobacco Use
    Per capita cigarette consumption
    Behavioral surveys on tobacco use
    Prevalence of smoking among adolescents
    Other uses of tobacco
    Attitudes, knowledge, and opinions on smoking
        Knowledge of the health effects of smoking
        Attitudes toward smoking by smokers

Smoking and Health
    Morbidity
    Overall mortality
    Lung cancer mortality

Tobacco Use Prevention and Control Activities
    Government actions
        Policies and executive structure
        Legislation
        School education
        Public information campaigns
        Taxes
    Nongovernmental actions

Summary and Conclusions

References

General Characteristics

Peru is a Spanish- and Quechua-speaking country occupying 1,285,215 km^2 in the Andes on the west coast of South America. In 1988, the estimated mid-year population was 21,269,000. Peru is one of the most economically depressed countries in the Region. There are dramatic cultural and economic disparities between Caucasians and Indians, between rich and poor persons, and between urban and rural dwellers. The average annual increase in gross domestic product (GDP) decreased from 3.9 percent in the period from 1965 to 1980 to 1.1 percent in 1980 to 1988 (World Bank 1989). Economic growth in the former period permitted a burgeoning middle class to adopt social customs and consumer habits similar to those of North Americans or Europeans. Economic depression during the 1980s increased poverty and changed the purchasing power of the middle class. Historically in Peru, more than 3 million Indians are and have been isolated from the national economy. With the increase in drug use and trafficking in the 1980s, coca leaf production and illegal commerce became important for participation in the economy. Coca leaf is also one of Peru's illegal agricultural exports.

During the 1980s, a severe economic recession resulted in a deterioration of both the formal and the informal economy, especially in urban areas. Inflation increased uncontrollably from 200 percent in 1985 to 2,775 percent in 1989, further affecting the purchasing power of the average Peruvian. Subsequently, unemployment levels in some areas rose to as much as 40 percent. Because of this economic crisis, Government revenue from income taxes also diminished radically. In fact, only 100,000 of the 21 million Peruvians declared any income at all in 1989. Paradoxically, public spending on defense to control growing domestic terrorism increased from 14 to 20 percent of GDP over the last 15 years. Health expenditures remained at approximately 5.5 percent of GDP during the same period (World Bank 1990).

In 1988, 39.1 percent of the population was younger than 15 years old, with only 3.7 percent 65 years or older. Thus, Peru maintains a rather young population, with a relatively high crude birth rate of 25/1,000 (Pinillos 1989). The high infant mortality rate (86/1,000 live births) suggests that infectious diseases and diseases characteristic of underdevelopment still dominate the mortality and longevity patterns in Peru (Table 1).

Table 1. Basic health and economic indicators, Peru, 1988

Indicator	Year	Level
Population	1988	21,269,000
% < age 15	1988	39.1
% ≥ age 65	1988	3.7
% urban	1988	69
Crude birth rate per 1,000 persons	1988	25
Crude mortality rate per 1,000 persons	1988	9
Infant mortality rate per 1,000 live births	1988	86
Life expectancy at birth	1988	62
GNP per capita ($US)	1988	1,300
GDP (millions $US)	1988	25,670

Sources: Pinillos, 1989; World Bank, 1990.

The Tobacco Industry

Agriculture

The land area used for growing tobacco in Peru increased from 2,435 ha in 1971 to 4,025 in 1976. This increase, combined with an increase in the yield of tobacco per ha from 0.98 to 1.37 MT during the same period, kept pace with the observed increase in domestic consumption during the 1970s (Table 2). However, tobacco production in 1984 was significantly less than that in 1976. By 1983, tobacco plantations accounted for only 0.1 percent of arable land (Agro-Economics, Ltd and Tabacosmos, Ltd 1987).

In 1988, two private companies grew tobacco in Peru: Tabacos del Perú with 960 ha and Hoja Peruana de Tabaco with 520 ha. These two companies reported consistent growth in recent years at the expense of small farmers or State-owned farms (Pinillos 1990). Rural inhabitants typically are hired by the tobacco companies to grow tobacco on small land parcels of approximately 0.5 to 1 ha. The tobacco companies guarantee purchase of the total harvest from these farmers. In 1983, tobacco industry sources reported that there were approximately 1,570 farmers growing tobacco (Agro-Economics 1987). With additional persons hired at harvest time, 3,500 full-time jobs were generated by tobacco growing in 1983, accounting for only 0.2 per-

Table 2. Production, imports, exports, and total domestic consumption of raw tobacco in MT, Peru, 1970–1989

Year	Production	Imports	Exports	Total domestic consumption
1970	2,580	60	586	3,078
1971	2,676	75	854	1,910
1972	3,360	5	2,220	3,285
1973	4,816	555	2,000	4,055
1974	5,264	730	2,500	2,880
1975	5,376	1,080	1,595	4,195
1976	4,510	619	868	4,231
1977	3,190	440	642	3,595
1978	2,860	465	425	3,720
1979	3,371	572	450	3,900
1980	4,500	870	300	4,200
1981	3,820	930	200	4,080
1982	3,930	900	100	4,289
1983	3,080	515	121	3,195
1984	3,080	716	129	3,278
1985	3,100	613	100	3,403
1986	3,100	667	111	3,417
1987	3,100	865	113	3,615
1988	3,100	850	101	3,600
1989	3,100	850	100	3,600

Source: United States Department of Agriculture (USDA), 1990.

cent of all agriculture employment (Pinillos 1990). Because of the alarming increase in coca production in Peru in the 1980s, the Government suggested that tobacco would be a good replacement crop for coca because it might be more profitable to the Government as a legitimate export product (Agencia EFE 1990).

In 1989, 80 percent of the harvested tobacco was flue cured using wood as a fuel; 20 percent was sunlight/air cured. The dominance of flue curing is related to the industrialization of agriculture in Peru. However, because of the heavy demand for wood fuel in this process, it may be linked to deforestation, a growing ecological problem in South America (Chapman 1990). Given an average 2 to 3 ha of forest needed to flue cure a single ton of tobacco, it is estimated that 6,200 ha of forest are harvested each year to support flue-cured tobacco production (Nichter 1991).

Production and Trade

As of 1990, the tobacco manufacturers in Peru included Tabacalera Nacional, S.A., a private Peruvian concessionaire of both R.J. Reynolds and Philip Morris International (60 to 70 percent of the total market); Compañía Tabacalera del Sur, a private

Peruvian company (12 to 14 percent of the total market); and Empresa Nacional de Tabacos, S.A., (ENATA), a State-run company (16 to 26 percent of the total market). These three companies together employed 802 persons, approximately 0.2 percent of all formally employed persons in 1983 (Agroeconomics, Ltd and Tabacosmos, Ltd 1987). In addition, small companies manufacture cigars and hand-rolled cigarettes.

Data on production, importation, exportation, and domestic consumption vary by source. According to data reported by the U.S. Department of Agriculture (USDA), the total production of manufactured cigarettes increased from 2,950 MT in 1970 to 4,200 MT in 1988 (2.95 to 4.2 billion cigarettes) (Table 2) (USDA 1990). However, according to data supplied by the Peruvian Government, cigarette production declined from 3.6 to 2.8 billion units from 1981 to 1985, increased to 4.5 billion in 1986, and declined to 4.0 billion by 1989 (Pinillos 1990). Such a decline would be expected as a result of the severe inflation in Peru during the 1980s that led to a subsequent reduction in individual purchasing power.

Legal importation of manufactured cigarettes into Peru is minimal, accounting for only 0.3 percent of total domestic consumption (Euromonitor

Consultancy [EMC] 1990). Since 1968, an unknown quantity of cigarettes, mainly U.S. brands, has been smuggled each year into Peru. However, this illegal trade probably represents no more than 5 percent of the total market (Pinillos 1990). Since 1989, Brazilian cigarettes have also been illegally imported and sold at low prices. No cigarette exports from Peru have been reported since 1984; in that year a trade deficit of $US2,881,000 for tobacco products was reported (Chapman 1990).

Tobacco Advertising and Promotion

Between 1981 and 1991, advertising of tobacco products was not permitted on radio and television before 9 p.m. (República del Perú 1981). In December 1991, this restriction was extended to 10 p.m. However, more than $US200,000 was spent on television advertising for low-tar cigarettes alone in 1986 (Euromoniter Consultancy 1990). In a study of smoking among university women in Lima, Gastiaburu observed that "cigarettes are offered to

consumers of both sexes through a well-planned daily television advertising campaign using stimulating, exciting, and elegantly dressed ladies and gentlemen, whose images and gestures are aimed at impressing and commercially impacting young adults and adolescents of both sexes" (Gastiaburu et al. 1985).

Tobacco Use

Per Capita Cigarette Consumption

Per capita cigarette consumption data are derived from population estimates (CELADE 1990) and total domestic consumption estimates from the USDA (1990), the Euromonitor Consultancy (1990), and the Government of Peru (Pinillos 1990). All three sources suggest that the annual per capita consumption of manufactured cigarettes among persons aged 15 and older was between 236 and 459 cigarettes during 1970 to 1989 (Table 3). Per cap-

Table 3. Total domestic consumption (DC) and per capita consumption (PCC) of cigarettes, according to three sources

| Year | USDA | | Government of Peru | | ERC | | | |
	DC	PCC	DC	PCC	DC	PCC	F	NF
1970	2,954	400						
1971	3,103	407						
1972	3,305	421						
1973	3,685	455						
1974	3,829	459						
1975	3,757	437						
1976	3,757	423						
1977	3,648	398						
1978	3,383	358	2,609.9	276				
1979	3,659	375	2,911.3	298				
1980	4,034	401	3,377.5	325				
1981	3,968	382	3,584.9	336				
1982	4,017	376	3,659.3	334	3,732	324	4,056	380
1983	4,010	364	3,228.3	287	3,299	287	3,586	326
1984	4,010	354	3,154.8	273	3,222	280	3,502	309
1985	4,120	353	2,797.4	236	2,862	249	3,111	266
1986	4,210	350	4,462.9	368	3,527	265	3,792	316
1987	4,210	341	4,078.3	328	3,534	266	3,800	307
1988	4,210	331	3,842.7	301			3,750	295
1989			3,990.4	305				

Millions of tons.
Government of Peru. Number in billions.
ERC = Euromonitor Consultancy, Statistics International Ltd. (1987); USDA = United States Department of Agriculture (1990), Number in billions.
PCC = Consumption by the population 15 yrs and over.
F = filtered; NF = nonfiltered.

ita cigarette consumption increased 9 percent between 1970 and 1975, and subsequently decreased 25 percent between 1976 and 1988, according to the USDA. According to the data provided by the Peruvian Government, the reduction between 1980 and 1989 was approximately 9 percent; however, if the unusual increase in consumption in 1986 reported by this source is excluded from the analysis, the decline in per capita consumption since 1985 would be 55.9 percent. According to the tobacco-industry-sponsored ERC data, per capita consumption decreased 22.4 percent overall between 1982 and 1988, with a 19 percent increase between 1985 and 1986. In 1986, the tobacco industry began the above-mentioned advertising campaign for low-tar cigarettes. These consumption patterns suggest that intensive advertising may have achieved at least a temporary increase in per capita cigarette consumption. Another and probably more important factor was a short-term economic reactivation and growth of over 8 percent in 1985 to 1986 (Vargas Llosa 1991).

The influence of a depressed economy is evident in the reduction in per capita consumption in the 1980s, with the exception of 1985 to 1986. Peru, Bolivia, and Haiti are reported to have the lowest per capita consumption in the Western Hemisphere; these nations also report the lowest per capita GNPs in the hemisphere. In 1989, a pack of 20 cigarettes cost $US0.92 on the average, and the average worker's wage was $US110. Therefore, a smoker of 10 cigarettes a day spent 12 percent of his or her wages on smoking.

Behavioral Surveys on Tobacco Use

Lima was included in the 1971 eight-city survey of smoking in Latin America (Joly 1977). This survey permits estimates of the prevalence of smokers, ex-smokers, and nonsmokers by sex and 15-year age groups. However, the data were collected so that only aggregate reports are possible for all eight cities on smoking status by educational level, occupation, opinions, attitudes, and knowledge. Compared with the other cities surveyed, the prevalence of smoking in Lima was the lowest reported for both men and women (Table 4): 33 and 6.3 percent, respectively. In addition, the male-to-female ratio of current smoking prevalence (5:2) was the highest among all eight cities.

More recently, several informative surveys of the general public and specific groups have been performed in Peru (Table 4). Tobacco use was included in a survey on drug use among persons 12 to 45 years old by the Health Division of the Police Force (SFP) in Lima and El Callao. Current smoking prevalence possibly was overestimated by this survey because "occasional use" was included in the

Table 4. Surveys on smoking and prevalence (percent) of adult smoking, Peru, 1970–1990

Survey	Year	Age	Coverage	N	Definition of smoker	Men	Women	Both
OPS	1971	15–74	Lima	1,966	>100 cig.			
					Current	33	6.3	19.2
					Ever	38.8	7.4	22.5
SFP	1979	12–45	Lima Metropol.	2,167	Daily	48.5	23.2	35.5
					Ever	62.7	34	47.9
POP[1]	1987	15–50	Lima	1,800	Current	68	40	53
					<3 cig/day	37	26	31
					≥3 cig/day	31	14	22
CEDRO	1989	12–50	Peru[2]	6,761	Ever	69	37	52
					At least 100 cig.	34	7	20
					Last month	41	13	26
			Lima	1,623	≥100 cig. Ever			26
Gallup	1988	18–35+	Lima	400	≥100 cig. Current	28	17	22

[1]Design not known. Market survey.
[2]Towns with more than 2,500 inhabitants (48%) of the country's population.

estimate of current smoking prevalence and because the port city of El Callao was included in the sample. This area has behavioral characteristics distinct from those of Lima. The prevalence of current daily smoking was 48.8 percent among men and 23.2 percent among women. This represents a relative increase in prevalence since 1971 of 46.9 percent in men and 268 percent in women. The male-female ratio of smoking prevalence in this survey was 2 to 1. However, the two surveys covered different age groups. The SFP survey found that 98 percent of women and 90.6 percent of men smoked between 1 and 10 cigarettes per day, with an average number of cigarettes smoked per day of 5.3 for women and 6 for men. By age group and sex, the highest smoking prevalence was among men and women 30 to 34 years old (78.6 percent and 59.6 percent, respectively). The average age of smoking initiation reported from this survey for men was 17.3 years (range 6 to 35 years) and among women 18.8 years (range 6 to 40 years).

In 1987, 8 years after the SFP survey, and 16 years after the Joly survey, a public opinion survey company (Peruana de Opinión Pública 1987) established for marketing purposes smoking prevalences among persons aged 15 to 50 years old in the city of Lima. Among men, 68 percent were current smokers and among women, 40 percent were current smokers. Compared with the 1979 Lima survey, smoking prevalence increased 40 percent among men and 72.4 percent among women. More than half of the smokers surveyed reported smoking fewer than three cigarettes a day. The ratio of men to women smokers was 2 to 1, similar to 1979. This survey reported the average age of starting to smoke at 16.2 years in men and 17.9 years in women.

In 1988, the American Cancer Society sponsored a survey of 400 Lima residents aged 18 to 35 and older, but the methodology and validity for this survey are questionable; nonetheless, 47 percent of men and 23 percent of women were classified as ever smokers (smoked at least 100 cigarettes in their lifetimes); 28 percent of men and 17 percent of women were current smokers in this survey (Gallup 1988).

The only national surveys on smoking are by the Center for Information and Education for the Prevention of Drugs (CEDRO) (1986, 1989). Complete data from the 1989 survey are available. The definitions of smoking status are comparable to the 1971 Joly survey (the prevalence of smoking sometime in the last month among persons who had smoked at least 100 cigarettes in their lifetimes is

Table 5. Surveys on smoking compiled by COLAT, and current smoking prevalence, Peru, 1990

Area surveyed	Age group	N	Prevalence		
			Men	Women	Both
Rural					
South	15–72	427			47.5
Urban					
(Lima)	15+	712	36.8	41.5	40.3
Adolescents	13–14	103			30.0

Source: Amorín, 1990.

considered to be "current smoking" on the CEDRO survey). Although the age group surveyed (12 to 50 years) was somewhat younger than the Joly survey, the prevalence of smoking sometime in the last month among both men and women was much higher in 1989 than in 1971 (41 percent and 13 percent, respectively). The 1989 CEDRO survey found an average age of initiation of 17.7 years. It was to be expected that the city of Lima would have a lower average age of initiation than urban Peru. In this city the average age of starting to smoke has declined by 1 year for both sexes compared with 1979.

Finally, Amorín (1990) coordinated a series of surveys on behalf of the Permanent National Antitobacco Commission (COLAT) (Table 5). These surveys provided data on tobacco use by rural and urban inhabitants, as well as some data on initiation of smoking and knowledge and attitudes toward smoking. Among 427 rural residents of Arequipa, Ica, Moquegua, and Tacna, aged 15 to 72 years, 47.5 percent were current smokers. Approximately one-third smoked "Hamilton" cigarettes, a Peruvian brand. The overwhelming majority (83.3 percent) smoked less than one pack per day. Among 653 Lima residents aged 15 years and older, 40.3 percent were current smokers; interestingly, more women than men were smokers in this population (41.5 vs. 36.8 percent). The leading brand for urban smokers was "Winston," and most smoked less than one pack of cigarettes per day.

As early as 1971 Joly noted that the prevalence of smoking was higher among those with higher educational attainment than among persons with lower educational attainment (e.g., less than high school). The 1979 SFP survey of Lima-Callao also reported a positive correlation between smoking prevalence and socioeconomic status. The CEDRO survey of cities larger than 2,500 inhabitants also confirmed this association (Table 6). The CEDRO

Table 6. Prevalence (percent) of ever smoking by educational attainment, Peru, 1979 and 1989

	Lima 1979	Urban Peru 1989
None	10	19
Primary	26	31
Secondary	50.6	52
Technical school	66	66
University	62.7	76

Sources: CEDRO, 1989; SFP, 1979.

survey also reported that 51.4 percent of smokers with low education had attempted to quit smoking, while only 38 percent of smokers with a university education had done so. The SFP survey reported that persons in high and intermediate socio-economic strata had higher smoking prevalences than did those in lower socioeconomic strata (Table 7). A survey by Albarran (1986) of 1,226 female private university students in Lima reported that 90 percent of these students were current smokers. Of these smokers, 42 percent smoked four or fewer cigarettes per day. This survey also lends credence to the notion of higher smoking prevalence among well-educated students of high socioeconomic status. The average age of initiation for these women was 14.7 years, much lower than the average age of initiation found in Lima by the 1987 Peruana de Opinión Pública survey (17.9 years for women).

It appears that there has been a significant increase in the prevalence of smoking in Peru, particularly among women, since 1971. The differences between men and women have diminished but continue to be significant. Generally low per capita consumption prevails (fewer than 10 cigarettes per day), and a large proportion of the popu-

lation smokes only occasionally. Persons with high educational attainment and with higher socio-economic status have higher smoking prevalence rates than those with less education and low socio-economic status. The association is significant, although it appears that these differences in smoking prevalence are becoming less apparent over time. The age of initiation may be decreasing somewhat in urban areas.

Prevalence of Smoking among Adolescents

The 1989 CEDRO survey included 419 persons in the 12- to 19-year age group. Among those aged 12 to 14 years, 6.3 percent had experimented with smoking, and among those aged 15 to 19, the percentage of experimenters increased to 42.8 percent. The survey found that 34 percent of respondents aged 12 to 19 years had smoked at some time and approximately 3.4 percent had smoked at least 100 cigarettes at the time of the survey.

The National Institute for Neoplastic Diseases (INEN) survey compared smoking among male adolescents from two socioeconomic strata (Rubini 1982). In a Lima public school, 41.5 percent of 1,311 male students surveyed had smoked at some time, and 13 percent smoked at the time of the survey. In a private school, 63.5 percent of 255 boys and girls surveyed had smoked at some time, and 28.6 percent smoked at the time of the survey. Thus, as for Peruvian adults, a higher prevalence of smoking was observed for students from a presumably higher socioeconomic background. In the private school, the male-to-female ratio for current smoking status was 14 to 1. The average age of initiation was 12.8 years among boys, whereas in the public school, it was 14 years. Of public schoolchildren, 5.2 percent reported beginning to smoke before age 10, whereas in the private school, 17.3 percent be-

Table 7. Prevalence (percent) of never, former, and current smoking by socioeconomic strata and cigarettes smoked per day, Lima and Callao, 1979

| | Never smokers | | Former smokers | | Current smokers (cigarettes/day) | | | | | | |
| | | | | | 1–10 | | 11–20 | | + 20 | | |
Stratum	n	%	n	%	n	%	n	%	n	%	TOTAL
High	16	37	5	11.6	18	41.8	3	7	1	2.3	43
Middle	287	44.7	78	12.2	255	39.7	21	3.3	1	0.2	642
Low	825	55.7	187	12.6	442	29.8	25	1.7	3	0.2	1,482
TOTAL	1,128	52	270	12.4	715	33	49	2.3	5	0.2	2,167

Source: Carbajal, 1980.

gan to smoke before age 10. In the private school, the average number of cigarettes smoked per day by smokers was 2.3, and in the public school, 2.6.

Other Uses of Tobacco

Pinillos collected data on pipe and cigar smoking in predominantly rural provinces in 1989 and 1990. Only 6 percent of 102 respondents smoked pipes or cigars (Pinillos 1989, 1990).

The increase in the use of the coca leaf to produce cocaine has led to an increase in the use of "basuco," or "pasta básica," which is an initial by-product in cocaine production and is mixed with tobacco in cigarettes known as "piticlines" (Gastiaburu 1985). The SFP survey (1979) found that all those who smoked this substance also smoked cigarettes. Smoking may be considered a gateway drug to cocaine use in this form (Jeri 1985).

Attitudes, Knowledge, and Opinions on Smoking

Knowledge of the health effects of smoking

Joly reported that in 1971 nonsmokers in Lima remained abstinent primarily because they "did not like it," followed by "health reasons" and "family influence." In reply to questions on the extent of concern for the possible health effects of smoking, the great majority of smokers answered "none." In the Pinillos survey, the most important reason to stop smoking was considered by 65.7 percent of respondents to protect health, by 7.5 percent to avoid unpleasant symptoms, and by 11.2 percent because of family pressure. In the INEN survey of adolescents in two schools, 95.8 percent of those surveyed thought smoking was harmful and 4.2 percent thought that it was not (Rubini 1982). In the women's college survey in Lima, the students were asked the reasons why they were smokers (Albarran 1986). The majority of respondents (81 percent) recognized some of the physiological effects of nicotine (i.e., greater concentration, a sensation of warmth or cooling, reduction of appetite, improvement of digestion, and relief from sleepiness and fatigue).

Attitudes toward smoking by smokers

Pinillos asked smokers if they would still be smoking in 5 years; 60.8 percent answered yes, 28.5 percent said probably not, and 8.8 percent answered probably yes. In this survey, 7.5 percent considered that an important reason to stop smoking was to avoid inconveniencing nearby persons.

Smoking and Health

As early as 1890 an item appeared in a Peruvian newspaper drawing attention to the dangers of tobacco: ". . . It has been proven that tobacco is very harmful for the heart. Irregularity of the pulse, palpitations, and angina pectoris are frequently caused by tobacco abuse" (Diario El Comercio 1990). Concern for the health consequences of smoking has increased in Peru, with more attention paid to national morbidity and mortality data on chronic diseases associated with smoking.

Morbidity

The city of Lima has maintained a cancer registry since 1968, and has published figures through 1978 (Parkin 1986). The small degree of under-registration supports the validity of the reported data. Lung cancer, with an age-adjusted incidence rate of 10.5/100,000, is the second most common cancer among males (after stomach cancer, 15.6/100,000). The lung cancer incidence rate among women was 3.5/100,000, and thus the male-to-female ratio of 2:9. This ratio is higher than that based on mortality data for Lima, which, as discussed below, has a higher proportion of under-registration for this diagnosis in men.

Rubini (1972) reviewed a series of 768 cases of bronchogenic carcinoma diagnosed in 1952 to 1969 from the INEN study (Table 8). A total of 617 patients in the series had histological verification. The average age of the patients was 57.9 years, with 64.7 percent aged 50 to 64 years. The male-to-female ratio was 3:3. Only four patients were Indians, and 91.4 percent were Caucasians and mestizos. According to smoking status, of 697 cases in which a history of smoking could be documented, 77 percent were smokers and 23 percent non-smokers. Exposure was considered as "having smoked at some time." Of the 537 lung cancer patients who were smokers, 47 percent smoked 21 or more cigarettes per day. Slightly more than half of the cases in nonsmokers were adenocarcinomas (which is usually not associated with smoking [WHO 1986]), whereas more than half of the cases in smokers were squamocellular carcinomas (which are associated with smoking).

Overall Mortality

According to the Pan American Health Organization (PAHO), underreporting of mortality in Peru approaches 50 percent (PAHO 1990). Most

Table 8. Distribution of bronchogenic carcinoma by histologic type and exposure to cigarettes in a series of 520 patients. Institute of Neoplastic Diseases, Lima, 1972

Histologic type	Nonsmokers		Smokers		All cases	
	N	(%)	N	(%)	N	(%)
Epidermoid	38	30.2	215	54.6	253	48.6
Anaplastic	6	4.8	30	7.6	36	6.9
Undifferentiated	15	11.9	83	21	98	18.8
Adenocarcinoma	65	51.6	65	16.5	130	25
Round cell	2	1.6	1	0.25	3	0.58
Total	126		394		520	

Source: Rubini, 1972.

mortality reports are for Lima and other urban areas. The mortality structure for urban areas is likely to be quite different from that for the rest of Peru. For example, it was estimated in 1983 that the life expectancy at birth was 58 years overall in Peru, while in Lima it was 67.3 years (PAHO 1986). Thus, proportionate mortality analyses will overrepresent urban areas. In analyzing national cause-specific rates, such as lung cancer, the reported rate would be minimized because the denominator includes the entire population and the numerator includes only urban areas. Given that there has been a higher prevalence of smoking and earlier acquisition of smoking by urban populations, lung cancer mortality rates may be very near the real rates. Those areas with significant underregistration of deaths are also areas with few lung cancer deaths.

Although only 7.4 percent of the deaths re-ported in Peru for 1982 were classified as "ill defined" (ICD-9 760–788), only 62.7 percent of the reported deaths were physician-certified in 1980. In Peru, where pulmonary tuberculosis is still very frequent (PAHO 1990), it is possible that deaths from lung cancer are misclassified as pulmonary tuberculosis. Because misclassification of cardiovascular disease deaths is common throughout the world, this category of smoking-related illness may also be difficult to analyze.

Infectious diseases were the most frequently registered cause of death between 1979 and 1985 (accounting for approximately 30 to 40 percent of all deaths) and cardiovascular diseases were second with 11 to 14 percent of all registered deaths (Table 9). The case of infectious diseases appears to be one of "minimum underrepresentation" (lack of rural reporting) and that of cardiovascular diseases and

Table 9. Deaths, mortality rates, and proportionate mortality for large groups of causes, Peru, 1979, 1983, and 1985

Cause and ICD code	1979			1983			1985
	Deaths	Rate*	%	Deaths	Rate*	%	%
Infectious diseases (ICD 001–134, 320, 460–466, 480–487)	37,319	195.7	41.8	34,450	172.3	36.9	30.5
Malignant neoplasms (ICD 140–209)	6,164	37.6	6.9	5,663	30.5	6.1	9.4
Cardiovascular disease (ICD 400–458)	10,116	60.8	11.3	11,009	60.5	11.8	14.5
Violence and accidents (ICD E810–E999)	4,694	27	5.3	5,734	29.5	6.1	6.9
Symptoms and ill-defined conditions (ICD 780–799)	7,370	38.4	8.3	6,542	31.5	7.0	
Other causes	23,610	127.5	26.4	29,892	149.7	32.0	38.3
All causes	89,273	487	100.0	93,290	474	100.0	

Sources: PAHO, 1986; 1990; Pinillos, 1989.
*Rate per 100,000 persons, adjusted for age.

Table 10. Deaths, mortality rates, and proportionate mortality for large groups of causes, Lima, 1962–1964

Cause and ICD code	Men Deaths	Men Rate*	Men %	Women Deaths	Women Rate*	Women %	Both Deaths	Both Rate*	Both %
Infectious diseases (ICD 001–138, 480–493)	472	62.7	19.5	297	38.8	15	768	50.7	17.5
Malignant neoplasms (ICD 140–205)	408	54.2	16.9	562	73.6	28.6	970	64	22.2
Cardiovascular diseases (ICD 330–334, 400–468)	690	91.7	28.6	489	64	24.9	1,179	77.8	27
Violence and accidents (ICD E810–E999)	328	43.6	13.6	83	10.9	4.3	411	27.1	9.4
Symptoms, senility, and ill-defined conditions (ICD 780–795)	47	6.3	1.9	34	4.5	1.7	81	5.4	1.9
Other causes	472	62.7	19.5	496	65	25.3	968	63.8	22.1
All causes	2,417	321.1	100	1,961	256.9	100	4,378	288.8	100

Source: Puffer and Griffith, 1968.
*Crude rate.

malignant tumors, one of "minimum overrepresentation" (almost total coverage of reporting in urban areas). Most infectious diseases occur in children, and deaths among children are underreported more than are deaths among adults.

A PAHO study of urban mortality in 12 cities (10 in Latin America) among persons aged 15 years and older in 1962 to 1964 (Puffer 1968) included Lima (Table 10). Although this analysis is now more than 25 years old, the mortality structure for Lima appeared to be that of a developed country, with a heavy burden of cardiovascular diseases and malignant tumors. Today, most mortality from smoking-related diseases is also concentrated in metropolitan Lima, just as is the largest proportion of the smoking population.

Lung Cancer Mortality

In the 1968 Puffer study of urban mortality, the lung cancer mortality rate was still fairly low (17.9/100,000 men and 5.5/100,000 women). Age-specific lung cancer mortality for men aged 45 to 54 years was 26.5/100,000, and was 67.1/100,000 for men aged 55 to 64 years. The rates among women in these age groups were 6.2/100,000 and 17.9/100,000, respectively. In 1968 (the year closest to the Puffer study) (Table 10), the lung cancer mortality rates for all of Peru were 7.4 and 23.1 per 100,000 among men and 2.2 and 6.4 per 100,000 among women, respectively, in those age groups. In 1972, 65 percent of total tobacco consumption was concentrated in Lima, and thus the higher

rates of lung cancer mortality in Lima are not surprising.

The lung cancer mortality rates for men and women aged 45 to 54 years increased from 1974 to 1989, although somewhat irregularly in women (Table 11). In addition, the male-female ratio appears to have declined, as expected from the increased prevalence of smoking among women between 1971 and 1989.

Tobacco Use Prevention and Control Activities

Government Actions

Policies and executive structure

The Government of Peru, through the Ministry of Health's Institute of Neoplastic Diseases (INEN), has taken an official stand on controlling in Peru the growing epidemic of diseases associated with smoking (PAHO 1987). Goals of the Ministry's national program include:

1. To establish and formalize an interdisciplinary commission to coordinate Government agencies and actions against tobacco.
2. To organize public education campaigns addressing the risks of smoking, the health benefits of not smoking, and to emphasize the rights of nonsmokers to breathe smoke-free air.
3. To strengthen antismoking legislation and policies addressing:
   a. nonsmoking in public places

Table 11. Lung cancer mortality among men and women, age groups 45–54 and 55–64, Peru, 1968–1983

Year	Total Deaths	Total Rate*	Men Deaths	Men Rate*	Women Deaths	Women Rate*
Age Group 45–54						
1968	39	4.8	30	7.4	9	2.2
1969	39	2.5	22	5.3	17	4.0
1970	48	5.5	30	7.0	18	4.1
1971	50	5.6	41	9.2	9	2.0
1972	41	4.5	26	5.7	15	3.3
1973	60	6.4	46	9.8	14	3.0
1974	Not available					
1975	48	4.9	Not available			
1976	Not available					
1977	55	5.2	44	8.4	11	2.1
1978	53	4.9	43	8.0	10	1.8
1979	73	6.3	Not available			
1980	68	5.7	45	7.6	23	3.9
1981	76	6.2	46	7.6	30	4.9
1982	64	5.1	48	7.7	16	2.5
1983	52	4.0	38	5.8	14	2.1
Age Group 55–64						
1968	75	14.5	58	23.1	17	6.4
1969	82	15.4	65	25.0	17	6.2
1970	90	16.3	68	25.4	22	7.8
1971	111	19.6	80	29.1	31	10.7
1972	82	14.1	61	21.6	21	7.0
1973	78	13.2	55	18.9	23	7.6
1974	Not available					
1975	74	11.9	Not available			
1976	Not available					
1977	102	15.2	74	22.4	28	8.2
1978	87	12.6	63	18.5	24	6.8
1979	117	15.8	Not available			
1980	113	14.9	87	23.6	26	6.7
1981	119	15.3	78	20.6	41	10.2
1982	110	13.8	80	20.6	30	7.3
1983	85	10.1	55	13.4	30	6.9

Source: PAHO database, unpublished data, 1991.

b. advertising of tobacco products

c. health warnings on cigarette packs

d. public service announcements on the health risks of smoking in the mass media

4. To develop formal educational programs involving school and health personnel as well as media resources.

5. To develop educational programs for persons affected by smoking-related illnesses because these persons may be most ready to change their behavior.

6. To support research on the economic costs of smoking and premature death due to smoking.

7. To support epidemiologic research on the relationship between smoking and specific disease entities such as heart disease and diabetes.

8. To work with international agencies to develop methods to control and prevent tobacco use.

9. To increase community participation in tobacco control activities.

10. To involve scientific and medical associations in further antitobacco program activities.

11. To improve data collection and analysis on both the behavioral aspects and outcomes of exposure to tobacco.

In pursuit of this program, Ministerial Resolution 499-88-SA established in December 1988, COLAT, a multisectoral and decentralized organization of community antismoking leaders. Activities of this organization as well as other interventions against smoking in Peru are described below.

Legislation

Several legislative interventions are reported in Peru, dating back rather early in the history of world-wide antitobacco actions. In 1970, a presidential decree mandated that the warning, "May be harmful to health," be placed on cigarette packages. This health warning was one of the first to appear on cigarettes manufactured in Latin America. In addition, the decree prohibited tobacco product advertisements before 8 p.m. on radio and television or at any public performance, so that children may be less likely to be influenced by these advertisements, and set fines for noncompliance (República del Perú 1970). In 1981, the tobacco advertising regulations were amended by another presidential decree so that advertisements must also include a health warning approved by the Ministry of Health; in addition, cigarette advertising on radio and television was prohibited before 9 p.m. In 1991, the time was moved back to 10 p.m. Indirect advertising (i.e., brand advertisement without mention of cigarettes) is also prohibited.

In 1985, the Ministry of Health prohibited smoking in all its administrative and health-care facilities (Ministry of Health 1985). No enforcement provisions were stipulated, however, and the compliance with this regulation is unreported. In 1987, school-based vendors were prohibited under a hygiene regulation from selling cigarettes on school premises (República del Perú 1987); this regulation provided for punishments against noncompliant vendors.

Recently, in November 1991, a new law was passed (Law No. 17235). This law bans smoking in all public and private enclosed areas. The local governments will enforce the law with monetary sanctions against violators. The new law also bans smoking in all public transportation facilities in the country (El Peruano 1991).

In 1991, the health warning on cigarette packages was changed to "Tobacco *is* harmful for your health" instead of "may be harmful" as in the past.

School education

In 1986 INEN and the Ministry of Education piloted a program of short informational presentations to schoolchildren aged 9 to 12 years. INEN now estimates that it reaches 50,000 children per year with this program. Efforts are being made to include antismoking information in the academic curricula of all primary schools (Pinillos 1990).

Public information campaigns

In 1985, Peru's "No Smoking Day" was established by the Ministry of Health and other groups interested in smoking. Initially, this day was December 5th each year, but since 1989 it has been celebrated simultaneously with the World Health Organization's No-Tobacco Day on May 31. Community and press interest in this event is particularly evident in Lima. Activities include parades, national radio reports on smoking and health, and publication of articles in national newsletters and journals of CEDRO, the Association of Lawyers, and the Lions Club. In 1990, antismoking posters were displayed in sports facilities (Pinillos 1990).

Taxes

Peru is somewhat unique among countries of the Americas in that a portion of its cigarette taxes is dedicated to anticancer, and hence, antitobacco, activities at INEN. Two categories of tax add 55 percent to the wholesale price of cigarettes. The first is the consumption tax, currently at 70 percent on unfiltered cigarettes containing domestic tobacco and at 95 percent on all other types of cigarettes. However, this tax rate represents a substantial reduction since 1987, when the rate was reduced from 326 percent by successive presidential and legislative decrees, in particular because the tax rate may have stimulated an illegal trade in cigarettes from other countries. The second tax is the general sales tax of 11 percent. Imported cigarettes are taxed additionally at 110 percent ad valorem. Most importantly, Law No. 23482, enacted in October 1982, earmarked 7 percent of the total taxes on light tobacco cigarettes for construction of a new Hospital for Neoplastic Diseases. This law was revised so that after the hospital was completed, the earmarked tax revenues were "preferably" to be allocated to the construction of cancer detection centers and cancer research.

In 1988, the State collected 8,225,587,000 Intis (approximately $US16,451,174) in cigarette taxes.

This amounted to 1.6 percent of total Government tax revenues. Total cigarette taxes continued to increase, to $US22,286,062, in 1990 (Pinillos 1990).

Nongovernmental Actions

COLAT includes several nongovernmental organizations (NGOs), such as the Peruvian Society of Internal Medicine, CEDRO, the Peruvian Cancer Society, the Association of Lawyers, the Archbishopric of Lima, the Lions Club, and the Rotary Club. The most active organization is CEDRO, which has included questions on smoking in two drug use surveys of urban Peru. It has also supported, as part of COLAT, community antismoking coalitions outside metropolitan Lima. CEDRO prepared a children's coloring book entitled, "Color While Caring for Your Health"; this book depicts cigarettes as an addictive drug. In addition, this organization joined with the Ministry of Education in 1989 in programs on drug abuse for secondary school teachers and students.

Smoking cessation classes and public information on the health consequences of smoking have been provided by other NGOs inside the COLAT structure. These include The Young Men's Christian Association and the Inca Union of the Seventh Day Adventist Church (Pinillos 1990). During 1991, monthly 1-week cessation classes were held at INEN by these groups.

Summary and Conclusions

Peru has one of the lowest rates of per capita cigarette consumption of countries in the Americas, but as in many other Latin American countries, urbanization and modernization have produced since the 1970s a gradual increase in cigarette consumption, particularly by women. Large differences in health status, predominant disease conditions, and smoking behavior are evident between urban and rural Peruvians. As a result of these differences, morbidity and mortality associated with smoking are concentrated in urban areas. Despite the serious social and economic problems affecting Peru in the 1980s, considerable legislative and organizational efforts against smoking have been made. One very important intervention has been the earmarking of 7 percent of cigarette taxes since 1982 for building and equipping a Cancer Institute in Lima and cancer centers around the country for treatment, detection, research, and control programs.

Based on the data presented in this report, the following conclusions can be drawn:

1. The prevalence of smoking among Lima residents decreased from 71.8 percent to 68 percent among men and increased from 13.7 percent to 40 percent among women between 1971 and 1987. The prevalence of smoking is highest among those with higher socioeconomic status and higher educational attainment. In 1990, approximately one-half of rural and urban residents were current smokers. Among urban residents, the prevalence of smoking was somewhat higher for women than for men.

2. Per capita consumption has varied according to economic conditions in Peru, and at 331 is one of the lowest in the Americas; however, the contribution of illegally imported cigarettes to per capita consumption has not been considered in this figure.

3. Cancer registry data from Lima suggest that the impact of smoking among men, as indicated by lung cancer mortality rates, is higher than among women. Rates have increased substantially since the late 1960s, however, in response to increasing trends in tobacco use. After infectious diseases, cardiovascular diseases are the second most common reported cause of death in Peru.

4. Considerable legislative, Government, and nongovernmental activities against tobacco exist in Peru. Peru has one of the few cigarette taxes of any country of the Americas dedicated to the control of cancer.

References

AGENCIA EFE. *Peru: Reemplazar cultivos de coca por tabaco es mas rentable*. Lima, 27 de febrero de 1990.

AGRO-ECONOMICS, LTD AND TABACOSMOS, LTD. *The Employment, Wealth, and Tax Benefits that the Tobacco Industry Creates*. Agro-economic Services Ltd., September 1987.

ALBARRAN, A.M. *El hábito de fumar cigarrillos, su costo, sus consecuencias y posibles soluciones*. Universidad Femenina del Sagrado Corazón. Lima, Perú: Departamento de Ciencias de la Comunicación, Area de Investigaciones, 1986.

AMORIN, E. *Encuestas coordinadas para COLAT*. In press, 1990.

CARBAJAL, C. et al. *Revista Sanidad de las Fuerzas Policiales* 44:1–38, 1980.

CEDRO. *Uso de drogas en las ciudades del Perú. Segundo Estudio Epidemiológico. Principales resultados*. Resumen de Investigación No. 4., Junio 1989.

CEDRO. *El consumo de tabaco en Perú*. Resumen de Investigacion. No. 5, Agosto de 1989.

CENTRO LATINOAMERICANO DEMOGRAFICO. *Boletín Demográfico*, Año XXIII, No. 45. Santiago, Chile, enero de 1990.

CHAPMAN, S., WONG, W.L. *Tobacco Control in the Third World—A Resource Atlas*. Penang, Malaysia: International Organization of Consumers Unions, 1990.

DIARIO El COMERCIO. *Sucedió hace un siglo*. 4 de enero de 1990.

EL PERUANO. *Normas Legales*. Ley No. 25357. 27 de noviembre de 1991.

EUROMONITOR CONSULTANCY (ERC). *The World Market for Tobacco: Strategy 2000*, Volumes I-II, agosto de 1989.

GALLUP ORGANIZATION. *The Incidence of Smoking in Central and Latin America*. Conducted for: American Cancer Society, GO 87333, Princeton, New Jersey: The Gallup Organization, 1988.

GASTIABURU, R., LACUNZA, E., INFANTES, V., KOSAKA, A., HONORES, F., APONTE, I. Tabaquismo y psicopatología. Características del tabaquismo en una población supuesta sana. *Revista de Sanidad de las Fuerzas Policiales* 46(1):64–68, 1985.

JERI, R.F. Los problemas medicos y sociales generados por el abuso de drogas en el Perú. *Revista de Sanidad de las Fuerzas Policiales* 46(1):36–44, 1985.

JOLY, D.J. *Encuesta sobre las características del hábito de fumar en América Latina*. Washington, D.C.: Organizacion Panamericana de la Salud. Publicación Científica No. 337, 1977.

MINISTRY OF HEALTH. *Resolución No. 576–85*. 3 de diciembre de 1985.

MINISTRY OF HEALTH. *Resolución Ministerial 449-88*. 5 de diciembre de 1988.

NICHTER, M., CARTWRIGHT, E. Saving the children for the tobacco industry. *Medical Anthropology Quarterly*, Fall, 1991.

PAN AMERICAN HEALTH ORGANIZATION. *Control del hábito de fumar. Segundo taller subregional. Area Andina.* Caracas, Venezuela, 16–21 de noviembre 1986. Technical Paper No. 6, 1987.

PAN AMERICAN HEALTH ORGANIZATION. *Health Conditions in the Americas—1986 Edition*. Washington, D.C.: Pan American Health Organization. Scientific Publication No. 500, 1986.

PAN AMERICAN HEALTH ORGANIZATION. *Health Conditions in the Americas—1990 Edition*. Washington, D.C.: Pan American Health Organization. Scientific Publication No. 524, 1990.

PAN AMERICAN HEALTH ORGANIZATION. Mortality Data Base. Unpublished tabulations, 1991.

PARKIN, D.M. *Cancer Occurrence in Developing Countries*. In Olivares, L., IARC Scientific Publication No. 75, pp. 185–187, Lyon, France: 1986.

PERUANA DE OPINION PUBLICA. Perfil básico de fumadores. Unpublished data, 1987.

PINILLOS, L. Country collaborator's report. Unpublished data. Washington, D.C.: Pan American Health Organization, 1990.

PINILLOS, L. *La salud en el Perú*. Estrategia de Gestión. Lima, 1989.

PUFFER, R.R., GRIFFITH, G.W. *Características de la mortalidad urbana*. Washington, D.C.: Pan American Health Organization. Scientific Publication No. 151, 1968.

REPUBLICA DEL PERU. *Decreto Supremo de la Presidencia de la Republica No.0079-70-SA*. 29 de abril de 1970.

REPUBLICA DEL PERU. *Decreto Supremo de la Presidencia de la Republica No. 002-81*. 21 de abril de 1981.

REPUBLICA DEL PERU. *Legislacion Artículo 1, Norma 16 del D.S. No. 002-81-OCI-OAJ*. 21 de abril de 1981.

REPUBLICA DEL PERU. *Decreto Supremo de la Presidencia de la Republica No. 026-87-SA*. 4 de junio de 1987.

RUBINI, D.C. *Carcinoma broncogénico*. Tesis de Doctor en Medicina. Lima: Universidad Peruana Cayetano Heredia. Mayo 1972.

RUBINI, D.C. *Hábito de fumar en niños*. Lima: Instituto Nacional de Enfermedades Neoplásicas, 1982.

TAYLOR, S.A. Tobacco and economic growth in developing nations. *Business in the Contemporary World*. Winter 1989.

U.S. DEPARTMENT OF AGRICULTURE. Tobacco, Cotton, and Seeds Division. Foreign Agricultural Service. Unpublished tabulations, April 1990.

VARGAS LLOSA, M. A fish out of water. *Granta* No. 36: 18, Summer 1991.

WORLD BANK. *World Development Report 1989*. New York: Oxford University Press, 1989.

WORLD BANK. *World Development Report 1990—Poverty*. New York: Oxford University Press, 1990.

WORLD HEALTH ORGANIZATION. *IARC Monographs on the Evaluation of Carcinogenic Risk of Chemicals to Humans*. Tobacco Smoking. 38:221–228. Lyon, France: IARC, 1986.

Puerto Rico

General Characteristics

The Tobacco Industry
    Agriculture
    Manufacturing
    Marketing

Tobacco Use
    Adult prevalence surveys
    Adolescent prevalence surveys

Smoking and Health
    Changes in adult mortality patterns
    Smoking-related mortality rates
    Cancer incidence
    Smoking-attributable mortality estimates
    Smoking-attributable economic costs

Tobacco Use Prevention and Control Activities
    Legislation and taxes
    Public information/education campaigns
    School education programs
    Government policies

Summary and Conclusions

References

General Characteristics

Puerto Rico is a tropical Caribbean island of approximately 9,100 km². Puerto Rico is a democratically self-governed Commonwealth of the United States, ruled since 1952 by the U.S. constitution. Four different political parties currently debate whether Puerto Rico is to remain a Commonwealth, become a State, or become an independent nation.

The estimated 1987 population was 3,293,872, with a population density of 941 inhabitants per square mile (Departamento de Salud 1987). Of this total, 66.8 percent is urban (Leon 1985), 26.7 percent is younger than 15 years of age, and 10 percent is 65 and older (Departamento de Salud 1989b). Life expectancy at birth was 74.7 years in 1988 (70.7 years for men and 78.9 years for women) (Departamento de Salud 1989b). In 1980, the infant mortality rate was 14.2/1,000 live births, a dramatic decline from the 1950 rate of 68/1,000 live births (Departamento de Salud 1989b) (Table 1).

The annual per capita income in Puerto Rico for fiscal year 1989 was $1,504, and the total gross commonwealth product was $4,894 million (Amato 1989).

The Puerto Rican economy depended for centuries on agriculture; the primary crops were tobacco, coffee, and sugar cane. Historically, State control over tobacco began in 1614 under the Spanish colonial regime (Gaztambide 1968). When the island became part of the United States, Puerto Rico industrialized rapidly, and agriculture began to decline. Because of increased demands for urban and industrial land development, a shrinking work force due to emigration, and increasing imports of foreign products, Puerto Rican agricultural output declined even further in the 1960s (Gaztambide 1968). In 1990, traditional crops such as sugar cane, coffee, and tobacco represented only 10 percent of the total agricultural output of the island. Large-scale production of farinaceous vegetables and citrus fruits was developed in their place (Amato 1989). The most dynamic sectors of the local economy are now manufacturing, construction, and tourism (Amato 1989). Puerto Rico is strongly linked to the United States through financial activities, health programs, and culture; millions of Puerto Ricans live in the New York City area and maintain strong ties to the island.

The Tobacco Industry

Agriculture

In 1988, there were 101 tobacco growers in Puerto Rico (0.5 percent of all 20,000 agricultural workers). During 1984 and 1985, 47.3 ha were planted with tobacco (0.03 percent of total arable land). At present an official Government program encourages farmers to substitute for tobacco other crops including coffee, citrus fruit, and farinaceous vegetables such as plantain, yucca, yams, and sweet potatoes (Santiago 1990). Production of unmanufactured tobacco has decreased significantly over the last decade (Table 2) because of lack of mechanization, because of a crop-damaging infestation with "blue mold," and because raw tobacco is more cheaply grown in and imported from the Dominican Republic and the Philippines. Prior to 1982, tobacco farmers benefited from price supports established by the U.S. Department of Agriculture (Turner 1982).

Manufacturing

In 1989, only one locally owned factory in Puerto Rico manufactured tobacco products, the Consolidated Cigars Corporation. This small private enterprise manufactures cigars containing locally grown tobacco, which are exported mainly to the United States; it has no relations with any of the multinational tobacco companies. However, cigarettes are manufactured locally in one plant owned by the mainland U.S.-based multinational corporation, R.J. Reynolds. Overall, fewer than 2,000 workers were employed in tobacco-related activities in 1989 (0.22 percent of the total labor force)

Table 1. Health and economic indicators, Puerto Rico, 1980s

Indicator	Year	Value
Population	1987	3,293,872
Percent <15 years old	1987	26.7
Percent ≥65 years old	1987	10.0
Percent urban	1985	66.8
Crude mortality rate per 1,000		
Infant mortality rate per 1,000		
live births	1987	14.2
Life expectancy at birth		
Men	1987	70.7
Women	1987	78.9
Average annual per capita		
income (in $US)	1989	1,504
Gross Commonwealth		
product (in $US)	1989	4,894,000

Table 2. Raw tobacco production, exportation, importation (in MT), manufactured cigarettes—total and adult per capita consumption, Puerto Rico, 1979–1989

Year	Production (MT)	Exportation (MT)	Importation (MT)	Total cigarette consumption	Per capita cigarette consumption
1979	955	3407	5931	3,600,000,000	2,700
1980	72	3843	5936	3,600,000,000	2,000
1981	227	4441	6128	3,600,000,000	2,070
1982	152	3583	4917	3,500,000,000	—
1983	437	2657	4003	3,500,000,000	2,015
1984	309	2248	4198	3,500,000,000	2,100
1985	198	2449	2710	3,400,000,000	2,040
1986	95	2881	3293	3,400,000,000	2,020
1987	68	2983	3347	3,400,000,000	2,064
1988	59	2106	2804	3,300,000,000	2,033

Source: Maxwell, 1989; Santiago, 1990.

(Departamento de Agricultura de Puerto Rico 1990). The local manufacturing of cigarettes in Puerto Rico has increased over the last decade from 1.8 million MT in 1979 to 2.84 million MT in 1987 (Santiago 1990). Total domestic cigarette consumption decreased from 3.6 billion in 1979 to 3,4 billion in 1987 (Table 2). However, because domestic cigarette production does not satisfy local demand, the island also imports manufactured cigarettes (more than 3,000 MT in 1987) (Santiago 1990).

Marketing

Promotion and advertising of tobacco products in Puerto Rico is widespread. Television and radio advertising of these products is prohibited by U.S. law, but all other mass media are used, including newspapers, magazines, billboards, and movies. In addition, sports and cultural events are heavily sponsored by tobacco companies. The distribution of free tobacco product samples is permitted. Information is not available on the monetary value of tobacco product advertising purchased by the multinational corporations in Puerto Rico. The Commonwealth Government does not have a separate price support program for tobacco product sales.

Winston cigarettes claimed 74 percent of the Puerto Rican market in 1989, and Salem cigarettes, 9.1 percent (Table 3). Both of these R.J. Reynolds products are manufactured on the island. The island is saturated with print media and outdoor advertising bearing the slogan, "Winston y Puerto Rico—no Hay Nada Mejor." Philip Morris imports their brands into Puerto Rico. These include Marl-

Table 3. Market share (%) for major cigarette brands, Puerto Rico, 1988

Cigarette brand	Market share
Winston	74.0
Salem	9.1
Marlboro	7.4
Merit	6.0

Source: Maxwell, 1989.

boro (the most popular brand in the continental United States of America) with 7.4 percent of the market, and Merit with 6 percent of the market (Maxwell 1989). Puerto Ricans show an overwhelming preference for filtered cigarettes (99.8 percent of total sales) (Maxwell 1989).

Cigarettes are sold in packages of 10 and 20. The 20-cigarette package, whether domestically produced or imported, is preferred by most Puerto Rican smokers. Its average price was $1.60 in 1989 (Santiago 1990). Cigarettes are also sold singly by street vendors and in packages in vending machines. Tobacco sales in Puerto Rico are modestly restricted because retail stores are required to have a municipal license to sell cigars and cigarettes. Also, a Commonwealth law restricts the sale of tobacco products to persons 18 years and older (Santiago 1990).

Tobacco Use

Data on cigarette consumption are available from the tobacco industry (Maxwell 1989) and from

Table 4. Surveys on tobacco use in Puerto Rico and prevalence (percent) of smoking among men and women, 1979–1989

Survey name	Year	Sample	N	Prevalence	
				Men	Women
Puerto Rico Fertility and Family Planning Assessment	1982	Women Aged 15–49	?		15
Hispanic Health and Nutrition Survey	1982–84	Puerto Ricans in New York Aged 20–74	1,220	39.8	30.3
PFCAMPR (Rullán et al.)	1989	Urban residents Aged ≥ 18 years	772	22.5	10.6

the Departamentos de Hacienda y de Comercio (Santiago 1990). Total per capita cigarette consumption in Puerto Rico was 1,364 for 1989 (Santiago 1989). Annual adult (not defined) per capita consumption declined from 3,100 in 1976 to 2,033 in 1988 (Maxwell 1989).

Adult Prevalence Surveys

In 1965 to 1968, 9,824 men aged 45 to 64 years were surveyed for cardiovascular disease risk factors. Among these men, 44 percent were current smokers, and the prevalence of smoking was significantly higher among urban than among rural men (Sorlie et al. 1982). A few studies that report the prevalence of smoking among adults in Puerto Rico have been conducted in the last decade (Table

4). Maxwell (1989) reported on the prevalence of ''smoking'' among men and women for each year from 1976 to 1988 (Figure 1). According to these surveys, the prevalence of smoking among men decreased from 63.5 percent to 57 percent while the prevalence of smoking among women increased from 36.5 percent to 43 percent.

In 1982, the Puerto Rico Fertility and Family Planning Assessment (PRFFPA) surveyed a representative sample of Puerto Rican women aged 15 to 49 years, obtaining information on smoking. This carefully performed survey of women of child-bearing age reported that only 15 percent were current smokers (defined as those who had smoked 100 cigarettes in their lifetimes and were smoking at the time of the survey) while 14 percent were former smokers (Becerra and Smith 1988). This level is less

Figure 1. Prevalence of ever smoking (%), by sex and year, Puerto Rico, 1976 to 1988

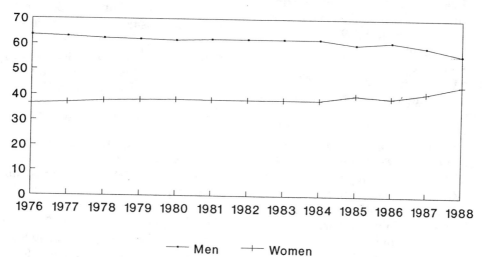

Source: Maxwell, 1989.

than half that reported by Maxwell for all women (unknown age group) in 1982 (38 percent).

In 1989, students of the Graduate School of Public Health of the University of Puerto Rico conducted a telephone survey on behavioral and attitudinal aspects of smoking among 772 men and women aged 18 years and older living in metropolitan San Juan. This survey also defined current smokers as those who had smoked at least 100 cigarettes in their lifetimes and were regular smokers at the time of the survey. Lifetime smoking prevalence was 34.3 percent overall. Of these, 55 percent (54.6 percent of men and 56.5 percent of women lifetime smokers) were not smoking (and may be considered former smokers) at the time of the survey. Therefore, current smoking prevalence was 22.5 percent among men and 10.6 percent among women. More than 50 percent of respondents reported their age at smoking initiation as 18 years or under. Most current smokers (89 percent) were aware that smoking is harmful to their health, and 77.1 percent expressed an intention to quit. Of lifetime smokers who had quit, most simply quit "cold turkey" (Rullán 1989). It is difficult to reconcile the large differences between the Maxwell reports and the data in the Becerra and Rullán reports. It may be that lifetime smokers were included in Maxwell's estimates, and that the prevalence of current smoking is actually far less than that reported by Maxwell.

Puerto Ricans living outside the Commonwealth (e.g., in the New York City area) were included in the Hispanic Health and Nutrition Examination Survey (HHANES) conducted in 1982 to 1984 by the U.S. National Center for Health Statistics. For this survey, 1,220 men and women aged 20 to 74 years were interviewed, and current smoking status was defined in a manner similar to the 1989 Rullán survey above. In New York, 39.8 percent of men and 30.3 percent of women were current smokers (Haynes et al. 1990). Again, these levels are far lower than those reported by Maxwell, lending additional evidence to the doubtful validity of the Maxwell estimates.

The proportions reported by the HHANES are remarkably higher for women aged 20 to 74 than for women aged 15 to 49 as reported by the PRFFPA above. The proportions reported for 1989 in San Juan by Rullán are much lower than the HHANES, but because the San Juan survey was telephone-based, substantial underreporting or selection bias may have occurred. Nonetheless, it is likely that Puerto Ricans living in New York smoke at higher rates than do those living on the island itself.

Adolescent Prevalence Surveys

Systematic surveillance of tobacco use among youth has not been established as yet in Puerto Rico. The only survey data available are those from a survey that was sponsored by a periodical (*El Nuevo Día*) and conducted in 1985. A total of 537 male and female adolescents aged 14 to 18 years living in northern urban areas were interviewed in their homes. According to a report from this survey, "the overwhelming majority (of those interviewed) do not have the habit of smoking cigarettes, although 60 percent of the young males and 55 percent of the young females knew someone who smoked marijuana" (Leal 1985). There are no other data on adolescent smoking for Puerto Rico.

Tobacco and Health

Changes in Adult Mortality Patterns

Deaths in Puerto Rico are recorded locally and reviewed by the Central Demographic Registry. The Oficina de Estadísticas de Salud del Departamento de Salud reported data for 1987: chronic diseases such as cancer, heart disease, and cerebrovascular diseases were the leading causes of death (Departamento de Salud 1989b) (Table 5).

Age-adjusted mortality rates for heart disease and cancer increased substantially between 1950 and 1987 (from 60/100,000 to 108/100,000 for cancer and from 105/100,000 to 190/100,000 for heart disease (Figure 2). These data, together with a declining overall mortality rate and a declining infant mortality rate (Figure 2), demonstrate the epidemiologic transition that has occurred in Puerto Rico since 1950. This transition is characterized by the emergence of chronic diseases as the population ages and as diseases due to infectious and childhood diseases decrease (Jamison 1991).

Smoking-related Mortality Rates

Five-year grouped mortality rates for all cancers and for the five leading causes of cancer death (stomach, prostate, esophagus, lung, and colon among men; colon, breast, uterus, lung, and stomach among women) increased from 1950 to 1987. Lung cancer represented 13.2 percent of all cancer-related deaths among men, and 9.4 percent among women in 1987 (Departamento de Salud 1989c).

Table 5. Leading causes of death in Puerto Rico, 1987

Cause of death	(ICD code)	Number of deaths	Proportion
Heart diseases	390–398, 402, 404–429	6,350	26.5
Malignant neoplasms	140–208	3,693	15.4
Cerebrovascular diseases	430–438	1,358	5.7
Pneumonia and influenza	480–487	1,297	5.4
All accidents	E800–949	1,173	4.9
Diabetes mellitus	250	1,108	4.6
Hypertension	401,403	776	3.2
Liver disease	571	765	3.2
Atherosclerosis	440	689	2.9
Chronic lung disease	490–496	686	2.9
Perinatal diseases	760–769	515	2.1
Homicides	E960–978	505	2.0
AIDS	042–044	472	2.0
Kidney diseases	580–589	413	1.7
Septicemia	038	293	1.2
Other causes		3,861	16.1

Cancer Incidence

Puerto Rico has maintained a cancer registry since 1950. Data from this source permit an analysis of time trends in the incidence of lung cancer that reflect the exposure of the population to smoking. Lung cancer is essentially caused only by smoking (attributable-risk percentage = 87 [U.S. Department of Health and Human Services 1989]). Among men, age-adjusted lung cancer incidence increased from 16.3/100,000 in 1973 to 18.1/100,000 in 1982. In 1987, lung cancer was the most common cancer diagnosis recorded among men by the cancer registry (Departamento de Salud 1989c).

Among women, age-adjusted lung cancer incidence increased from 5.4/100,000 in 1973 to 6.3/100,000 in 1982. However, overall cancer incidence decreased slightly after 1975. This decrease may indicate improved treatment and screening for such diseases as cervical and breast cancer, and a

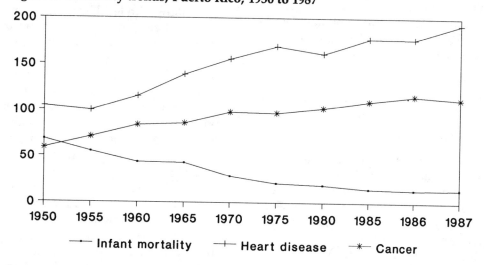

Figure 2. Mortality trends, Puerto Rico, 1950 to 1987

Source: Vital Statistics and Health Facilities Unit.

decrease in stomach cancer incidence similar to that experienced in other areas of the Americas. Lung cancer now ranks sixth among cancers in women and accounted for 4 percent of all new cancers among women in 1987 (Departamento de Salud 1989c).

Smoking-attributable Mortality Estimates

Personnel of the Department of Health of Puerto Rico, together with those of the U.S. Centers for Disease Control (CDC), estimated smoking-attributable deaths for diseases in 24 diagnostic categories including cancers, cardiovascular diseases, chronic lung diseases, ulcers, and selected pediatric conditions (Dietz 1991). This study found that 2,468 of the total 21,499 deaths (11.5 percent) in 1983 were caused by smoking. These deaths resulted in 19,445 years of potential life lost before the age of 75 years. Smoking-attributable mortality was four times higher than the number of deaths caused by homicides, suicides, or road accidents combined in Puerto Rico in 1983.

Smoking-attributable Economic Costs

In addition to smoking-attributable mortality, Dietz and coworkers (1991) estimated the direct costs of smoking-related health care in Puerto Rico for 1983. According to utilization data supplied by the Departamento de Salud and attributable-risk percentage estimates developed using data from the U.S. National Health Interview Survey, an estimated $55.9 million was spent on health care for neoplasms, cardiovascular disease, and chronic lung diseases caused by smoking in Puerto Rico. This is equivalent to 10 percent of the total health budget of the island. Most of the smoking-related health care expenses (69 percent) were for diseases among men (Dietz 1991).

Interventions against Tobacco Use

Legislation and Taxes

In Puerto Rico, the total tax on a package of 20 cigarettes, whether manufactured locally or imported, was $0.63 in 1989 (Departamento de Hacienda 1989). Total tobacco tax revenues were $72,445 million in 1979 and $97,889 million in 1989 (Departamento de Hacienda 1989). In 1989, cigarettes generated an estimated 3 percent of total Commonwealth revenue. Tax is 39.4 percent of the total retail cost of a pack of cigarettes ($1.60 on average

in 1989). The average wage in Puerto Rico is $5.73 an hour, and the average laborer works 38.5 hours a week. Thus, if the average worker smoked one pack of cigarettes per day, he or she would spend $11.20 a week on cigarettes, or 5 percent of the weekly salary. This is quite a low proportion compared to similar expenditure estimates for other parts of Latin America and the Caribbean.

According to U.S. Federal Law #98–474 (Comprehensive Smoking Education Act of October 12, 1984), four rotating health warnings must appear on cigarette packs sold in Puerto Rico, just as on the U.S. mainland (Rigau 1987). These warnings are:

SURGEON GENERAL'S WARNING: Smoking Causes Lung Cancer, Heart Disease, Emphysema, and May Complicate Pregnancy.

SURGEON GENERAL'S WARNING: Quitting Smoking Now Greatly Reduces Serious Risks to Your Health.

SURGEON GENERAL'S WARNING: Smoking by Pregnant Women May Result in Fetal Injury, Premature Birth, and Low Birth Weight.

SURGEON GENERAL'S WARNING: Cigarette Smoke Contains Carbon Monoxide.

A few statutes and regulations restrict smoking in public places in transportation facilities in Puerto Rico. The U.S. Federal law banning smoking on domestic flights lasting less than 6 hours also applies to flights between Puerto Rico and cities on the U.S. mainland (Calero 1990). At the Commonwealth level, smoking is prohibited in theaters and elevators. There are no prohibitions on smoking in schools, restaurants, Government offices, other public transportation facilities, or health care facilities. However, at the local level, smoking is restricted by law in some public places in San Juan (Dietz 1991) and by regulation in some private offices, Government buildings, and some hospitals in several different locales (Santiago 1990).

A coalition of the Puerto Rican Lung Association, the Puerto Rican Heart Association, and the Puerto Rican chapter of the American Cancer Society lobbies constantly for increased restrictive clean indoor air legislation. In 1989, three bills sympathetic to this coalition were submitted to the legislature by Commonwealth legislators. These would endow the Secretary of Health with the authority to enforce provisions of the laws and would impose civil penalties such as fines for violations of the smoking restrictions. None of these bills was approved in 1989, but they were reintroduced by the coalition in 1990. Coalition actions such as these have been effective in the enactment of hundreds of laws restricting smoking in public places in the United States (USDHHS 1989).

Public Information/Education Campaigns

In addition to the legislative attempts listed above, several organizations have attempted to educate Puerto Ricans about the harmful effects of smoking on health. The Puerto Rican Lung Association focuses on preventing smoking among children and adolescents and on providing smoking cessation programs (Miller 1989). This organization has also pursued restrictive worksite smoking policies directly with private companies and Government agencies. In 1989, the Association sponsored nine smoking cessation clinics benefiting 111 smokers. In September 1989, the Association conducted a workshop for health professionals to train them in behavior modification techniques for smoking cessation. The self-help smoking cessation program, "Freedom from Smoking in 20 Days," which is widely available to the public, has also been supported by the Association. Finally, antismoking messages for the print media, radio, and television are a major component of Association activities; these messages are developed by the U.S. American Lung Association and are translated into Spanish for use in Puerto Rico and other Latin American countries.

Every year, "No Smoking Day" is celebrated in February. Included in this activity are health fairs, distribution of educational material, aerobics classes, and pulmonary function tests. All these activities are also supported by both Government and private sector agencies.

The American Cancer Society (Puerto Rico chapter) has had several public education programs on smoking and health. At the community level, the Society sponsors presentations with the theme, "Deja los cigarrillos y vive más." An average of 16 presentations per month throughout the island is reported. At the professional level, the Society frequently sends smoking-related literature to health care personnel. In the private sector, worksite smoking cessation clinics are offered to employees under the "Smart Move" program developed by the national organization. Since 1987, the American Cancer Society has sponsored each November in association with the "Great American Smokeout,"

a public information campaign called "Descubre a Puerto Rico libre de humo," that includes television and radio announcements. Also, smoking cessation classes for the general public are sponsored with the support of the Puerto Rico Department of Health.

Finally, just as in many other Caribbean nations, the Puerto Rican Seventh Day Adventist Church has offered since 1955 the "Five-Day Plan to Quit Smoking" (Santiago 1990).

School Education Programs

Antismoking education is not part of the official school curriculum, but the Puerto Rican Lung Association sponsors several educational activities in schools. These include a system-wide "No Smoking Day" and antismoking speech and poster contests (Calero 1990). In 1989, an antismoking information campaign was carried out by the Association that reached 672,837 students attending daytime schools and 138,440 attending vocational schools. In addition, 12 universities conducted antismoking activities that reached approximately 127,000 students (Miller 1989). The American Cancer Society provides educational presentations for grade 7 and above using the teaching module entitled, "Cancer, a disease that can be avoided, prevented and cured." This program reached an estimated 85 percent of the public schools and 30 percent of the private schools of Puerto Rico.

Government Policies

The Government of Puerto Rico has no formal tobacco prevention and control program. Although no personnel or financial resources are specifically dedicated to tobacco prevention and control, the Department of Health collaborates with the voluntary agencies as cited above (Santiago 1990).

Two insurance companies (Cooperative of Life Insurance of Puerto Rico and Blue Cross of Puerto Rico) offer a one-third discount on life insurance premiums for nonsmokers (Santiago 1990).

Summary and Conclusions

Tobacco agriculture at one time was an important economic activity in Puerto Rico. However, by 1990, only one indigenous cigar manufacturer survived, and only a few farmers made their living from growing tobacco. The multinational corporations, in particular R.J. Reynolds, have saturated the island with advertisements and promotion, utilizing themes that identify particular brands as almost a national symbol.

To date, the Government of Puerto Rico has not designated tobacco use as the most important cause of death in Puerto Rico. Smoking was responsible for more than one-tenth of all deaths in Puerto Rico in 1983, and cancer registry data show an increasing burden of mortality due to lung cancer among both men and women; this particular disease is an indisputable marker of population exposure to smoking. The exact measurement of exposure is somewhat difficult, with a lack of survey data representative of the Commonwealth as a whole. Reported adult per capita cigarette consumption shows that exposure may be decreasing in Puerto Rico. The uptake of smoking by adolescents is unknown in Puerto Rico. Fortunately, various voluntary groups, including the Puerto Rican chapters of the Lung Association, the Cancer Society, and the Heart Association, have mounted vigorous antismoking campaigns that are quite visible. The effect of these activities, which are supported by the Department of Health, may be reflected in declining per capita cigarette consumption figures.

The data presented above support the following conclusions on smoking and health in Puerto Rico:

1. Indigenous tobacco agricultural and manufacturing activities in Puerto Rico have declined over the last several decades. The multinational tobacco corporations are active both in the local manufacture of cigarettes and in the promotion of tobacco among Puerto Ricans.
2. The prevalence of smoking among men has probably declined over the last two decades in Puerto Rico, while the proportion of women smokers has apparently increased. Women of child-bearing age display a lower prevalence of smoking than does the general female population. Male and female Puerto Rican residents of the New York area are reported to smoke at higher rates than do those remaining in Puerto Rico.
3. Almost 2,500 deaths were attributable to smoking in 1983 in Puerto Rico. This is equivalent to 11.5 percent of all deaths in that year, and accounted for 19,445 years of potential life lost. Lung cancer mortality and incidence rates have increased steadily from 1950 to 1987, indicating an increasing burden of smoking-related disease among Puerto Ricans.
4. Voluntary organizations including the Puerto Rican Lung Association and Cancer Society are the primary foci of antismoking activities for the Commonwealth of Puerto Rico. To date, there is no official Government tobacco use prevention and control program.

References

AMATO, A. *Progreso en Puerto Rico.* Banco Popular de Puerto Rico, Departamento de Estudios Económicos 25(3), 1989.

BECERRA, J., SMITH, J. Maternal smoking and low birth weight in the reproductive history of women in Puerto Rico. *American Journal of Public Health* 78: 268–272, 1988.

CALERO, M.S. Cero fumar en los vuelos de seis horas. *Periódico El Mundo,* 24 February 1990.

DEPARTAMENTO DE HACIENDA. *Datos seleccionados sobre cigarrillos tributables y exentos, años fiscales 1963 a 1989.* Departamento de Hacienda, Oficina de Asuntos Económicos y Financieros, 1989.

DEPARTAMENTO DE SALUD. *Informe anual de estadísticas vitales 1985.* Departamento de Salud, Secretaría Auxiliar de Administración, Oficina de Planificación, Evaluación e Informes: San Juan, Puerto Rico. June 1987.

DEPARTAMENTO DE SALUD. *Informe estadístico de facilidades de salud hospitales 1985–1986.* Departamento de Salud, Administración de Facilidades y Servicios de Salud, Oficina de Estadísticas de Salud: San Juan, Puerto Rico. October 1989a.

DEPARTAMENTO DE SALUD. *Informe anual de estadísticas vitales 1987.* Departamento de Salud, Administración de Facilidades y Servicios de Salud, Oficina de Estadísticas de Salud: San Juan, Puerto Rico. December 1989b.

DEPARTAMENTO DE SALUD. *Cáncer en Puerto Rico 1987.* Departamento de Salud, Registro Central de Cáncer. San Juan, Puerto Rico, 1989c.

DEPARTAMENTO DE SALUD. Médicos activos en Puerto Rico durante el primer registro de profesionales. *Boletín Estadístico,* Año V No. 59, July 1985. Departamento de Salud, Administración de Facilidades y Servicios de Salud, Sistema cooperativo de Estadísticas de Salud: San Juan, Puerto Rico.

DIETZ, V.J., NOVOTNY, T.E., RIGAU-PEREZ, J.G., SHULTZ, J.M. Smoking-attributable mortality, years of potential life lost, and direct health care costs for Puerto Rico, 1983. *Bulletin of PAHO* 25(1), 1991.

GAZTAMBIDE, J. La historia del tabaco en Puerto Rico. *Revista de Agricultura de Puerto Rico.* Departamento de Agricultura, July 1968.

HAYNES, S.G., HARVEY, C., MONTES, H., COHEN, B.H. Patterns of cigarette smoking among Mexican-

Americans, Puerto Ricans, and Cuban-Americans aged 20–74 years in the United States: Results from the Hispanic Health and Examination Survey, 1982–1986. In press, *American Journal of Public Health,* 1990.

JAMISON, D.T., MOSLEY, W.H. Disease control priorities in developing countries: health policy responses to epidemiological change. *American Journal of Public Health* 81(1):15–22, January 1991.

LEAL, G. Una juventud idealista, religiosa y bebedora. (Resultados de la encuesta encomendada por *El Nuevo Día* a la firma Human Communications) *El Nuevo Día,* 20 June 1985, pp. 52–54.

LEON, L. *Perfil demográfico de la población de Puerto Rico: 1980.* Centro de Datos Censales, Universidad de Puerto Rico. September 1985, p. 11.

MAXWELL, J.C. *International Tobacco 1988: Part Two,* The Maxwell Consumer Report. Industry Update, No. 38, June 30, 1989, WFS-2758.

MILLER, A. *Informe Anual: Asociación Puertorriqueña del Pulmón 1988–1989.* pp. 10–14. San Juan, Puerto Rico, 1989.

RIGAU, J. El tabaquismo y la salud. Progreso hacia los objetivos nacionales de salud para 1990 (XII). Departamento de Salud, *Los Objetivos de Salud para Estados Unidos en 1990 y su aplicación para Puerto Rico.* 1987.

RULLAN, J., SANTIAGO, A., APONTE, J., BONILLA, N., et al. Tendencias en el hábito de fumar cigarrillos en la población del área metropolitana de Puerto Rico. Universidad de Puerto Rico, Recinto de Ciencias Médicas, Escuela Graduada de Salud Pública, 1989 (Unpublished).

SANTIAGO, A. Country Collaborator's Report (Unpublished). Pan American Health Organization: Washington, D.C., 1990.

SERVICIOS DE SALUD DE PUERTO RICO. *San Juan: Asociación de Hospitales de Puerto Rico,* publicación del XXIV Congreso Mundial de Hospitales, May 1985.

SORLIE, P.D., GARCIA-PALMIERI, M.R., COSTAS, R., et al. Cigarette smoking and coronary heart disease in Puerto Rico. *Prev Med* 11:304–316, 1982.

TURNER, H. Tobacco: Island industry, burned by law, is up in smoke. *The Sunday San Juan Star.* Vol. No. 306, September 5, 1982.

U.S. DEPARTMENT OF HEALTH AND HUMAN SERVICES. *Reducing the Health Consequences of Smoking—25 Years of Progress.* A Report of the Surgeon General. U.S. Department of Health and Human Services, U.S. Public Health Service, Centers for Disease Control, Center for Chronic Disease Prevention and Health Promotion, Office on Smoking and Health. DHHS Publication No. (CDC) 89–8411, 1989.

Suriname, Aruba, and the Netherlands Antilles

General Characteristics

This chapter will describe tobacco and health issues for the Netherlands Antilles, Aruba, and Suriname. Aruba is an island located 24 km north of Venezuela. Suriname, the former Dutch Guyana, is on the northern mainland of South America between Guyana and French Guiana. The Netherlands Antilles include the islands of Curaçao and Bonaire (also north of Venezuela) and the Windward islands of Saba, St. Eustatius, and St. Maarten in the Antillean archipelago east of Puerto Rico. The populations range from 1,029 on Saba to 352,041 in Suriname.

Until the 1980s, the economy of Suriname was based mainly on bauxite mining, which accounted for 75 percent of export earnings (Pan American Health Organization [PAHO] 1990). Agriculture and food processing accounted for the balance of exports and included rice, bananas, palm oil, citrus fruits, and lumber. Until 1982, economic aid from the Netherlands accounted for 10 percent of the gross national product (GNP) of Suriname. This aid was discontinued subsequent to a military coup in 1980. The coup was followed by an economic crisis further exacerbated by a decrease in the world price of bauxite and a 45 percent decline in mining. This decline in exports that generate foreign exchange resulted in severe curtailment of imports. As a result, there has been little economic growth in Suriname since 1981. The estimated per capita gross domestic product was $US2,500 in 1982 and $US2,757 in 1987 (PAHO 1990).

The economies of Aruba and the Netherlands Antilles are based mainly on oil production and tourism. The drop in oil prices in the early 1980s contributed significantly to a deep recession with high inflation during 1982 to 1985. Despite this economic downturn, the per capita GNP in 1987 was $US10,000, due in part to an increasingly vibrant tourist trade in these islands (PAHO 1990).

Population Dynamics

The 1980 census estimated Suriname's population at 352,041. Most (95 percent) of the population, a mixture of Creole, Javanese, Hindostani, and Chinese ethnic groups, lives along the flat coastlands. The remaining population of Amerindian and Bush Negroes is scattered throughout the mountainous and forested interior. The population is largely youthful, with more than 50 percent aged

under 20 years. However, 1987 population estimates suggest a disproportionately larger number of females than males in the 25 to 44 year age group. This may be the result of large-scale emigration of young men seeking employment and educational opportunities in the Netherlands in 1975 (the year of independence) and again after the revolution in 1980 (PAHO 1990).

According to the 1981 Netherlands Antilles census, 28.9 percent of the population was under 15 years of age while 6.5 percent was 65 years or older. The population is ethnicly mixed, composed of Blacks, Europeans, and Amerindians. Although there are no known figures on internal migration, significant emigration from Aruba took place during 1985 to 1987 after the closing of an oil refinery, resulting in a population decline from 1984 to 1987. By 1988, the population was increasing at an estimated yearly growth rate of 1.5 percent. Curaçao and Bonaire also experienced declining populations in recent years, while the populations have been growing in St. Maarten, St. Eustatius, and Saba (PAHO 1990).

Health Indicators

Health services in Suriname are provided through a well-established network of primary care facilities both in the interior and on the coast. Suriname has two private and three public hospitals. Vertical programs, such as malaria eradication, have been successfully integrated into the delivery of primary health care.

The populations of Aruba and the Netherlands Antilles are served by 35 establishments, including a general hospital on each island, as well as specialist institutions, i.e., pediatric, maternity, and psychiatric hospitals. All hospitals except the psychiatric hospital are private on Curaçao.

The difference in the economies of Suriname and of Aruba and the Netherlands Antilles is reflected in the health status of the populations (Table 1). For example, the infant mortality rate for Aruba and the Netherlands Antilles fell from 23.8 per 1,000 live births in 1981 to 11.8 in 1988, while that for Suriname was 26.7 per 1,000 live births in 1987. The consistent departure of medical personnel from Suriname may account in part for the higher death, birth, and fertility rates and the lower life expectancies in this former Dutch colony compared with Aruba and the Netherlands Antilles.

Table 1. Health indicators, Suriname, Aruba, and the Netherlands Antilles, 1987

Health indicator	Suriname	Aruba and Netherlands Antilles
Crude birth rate	25.0	17.5
Fertility rate (per 1,000 women aged 15–44)	128.4	73.5
Crude mortality rate	6.1	5.4
Infant mortality rate	26.7	11.8
Life expectancy at birth		
(male)	63.6	71.1
(female)	71.7	75.8

Source: PAHO, 1990.

The Tobacco Industry

Agriculture and Manufacturing

Despite substantial agricultural activities, no tobacco is grown in Suriname, Aruba, or the Netherlands Antilles. In 1989, two tobacco factories imported 422,000 kg of tobacco into Suriname, using scarce foreign exchange to purchase this raw material. These factories manufactured a total of 528 million cigarettes under license to the British American Tobacco Company, the only cigarette manufacturing company operating in Suriname. Production of cigarettes increased steadily from 1980 to 1986, but subsequent reported production has fluctuated widely (Figure 1).

Marketing

In Suriname, the local brand Tacoma accounted for 95 percent of the legitimate market for cigarettes in 1990. The imported brands, Morello, Skwala, and Mix, accounted for the remaining 5 percent. Cigarettes are available for sale in packs of 20, which retail for approximately $US2. Although most of the cigarettes manufactured domestically are consumed by Surinamese, some cigarettes are smuggled to Guyana. The illegal nature of the trade makes it difficult to estimate its magnitude (Bakker 1990).

Marlboro cigarettes are manufactured in Aruba by the Superior Tobacco Company under license to the Philip Morris Company. This brand accounts for 95 percent of the cigarette market. In 1989, 150 million cigarettes were produced in Aruba, with 78 million of these exported to Curaçao. Imports of cigarettes fluctuate markedly, in part due to seasonal fluctuations in tourist purchases of duty-free goods (Vorst 1990).

In the Netherlands Antilles, yearly per capita

Figure 1. Cigarette production, in millions, Suriname, 1980–1989

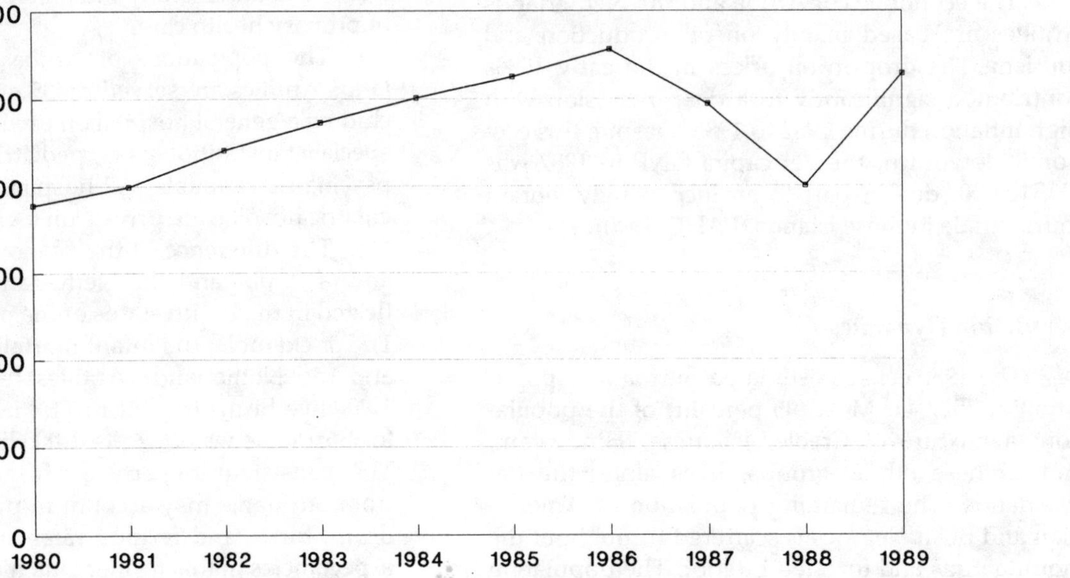

Source: Bakker, 1990.

consumption for persons 15 years of age and older was estimated at 2,080 cigarettes in 1987 (Euromonitor Consultancy 1989). While illegal trade in cigarettes cannot be documented easily, the Netherlands Antilles and Aruba are believed to be important transhipment points for this trade to Colombia, a country that currently prohibits imports of cigarettes (U.S. Department of Health and Human Services [USDHHS] 1992). It has been estimated that smuggled cigarettes account for approximately 40 percent of the cigarette market in Colombia (Nares 1991).

Tobacco Use

Consumption

Because many Surinamese receive cigarettes from relatives living abroad, data on cigarette production, import, and export may grossly underestimate domestic consumption of tobacco products. In the Netherlands Antilles and Aruba, cigarette import data cannot be used to estimate accurately domestic consumption because of increasing duty-free purchases by tourists (Lagro 1990) and the above-mentioned illegal trade in tobacco products. Thus, behavioral surveys may provide more meaningful information on tobacco use in these areas.

Survey Data

A few scattered surveys of adults and youth have been performed in the last 10 years in Suriname and Aruba; none are available from the Netherlands Antilles. In 1985, 1,038 pregnant women aged 15 to 48 years who visited selected health centers in the urban areas of Paramaribo and Wanica were surveyed for health risk factors (Bakker 1990). Of all women surveyed, 26.2 percent were regular smokers of at least one cigarette per week. Approximately 10 percent were former smokers (i.e., had not smoked in 3 or more months before the survey). The prevalence of regular smoking varied by ethnic background: 38 percent of Creole and Hindostani young women were current smokers compared with 20 percent or less among East Indians and Bush Negroes. Most (85 percent) of these current smokers smoked less than one pack of 20 cigarettes per week. Among the overall population surveyed, the mean age of initiation (i.e., when the first cigarette was smoked) was 18.3 years.

In 1987 and 1988, drug and alcohol use was surveyed among schoolchildren aged 10 to 19 years in three urban centers and four rural areas in Suriname (Bakker 1990). Of surveyed students, 36 percent of boys and 12 percent of girls reported ever having smoked cigarettes. The prevalence of ever smoking was slightly higher among students in rural areas than among students in urban areas. As in the previously mentioned study, the prevalence of ever smoking was higher among Javanese (29 percent) and Creoles (25 percent) than among Hindostanis (18 percent). Students were also asked about their knowledge of the health effects of smoking. Of the total sample, 66 percent reported that they did not know smoking was associated with reduced life expectancy, and 50 percent were aware that smoking was associated with lung cancer.

In 1989, a 1 percent random sample of the Aruban population 15 years and older was surveyed for risk factors for cardiovascular disease including cigarette smoking (Vorst 1990). The final sample consisted of 270 males and 353 females. Of these, 32 percent of men and 13 percent of women were classified as smokers and 17 percent of men and 6 percent of women as ex-smokers (no other definitions for categories of smoking are available).

In 1988, 339 adolescents in Aruba aged 13 to 21 years from 13 of Aruba's 25 secondary schools were surveyed for drug and alcohol use (Vorst 1990). Because this survey was part of a larger standardized survey of Dutch and European youth for drug and alcohol use in 1987, comparisons between island and European youth were possible (Hubert 1988). For this survey, lifetime history of smoking was defined as having smoked 20 or more cigarettes. The survey did not select a random sample of students, but sufficient numbers from each age group were selected to represent three age strata: 13 to 15, 16 to 17, and 18 to 21 years. The response rate was 100 percent for this school-based, self-administered questionnaire survey. Of the total sample, 67 percent (72 percent of boys and 61 percent of girls) reported lifetime use of cigarettes. Of these, 18 percent had smoked 20 times or more in the past 30 days. Prevalence of smoking among boys in this group was twice as high as among girls (23.9 vs. 11.9 percent). Both boys and girls had tried their first cigarette at the same mean age, 13.2 years. The percentage of lifetime use of cigarettes increased from 53.8 percent among youth aged 13 to 15 to 75.6 percent among youth aged 18 to 21. Youth on Aruba were found to have a higher prevalence of lifetime use of cigarettes than did European Dutch youth in the same age group (67 vs. 53.5 percent).

Smoking and Health

Because of the small numbers of deaths in these islands and countries, mortality data cannot be analyzed with respect to smoking-attributable fractions. However, proportionate mortality analyses where cause of death has been specified on the death certificates may help to understand the current disease impact of tobacco in these small countries and dependencies. Medical certification of cause-of-death coverage (and thus data quality) is extremely variable from year to year and region to region in Suriname. Because of the general decline in health monitoring, noncertification of deaths even in hospitals increased to 25 percent in 1989 (Bakker 1990). Of the 2,427 deaths recorded in 1985 in Suriname, ill-defined causes accounted for 15 percent. However, in Aruba and the Netherlands Antilles, mortality registration has improved in recent years so that in 1989 only 5.3 percent of deaths were classified as ''ill defined'' (Vorst 1989). In 1981, 6.1 percent of deaths on Curaçao were ''ill defined'' (PAHO 1990).

The five leading causes of death in Suriname, Aruba, and the Netherlands Antilles (Curaçao) appear to be ranked similarly, with cardiovascular disease and neoplasms in first and second place respectively in each area (Table 2). Thus, these populations have already begun to demonstrate the epidemiologic transition in the expression of diseases that is more characteristic of developed countries (Jamison and Mosley 1991). The patterns of mortality due to selected smoking-related diseases

(bronchitis, emphysema, and asthma; pneumonia and influenza; cancer of the lung; cancers of the lip, oral cavity, and pharynx; cerebrovascular disease; and ischemic heart disease) differ markedly between Suriname and the Netherlands Antilles. Detailed cause-specific mortality data are not available for Aruba (Table 3). The age-adjusted mortality rates for these smoking-related diseases are in general higher than in the United States; exceptions are cancers of the lung, lip, oral cavity, and pharynx. The age-adjusted mortality rate (per 100,000 persons) for chronic lung disease (ICD 490–493) is higher in Suriname than in either the Netherlands Antilles or the United States. The age-adjusted cerebrovascular disease mortality rate is higher in both Suriname and the Netherlands Antilles than in the United States. Of additional interest is a comparison of the age-adjusted mortality rates for infectious diseases (ICD 001–139) for the United States, the Netherlands Antilles, and Suriname. For the latter two, infectious disease mortality is substantially higher (10.3 and 34.7 per 100,000 persons, respectively) than for the United States (5.4 per 100,000 persons). Thus, the attention of the medical system is drawn toward the large group of infectious diseases that accounts for higher mortality rates, especially among younger persons.

These patterns suggest that risk factors other than smoking may have a relatively greater effect on cardiovascular disease and nonmalignant lung diseases in Suriname and the Netherlands Antilles than in the United States. In the United States, cigarette smoking has been more common than in

Table 2. Leading causes of death in Suriname, Aruba, and the Netherlands Antilles (Curaçao), according to proportional mortality (percent) of defined causes of death, 1980s

Cause of death	Suriname		Aruba		Netherlands Antilles (Curaçao)	
	No.	%	No.	%	No.	%
All causes	2,275	100.0	337	100.0	1,075	100.0
Ill-defined conditions	369	16.2	28	5.3	66	6.1
Deaths, defined causes	1,906		309		1,009	
Cardiovascular diseases	562	29.5	125	40.5	330	32.9
Neoplasms	169	9.9	73	23.6	236	23.4
Accidents	163	9.6	28	9.1	49	4.9
Cerebrovascular diseases	154	8.1	NA	NA	93	11.6
Endocrine and metabolic diseases	86	4.5	27	8.7	NA	NA
Perinatal conditions	135	7.1	6	1.9	74	7.3

Source: PAHO, 1990; Vorst, 1990.

Table 3. Number of deaths (N) and age-adjusted mortality rates (M.R.) per 100,000 persons for selected tobacco-related diseases, Suriname, Netherlands Antilles, and the United States, last available year

Cause and ICD code	Suriname (1985)		Netherlands Antilles (1981)		U.S.A. (1987)	
	N	M.R.	N	M.R.	N	M.R.
Bronchitis, emphysema, asthma (490–493)	64	15.0	15	6.7	22,424	3.3
Pneumonia and influenza (480–487)	89	21.2	24	8.1	69,225	9.1
Ischemic heart disease (410–414)	203	47.6	62	24.0	512,138	67.2
Cerebrovascular disease (430–438)	154	34.4	93	35.3	149,835	18.7
Cancer of the lung (162)	14	3.2	24	10.1	130,009	21.2
Cancers of lip, oral cavity, and pharynx (140–149)	3	0.7	8	3.3	7,968	1.4

Source: PAHO, 1990.

Suriname and the Netherlands Antilles over the last several decades; thus, the lung cancer mortality rate is much higher.

Tobacco Use Control and Prevention Activities

Government Activities

Of the average retail price of $US2 per pack of 20 cigarettes in Suriname, 55 percent is tax, and this tax generates revenues of approximately $US25.4 million per year. In Aruba, 64 percent of the $US1.50 price per pack of 20 cigarettes is tax, producing annual revenues exceeding $US2 million.

No health warnings are required on cigarette packs in any of the political entities, although a warning is required on cigarette packages produced in the Netherlands. No regulations have been implemented to control tar and nicotine yield. The advertisement or promotion of tobacco products is not restricted in any of the areas.

Moderate activity against tobacco by the Government of Suriname is reported. In addition to the surveys mentioned above, the Government allocates $US6,000 each year for tobacco control. Specific details of this program were not reported, but Government activities include a 1986 Ministry of Health decree restricting smoking in health facilities. Most smoking intervention programs have been initiated by nongovernmental agencies. The

National Council Against Drug Abuse, the Association of Heart Disease Patients, the Association for Physical Fitness, the Medical Association of Suriname, and the Seventh Day Adventist Church have organized antismoking activities, educational programs, and smoking cessation classes. Other interventions include public service announcements on television and in the daily newspapers that have publicized the health effects of tobacco on smokers and on the unborn child. In addition, the health consequences of environmental tobacco smoke have been publicized. The Teachers' Union of Suriname has collaborated with the Ministry of Health in a joint project to train teachers to educate children against smoking. The implementation of this educational effort has not yet been described. Suriname appears to have several components of a functional antitobacco program in place.

Nongovernmental Activities

In Aruba, national regulations restrict smoking in schools and on buses. In addition, voluntary restrictions on smoking in health care facilities, theaters, and elevators are reported (Vorst 1990). However, there is no formal programmed antismoking campaign in Aruba and the Netherlands Antilles. Public information on tobacco and health is presented as part of regular health education programs in both the electronic and print media. Antismoking messages are a component of health education messages targeted at reducing cardiovascular disease. Both the medical and nursing associations of Aruba participate in inpatient consultations for smoking cessation. In contrast to Suriname, religious organizations do not appear to offer cessation programs to Arubans. Thus, the populations of Aruba and the Netherlands Antilles have had at least some exposure to antismoking information through messages from health care personnel, through modest restrictions on smoking in selected public places, and from the media.

Summary and Conclusions

Survey data for pregnant women in Suriname indicate that 26.2 percent of this high-risk group are regular smokers. While no data on other adults are available, it is likely that the prevalence of regular smoking is much higher among men and nonpregnant women. Of adults aged 15 years and older on Aruba, 32 percent of men and 13 percent of women are current smokers. The mean age of initiation among pregnant women in Suriname is 18.3 years, but the mean age of initiation reported by Aruban students aged 10 to 19 years was 13.2 years. The lifetime prevalence of smoking among Aruban youth is higher than that among youth in the Netherlands (67 vs. 53 percent). Knowledge of the health consequences of smoking appears to be minimal among Surinamese students. Educational programs are not yet widely available to schoolchildren or to the general public in all of the Dutch colonies and former colonies.

Age-adjusted mortality rates for malignant neoplasms, including lung and upper airway cancers, are higher for Suriname and the Netherlands Antilles than those for several other Caribbean populations. Thus, the epidemic of tobacco-related illnesses familiar to Canada and the United States may be possible for these small countries in the future. The age-adjusted mortality rate for infectious diseases is still higher in Suriname and the Netherlands Antilles than are rates for the chronic illnesses associated with tobacco; therefore, the attention of Ministries of Health has not yet focused strongly on smoking as a health risk factor. In Suriname, scarce Government funding has been allocated to tobacco control, but hard currency that is even scarcer has been used to purchase tobacco for the manufacture of cigarettes in Suriname. It is unlikely that the profits realized by this enterprise can overcome the future costs of tobacco use. Fundamental channels for tobacco control have been es-

tablished in all of the current and former Dutch colonies, and these channels may permit effective tobacco control activities in the future.

Based on the data presented in this report, the following conclusions can be made:

1. The impact of smoking in Suriname, Aruba, and the Netherlands Antilles is at present low, but mortality patterns suggest the chronic diseases associated with tobacco will increase substantially in the future.

2. Behavioral surveys are more important than consumption data for islands such as Aruba where consumption data are inaccurate. These inaccuracies arise from large duty-free purchases of tobacco by tourists and through a substantial illegal trade in cigarettes.

3. The exposure of populations to tobacco on Aruba is similar to that for men in developed countries. Among youth, the prevalence of smoking may be higher on Aruba than in the Netherlands. Of pregnant women in Suriname, 26.2 percent are smokers.

4. Basic structures for the prevention and control of tobacco use are in place in these islands and nations, but little funding for this activity has been designated.

References

BAKKER, W. Country Collaborator's Report, Aruba. Pan American Health Organization, unpublished data, 1990.

EUROMONITOR CONSULTANCY. *The World Market for Tobacco: Strategy 2000*, Volume Two. London, England, August 1989.

HUBERT, J., DRIESSEN, F.M.H.M. *Results of a Drug Use Survey Among Students of Secondary Education on Aruba.* Department of Social Medicine, Free University, Amsterdam, 1988.

JAMISON, D.T., MOSLEY, H. Disease control priorities in developing countries: health policy responses to epidemiological change. *American Journal of Public Health* 1991 81(1):15–22.

LAGRO, M., PLOTKIN, D. *The Suitcase Traders in the Free Zone of Curaçao.* United Nations Economic Commission for Latin America and the Caribbean. Catalogue No. LC/L.587 (MDM.11/6), Port-of-Spain, Trinidad and Tobago, August 28, 1990.

MINISTRY OF EDUCATION, SURINAME. Roken onder Scholieren in Suriname, 1987–88, Ministry of Education, unpublished data.

NARES, P. Cigarette smuggling continues, and problem may worsen. *Tobacco International* 193(7):19–20, 15 April 1991.

PAN AMERICAN HEALTH ORGANIZATION. *Health Conditions in the Americas, 1981–1984.* Vols. 1,2. Pan American Health Organization, Pan American Sanitary Bureau, Regional Office of the World Health Organization. Scientific Publication No. 500, 1986.

PAN AMERICAN HEALTH ORGANIZATION. *Health Conditions in the Americas, 1990 Edition,* Volume 2. Pan American Health Organization, Pan American Sanitary Bureau, Regional Office of the World Health Organization. Scientific Publication No. 524, 1990.

ROKEN ONDER SWANGEREN, 1985, Ministry of Health, unpublished data.

UNITED NATIONS ECONOMIC COMMISSION FOR LATIN AMERICA AND THE CARIBBEAN. Selected Statistical Indicators of the Caribbean Countries, Volume 2. LC/CAR/G.293. 1990.

U.S. DEPARTMENT OF HEALTH AND HUMAN SERVICES. *Smoking and Health in the Americas. A Report of the Surgeon General.* Atlanta, Georgia: U.S. Department of Health and Human Services, Public Health Service, Centers for Disease Control, National Center for Chronic Disease Prevention and Health Promotion, Office on Smoking and Health; 1992; DHHS Publication No. (CDC) 92-8419.

VORST, F.A. Country Collaborator's Report, Aruba. Unpublished data, Pan American Health Organization, Aruba, 1990.

Trinidad and Tobago

General Characteristics

The Tobacco Industry
    Agriculture
    Manufacturing
    Marketing

Tobacco Use
    Consumption data
    Survey data

Smoking and Health

Tobacco Use Prevention and Control Activities

Conclusions

References

General Characteristics

Trinidad and Tobago is a two-island State situated at the southernmost end of the Caribbean archipelago. Trinidad is 11 km from the northeastern coast of Venezuela and about 10 degrees north of the equator. It has an area of 4,828 km². Tobago, with an area of 300 km², lies 30 km northeast of Trinidad (Trinidad and Tobago Central Statistical Office 1983).

The estimated 1988 mid-year population was 1,211,539 and is projected to reach 1.6 million by the end of the century (Trinidad and Tobago Central Statistical Office 1989). At the time of the 1980 census, 34 percent of the population was under 15 years of age; 23 percent was aged 15 to 24 years; 25 percent was 25 to 44 years; 13 percent was 45 to 64 years; and 5.6 percent was 65 years and older. In 1980, women aged 15 to 49 years accounted for 51.0 percent of the total female population and the total fertility rate was 3.1 births per woman.

People of African and Asian Indian descent comprise the two major ethnic groups, accounting for 40.8 percent and 41.0 percent of the total population, respectively; the remainder are of Mixed, European, Chinese, and Syrian-Lebanese origins (Trinidad and Tobago Central Statistical Office 1989).

The 1980 census data indicate that 63 percent of the population over 5 years old had attained primary level education while an additional 32 percent had attained a secondary or higher level of education.

National revenue derives principally from the petroleum industry, which provided 27 percent of gross domestic product (GDP) (1985 constant prices) in 1988 (Trinidad and Tobago Central Statistical Office 1989). During the 1980s, the economy of Trinidad and Tobago deteriorated because of a collapse in oil prices and a high foreign debt. From 1980 to 1988, the decline in economic growth caused a 7.3 percent average annual decrease in the per capita gross national product (GNP). In 1988, the per capita GNP was $US3,350 (The World Bank 1989), and 22 percent of the labor force was unemployed (Central Statistical Office 1989).

During 1979 to 1987, the birth rate decreased from 27.9 to 24.1 per 1,000 population. The crude death rate remained at 6.6 per 1,000 population, but the infant mortality rate decreased 36 percent between 1979 and 1987 to 11.4 per 1,000 live births. In 1980, life expectancy at birth was 66.9 years and 71.6 years for males and females, respectively (Trinidad and Tobago Central Statistical Office 1989).

The population and vital statistics presented above show that the age structure of Trinidad and Tobago is that of a young population. Although the birth rate and total fertility rate appear to be declining, decreasing infant mortality and extended life expectancy at birth have resulted in large cohorts of children (34 percent under 15 years) and young adults (23 percent aged 15 to 24 years). As these groups age, a considerable proportion of the total population will become susceptible to the chronic non-communicable diseases, including tobacco-related diseases such as heart disease, cerebrovascular disease, cancer, and chronic obstructive lung disease.

The Tobacco Industry

The West Indian Tobacco Company (WITCO) Ltd., a private company incorporated in the Republic of Trinidad and Tobago, is the only tobacco company currently operating in Trinidad and Tobago (WITCO 1983, 1984, 1986, 1989, 1990). At the end of 1989, British American Tobacco (BAT) Company Ltd., which is registered in the United Kingdom, was the largest single shareholder, controlling 47 percent of the issued shares of WITCO Ltd. (WITCO 1990; Milne 1990).

Agriculture

There are currently 29 farmers contracted by WITCO, growing tobacco on 40 ha of flat lands in central Trinidad (Milne 1990; Trinidad and Tobago Central Statistical Office 1990). In 1989, tobacco occupied 0.04 percent of total croplands in Trinidad and Tobago and the tobacco industry employed 0.09 percent of all farmers, or 0.07 percent of all employed persons (Trinidad and Tobago Central Statistical Office 1986 and 1989). Two types of Virginia tobacco, Speights G28 and K326, are grown from seeds imported from Venezuela. WITCO assists farmers with machinery and other items necessary for cultivation and buys all the leaf they produce (Milne 1990). Domestic production yielded 15 percent of the tobacco needed for manufacturing in 1989, and WITCO has reported plans to increase the acreage under cultivation to double local leaf production within the next 5 years (Milne 1990). The company also embarked on a diversification project in floriculture in 1989 and in 1990 began exporting orchids.

Manufacturing

From 1979 through 1988, average annual imports of unmanufactured tobacco (986,773 kg) greatly exceeded both annual domestic production (57,660 kg) and annual exports (3,289 kg) (Trinidad and Tobago Central Statistical Office 1980, 1981, 1982, 1983, 1984, 1985, 1986, 1987, 1988, 1989). Imports were much lower in 1988 than in 1980, while domestic production increased by 400 percent during this period (Figure 1).

The numbers of cigarettes produced, traded, and consumed annually during the decade 1979 to 1988 were calculated using data on overseas trade and conversion factors provided by the Production Division of WITCO [73.3 percent of the weight of 1 cigarette = tobacco; 1 kg of tobacco = 1,350 cigarettes] (Trinidad and Tobago Central Statistical Office 1980, 1981, 1982, 1983, 1984, 1985, 1986, 1987, 1988, 1989; WITCO 1990). In contrast to unmanufactured tobacco, annual production of manufactured cigarettes was greater than either imports or exports of manufactured cigarettes (Figure 2). Domestic cigarette production was significantly lower in 1988 than in 1983. Imports fell by 87 percent and exports increased 80 percent; however, the rise in exports was not associated with a positive effect on balance of trade.

Annual costs including base costs, insurance, and freight of imports and annual free on-board earned income from exports of unmanufactured tobacco were calculated by summing the monies for the various categories of this commodity (Economic and Social Council of the United Nations 1975), and the trade balance (i.e., the difference between export earnings and import costs) was calculated for the decade 1979 to 1988 (Trinidad and Tobago Central Statistical Office 1980, 1981, 1982, 1983, 1984, 1985, 1986, 1987, 1988, 1989). During this period, the Trinidad and Tobago dollar (TT$) was devalued against the U.S. dollar ($US) on two occasions. The value of the trade balance in $US was calculated using information provided by the Foreign Exchange Department of the Central Bank (Central Bank of Trinidad and Tobago 1990).

Figure 3 shows that for every year of that decade, there was a negative balance of trade on unmanufactured tobacco and manufactured cigarettes. The 10-year deficit on unmanufactured tobacco was TT$105,822,400 ($US39,057,421). The deficit for manufactured cigarettes was TT$32,841,591 ($US13,277,320). Throughout the 1980s, the cost of importation of these tobacco products was estimated at $US52 million (approximately $US5 million per year). This estimate does not include the cost of repatriating dividends or im-

Figure 1. Unmanufactured tobacco, in thousands of kgs, Trinidad and Tobago, 1979–1988

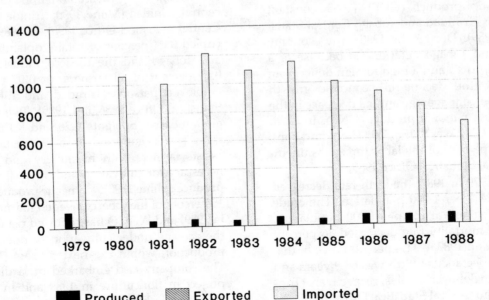

Figure 2. Manufactured cigarettes, in millions, Trinidad and Tobago, 1979–1988

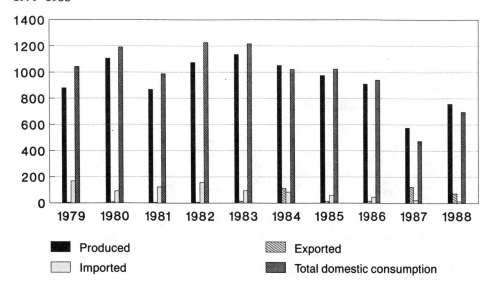

- ■ Produced
- ▨ Exported
- ▫ Imported
- ▨ Total domestic consumption

Figure 3. Trade balance on tobacco, Trinidad and Tobago, 1979–1988

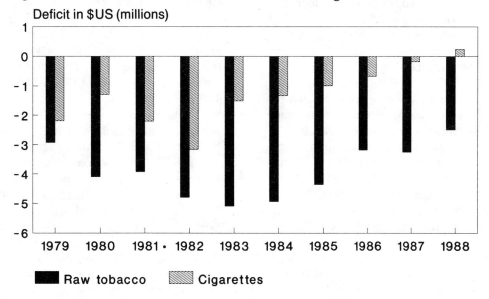

- ■ Raw tobacco
- ▨ Cigarettes

Trade balance = export earnings - import costs

porting materials such as pesticides, fertilizers, paper, and machinery, which are used in the production of tobacco products.

Marketing

Tobacco products are advertised in print and by the electronic media. They are promoted on billboards and posters; preceding films in theaters; and at sports, concerts, and other cultural events.

The most popular brands of cigarettes sold in Trinidad and Tobago are du Maurier, Broadway, Mt. d'Or, Benson & Hedges, and State Express 555, all manufactured locally by WITCO Ltd. (WITCO 1983, 1984, 1986, 1989, 1990; Milne 1990). The cigarette brands imported most commonly are Pall

Figure 4. Market for imported cigarettes (percent of cigarette market), Trinidad and Tobago, 1979–1988

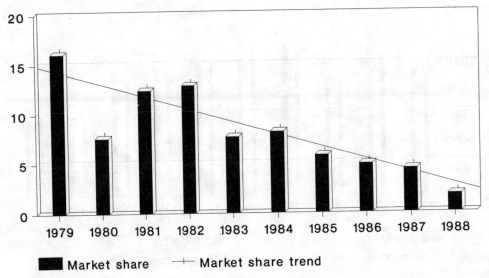

Mall, Kent, and John Players from the United States and Benson & Hedges Mayfair (mentholated) from Barbados (Beckles 1990a). During 1979 through 1988, consumption of imported manufactured cigarettes accounted for a steadily declining proportion of total annual domestic consumption (16.1 percent in 1979 and 1.8 percent in 1988) (Figure 4). This decline may have occurred as a result of either less disposable income among consumers or less foreign exchange available to importers. Thus, as the sole tobacco company operating in Trinidad and Tobago, WITCO Ltd. dominates the market, currently commanding more than 95 percent of market share (WITCO 1990; Milne 1990). There is no evidence of illegal trade in tobacco products in Trinidad and Tobago (Beckles 1990a).

Cigarettes are sold singly and in packs of 20 and 10. The cost of a packet of 20 locally manufactured cigarettes ranges from TT$3.50 to TT$5.00 ($US0.82 to $US1.18) (Beckles 1990a). The average weekly wage for employed persons in Trinidad and Tobago is TT$674.64 (Trinidad and Tobago Central Statistical Office 1988). Thus, the average worker would need to work 15 minutes to earn the average price of TT$4.29 for one pack of 20 locally manufactured cigarettes.

WITCO actively promotes its brands of cigarettes by sponsoring sports and cultural events and projects, such as the WITCO Sports Foundation—Sportsman and Sportswoman of the Year, awarded annually since 1964; the WITCO Sports Hall of Fame; the Benson & Hedges Caribbean Creole Championship, a horse race; the annual international Benson & Hedges Golf Tournament; the du Maurier Great Race to Tobago, an annual powerboat race; the WITCO Desperadoes Steelband (sponsored since 1964); and the WITCO Pan Innovation Award (since 1988) (WITCO 1983, 1984, 1986, 1989, 1990).

The tobacco industry in Trinidad and Tobago is not characterized by a high degree of vertical integration and the country is not self-sufficient in leaf production. Tobacco leaf, materials, and machinery needed for the manufacture of cigarettes must be imported. During 1979 to 1988, earnings from exports did not offset the cost of these imports. Thus, the industry does not contribute to a strengthening of the economy. Although the Government derives excise, purchase, corporate, and other taxes from the industry, these revenues have been generated by the domestic economy; that is, money has been transferred from one segment of the economy to another. No data are available to indicate the extent of direct and indirect costs that result from the personal and social effects of tobacco use.

Tobacco Use

Consumption Data

Of the total tobacco consumed in Trinidad and Tobago, 99.8 percent is in the form of manufactured

Figure 5. Per capita cigarette consumption* Trinidad and Tobago, 1979–1988

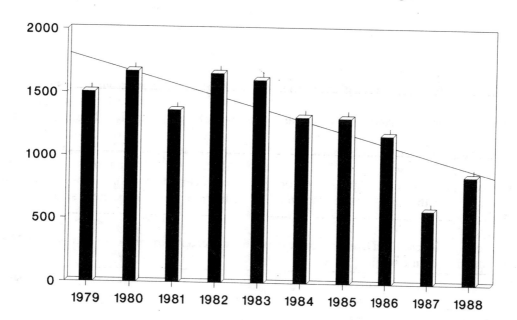

* per person aged 15 years or older

cigarettes; other forms of tobacco account for the remaining 0.2 percent (Beckles 1990a).

Although there was a net decline in domestic cigarette consumption over the decade 1979 to 1988, total domestic consumption increased by 18 percent, from 1,043 million in 1979 to 1,228 million cigarettes in 1982, and then decreased by 43 percent to 697 million in 1988 (Figure 2). The 1989 WITCO annual report indicated that total domestic consumption further declined by 3.6 percent. This decrease in sales may be linked to the marked decline in disposable income experienced by many individuals following the economic recession of the 1980s. Consumption per person aged 15 years and older declined at an average of 4 percent per year (1,506 for 1979 and 853 for 1988) (Figure 5).

Survey Data

The St. James Cardiovascular Disease Study (1977 through 1986) assessed the distribution and relation of risk factors associated with cardiovascular disease, including smoking, among adults aged 35 to 69 years, who were residents of the urban district of St. James (Miller, 1989; Beckles, 1990b). Of the target population, 92 percent (1,264 men and 1,030 women) responded to questionnaires on smoking status.

Ever smokers were defined as individuals who had ever smoked as much as one cigarette per day for 1 year or more or who had smoked pipes or cigars for 1 year or more. Current smokers were defined as individuals who were smoking at the time of the survey. Ever smokers with a history of having stopped prior to the survey were classified as ex-smokers. Persons who had either smoked less than one cigarette per day for at least 1 year or had never smoked at all were classified as nonsmokers. Never smokers were persons who denied any history of smoking.

Very few men reported smoking a pipe and none smoked cigars; women smoked cigarettes only. The prevalence data reported refer to cigarette use only.

Of the 2,294 respondents, 37 percent had a history of smoking, with 27 percent current and 10 percent ex-smokers. Prevalence of current smoking was five times higher among men than among women (42 vs. 8 percent); three times as many men as women were former smokers (15 vs. 5 percent). The gender differential in prevalence was seen in all age and ethnic groups (Table 1).

Current cigarette smoking was more frequent among younger than among older adults (Table 2). Of all men aged less than 55 years, 50 percent were current smokers compared with 35 percent of those aged 55 to 64 and 26 percent of those aged 65 years and older. The proportions of current smokers among women aged 35 to 44, 45 to 54, 55 to 64, and 65 or older were 13, 9, 6, and 5 percent, respectively (Miller, 1989).

The prevalence of cigarette smoking was similar in all ethnic groups (Table 1). After adjusting for the age distribution differences across groups, the prevalence among African, Asian Indian, and European males, and men of Mixed ethnicity was 39, 46, 37, and 40 percent, respectively; among women, prevalence in the same groups was 7, 8, 14, and 10 percent, respectively.

Male smokers also reported higher rates of heavy cigarette smoking than did female smokers

(Table 3): 48.2 percent of male smokers vs. 21.2 percent of female smokers reported smoking 20 or more cigarettes per day.

After adjusting for age, the percentage of Asian Indian and European male smokers who smoked more than 20 cigarettes per day (51.8 and 71.7 percent, respectively) was higher than that for men of African and Mixed origins (43.4 and 43.1 percent, respectively) (Table 3). The proportion of heavy cigarette smoking among women of European descent was higher than that for women of African, Asian Indian, or Mixed ethnicity (Table 3). However, the proportion of heavy smokers among all women was extremely small (1.7 percent over-

Table 1. St. James Cardiovascular Disease Study. Prevalence (percent) of smoking adults aged 35–69 at entry, by gender and ethnic origin

Population		Current smokers	Ex-smokers	Never smokers	Sample size
Total adults		26.8	10.3	62.9	2,294
Men		42.1	15.1	42.8	1,264
Women		8.0	4.5	87.5	1,030
Ethnicity*					
African	M	39.4	14.5	46.1	498
	F	7.1	3.7	89.2	382
Indian	M	46.1	11.3	42.6	381
	F	7.6	2.9	89.5	315
European	M	36.7	0	28.4	118
	F	14.2	0	77.5	49
Mixed	M	39.9	16.4	43.7	250
	F	9.9	7.1	83.0	263

*Age-adjusted to the total study population by the direct method.

Table 2. St. James Cardiovascular Disease Study. Prevalence (percent) of smoking in the study population, by age and gender

Population		Current smokers	Ex-smokers	Never smokers	Sample size
Age group					
35–44	M	49.8	10.3	39.9	343
	F	12.6	2.9	84.5	239
	T	34.6	7.1	58.3	582
45–54	M	49.6	9.7	40.7	371
	F	8.5	5.1	86.4	316
	T	30.8	7.5	61.7	687
55–64	M	35.0	19.3	45.7	383
	F	5.9	4.6	89.5	305
	T	22.1	12.8	65.1	688
≥65	M	25.8	27.5	46.7	167
	F	4.7	5.3	90.0	170
	T	15.1	16.3	68.6	337

Table 3. Percentage of all respondents and percentage of smokers reporting 1 to 19 and 20 or more cigarettes smoked per day, aged 35 to 69 at entry, by sex and ethnic origin*

Population	(Percentage smoking)			
	All	1–19 Cigarettes/day (Smokers)	>19 All	Cigarettes/day (Smokers)
Both sexes	14.8	(55.2)	12.0	(44.8)
All men	21.8	(51.8)	20.3	(48.2)
African	22.3	(56.6)	17.1	(43.4)
Asian Indian	22.2	(48.2)	23.9	(51.8)
European	10.4	(28.3)	26.3	(71.7)
Mixed	22.7	(56.9)	17.2	(43.1)
All women	6.3	(78.8)	1.7	(21.2)
African	5.3	(74.7)	1.8	(25.4)
Asian Indian	6.4	(84.2)	1.2	(15.8)
European	9.0	(63.4)	5.2	(36.6)
Mixed	8.0	(80.8)	1.9	(19.2)

Source: St. James Cardiovascular Disease Study (Miller, 1989).
*Age-adjusted to the total study population by the direct method.

all), and thus the population exposure to cigarettes for this group is minimal. Nonetheless, among smokers, very few smoke more than 20 cigarettes per day.

Data on the prevalence of smoking among adolescents was obtained from a survey conducted in 1985 among secondary school students (Remy 1985). Information on smoking was obtained by questionnaire in a 2.2 percent nationally representative sample of 2,292 students (993 males and 1,199 females). The response rate for this survey was 92.6 percent. Respondents were classified as ever smokers and never smokers. Ever smokers were then categorized as lifetime, annual, and monthly cigarette smokers. Lifetime smokers were those who had ever smoked cigarettes; annual smokers were adolescents who had smoked cigarettes in the 12 months preceding the survey; monthly users were those respondents who had smoked cigarettes in the 30 days preceding the survey.

Of all adolescents aged 11 to 19 years, 46 percent reported having smoked cigarettes sometime in their lives. The overall annual prevalence and monthly prevalence were 17 and 7 percent, respectively. Of the monthly users, 7 percent reported smoking daily compared with 10 percent who smoked cigarettes more than three times per week and 20 percent who smoked once per week; 63 percent smoked less than once per week. The annual prevalence among adolescent boys was almost twice as high as among adolescent girls (22 vs. 11.5 percent).

The two surveys described provide only a limited assessment of the prevalence of tobacco use in Trinidad and Tobago. Additional surveys need to be performed to obtain a comprehensive understanding of the dimensions of tobacco use and to identify high-risk groups. Questions on beliefs and attitudes concerning tobacco were not asked on these surveys. Even though the criteria used to categorize smoking status in the two surveys were not strictly comparable, the sharp increase in prevalence of regular cigarette smoking that occurred between adolescence and age 35 suggests that young adults are a high-risk group for uptake of tobacco use. Data are needed on the prevalence and patterns of tobacco use among young adults in the group aged 20 to 34 years. Prevalence estimates from the St. James Study reflect the situation that existed between 1977 and 1981 while those from the student survey refer to 1985; there is a need to ascertain longitudinal trends among adolescents and adults in Trinidad and Tobago. Data are also needed on the attitudes, awareness, and opinions of various groups in relation to tobacco use and other substances of abuse so that determinants of smoking behavior can be identified and targeted for intervention.

Smoking and Health

Since the early 1960s, cardiovascular diseases and malignant neoplasms (cancers) have ranked as the most important causes of death in Trinidad and

Tobago (Trinidad and Tobago Central Statistical Office 1968; Abdulah 1985). By 1987, the five leading causes of death were heart disease (ICD9:390–429), malignant neoplasms (ICD9:140–208), cerebrovascular disease (ICD9:430–438), diabetes mellitus (ICD9:250) and accidents (ICD9:E800–E949, E980–E989), accounting for 26.5, 13.4, 12.4, 11.1, and 6.5 percent of total deaths, respectively (Trinidad and Tobago Central Statistical Office 1990). During 1971 to 1986, coronary heart disease (ICD9:410–414) accounted for an increasing proportion of deaths due to heart disease (51 percent in 1971 vs. 66 percent in 1986), while deaths due to cancer of the lung (ICD9:162) contributed to 8 and 10 percent of total cancer deaths in 1971 and 1986 respectively (Pan American Health Organization [PAHO] 1974, 1982, 1990a). In 1986 and 1987, symptoms and ill-defined conditions accounted for 2.4 and 2.2 percent of total deaths, respectively. Thus, under-registration is not a significant problem with mortality data in Trinidad and Tobago (Trinidad and Tobago Central Statistical Office 1990; PAHO 1990).

The 1989 U.S. Surgeon General's Report states that certain diseases are causally related to smoking, including coronary heart disease; cerebrovascular disease; chronic obstructive lung disease; and cancers of the lung, stomach, cervix, lip, oral cavity, pharynx, larynx, esophagus, pancreas, bladder, and kidney (United States Department of Health and Human Services [USDHHS]

1989). Table 4 shows that in Trinidad and Tobago, during 1983 to 1987, coronary heart disease and cerebrovascular disease were the principal smoking-related diseases contributing to mortality in adults aged 35 years or older, accounting for one-third of all deaths in either sex. Deaths attributed to chronic obstructive lung disease were two and one-half times more common among men than women (3.0 vs. 1.2 percent, respectively). Among men, cancers of the lung and stomach were the principal smoking-related cancers, together accounting for 61 percent of deaths due to this group of cancers. Among women, 57 percent of deaths due to smoking-related cancers were attributed to cancers of the cervix and stomach. Death from lung cancer was three times more common among men than among women (1.9 vs. 0.6 percent of all deaths, respectively) (Table 4).

Although these observations result in part from changes in diagnostic, certification, and nosologic practices, data from the St. James Study confirm the significance of cardiovascular diseases and cancers in the local population, at least in urban areas (Beckles, 1986). National cause-specific mortality data should be interpreted with caution because autopsy rates are low, especially for the elderly, for middle-aged women, and for individuals who die at home (Trinidad and Tobago Ministry of Health 1986; Beckles 1990c). Sufficient inequality exists within the country concerning availability, accessibility, and use of diagnostic facil-

Table 4. Number of deaths and proportional mortality (percent of total deaths) due to smoking-related diseases among adults aged 35 years and older. Trinidad and Tobago, 1983–1987

Cause	Men		Women		Both	
	N	(%)	N	(%)	N	(%)
All causes	17,590	(100.0)	15,416	(100.0)	33,006	(100.0)
Ill-defined causes	371	(2.1)	417	(2.7)	788	(2.4)
Coronary heart disease (410–414)	3,714	(21.1)	2,785	(18.1)	6,499	(19.7)
Other heart disease (390–398, 401–405 415–417, 420–429)	1,665	(9.5)	1,575	(10.2)	3,240	(9.8)
Cerebrovascular disease (430–438)	2,349	(13.4)	2,338	(15.2)	4,687	(14.2)
Other circulatory diseases (440–448)	305	(1.7)	198	(1.3)	503	(1.5)
Chronic obs. lung diseases (490–492,496)	533	(3.0)	182	(1.2)	715	(2.2)
Other resp. diseases (010–012, 480–487,493)	653	(3.7)	504	(3.3)	1,157	(3.5)
Cancer, stomach (151)	294	(1.7)	182	(1.2)	476	(1.4)
Cancer, lung (162)	334	(1.9)	96	(0.6)	430	(1.3)
Cancer, cervix (180)	—	(—)	258	(1.7)	258	(n.a.)
Cancer, all other smoking-related	404	(2.3)	240	(1.6)	644	(2.0)

ities before and after death to warrant cautious evaluation of cause-of-death data for particular population subgroups. No procedure exists for systematic querying of cause-of-death statements that are part of the national mortality data system.

No specific data are available on trends in mortality from smoking-related diseases or on trends in tobacco use. In the St. James Study, blood pressure and hypertension, blood glucose and diabetes, total cholesterol, and LDL- and HDL-cholesterol levels were independent predictors of risk of fatal and nonfatal cardiovascular disease (Beckles, Miller, et al. 1986; Beckles, Miller, et al. 1990b). Neither smoking status nor daily cigarette consumption was predictive of risk of coronary disease in men. The low prevalence of smoking among women precluded a search for a relationship.

Tobacco Use Prevention and Control Activities

Customs and excise revenue earned from cigarettes was first listed as a separate line item in the national Estimates of Revenue in 1988. Total national cigarette tax revenues were TT$41.25 million and TT$44.5 million in 1988 and 1989, respectively (Trinidad and Tobago Ministry of Finance 1989). In 1988, tobacco contributed 1.3 percent of total excise taxes or 1.1 percent of total national taxes. A value-added tax of 15 percent is paid on each pack of cigarettes.

The Children Act, Chap. 46:01 of the Laws of Trinidad and Tobago, prohibits the sale of tobacco products to individuals aged 16 years or younger (Laws of Trinidad and Tobago 1981a). However, a survey of secondary school students indicated that the provisions of the Children Act are not enforced strictly (Remy 1985).

No laws have been enacted that restrict advertising or require health warnings on cigarette packs. However, the Trinidad and Tobago Bureau of Standards, a statutory body established under the authority of the Standards Act, No. 38 of 1972, has declared standards for advertising and labeling of tobacco products (Laws of Trinidad and Tobago 1981a, 1981b; Trinidad and Tobago Bureau of Standards 1977, 1984, 1989). These standards were based on the ''Code of Advertising Practice (1969)'' of the Advertisers' Association (ASA) of Trinidad and Tobago and were developed in cooperation with other agencies.

Standards TTS 21 20 500–Part I:1977 and TTS 21 10 500–Part III:1989 stipulate that advertisements

for free samples of cigarettes shall appear only in the trade press; packets of cigarettes shall not contain coupons or trading stamps; and advertisements and promotions for tobacco may not be directed at audiences that include children or persons younger than age 18. These standards require advertisements and cigarette packs to show the following health warning:

''The Minister of Health Advises that Smoking Can Be Dangerous to Your Health''

In 1989, the phrase ''can be dangerous'' was replaced by ''is dangerous.'' Further, TTS 21 20 500–Part III:1984 and TTS 21 10 500–Part II:1984 contain regulations for tar and nicotine yields in cigarettes. These standards require the label of each retail package to carry the tar group designation as specified in the standard. The standards also specify the typeface and size of letters to be used in statements of tar group or nicotine averages shown in advertisements. However, the local manufacturer has failed so far to comply with the standards for labeling of packages of locally manufactured cigarettes (Beckles 1990a).

Although compliance with these standards is voluntary, the Standards Act empowers the Bureau to recommend to the Minister responsible that any standard be made compulsory if self-regulation is ineffective (Laws of Trinidad and Tobago 1981b). In early 1990, the Minister gave notice of his intention to declare TTS 21 10 500–Part II:1989 a compulsory standard (Trinidad and Tobago Gazette 1990).

There are no laws restricting smoking indoors or on public transportation (Laws of Trinidad and Tobago 1981c, 1985; University of the West Indies 1987). However, administrative and voluntary restrictions on smoking are in effect in schools, in health care facilities, and in places of business. The national airline, British West Indian Airways (BWIA), has recently adopted a regulation prohibiting smoking on commercial flights of one and one-half hours or less (BWIA 1990).

Smoking prevention education is included in the syllabus of a general health education program (Trinidad and Tobago Ministry of Education 1988, 1985a, 1985b). The curriculum is introduced at the primary school level (ages 6 through 11) and continues through the junior and senior high school levels (ages 12 through 17). The effectiveness of the program has not been evaluated formally, but personnel at the Ministry of Education report that students can be examined on this portion of the syllabus, and that the students' performance in these examinations is of a high standard.

Nongovernmental organizations engage in limited prevention and control activities. The Trinidad and Tobago Cancer Society sponsors a Smoke-out Day during the Society's annual Cancer Week (Trinidad and Tobago Cancer Society 1990). The Society also supplies antismoking materials and "No smoking" signs, lectures to groups and organizations when invited, and has plans to lobby the Government to enact legislation to ban smoking in public. Upon request by community residents, the Seventh Day Adventist Church sponsors smoking cessation clinics (Beckles 1990a).

Conclusions

1. During 1979 to 1988, consumption of cigarettes in Trinidad and Tobago declined sharply. In 1988, total per capita consumption of manufactured cigarettes (575 per person) was 42 percent lower than the global average and the rate for adults (854 per person 15 years and older) was 70 percent lower than the rate observed in Canada (Kaiserman and Allen 1990a, 1990b).

2. Data from surveys of tobacco use conducted in Trinidad and Tobago indicate that prevalence of cigarette smoking was higher among adolescent males and older adult males (35 years or older) than among females of similar ages. Approximately one of every two adult males had a history of daily cigarette smoking and one in every five smoked 20 or more cigarettes per day. Only 1.2 percent of adolescents surveyed smoked three or more times per week but almost half of them had smoked cigarettes at some time in their lives. These data together with the high prevalence noted among adults aged less than 55 years suggest that, as elsewhere, young adults in Trinidad and Tobago are at high risk for uptake of cigarette smoking. The low prevalence of smoking among adolescents provides an opportunity for prevention and control of a potential epidemic of tobacco use.

3. Chronic diseases (heart disease, cerebrovascular disease, cancer) are the largest contributors to mortality in Trinidad and Tobago. As the large young cohort ages, the burden of these conditions on the health of the susceptible population can be expected to increase unless efforts are made to reduce the high prevalence of cigarette smoking and other major risk factors.

4. A limited infrastructure exists to support prevention and control of tobacco use in Trinidad and Tobago. Nongovernmental and health professional organizations are currently engaged in some limited antismoking activities.

References

ABDULAH, N. (ed.) Trinidad and Tobago 1985. A Demographic Analysis. UNFPA Project No: TRI/84/PO2. Caricom 1985.

BECKLES, G.L.A. Country Collaborator's Report, Trinidad and Tobago. Pan American Health Organization, unpublished data, 1990a.

BECKLES, G.L.A. The St. James Cardiovascular Disease Study. Autopsy frequency in an urban population in Trinidad. Unpublished data, 1990c.

BECKLES, G.L.A., MILLER, G.J., et al. The St. James Cardiovascular Disease Study: Cigarette smoking. Unpublished data, 1990b.

BECKLES, G.L.A., MILLER, G.J., KIRKWOOD, B.R., ALEXIS, S.D., et al. High total and cardiovascular disease mortality in adults of Indian descent in Trinidad: Unexplained by major coronary risk factors. *Lancet*. i: 1298–1301, 1986.

BRITISH WEST INDIAN AIRWAYS. Ground Services Division. Piarco. Trinidad and Tobago 1990.

CENTRAL BANK OF TRINIDAD AND TOBAGO. Foreign Exchange Department, Eric Williams Plaza, Port of Spain, Trinidad and Tobago 1990.

ECONOMIC AND SOCIAL COUNCIL OF THE UNITED NATIONS. Standard International Trade Classification, 2nd Revision. Statistical Papers Series M, No. 34, Rev.2. United Nations, New York, 1975.

KAISERMAN, M.J., ALLEN, T.A. Global per capita consumption of manufactured cigarettes—1988. *Chronic Diseases in Canada* 11(4): 56–57, July, 1990a.

KAISERMAN, M.J., ALLEN, T.A. Trends in Canadian tobacco consumption, 1980–1989. *Chronic Diseases in Canada* 11(4): 54–55, July, 1990b.

LAWS OF TRINIDAD AND TOBAGO. Chronological and Alphabetical Lists of Ordinances and Acts, 1832–1983. Compiled by the Law Commission. Government Printery. Trinidad and Tobago, 1985.

LAWS OF TRINIDAD AND TOBAGO. Revised Edition. The Children Act, Chapter 46:01. Government of Trinidad and Tobago, 1981a.

LAWS OF TRINIDAD AND TOBAGO. Revised Edition.

The Standards Act, Chapter 82:03. Government of Trinidad and Tobago, 1981b.

LAWS OF TRINIDAD AND TOBAGO. Revised Edition. Index. Compiled by Hewitt, A.R. Government of Trinidad and Tobago, 1981c.

MILLER, G.J., BECKLES, G.L.A., MAUDE, G.H., CARSON, D.C., et al. Ethnicity and other characteristics predictive of coronary heart disease in a developing community: Principal results of the St. James Survey, Trinidad. *International Journal of Epidemiology* 18(4):808–817, 1989.

MILNE, A. Productivity rises at WITCO with local staff—Walker. *Sunday Express.* February 4, 1990, pp. 23–25.

PAN AMERICAN HEALTH ORGANIZATION. *Health Conditions in the Americas.* Scientific Publication No. 287. Pan American Sanitary Bureau. Washington D.C., 1974.

PAN AMERICAN HEALTH ORGANIZATION. *Health Conditions in the Americas. 1990 Edition* Scientific Publication No. 427. Pan American Sanitary Bureau. Washington D.C., 1982.

PAN AMERICAN HEALTH ORGANIZATION. *Health Conditions in the Americas, 1990 Edition.* Scientific Publication No. 524. Pan American Sanitary Bureau. Washington D.C., 1990.

REMY, L.F. Summary Report of Survey on Drug Use among the Secondary School Students in Trinidad and Tobago. Ministry of Health, 1985.

TRINIDAD AND TOBAGO BUREAU OF STANDARDS. Requirements for Advertising. General: TTS 21 20 500 PART I : 1977. Trinidad and Tobago Standard. 1977.

TRINIDAD AND TOBAGO BUREAU OF STANDARDS. Requirements for Advertising. Advertising of Tobacco Products: TTS 21 20 500 PART III : 1984. Trinidad and Tobago Standard. 1984.

TRINIDAD AND TOBAGO BUREAU OF STANDARDS. Requirements for Labelling. Part II—Labelling of Retail Packages of Cigarettes: TTS 21 10 500 PART II: 1989. Compulsory Trinidad and Tobago Standard [Proposed]. 1989.

TRINIDAD AND TOBAGO CANCER SOCIETY. Planned antismoking campaign for 1990. Trinidad and Tobago, 1990.

TRINIDAD AND TOBAGO CENTRAL STATISTICAL OFFICE. Agricultural Census, 1982. Office of the Prime Minister. 1986.

TRINIDAD AND TOBAGO CENTRAL STATISTICAL OFFICE. Agricultural Statistics Unit. Office of the Prime Minister. Unpublished data, 1990.

TRINIDAD AND TOBAGO CENTRAL STATISTICAL

OFFICE. Annual Statistical Digest 1981. Central Statistical Office, Ministry of Finance. No. 28, 1983.

TRINIDAD AND TOBAGO CENTRAL STATISTICAL OFFICE. Annual Statistical Digest 1988. Central Statistical Office, Office of the Prime Minister. No. 35, 1989.

TRINIDAD AND TOBAGO CENTRAL STATISTICAL OFFICE. Continuous Survey of Business Establishments. Office of the Prime Minister. Unpublished data, 1989.

TRINIDAD AND TOBAGO CENTRAL STATISTICAL OFFICE. Economic Indicators Unit. Office of the Prime Minister. Unpublished data, 1988.

TRINIDAD AND TOBAGO CENTRAL STATISTICAL OFFICE. Overseas Trade, Part A 1979. Ministry of Finance. 1980.

TRINIDAD AND TOBAGO CENTRAL STATISTICAL OFFICE. Overseas Trade, Part A 1980. Ministry of Finance. 1981.

TRINIDAD AND TOBAGO CENTRAL STATISTICAL OFFICE. Overseas Trade, Part A 1981. Ministry of Finance. 1982.

TRINIDAD AND TOBAGO CENTRAL STATISTICAL OFFICE. Overseas Trade, Part A 1982. Ministry of Finance. 1983.

TRINIDAD AND TOBAGO CENTRAL STATISTICAL OFFICE. Overseas Trade, Part A 1983. Ministry of Finance. 1984.

TRINIDAD AND TOBAGO CENTRAL STATISTICAL OFFICE. Overseas Trade, Part A 1984. Ministry of Finance. 1985.

TRINIDAD AND TOBAGO CENTRAL STATISTICAL OFFICE. Overseas Trade, Part A 1985. Ministry of Finance. 1986.

TRINIDAD AND TOBAGO CENTRAL STATISTICAL OFFICE. Overseas Trade, Part A 1986. Office of the Prime Minister. 1987.

TRINIDAD AND TOBAGO CENTRAL STATISTICAL OFFICE. Overseas Trade, Part A 1987. Office of the Prime Minister. 1988.

TRINIDAD AND TOBAGO CENTRAL STATISTICAL OFFICE. Overseas Trade, Part A 1988. Office of the Prime Minister. 1989.

TRINIDAD AND TOBAGO CENTRAL STATISTICAL OFFICE. Population and Births 1986. Population and Vital Statistics 1987. Office of the Prime Minister. 1990.

TRINIDAD AND TOBAGO CENTRAL STATISTICAL OFFICE. Population and Vital Statistics Report 1963–64. Ministry of Finance. 1968.

TRINIDAD AND TOBAGO GAZETTE. Legal Notice No. 81. Legal Supplement, Part B. 29:115. April 26, 1990.

TRINIDAD AND TOBAGO MINISTRY OF EDUCATION. Primary School Syllabus. Social Studies and Family Life Education. Republic of Trinidad and Tobago, September 1988.

TRINIDAD AND TOBAGO MINISTRY OF EDUCATION. First Cycle of Secondary Education. Social Studies. Forms I—III(JSS). June 1985a.

TRINIDAD AND TOBAGO MINISTRY OF EDUCATION. Social Studies. Forms IV—V. 1985b.

TRINIDAD AND TOBAGO MINISTRY OF FINANCE. Estimates of Revenue for the year ending December 31, 1989. Government Printery. Trinidad and Tobago, 1989.

TRINIDAD AND TOBAGO MINISTRY OF HEALTH. Pathology Department, Port of Spain General Hospital. Unpublished data, 1986.

U.S. DEPARTMENT OF HEALTH AND HUMAN SERVICES. *Reducing the Health Consequences of Smoking: 25 Years of Progress. A Report of the Surgeon General.* U.S. Department of Health and Human Services, Public Health Service, Centers for Disease Control, Center for Chronic Disease Prevention and Health Promotion, Office on Smoking and Health. DHHS Publication No. (CDC) 89–8411, 1989.

UNIVERSITY OF THE WEST INDIES. Consolidated Index of Statutes and Subsidiary Legislation to January 1, 1987. Compiled by the Faculty of Law Library, University of the West Indies, Barbados. Government Printery, Trinidad and Tobago, 1987.

WEST INDIAN TOBACCO COMPANY LIMITED. Annual Report 1982. Texprint Ltd. Trinidad and Tobago, 1983.

WEST INDIAN TOBACCO COMPANY LIMITED. Annual Report 1983. Texprint Ltd. Trinidad and Tobago, 1984.

WEST INDIAN TOBACCO COMPANY LIMITED. Annual Report 1985. Texprint Ltd. Trinidad and Tobago, 1986.

WEST INDIAN TOBACCO COMPANY LIMITED. Annual Report 1988. Texprint Ltd. Trinidad and Tobago, 1989.

WEST INDIAN TOBACCO COMPANY LIMITED. Annual Report 1989. Texprint Ltd. Trindad and Tobago, 1990.

THE WORLD BANK. *The World Bank Atlas 1989.* Washington, D.C.: International Bank for Reconstruction and Development/The World Bank, November 1989.

United States Virgin Islands

General Characteristics

The Tobacco Industry

Tobacco Use
    Adult tobacco use
    Hurricane Hugo health assessment
    Adolescent tobacco use
    Brand preference

Smoking and Health

Tobacco Use Prevention and Control Activities
    Policies and laws
    Public information/education campaigns
    School education programs
    Private voluntary group activities

Summary

Conclusions

References

General Characteristics

The United States Virgin Islands (USVI) is the westward most group of islands in the Lesser Antilles, comprising three main islands—St. Croix (84 mi²), St. Thomas (32 mi²), and St. John (20 mi²)—and 60 smaller islands and cays. The United States has controlled the USVI since the early part of the 20th century, originally to improve strategic defense of the Panama Canal. Formerly, the USVI was a Danish colony. U.S. citizenship was granted to the residents of the Islands in 1927, and the Islands were placed under the jurisdiction of the U.S. Department of Interior as an organized but unincorporated territory. Since 1954 the legislative authority of the USVI has been the 15–member unicameral Legislature of the U.S. Virgin Islands. It enjoys most of the powers held by State legislatures of the United States (USVI Legislature 1983). There has been an active effort to establish home rule in the Islands, but a majority of registered voters did not approve a recent referendum as required by law for passage of this initiative.

The U.S. Government defines a population of under 50,000 as rural for purposes of funding community health centers. Each individual island of the USVI would be considered rural under this definition. However, St. Thomas and St. Croix both have defined cities, and Charlotte Amalie on St. Thomas is a hub of tourist trade with cosmopolitan influences and urban problems of poverty and crowding. In 1960, the population of the USVI was estimated to be 32,099; by 1980, the USVI population was 96,569 with a geometric growth rate of 5.7 percent per year. The estimated 1990 population is 113,000. In 1989, the population was 80.2 black and 17.0 percent white; among these groups, 18.0 percent declared Hispanic origin.

The proportion of native-born residents declined by almost half from 1960 to 1980 (83 vs. 44.7 percent). Of whites in the territory, the majority (58.8 percent) were born in the United States. Of blacks, the majority (52.2 percent) were born on other Caribbean islands.

The life expectancy at birth in the USVI is approximately 76 years (USVI Department of Health [USVIDOH] 1988). The infant mortality rate (IMR) varies from year to year; for example, the IMR was 19.2 per 1,000 live births in 1987 and 12.5 per 1,000 live births in 1988. This represents a marked decrease from the 1984 rate of 23.2 per 1,000 but still exceeds the U.S. infant mortality rate of 10.1 per 1,000 live births (USVIDOH 1988; U.S. Department of Health and Human Services [USDHHS] 1990). However, the IMR reflects a better health status for USVI blacks than for blacks in the rest of the United States, with an IMR of 17.9 per 1,000 live births in 1987 (USDHHS 1990) (Table 1). Reasons for the decline in infant mortality, if sustained, include improved control of childhood infectious diseases and improved childbirth practices.

The gross domestic/territorial product (GTP) was US$1,246 million in 1988 and the GTP per capita was $11,755 (USVI Industrial Development Commission 1990). This level would rank the USVI among the high-income economies of the world (World Bank 1990), but because of a serious maldistribution of income, the per capita GTP figure may not represent the true economic conditions in the USVI. For example, fewer than 60 percent of the population graduated from high school, and only 15.3 percent have postgraduate training. In fiscal year (FY) 1990, the largest percentage (23.0) of the population earned less than $10,000. However, with a nearly 10–fold increase in tourist visits from 1960 to 1980 and an 11–percent growth rate in personal income, it is clear there was significant economic growth in the USVI over the last 20 years. The impact of inflation softened but did not invalidate these indices of growth and development (Jones-Hendrickson 1990).

More than 70 percent of the population is younger than 35 years of age, 13 percent is under 5 years, and only 4 percent is aged 65 and older (Christian 1988). The USVI has an increasing fertility rate, a low IMR, and significant immigration of young persons seeking better economic opportunities. Compared with other Caribbean islands, health conditions in the USVI are good, but they differ significantly from the U.S. mainland. Many of the infectious diseases in the USVI have come under control, and now the leading causes of death are heart disease (40 percent of total deaths), cancer

Table 1. Health and economic indicators, U.S. Virgin Islands, 1988

Population (estimated 1990)	113,000
Percent less than age 5	13
Percent age 65 or older	4
Infant mortality rate (per 1,000 live births)	12.5
Birth rate per 1,000	21.6
Crude death rate per 1,000	5.0
Per capita gross territorial product	US$11,755

Source: USVI Industrial Development Commission, 1990.

(11 percent), perinatal conditions (7 percent), diabetes (5 percent), and accidents (5 percent) (USVIDOH 1988).

In keeping with the U.S. Public Health Service's 1990 Health Objectives for the Nation (USDHHS 1980), the USVI regionalized the health care system to provide access to the entire population by the year 1990. Each regional district is to establish a primary care model that permits an integrated approach to health care. This integration would encourage interventions such as smoking cessation through primary care channels. In 1987, the Division of Prevention, Health Promotion, and Protection (DPHPP) was created to provide the administration and management to accomplish this integration. This comprehensive health care system emphasizes education, early detection, competent care, and outreach services. The DPHPP includes health education and chronic disease prevention in its mandate as well as standard public health activities such as immunization services, sexually transmitted disease control, HIV/AIDS interventions, and social services. The percent of the Health Department's budget of U.S. funds decreased from 35 percent in the early 1970s to less than 18 percent in 1990 (USVIDOH 1991). More than 60 percent of the budget for health-related activities is allocated for the operations of the hospitals.

Since colonial times, the USVI economy has been a satellite to the global trade of the United States. The islands possess both a strategic geographic location between North and South America and a stable political environment. However, because of extreme resource scarcity almost all goods are imported. The islands have depended on a single economic product, tourism, since the early 1960s when Cuba was closed to U.S. vacationers. Luxury and recreational items such as jewelry, perfumes, cigarettes, and alcohol are widely sold duty-free items, and these items often serve as advertisements for travel to the USVI. The tourist industry has caused a de-emphasis on indigenous agriculture and has infused U.S. habits and consumption patterns through exposure to advertisements and tourists (McElroy 1974).

The Tobacco Industry

In 1680, 50 estates on St. Thomas engaged in tobacco cultivation. Under Danish rule, tobacco was used to pay fines for such crimes as working on Sundays and leaving the island without the Governor's permission (Taylor 1888). Throughout the West Indies, tobacco was found to be an unsound economic staple. The tobacco grown on Barbados and in the Leeward Islands was of poor quality and could not compete with Virginian tobacco. Sugar emerged as the obvious substitute crop; unlike tobacco, it could be grown in the tropics using unskilled labor without exhausting the soil (Parry 1981).

During the American Revolution, North American tobacco became an essential commodity in trade between the continent and the islands. In 1767, Oldenthorp observed that despite the ease of growing tobacco in the USVI, the residents planted only enough tobacco for their own personal consumption (Oldenthorp 1987). During the slave trade from Africa to the Caribbean, a weekly pipeful of tobacco was added to the slaves' diets. Prior to slave auctions, slaves were prepared for this event (in addition to being fed, shaved, and clothed) with a new pipe filled with tobacco. The nicotine in tobacco possibly functioned as a stimulant, so that those who appeared stronger and more confident could be sold at a higher price (Oldenthorp 1987). In the 1800s, tobacco commonly was imported for consumption by planters, land owners, and slaves (Edwards 1801). There is currently no tobacco cultivated in the USVI. All tobacco products are imported.

At present, tobacco products are heavily promoted in the USVI. Cigarette companies frequently feature full-page print media advertisements with coupons for nontobacco items such as tee shirts, visors, and waistpacks. Local horse races are also sponsored by the parent companies. In addition, logo-bearing items such as hats, umbrellas, and drinking containers are provided free during Carnival. Promotion of cigarettes is not allowed on television or radio in accordance with U.S. law, the Public Health Cigarette Smoking Act of 1969 (USDHHS 1989).

The USVI has no sales tax. Only an excise tax is levied on goods brought into the Territory. In FY 1988, the value of tobacco products was $583,187.00 (Table 2), and the excise tax on these products was 4 percent ($23,327.48).

Tobacco Use

There are no tobacco industry or U.S. Government records for tobacco consumption and importation for the USVI. Because of the large tourist trade in duty-free goods, these data would not provide useful information on USVI residents' consumption patterns. However, from 1988 to 1991,

Table 2. Tobacco imported into the U.S. Virgin Islands, 1988

Type	Quantity	Value ($)
Cigarettes	1,262*	549,273
Cigars	673,000	25,274
Chewing tobacco, snuff	900,000	2,160
Manufactured tobacco	7,027,000	6,480

Source: USVI Department of Economic Development and Agriculture FY 1988.

*million packs

four surveys were conducted that provide consistent data on the prevalence of smoking for Territorial residents (Figure 1). Three of the surveys were conducted via face-to-face interviews, and one was conducted by telephone utilizing the Behavior Risk Factor Surveillance System questionnaire from the Centers for Disease Control (CDC).

Adult Tobacco Use

In 1988 the Virgin Islands Department of Health conducted face-to-face interviews with 1,506 persons in households on all three islands using a complex probability sample with a multistage design. In addition to other health-related queries, individuals were asked if they smoked. Overall, 12.9 percent indicated that they currently smoked. The highest prevalence of current smoking (16.5 percent) was among persons aged 35 to 44 years followed by that among persons aged 25 to 34 years (16.1 percent). The lowest prevalence (7.1 percent) was found among those aged 65 years and older. The prevalence of smoking among persons aged 18 and older stratified by island of residence was 15.5 percent on St. Croix, 9.9 percent on St. Thomas, and 14.5 percent on St. John. Respondents were also asked where they were born. Those born in the United States reported a prevalence of current smoking three times higher (19.6 percent) than those born on the islands (approximately 6.2 percent); those born in Puerto Rico also had a much higher prevalence of current smoking (15.6 percent) than those born in the USVI.

The USVI participated in the CDC's Behavioral Risk Factor Surveillance System (BRFSS) in 1989 by conducting a point-in-time survey. Questions on smoking are included in this standardized questionnaire. In 1989, 1,410 households (individuals) were surveyed by telephone using a multistage cluster design based on the Waksburg Sam-

Figure 1. Adult current smoking prevalence (percent), U.S. Virgin Islands, 1988–1990

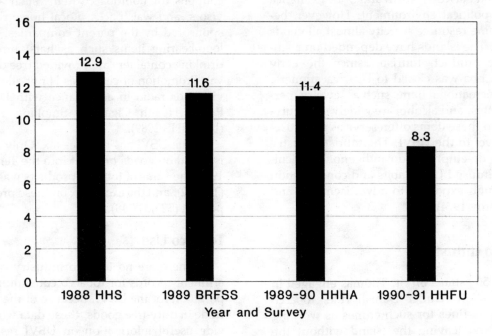

See text for survey names.

pling Method for Random Digit Dialing. Overall, the prevalence of current cigarette smoking among those with telephones in the USVI was 11.6 percent; 9.2 percent were former smokers, and 78.5 percent had never smoked (or had smoked fewer than 100 cigarettes in their lifetimes) (Table 3). Men had a statistically higher prevalence of smoking compared with women (14.6 vs. 9.1 percent), but 62 percent of women and only 40 percent of men smoked fewer than 20 cigarettes per day (Table 4). Men had a higher prevalence of former smoking than women (11.3 vs. 7.5 percent), indicating a slightly greater tendency to quit (Table 3).

Table 3. Current smoking prevalence (percent), by sex, age group, educational attainment, income, and race, U.S. Virgin Islands, 1989

Variable	Current smoking	Former smoking
Sex		
Male	14.6	11.3
Female	9.1	7.5
Both	11.6	9.2
Age group		
18–24	5.9	
25–34	13.9	
35–44	15.4	
45–54	10.3	
55–64	9.4	
65+	11.0	
Educational attainment		
9th grade	6.0	
Some hs	16.3	
Hs graduate	7.8	
Tech/tech grad	5.6	
Some college	15.5	
College grad	15.9	
Postgrad	22.9	
Income		
< 10,000	10.3	
10–14,000	9.6	
15–19,000	15.8	
20–24,000	9.3	
25–34,000	11.4	
35–50,000	17.1	
> 50,000	21.1	
Race		
Blacks	6.9	
Whites	29.3	
Hispanics	16.4	

Source: Christian, 1990.

Table 4. Cigarettes smoked per day, Behavioral Risk Factor Survey, U.S. Virgin Islands, 1989

No. of cigarettes		Percentage of respondents
0	cigarettes per day	88.4
1–20	cigarettes per day	8.9
21+	cigarettes per day	1.7

Source: Christian, 1990.

In contrast to the pattern in the mainland U.S. population, the prevalence of smoking among whites is higher than among non-whites (largely blacks and Hispanics) in the USVI (29.3 percent among whites, 6.9 percent among blacks, and 16.4 among Hispanics). According to these data, whites were almost twice as likely as Hispanics and four times as likely as blacks to be smokers.

Among men, those aged 65 and older had the highest prevalence of smoking (19.8 percent), followed by those aged 35 to 44 (19.1 percent), 25 to 34 (17.6 percent), and 18 to 24 years (5.2 percent). Women aged 35 to 44 had the highest prevalence of current smoking (12.5 percent), and women aged 65 and older had the lowest (4 percent).

In general, the prevalence of smoking was positively associated with level of educational attainment. The highest prevalence was found among those with college and post-graduate education (Table 3). However, those with "some high school" had a prevalence of current smoking very similar to that for those with at least some college education. This pattern may also be reflected in the prevalence of smoking by income level. With the exception of persons earning $US15 to $US20 thousand per year, the prevalence of current smoking was positively associated with income. The prevalence of smoking was higher among unmarried than married persons (33.1 vs. 8.8 percent).

Hurricane Hugo Health Assessment

After Hurricane Hugo ravaged the USVI in September 1989, the Department of Health conducted a population-based survey on health status (Christian 1990). A 2 percent sample of the population was drawn using a list of water and electric consumers on the three main islands. A total of 727 individuals (549 women and 178 men) were interviewed in person. Questions on smoking included in this health assessment were adapted from the

BRFSS conducted a month before the hurricane. The rationale for this survey was to measure changes in health behavior after a disaster and to compare these data with data from the recently performed BRFSS telephone survey (Table 3). Persons interviewed in the original post-hurricane assessment and some additional respondents were interviewed 8 to 12 months later.

The surveys showed that before the hurricane, 10.6 percent of those interviewed were smokers; 3 to 5 months after the storm 11.4 percent were smokers. One year after the hurricane, 8.3 percent were smokers (Christian 1991).

Adolescent Tobacco Use

The 1988 household study also interviewed children and adolescents. No children aged 11 years or younger smoked. Among those aged 12 to 17 years, only 0.6 percent admitted smoking. Surveys of tobacco use by high school students were planned by the American Cancer Society, St. Croix Chapter, for the spring of 1991.

Brand Preference

Through a telephone survey of wholesalers, distributors, large supermarkets, pharmacies, and liquor stores the most popular brands of cigarettes and their average prices were ascertained. In addition, the total revenues derived from tobacco products were estimated. Respondents were asked to rank the five most popular brands of cigarettes sold or distributed in their company or store. Marlboro was the most popular brand with 19.4 percent of the market (Table 5). The average price of a pack of cigarettes was US$1.50. The most popular pack size contains 20 cigarettes. Based on data provided by all businesses surveyed, cigars account for approximately 4.3 percent of tobacco products sold in the USVI. Very small percentages of tobacco sold in the islands are pipe tobacco (2.3 percent) and smokeless tobacco (2.1 percent) (Hatcher 1991).

Table 5. Most popular brands of cigarettes in USVI in ranking order, 1990

Rank	Brand
1	Marlboro
2	Kools
3	Winston
4	Benson & Hedges, Newport, Salem
5	Merit

Source: Hatcher, 1991.

Smoking and Health

The mortality pattern of the USVI is similar to that of the United States. Cardiovascular diseases (CVD) and cancer are the leading causes of death. Of total mortality, 21.9 percent is CVD and 17.4 percent is cancer. Both sexes experienced increases in cancer mortality rates during 1982 to 1987. Male cancer mortality rates were consistently higher than female cancer mortality rates each year during this period (USVIDOH 1988). Overall, smoking-related illnesses accounted for 39.3 percent of all deaths.

CVD also accounts for the largest percentage of visits to the ambulatory health care system, with hypertension as the most common diagnosis (Christian 1990).

Tobacco Use Prevention and Control Activities

Policies and Laws

Laws that restrict smoking at the worksite may be effective in reducing cigarette consumption (Borland 1990). In 1985, a law was passed by the Virgin Islands' Legislature (Act #5125) that requires private employers, Government offices, and restaurants to make accommodations for nonsmoking areas. The Police Department and the Consumer Services Administration enforce this law, and appropriate penalties are assessed for noncompliance. The Virgin Islands Code, Subchapter XIII, section 892–895, states that each employer who operates an office shall adopt and maintain a written smoking policy and that all owners of restaurants shall designate and maintain at least 30 percent of their seating as nonsmoking areas. Penalties for employers or restauranteurs who fail to bring the office workplace or restaurant into compliance within 30 days of such order shall have their business license suspended for 1 month. This provision extends to all government buildings. The term "office workplace" extends to any building, structure, or enclosed area in which business of a clerical, professional, or administrative nature is performed. This law, classified in the 1989 Report of the U.S. Surgeon General, ranks as an "extensive" clean-indoor-air law (USDHHS 1989).

The American Lung Association of the Virgin Islands is seeking to amend Act #5125. If the new bill is signed into law, responsibility for enforcement would be transferred from the Police Department to the Department of Licensing and Consumer Affairs. The percentage of nonsmoking seating areas in restaurants would be increased from 30 to 70 percent. The bill also calls for licensing of tobacco vendors and prohibits cigarette vending machines.

In September 1991, the USVI Legislature's Operations Committee approved legislation banning smoking in government buildings, including hospitals. This legislation calls for fines of $100–300 as well as job suspension for recurrent offenses. The legislation has been submitted to the full Senate and the governor for action (Lohr 1991).

Minors have easy access to cigarette products because there are no restrictions on sales to minors or on access to vending machines. Cigarettes are sold in all grocery stores and pharmacies. The U.S. Secretary of Health and Human Services has recommended model legislation banning the sale of tobacco to persons younger than age 18 (Sullivan 1990). No actions on this model legislation have as yet been taken in the USVI.

As a territory of the United States all Federal Codes that relate to smoking are applied in the USVI. These include restrictions on television and radio advertisements, prohibition of smoking on flights up to 6 hours in length, and prohibition of all smoking in Department of Health and Human Services buildings (USDHHS 1989).

Public Information/Education Campaigns

Since 1980, the USVI Department of Health has celebrated the yearly Great American Smokeout sponsored by the American Cancer Society. Local public service announcements on quitting smoking and on the risks of smoking during pregnancy appear in the electronic media. In Fall, 1991, the American Cancer Society—St. Croix Chapter—was to sponsor a song-writing contest to promote nonsmoking among youth.

School Education Programs

The Department of Education has adopted in their revised health curriculum a unit on smoking and prevention activities related to cardiovascular health (USVI Department of Education 1991).

Private Voluntary Group Activities

The American Lung Association of the Virgin Islands was established in 1954 and now sponsors quit-smoking clinics. The Association hosts a 15-minute weekly radio program in addition to disseminating public service announcements and other information to the media. The Association

sponsors an annual fund-raising luncheon to promote lung health and to sensitize the population to the health consequences of smoking. Board members consist of volunteers from all three main islands. The actions of the American Cancer Society were described above in conjunction with media campaigns.

Summary

The USVI has the lowest prevalence of smoking documented in the Americas. The prevalence of smoking for the 1989 BRFSS was 11.6 percent; the 1988 Household Survey reported a current smoking prevalence of 12.9 percent; and the Hurricane Hugo Health Assessment (1989–1990) and the Hurricane Hugo Health Assessment Follow-up (1990) reported prevalences of 11.4 percent and 8.3 percent respectively.

In the United States the best single predictor of smoking is educational status (that is, those with the least educational attainment have a higher current smoking prevalence than those with the highest educational attainment) (USDHHS 1989). By contrast, in the USVI, those with 12 or more years of education were almost twice as likely to smoke than were those with less education.

In the BRFSS 23 percent of persons with a post-graduate degree were smokers and only 6 percent of those with less than a ninth grade education were smokers. In addition, the USVI has a pattern opposite that of the United States with regard to smoking and income status. The prevalence of current smoking is highest among those in higher income categories, especially in the level of US$50,000 or more. On the U.S. mainland, the highest percentage of smokers is found in the lower income group (USDHHS 1989). The prevalence of smoking among USVI men is higher than among women (14.6 vs. 9.1 percent).

Blacks on the U.S. mainland have a higher rate of current smoking than do whites while in the USVI, 29.3 percent of whites and only 6.9 percent of blacks are smokers. The majority of USVI whites were born in the continental United States. The high prevalence rate of smoking among this group may contribute adversely to behavioral patterns and mortality outcomes for the USVI as a whole. The behavior of groups with higher social standing may diffuse into populations who wish to emulate them. The health consequences of this behavior will be more of a burden to those with the least resources, and thus, groups who have not yet experienced high levels of tobacco use should be educated about the risks in order to prevent future disease outcomes. This pattern of higher prevalence among higher socioeconomic status groups is akin to that found in other developing nations of the Americas. It is evident that even though the prevalence of current smoking is low in the USVI, the same social norms that have decreased cigarette smoking in the U.S. mainland do not operate in the USVI.

Conclusions

1. The prevalence of smoking in the USVI is the lowest documented in the Americas. However, the population of the USVI is young, and the highest smoking levels are found among those with the most education and personal income. Promotion of cigarettes in the print media and through concerts and horse races is pervasive, and young people may be prone to initiate smoking in increasing numbers, in a manner similar to their counterparts in other developing countries in the Americas.

2. There is currently no law restricting minors' access to tobacco through vending machines, food stores, pharmacies, and large department stores, all of which are easily accessible to young persons. The USVI has what appears to be an extensive law limiting nonsmokers' exposure to environmental tobacco smoke, but the extent of compliance with this law is unknown. Plans by private voluntary groups and the Legislature to strengthen the law are pending.

3. USVI residents born outside the Islands, including teachers, may serve as role models who could influence health habits, either positively or negatively. These residents have a higher prevalence of smoking than those born in the USVI.

4. The low prevalence of smoking among women is thought to be culturally related. In the past, Caribbean women did not frequent bars or other places where smoking is common. This may account for the exceedingly low rate among women aged 65 and older and the overall low rate among USVI women. As USVI women assume greater involvement in the work force, the prevalence of smoking is likely to increase.

5. It appears that financial independence is linked to higher current smoking prevalence because these rates increase substantially beginning at age 25. Smoking cessation programs in the workplace may impact this group.

6. The aggressive marketing by tobacco companies needs to be restricted in the USVI. The enforcement and strengthening of laws on smoking in public places need to be addressed in addition to creating those that will restrict access to tobacco by young persons.

7. An infrastructure for effective tobacco-use prevention and control is in place in the USVI. This infrastructure includes school education, legislation to restrict smoking in public places, and active private voluntary groups. Additional taxation, laws restricting access to tobacco by young persons, bans on cigarette vending machines, and restrictions on tobacco product advertising are needed.

References

BORLAND, R. Effects of workplace smoking bans on cigarette consumption. *American Journal of Public Health* 80(2):178–180, February 1990.

CHRISTIAN, C. *An Analysis of Health Care in the US Virgin Islands*. USVI Department of Health, 1988.

CHRISTIAN, C. *Hurricane Hugo Health Assessment*, USVI Department of Health, 1990, pp. 16–21.

CHRISTIAN, C. *Hurricane Hugo Health Assessment Follow Up*, USVI Department of Health, 1991 (in press).

EDWARDS. On Sugar Plantation, 1801.

HATCHER, A.T. The most popular brands of cigarettes smoked in the U.S.V.I. VIDOH/HP, 1991.

JONES-HENDRICKSON, S.B. *A Profile of Frederiksted, St. Croix, U.S. Virgin Islands*. The Caribbean Research Institute, University of the Virgin Islands, 1990, pp. 3–4.

LOHR, L. $100 for smoking in govt bldg. *The St. Croix Avis*, Thursday, September 12, 1991, No. 211, p. 3.

MCELROY, J. *The Virgin Islands Economy: Past Performance, Future Projections, Planning Alternatives*. Caribbean Research Institute, College of the Virgin Islands, 1974, p. 3.

OLDENTHORP HIGHFIELD, A., BARAC, V. (eds). *Oldenthorp's History of the Mission of the Evangelical Brethren of the Caribbean Islands of St. Thomas, St. Croix, and St. John*, edited by Johann Jakob Bossard. Originally published 1770; English translation 1987.

PARRY, S. *A Short History of the West Indies*, 3rd edition, 1981.

SULLIVAN, L.W. Statement of Louis W. Sullivan, M.D., Secretary of Health and Human Services, before the Committee on Finance, U.S. Senate, May 24, 1990.

TAYLOR, C.E. Leaflets from the Danish West Indies: descriptive of the social, political, and commercial conditions of these islands, 1888.

U.S. DEPARTMENT OF HEALTH AND HUMAN SERVICES. *Healthy People 2000.* U.S. Department of Health and Human Services, Public Health Service. DHHS Publication No. (PHS) 91–50213. September 1990, p. 366.

U.S. DEPARTMENT OF HEALTH AND HUMAN SERVICES. *Reducing the Health Consequences of Smoking: 25 Years of Progress. A Report of the Surgeon General.* U.S. Department of Health and Human Services, Public Health Service, Centers for Disease Control, Center for Chronic Disease Prevention and Health Promotion, Office on Smoking and Health. DHHS Publication No. (CDC) 89–8411. January 1989.

U.S. DEPARTMENT OF HEALTH AND HUMAN SERVICES. *Promoting Health, Preventing Disease: Objectives for the Nation.* U.S. Department of Health and Human Services, Washington, D.C., Fall 1980.

USVI DEPARTMENT OF ECONOMIC DEVELOPMENT AND AGRICULTURE. Unpublished data, 1988.

USVI DEPARTMENT OF EDUCATION. Curriculum document, 1991.

USVI DEPARTMENT OF HEALTH. Unpublished data, Budget Director's Office, 1991.

USVI DEPARTMENT OF HEALTH. *V.I. Vital Statistics 1982–1987.* Virgin Islands Department of Health, December 1988.

USVI INDUSTRIAL DEVELOPMENT COMMISSION. Business Guide, 1990.

USVI LEGISLATURE. *The History of the Legislature of the United States Virgin Islands.* Amalie Printing, Inc., January 1983, pp. 28–29.

WORLD BANK. *World Development Report 1990—Poverty.* Oxford University Press: New York, 1990.

Uruguay

General Characteristics

The Tobacco Industry
  Agriculture
  Tobacco manufacturing
  Advertising and marketing
  Taxes

Tobacco Use
  Per capita cigarette consumption
  Surveys on tobacco use: limitations and results
  Prevalence of smoking among adolescents
  Attitudes and opinions toward smoking

Smoking and Health

Tobacco Use Prevention and Control Activities
  Government action
    Executive structure
    Legislation
    Education
  Action by nongovernmental agencies
    Campaigns and services

Summary and Conclusions

References

General Characteristics

Uruguay is a republic of 186,925 km² located south of Brazil on the Atlantic coast of South America. The country has had a democratic form of government since 1985. Compared with other countries of the Americas, Uruguay is 13th largest in land area and 21st largest in population. Uruguay has a predominantly European culture, with almost all residents claiming heritage from Spain or Italy. In 1990, 86 percent of the 3,094,000 inhabitants lived in urban settings. The population structure is similar to that of developed countries, with 74 percent aged 15 or older (Table 1).

Uruguay's per capita gross national product (GNP) ($US2,470 in 1988) is ranked among the upper-middle-income countries (World Bank 1990), but this relatively affluent country has also experienced the economic pressures of the 1980s. The per capita gross domestic product (GDP) growth rate was −1.3 percent during 1980 to 1987 (World Bank 1989). Uruguay is similar to almost all other Latin American countries in having a very high rate of inflation (54.5 percent per year from 1980 to 1987) and a foreign debt that exceeds one-half of the GDP ($US3,825 million in 1988) (World Bank 1990).

Despite these economic difficulties, Uruguay maintains very satisfactory social and health indicators, among the best in the Americas. Life expectancy at birth was 72 years in 1988; infant mortality was 20/1,000 live births. Literacy is 95.0 percent for the population aged 15 years and older (Table 1).

Table 1. Health and economic indicators, Uruguay, 1980s

Indicator	Level
Population (1988)	3,100,000
Urban (%) (1988)	86.0
Percentage aged < 15 years (1988)	26.2
Life expectancy at birth (1988)	72
Literacy (%), aged 15 and older (1985)	95.0
Infant mortality (per 1,000 live births, 1986)	23
Total fertility per 1,000 women	2.4
Crude mortality rate (per 1,000 persons)	10
Per capita gross national product (1988)	$US2,470
Annual inflation rate (%) (1980–1987)	54.5

Sources: World Bank, 1989; World Bank, 1990.

The Tobacco Industry

Agriculture

In 1988, approximately 1,000 ha (0.01 percent of total arable land) were used for tobacco growing (Encyclopedia Britannica 1989; Silva Sosa 1990). About 3,000 rural workers in 5 of the country's 19 departments are involved in tobacco agriculture. The Government does not regulate the price of tobacco or provide special assistance to tobacco growers. However, in 1985, import duties were waived on agricultural goods used in tobacco farming. This action also benefitted producers and growers through special financing by the Banco de la República Oriental del Uruguay for Virginia and Burley tobacco, types of tobacco used in exports (Pan American Health Organization [PAHO] 1986). The tobacco industry is represented by its trade organization, the Asociación de Fabricantes e Importadores de Tabacos y Cigarrillos (AFITYC). Nongovernmental organizations have attempted to convert land intended for tobacco farming to strawberry farming, but no formal crop substitution programs have been established.

Three sources for data on tobacco production, tobacco exports, tobacco imports, and tobacco consumption are available: the U.S. Department of Agriculture (USDA) (1990), the Uruguayan Government (Silva Sosa 1990), and the tobacco industry (AFITYC 1989 and ERC 1988). Although various sources report discrepant data, similar trends are evident in all three sources. The USDA reports a slight decline in annual leaf tobacco production from 1,587 MT to 1,400 MT over the decade from 1979 to 1989 (Table 2). Data on tobacco exportation are available for years beginning in 1984, and levels vary between 23 MT in 1987 and 460 MT in 1989. AFITYC reports that tobacco exports are "negligible" (PAHO 1986). According to the USDA, import tonnage of tobacco has been approximately twice that of production, declining from 3,500 MT in 1979 to 2,700 MT in 1989 (USDA 1990). However, AFITYC reports that 60 percent of the tobacco consumed in Uruguay is domestically produced while 40 percent is imported (AFITYC 1989).

Total domestic consumption decreased from 4,750 MT in 1979 to 3,500 MT in 1989 according to USDA 1990 data. However, according to the tobacco industry, total consumption declined from 3,900 MT in 1982 to 3,500 MT in 1988 (ERC 1988), and according to the Uruguayan Government, total consumption declined from 3,369 MT in 1984 to 3,051 MT in 1988 (Silva Sosa 1990). Consumption of

Table 2. Unmanufactured tobacco production, exportation, importation, and total domestic consumption (in metric tons), Uruguay, 1979–1989

Year	Production	Exports	Imports	Total consumption
1979	1,587	0	3,500	4,750
1980	1,487	0	3,724	4,940
1981	1,365	0	2,618	4,700
1982	1,808	0	3,500	3,700
1983	1,400	0	1,334	3,500
1984	1,400	399	2,545	3,489
1985	1,400	117	1,100	2,081
1986	1,400	98	2,800	3,900
1987	1,400	23	2,700	3,800
1988	1,400	468	2,749	3,500
1989	1,400	460	2,700	3,500

Source: USDA, 1990.

tobacco obtained through illegal trade or duty-free shops is not measured by any of these sources, and therefore, the actual tobacco consumption is probably significantly higher than reported.

Tobacco Manufacturing

The tobacco market in Uruguay is controlled by three major tobacco manufacturing companies: Monte Paz, La Republicana, and Abal Hermanos. The first two companies are joint ventures or subsidiaries of the British-American Tobacco (BAT) Company, and the third is a licensee of Philip Morris; Monte Paz alone holds three-fourths of the tobacco market.

According to the USDA, production of manufactured cigarettes increased from 3.54 billion in 1978 to 3.9 billion in 1988 (USDA 1990). According to Uruguayan Government sources, production was considerably less (3.05 billion) in 1988. Yearly imports of manufactured cigarettes declined from 50 million in 1978 to 40 million in 1988 (with an extremely high level of 126 million MT reported for 1979); yearly exports remained at approximately 2 million (Table 3) (USDA 1990). In 1984, the last year for which data are available, Uruguay suffered a $US3,706,000 deficit trade balance for tobacco products. The decline in tobacco imports may have decreased this negative balance somewhat, but special exemptions for tobacco production equipment and materials in 1985 undoubtedly increased the negative trade balance for the industry as a whole.

Loose-cut tobacco used in hand-rolled cigarettes was approximately 20 percent of all tobacco consumed in 1988. However, this figure is likely to be an overestimate given the unmeasured illegal or duty-free sales of cigarettes in Uruguay. Pipes accounted for less than 1 percent, and cigars for less than 0.1 percent of all tobacco consumed (Silva Sosa 1990).

In 1988, the AFITYC reported that 700 industrial workers were employed directly or indirectly in cigarette manufacturing; this is equivalent to less than 0.5 percent of the total industrial work force (211,600 persons in 1986) (AFITYC 1989; Encyclopedia Britannica 1989). This same source estimated

Table 3. Manufactured cigarettes—production, exports, imports, in millions, and yearly per capita consumption for persons aged 15 and older, Uruguay, 1979–1989

Year	Production (millions)	Exports (millions)	Imports (millions)	Total consumption (millions)	Per capita consumption (per person age ≥ 15 years)
1978	3,548	5	50	3,593	1,720
1979	3,593	5	126	3,714	1,771
1980	3,608	2	60	3,666	1,741
1981	3,650	2	24	3,672	1,738
1982	3,700	2	25	3,723	1,755
1983	3,750	2	25	3,773	1,772
1984	3,750	2	25	3,773	1,765
1985	3,850	2	35	3,883	1,816
1986	3,900	2	40	3,938	1,835
1987	3,900	2	40	3,938	1,822
1988	3,900	2	40	3,938	1,809

Sources: USDA, 1990; CELADE, 1990.

that 500 persons were employed in wholesale distribution of tobacco and that 16,000 persons were involved directly or indirectly in retail tobacco sales.

Advertising and Marketing

In 1987, the Philip Morris licensee/joint venture spent an estimated $US700,000 on advertising (Philip Morris, Inc. 1988). The amount spent by the BAT companies is unknown. Tobacco advertising is permitted and used on television and radio, in movies, and in print media, but not on transport posters. Other types of tobacco product promotion in Uruguay are widespread, including: distributing free cigarette samples on airplanes and at public performances, sponsoring cultural and sporting events, distributing free shopping bags that feature brand names or logos, and exchanging empty cigarette packs for tickets to cultural and sporting events (in particular, a series of dances involving youth groups sponsored by Casino cigarettes) (Silva Sosa 1990). All types of advertising must bear a health warning (see section on legislative actions below).

Several different pack sizes are available to accommodate the purchasing power of consumers of different economic capability; these include packs of 10, 18, 20, 27, and 50 cigarettes. The lowest price for one pack of a domestic brand of cigarettes ranges from N$450 to N$750 ($US1.10) in 1990. The best-selling imported brand is more than double this price (N$700 to N$1,800; $US2.30). Based on an average family income and an average price for imported cigarettes, one smoker consuming one pack of cigarettes per day would use approximately 10.3 percent of family income. Cigarettes are available from vending machines in Uruguay, but there is a national restriction prohibiting sales of tobacco to persons younger than 18 years (see section on legislation below) (Silva Sosa 1990).

Of the total retail price of a package of cigarettes, 60 percent is national excise taxes, 18 percent is returned to growers, 15 percent is spent on marketing, 5.5 percent is wages, and 1.5 percent is manufacturers' profits (AFITYC 1989).

Taxes

In 1988, taxes on tobacco products were N$20 billion ($US60 million) according to unverified tobacco industry sources, or approximately 5 percent of Uruguay's overall tax revenue (AFITYC 1989). Taxes on imported tobacco and cigarettes range from approximately 10 to 20 percent *ad valorem*, depending on the type of product. As with many other countries of the Americas, taxes on tobacco products are the most readily collected of all taxes. However, cigarettes are also one of the most readily traded item on the black market. Although difficult to document, an extensive illegal trade in cigarettes manufactured in Uruguay's neighboring countries—Brazil, Argentina, and Paraguay—is reported (Silva Sosa 1990). Almost all cigarettes (80 to 90 percent) produced in Uruguay for export are returned to the country as contraband. These cigarettes are sold domestically at prices 30 to 40 percent lower than the legitimate prices because no national excise taxes are paid.

Tobacco Use

Per Capita Cigarette Consumption

Interestingly, AFITYC reported a decline in the per capita consumption of cigarettes from 1979 to 1985 (PAHO 1986), but calculations based on USDA data show an increase in the per capita cigarette consumption during 1979 to 1988 (Table 3). A decreasing trend in per capita consumption is also reported for the other countries of the Southern Cone subregion (Argentina, Brazil, Chile, and Paraguay). In these countries, the downward trend could be partially explained by the adverse economic conditions which also affected Uruguay in the 1980s. However, the illegal trade in cigarettes may be substantial, with cigarettes entering Uruguay from three other countries and also reentering as tax-free domestic products. The World Health Organization also reported that adult per capita cigarette consumption increased 14 percent from 1970 to 1985 in Uruguay (Chapman 1990). Thus, it is most likely that tobacco consumption has increased in Uruguay in the 1980s; deteriorating economic conditions have forced alternative supply sources for both foreign and domestically produced cigarettes.

Surveys on Tobacco Use: Limitations and Results

Several surveys on adult and adolescent tobacco use have been conducted in Uruguay (Table 4). Each of these surveys has methodological limitations that preclude generalizations to the entire country; most were conducted in the capital city, Montevideo. Several of these surveys addressed health professionals because of the likelihood that this group would be most responsive to a health-

Table 4. Surveys of tobacco use, Uruguay, 1970s and 1980s

Author	Year	Target group	Age group	N
Saralegui	1974	Ministry of Health employees	Adults	1,061
Unknown	1975	Adolescent schoolchildren	12–18	10,496
Gallup	1978	Montevideo residents	Adults	?
Kasdorf	1984	Montevideo residents	18 and older	396
Pérez-Moreira	1985	Ministry of Health employees	18 and older	525
Gallup	1988	Urban residents	16–50 and older	799
Ruocco	1989	Fourth-year medical students	22–26	479

Table 5. Prevalence (percent) of regular daily smokers and ex-smokers among Ministry of Health employees by sex, Uruguay, 1978

	Prevalence		
Sex	Regular smokers	Ex-smokers	N
Men	60	18	382
Women	32	5	679
Both	42.1	9.7	1,061

Source: Saralegui, 1981.

related survey and also because this group may be more prone to changes in tobacco use.

In 1974, Saralegui interviewed a nonrepresentative convenience sample of 1,061 Ministry of Public Health employees in Montevideo (Table 5). Overall, 42.1 percent were current smokers (daily and occasional combined). The prevalence of smoking was almost twice as high among men as among women (62 vs. 32 percent), but the prevalence of former smoking was also higher among men than among women (18.0 vs. 5.0 percent). Thus, almost 80 percent of male health ministry employees and approximately 37 percent of female health ministry employees had smoked at some time during their lives. It can be assumed that these levels were probably similar to those in the general population of educated persons in Montevideo prior to the widespread changes in tobacco use evident in developing countries during the 1970s and 1980s.

Results of a 1985 follow-up survey of 525 Ministry of Public Health employees (Pérez-Moreira 1985) can be compared to the 1974 Saralegui survey. The prevalence of smoking for this convenience sample of professional and nonprofessional health workers was 44.8 percent overall, with a substantial decrease in the prevalence of smoking among men (45.1 percent) and a substantial increase in the prevalence of smoking among women (44.6 per-

cent) (Table 6). Between 1975 and 1985, the prevalence of former smoking among men increased to 24.7 percent, and among women to 17.9 percent. By 1985, 80 percent of men and 72 percent of women had smoked at some time in their lives. The prevalence of smoking among female health workers was nearly the same as that among males, but the increase in the prevalence of ever smoking among women since 1974 suggests that in one decade the initiation rate of smoking for women more than doubled. In 1985, there were no differences in the prevalence of smoking by job categories (university, administrative, and other) (PAHO 1986). Of male smokers, 21.9 percent smoked more than 20 cigarettes per day; of women, only 6.2 percent smoked more than 20 cigarettes per day. These differences in exposure may have implications for the relative incidence of smoking-related disease among men and women. However, it must be noted that the sampling frames for these two surveys differed and the surveys may not have been representative of all health ministry employees.

Table 6. Prevalence (percent) of regular daily smokers and ex-smokers among Ministry of Health employees, by sex and job type, Uruguay, 1985

	Prevalence		
Category	Regular smokers	Ex-smokers	N
Sex			
Men	45.1	24.5	162
Women	44.6	17.9	136
Job type			
University	46.3	20.0	80
Administrative	44.4	20.2	376
Other	44.9	18.8	69
Total	44.8	20.0	525

Source: Perez-Moreira, 1985.

Table 7. Prevalence (percent) of urban residents reporting current cigarette smoking, by number of cigarettes smoked per day, Uruguay, 1978

Category of response	%
Total current cigarette smoking	47
Percentage of current smokers who:	
Smoke infrequently	23.4
Smoke <5 cigarettes/day	10.6
Smoke 5–9 cigarettes/day	19.2
Smoke 10–19 cigarettes/day	36.5
Smoke ≥ 20 cigarettes/day	10.6
Smoke other tobacco type	1

Source: Gallup Organization, 1978.

In 1978, the Gallup Organization surveyed urban adults in the capital, but detailed methodologic information is not available for this survey. The prevalence of regular and occasional smoking among both men and women was 42.1 percent (Table 7). Of these, almost 90 percent smoked fewer than 20 cigarettes per day, and only one percent smoked pipes or cigars. In 1988, the Gallup Organization, on behalf of the American Cancer Society, surveyed 799 urban residents aged 18 to 50 years and older (Table 8). Overall, 32 percent of respon-

Table 8. Prevalence (percent) of current and ex-smokers by sex, age group, and social class, urban adults age 18–50+, Uruguay, 1988

Category	Current smokers	Ex-smokers	N
Total	32	16	799
Men	44	25	343
Women	23	9	456
Age group			
Men 16–21	50	0	24
22–34	55	12	94
35–49	60	19	80
50+	26	42	145
Women 16–21	18	3	28
22–34	36	9	111
35–49	30	17	109
50+	12	7	208
Social class			
Upper	22	19	127
Middle	32	15	469
Lower	36	18	203

Source: Gallup Organization, 1988.

dents were current smokers (44 percent among men and women, respectively). The peak prevalence for men (60 percent) was found in the age group 35 to 49 years old, and for women, among those aged 22 to 34 years (36 percent). The prevalence of smoking was inversely related to social class in this survey.

Kasdorf (1984) surveyed 396 Montevideo residents aged 18 years and older using a random household cluster sampling method. The overall prevalence of current smoking was 40 percent, slightly lower than that (44.8 percent) reported by Pérez-Moreira in 1985 for Ministry of Public Health employees (Table 9). Among men, the prevalence of current smoking was 49 percent, and among women, 31 percent. Among all respondents, prevalence was highest among persons in the upper socioeconomic stratum (50 percent) and middle socioeconomic stratum (52 percent) compared with persons in the lowest socioeconomic stratum (25 percent). Thus, the prevalence of current smoking in the general population of middle- or upper-class residents of Montevideo was somewhat higher than that among presumably middle- and upper-socioeconomic-status employees of the Ministry of Public Health.

The proportion of ex-smokers among men (35 percent) reported by Kasdorf was remarkably high. Among male smokers, 17 percent smoked more than one pack per day; among female smokers, only 7 percent smoked more than one pack of cigarettes per day.

Data from a 1989 survey of fourth-year medical students aged 22 to 26 years in Montevideo suggest that the prevalence of smoking among health professionals may be decreasing as it has in other developed countries. Of all respondents, only 36.3 percent had ever smoked, and of these, one-third had already quit smoking (Ruocco 1989).

In summary, although the surveys reported here are not representative, some conclusions may be made regarding smoking among certain groups in Uruguay. The overall trend in smoking prevalence among those who might be considered opinion leaders in health matters (i.e., Ministry of Public Health employees and medical students) appears to be downward. It is not clear whether the prevalence of smoking is higher among persons in upper than among those in lower socioeconomic classes in the general population, as has been seen in other countries of the Americas with substantial European cultural traditions. In addition, the per capita consumption data for Uruguay suggest that overall tobacco use is increasing. Given the proba-

Table 9. Prevalence (percent) of regular, occasional, and ex-smokers, by sex, age group, and socioeconomic status, Montevideo, 1984

Category	Regular smokers	Ex-smokers	Occasional smokers	Never smoked	N
Total	40	29	12	19	396
Men	49	35	9	7	186
Women	31	23	14	32	210
Age group					
18–29	35	18	20	27	99
30–49	52	23	9	16	147
50+	33	39	11	17	150
Socioeconomic status					
Highest	50	16	12	21	48
Middle	52	19	15	16	190
Lowest	25	40	19	15	158

Source: Kasdorf, 1984.

ble increase in illegal sales of tobacco associated with the increased economic disruption in the 1980s, it is likely that tobacco use has in fact increased substantially, especially among women, during the 1980s. Indeed, a PAHO report on 5,169 women aged 15 to 49 years who were surveyed six months prior to giving birth showed a 44–percent prevalence of current smoking. This level was the highest among the nine countries surveyed for that report (PAHO 1987).

Prevalence of Smoking among Adolescents

The single study available on smoking among adolescents was performed in 10 Montevideo secondary schools in 1975 (Silva Sosa 1990) (Table 10). Although the sample size for this survey was large (n=10,496), no information on the methodology used is available. The prevalence of smoking among students aged 12 to 18 years (37 percent among boys and 35 percent among girls) was approximately 10 percentage points lower than that reported for adult employees of the Ministry of Public Health in 1974 (Saralegui 1981; Table 5).

Using information on age of initiation of smoking from several of the above surveys, conclusions about smoking by Uruguayan youth may be drawn. Kasdorf (1984) reported that 21 percent of men and 30 percent of women began to smoke before age 15 and that most (63 percent) reported beginning to smoke between 16 and 18 years of age. Pérez-Moreira (1985) reported that 27.4 percent of male health ministry employees and 14.8 percent of female health ministry employees began smoking before age 15. Ruocco (1989) reported that 32 per-

Table 10. Prevalence of smoking (percent) among adolescents, age 12–18, 10 high schools, Montevideo, Uruguay, 1975

Category	%	N
Boys	37	4,206
Age 12	22	
12–16	33	
17–18	50	
Girls	35	6,290
Age 12	17	
12–16	32	
17–18	45	

Source: Silva Sosa, 1990.

cent of medical students of both sexes began smoking before age 15 and that the modal age of initiation for these students was 15 to 16 years. Thus, as in other industrialized countries, Uruguayans most often begin to smoke in their middle teenage years. It is apparent that rates for ever smoking rapidly increase to levels above 50 percent shortly after age 15. Young women exhibited a major increase in the initiation of smoking in the 1980s.

Attitudes and Opinions toward Smoking

Survey data on attitudes and opinions toward smoking are scant. Kasdorf (1984) reported that of all Montevideo residents surveyed, 35 to 49 percent tried to quit smoking, 24 to 32 percent wanted to quit, and 12 to 28 percent had no opinion regarding quitting. In addition, 73 to 87 percent agreed that smoking is harmful; only 8 to 16 percent were indifferent to the potential harmfulness of smoking. In 1978, urban residents were asked by the Gallup Organization if cigarette sales should be prohibited. Only 19 percent of the sample answered yes (Gallup 1978).

Smoking and Health

Excellent mortality data are available for Uruguay. Only 5.9 percent of deaths were classified as "signs, symptoms and ill-defined conditions" (ICD 780–796) in 1987 (PAHO 1990), and nearly 100 percent of deaths are medically certified. Given the extensive population exposure to tobacco in Uruguay, the disease impact of tobacco use on this heavily exposed population would be expected to be significant. The five leading causes of death in Uruguay are heart disease, malignant neoplasms, cerebrovascular disease, accidents, and influenza and pneumonia (PAHO 1990). Of these diseases, four can be associated with smoking.

To understand the relative impact of smoking on selected causes of death in Uruguay, it is helpful to compare age-adjusted mortality rates for cancer of the trachea and bronchus, cerebrovascular disease, and ischemic heart disease for countries of the Americas in which the epidemic of tobacco use may be considered mature and for which there are adequate national mortality data (i.e., United States, Cuba, and Canada) (Table 11). The overall age-adjusted lung cancer mortality rate for Uruguay (16.0/100,000) ranks third among all countries of the Americas (PAHO 1990), but for men, the rate (32.0/100,000) is identical to that of the United States and Canada, and somewhat higher than that for Cuba (23.5/100,000). For women, the lung cancer mortality rate (2.5/100,000) is still quite low compared with the United States, Canada, and Cuba. These data suggest that the exposure to smoking among men is mature, ranking among the most exposed countries, but that among women, exposure is still rather low.

Age-specific mortality rates for lung cancer among male Uruguayans show an increasing trend among all age groups; age-specific lung cancer mortality rates for women do not show these trends. Ischemic heart disease mortality rates increased among men for all age groups until 1980; thereafter, mortality rates decreased for men, but there was no apparent trend in ischemic heart disease mortality rates observed among women (Table 12). The control of other risk factors such as hypertension may have augmented the effects of declining per capita cigarette consumption among

Table 11. Age-adjusted mortality rates for cancer of the trachea, bronchus, and lung; ischemic heart disease; and cerebrovascular disease; Uruguay, Canada, the United States, and Cuba, most recent year available

Condition/country	Age-adjusted mortality		Rate/100,000
	Men	Women	Total
Cancer of the trachea, bronchus, and lung (ICD-9 162)			
Uruguay*	32.0	2.5	16.0
Canada**	32.6	11.9	21.1
United States*	32.0	12.9	21.2
Cuba**	23.5	8.7	16.2
Ischemic heart disease (ICD-9 410–414)			
Uruguay*	63.7	31.9	46.5
Canada**	90.3	43.3	64.8
United States*	91.2	47.8	67.2
Cuba**	93.5	68.4	81.3
Cerebrovascular disease (ICD-9 430–438)			
Uruguay*	43.2	41.4	32.8
Canada**	19.0	17.9	18.5
United States*	19.3	18.1	18.7
Cuba**	32.5	32.5	32.5

Source: PAHO, 1990.

  * 1987

  ** 1988

Table 12. Trends in age-specific mortality rates (per 100,000 persons) for selected smoking-related diseases, Uruguay, 1955–1984

Cancer of trachea, bronchus, and lung

Year	Men, by age group				Women, by age group			
	35–44	45–54	55–64	65–74	35–44	45–54	55–64	65–74
1955–59	8.9	52.2	140.6	219.5	1.2	5.1	8.8	25.6
1960–64	12.2	59.9	148.5	259.2	1.6	3.4	10.9	29.3
1965–69	12.5	57.7	156.9	313.6	1.0	4.5	9.4	25.0
1970–74	11.7	63.7	157.9	309.5	1.0	4.8	12.7	22.1
1975–79	15.7	71.7	173.2	331.3	1.1	5.7	13.2	26.4
1980–84	18.5	84.8	194.2	330.0	2.3	5.1	11.6	25.0

Ischemic heart disease

Year	Men, by age group				Women, by age group			
	35–44	45–54	55–64	65–74	35–44	45–54	55–64	65–74
1955–59	26.9	122.5	371.3	813.5	36.5	146.8	453.3	
1960–64	34.3	142.6	443.0	969.3	12.2	42.1	167.0	537.7
1965–69	31.9	135.8	444.9	1,156.1	8.3	39.6	166.5	600.0
1970–74	38.2	151.4	442.8	1,133.6	7.0	37.3	173.0	625.8
1975–79	38.6	152.2	442.3	1,037.3	8.6	32.6	133.8	482.6
1980–84	26.0	121.4	353.0	793.3	5.7	28.1	103.4	378.1

Bronchitis, chronic and unspecified, emphysema, and asthma

Year	Men, by age group				Women, by age group			
	35–44	45–54	55–64	65–74	35–44	45–54	55–64	65–74
1955–59	2.4	11.6	41.8	107.3	1.2	3.7	8.8	27.1
1960–64	2.2	14.1	52.2	124.2	1.1	4.8	10.0	20.9
1965–69	4.2	12.7	53.4	157.5	2.6	5.1	15.4	35.5
1970–74	5.6	16.8	60.8	161.4	4.0	6.0	17.5	39.3
1975–79	3.9	15.9	61.6	174.7	3.8	4.6	14.0	34.8
1980–84	3.5	11.6	41.4	114.4	3.4	7.9	15.1	31.5

Uruguayan men in recent years. Chronic lung disease mortality rates began decreasing for men and women aged 55 and older in 1980. These mortality trends indicate that smoking among women has not yet produced the burden of disease that is demonstrated by the lung cancer and chronic lung disease mortality rates for men.

The age-adjusted lung cancer mortality rate for men has increased substantially from 1953 to 1987, but the age-adjusted rate for women is relatively unchanged. Age-adjusted rates for mortality due to oropharyngeal cancer show similar patterns (Figures 1 and 2).

Smoking-attributable risk* calculations may be performed using Uruguayan mortality data, relative risk estimates for mortality due to selected smoking-related diseases (U.S. Department of Health and Human Services [USDHHS] 1989), and estimates of the prevalence of current smoking and former smoking by age group and sex from the 1988 Gallup survey mentioned above. Software designed by the U.S. Centers for Disease Control was used to facilitate these calculations (Shultz 1991). The prevalence in Uruguay of current and former smoking for men and women aged 35 to 64 and 65 and older and the number of deaths for selected smoking-related diseases by five–year age groups for persons 35 to 75 and above were used in the calculations. Mortality data were provided by the Statistics Division, Ministry of Public Health, for 1987. The relative risk estimates are those reported in the 1989 Report of the U.S. Surgeon General for the U.S. population (USDHHS 1989).

---

* Attributable risk = $p(rr-1)/p(rr-1)+1$, where p = prevalence of smoking, rr = relative risk of death due to smoking-related disease.

Figure 1. Age-adjusted lung cancer mortality rates (per 100,000 persons) by sex and period, Uruguay, 1953–1987

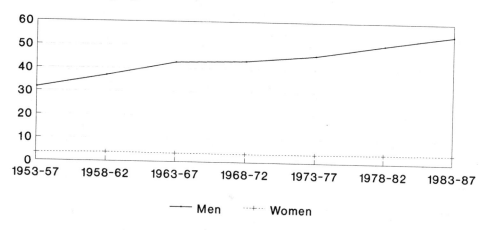

Source: Unpublished data De Stefani, 1991.

Figure 2. Age-adjusted oropharyngeal cancer mortality rates (per 100,000 persons) by sex and period, Uruguay, 1953–1987

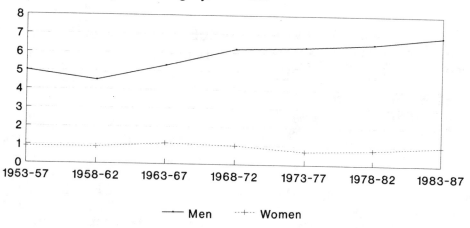

Source: DeStefani, 1991.

An estimated 5,077 Uruguayan deaths were attributable to smoking in 1987 (Table 13). Based on this estimate, 17 percent of all 29,882 deaths in Uruguay could be postponed or prevented if smoking were to be eliminated. These deaths accounted for 48,171 years of potential life lost before age 75 for Uruguayan smokers.

Several case-control studies reported by researchers in Uruguay have attempted to quantify the risks of tobacco use (particularly *tabaco negro*) for various cancers. De Stefani (1990a) reported that *tabaco negro* and alcohol interacted in a multiplicative way to increase the risk of esophageal cancer (odds ratio [OR] 22.6) among *mate* drinkers (*mate* is

Table 13. Smoking-attributable mortality and years of potential life lost (YPLL), Uruguay, 1987

Diagnosis	ICD-9 Code	Smoking-attributable mortality	Smoking-attributable YPLL*
Cancers			
Lip, oral cavity, and pharynx	140–149	101	1,167
Esophagus	150	254	1,779
Pancreas	257	77	611
Larynx	161	121	1,141
Lung	162	1,036	10,113
Cervix	180	18	352
Bladder	189	78	507
Kidney	188	44	532
Cardiovascular diseases			
Ischemic heart disease	410–414	912	8,509
Atherosclerosis	440–444	572	2,379
Other cardiovascular disease	390–394,401–405, 415–417,420–429	574	3,841
Respiratory diseases			
Chronic lung diseases	490–491,496	294	2,128
Pneumonias and other lung diseases	010–012,480–487,493	144	600
Perinatal diseases	760–766,768–779	105	7,829
Total		5,077	48,171

* Before age 75

a hot herbal drink favored by many Uruguayans). The risk for tongue cancer among smokers overall is 29.4 (95 percent confidence limits [CL] 3.7, 234.2) compared with nonsmokers. The tongue cancer risk for *tabaco negro* users compared with *tabaco rubio* users was 4.0 (Oreggia 1991). De Stefani also reported a significantly elevated OR for gastric cancer for male smokers compared with male nonsmokers (OR 2.7, 95 percent CL 1.3, 5.5) (De Stefani 1990b). In 1987, De Stefani reported that the OR for laryngeal cancer among *tabaco negro* smokers was 35.4 (95 percent CL 20.8, 60.3) compared with nonsmokers and 14.7 (95 percent CL 7.8, 27.6) for *tabaco rubio* smokers compared with nonsmokers (De Stefani 1987). Finally, De Stefani (1991) reported a significantly elevated risk for bladder cancer among male smokers compared with male nonsmokers (OR 11.9; 95 percent CL 3.3, 42.2).

The impact of smoking in Uruguay is substantial. Because the mortality rates for lung cancer and cardiovascular disease for men and women aged 35 and above have not stabilized or shown declines in recent decades, it is clear that the future disease impact of tobacco will increase in Uruguay. The excellent mortality data provided in Uruguay permit continued trend analyses and surveillance of tobacco-related diseases.

Tobacco Use Prevention and Control Activities

Government Action

Executive structure

The Ministry of Health of Uruguay issued a resolution on July 27, 1988, creating an Office on Smoking Control. As of 1990, the Director of this Office also chaired an interagency committee of government and nongovernment organizations. The Office did not have its own independent budget, but it utilized resources earmarked for epidemiology and also general health department funds. Six employees staffed the Office on Smoking Control. In 1990, the newly elected Government declared tobacco control one of the 12 priority areas for the Ministry of Public Health. This effort was included under the general area of "Toxic Habits," in conjunction with illicit drugs and alcohol.

Legislation

Numerous legislative actions exist to control tobacco use in Uruguay. Smoking has been prohibited in health facilities since 1977 (Orden de Ser-

Table 14. Tar and nicotine yields (mg per cigarette), five most popular brands of filtered cigarettes, Uruguay, 1988

Brand and type	Tar	Nicotine
Nevada	17.1	1.13
Casino 80 mm	16.1	1.45
Coronado 80 mm	15.6	1.00
Fiesta	13.3	1.27
Marlboro Box	15.7	1.01

Source: Silva Sosa, 1990.

vicio No. 3904, amended May 30, 1989). On August 12, 1981, Government Decree No. 407/981 banned smoking and advertising and promotion of tobacco products on interstate public transportation. Smoking is also banned by decree in government buildings. Local regulations prohibit smoking in theaters and at certain private worksites, especially those with combustible materials. Smoking is prohibited in all schools and in elevators (Silva Sosa 1990).

Nicotine and tar yields of cigarettes manufactured in Uruguay must be reported by the tobacco companies each year (Law No. 15.361, dated December 14, 1982, as amended by Law No. 15.656 of October 15, 1984). However, limits have not been set for the nicotine and tar yields in cigarettes. Tar and nicotine yields for the five most popular brands sold in Uruguay are comparable to yields for cigarettes sold in the United States and in other countries of the Americas (Table 14) (U.S. Federal Trade Commission 1988).

Law No. 15.656 and decree 263/983 dated July 22, 1983, provide regulations for package warnings about the harmful effects of smoking and on the sale of cigarettes to minors. The mandatory package warning also appears on advertising posters; it reads "Warning: Smoking is Harmful to Your Health. Ministry of Public Health." Cigarettes may not be sold at schools or to children under age 18 years. The extent to which these restrictions are enforced is unknown, and no recent data exist on adolescent tobacco use to determine the outcome of this restriction.

No other restrictions on tobacco product advertising are reported. However, the Commission on Hygiene and Assistance of the lower legislative chamber discussed an additional legislative project on tobacco control in 1991. This effort included prohibitions on smoking in health care facilities, in public offices, and in public transport vehicles. It also called for increased restrictions on tobacco product advertising.

Education

The Ministry of Public Health's Smoking Control Office has developed several public information and education activities, including a public television program entitled "To Live in Health," 5-second health warnings to be shown during tobacco commercials, antismoking posters, and a public information booklet entitled "Tobacco and Its Consequences" (Silva Sosa 1990).

Mandatory education to prevent tobacco use begins in the third year of primary school. In the fourth grade, specific behavioral skills training and information on the health consequences of smoking are presented. In the fifth grade, additional antitobacco education includes consideration of environmental tobacco smoke and its effects (Silva Sosa 1990).

Action by Nongovernmental Agencies

Campaigns and services

Nongovernmental organizations (NGO) have been very active against tobacco use in Uruguay; listed below are examples reported by Silva Sosa (1990). In particular, the activities of the Liga Uruguaya de Voluntarios de Educación para Prevención y Control del Cáncer (LUVEC), the International Organization of Consumers Unions (IOCU), and the Medical Association of Uruguay have been visible in antitobacco programs. Examples of specific NGO actions include the following:

- The newspaper *La República* has published several articles on smoking and health.
- The Medical Association of Uruguay publishes a newsletter ("Noticias") on behalf of the Ministry of Public Health's Smoking Control Program.
- Physicians of the Faculty of Medicine have established a Commission on the Control of Tobacco Use and a smoking cessation clinic at the University Hospital.
- LUVEC volunteers work with the Ministry of Health to disseminate information on the health consequences of tobacco use through public education activities; LUVEC also has an adolescent subgroup.
- The Seventh Day Adventist Church sponsors free smoking cessation clinics that are open to the public (the "Ma-Pa" Clinic), as well as public information campaigns on the health consequences of smoking.
- The Pablito Baez Foundation in Maldonado engages in health promotion activities that include tobacco control.

- Some private smoking cessation clinics in Uruguay are available to smokers.
- The Ecologist Party (political) works with the Ma-Pa clinic in lobbying for clean indoor air policies.
- The World Health Organization's World No-Tobacco Day activities are organized each year by the International Organization of Consumers Unions.

Summary and Conclusions

In summary, Uruguay has several Government and nongovernmental programs that promote antitobacco education and policies. Evaluations of these actions are hampered by the lack of data systems that track behavior changes.

Data on per capita consumption and limited survey data suggest that tobacco use has increased in the 1970s and 1980s; in fact, Uruguay may have one of the highest rates of tobacco use in the Americas. Tobacco prevention and control have increased in the late 1980s, but because the population's exposure to tobacco has been extensive, at least among men, the disease impact of tobacco use in Uruguay is significant and likely will increase in the near future.

Based on these data, the following conclusions can be drawn:

1. Tobacco agriculture and cigarette manufacturing were relatively stable during the 1980s. According to industry sources, imported tobacco, however, accounted for approximately 40 percent of total domestic consumption. Expenditures for these imports contribute to Uruguay's massive external debt. Illegal trade in cigarettes is extensive.
2. Behavioral data on tobacco use are scant, but data on per capita cigarette consumption suggest an upward trend in consumption during the last decade. Although Uruguay's health indicators are similar to those of developed countries in the Americas, the downward trend in per capita cigarette consumption demonstrated by those countries is not evident in Uruguay.
3. Smoking was responsible for an estimated 17 percent of all mortality in Uruguay for 1987. The age-adjusted mortality rate for lung cancer is among the highest in all of the Latin American countries; this rate has shown an upward trend for men but not women. The disease impact of smoking is likely to increase in the future.
4. Legislation to control tobacco use in Uruguay includes one of the few national laws to restrict sales to minors.

References

ASOCIACION DE FABRICANTES E IMPORTADORES DE TABACOS Y CIGARRILLOS. *La agroindustria del tabaco en el Uruguay*. Pamphlet. Montevideo, 1989.

CENTRO LATINOAMERICANO DE DEMOGRAFIA. *Boletín Demográfico* 23 (45). Santiago, Chile, January 1990.

CHAPMAN, S., WONG, L.W. *Tobacco Control in the Third World—A Resource Atlas*. Penang, Malaysia: International Organization of Consumers Unions, 1990.

DE STEFANI, E., CORREA, P., OREGGIA, F., et al. Risk factors for laryngeal cancer. *Cancer* 60(12):3087–3091, 1987.

DE STEFANI, E., CORREA, P., FIERRO, L., et al. Alcohol drinking and tobacco smoking in gastric cancer—a case control study. *Rev Epidem et Santé Publ* 38:297–307, 1990a.

DE STEFANI, E., MUNOZ, N., ESTEVE, J., et al. *Mate* drinking, alcohol, tobacco, diet, and esophageal cancer in Uruguay. *Cancer Research* 50:426–431, 1990b.

DE STEFANI, E., CORREA, P.L., FIERRO, L. et al. Black tobacco, *mate* and bladder cancer. *Cancer* 67(2):536–540, 1991.

ENCYCLOPEDIA BRITANNICA. *Yearbook 1989*. Chicago: Encyclopedia Britannica, 1989.

ERC INC. *The World Cigarette Market*. The 1988 International Survey. Suffolk: ERC Statistics International, Limited, 1988.

GALLUP. *The International Gallup Polls*. Princeton, New Jersey: The Gallup Organization, Inc., 1978.

GALLUP. *The Incidence of Smoking in Central and Latin America*. Princeton, New Jersey: The Gallup Organization, Inc., 1988.

KASDORF, H. *Estudio por muestreo del hábito de fumar en el área urbana de Montevideo—1984*. Montevideo: Typescript, 1984.

OREGGIA, F.L., DE STEFANI, E., CORREA, P.L., FIERRO, L. Risk factors for cancer of the tongue in Uruguay. *Cancer* 67(1):180–183, 1991.

PAN AMERICAN HEALTH ORGANIZATION. *Control del hábito de fumar. Taller Subregional para el Cono Sur Y Brasil*. Technical Paper No. 2. Washington, D.C.: Pan American Health Organization, 1986.

PAN AMERICAN HEALTH ORGANIZATION. *Health Conditions in the Americas, 1990 Edition*. Scientific Publication No. 524. Washington, D.C.: Pan American Health Organization, 1990.

PAN AMERICAN HEALTH ORGANIZATION. Tabaquismo y embarazo: hay que ayudar a parar. *Salud Perinatal—Boletín del Centro Latinoamericano de Perinatología y Desarrollo Humano* 2(7):67, 1987.

PEREZ-MOREIRA, L.P., GARRIDO, M. *Prevalencia del hábito de fumar entre funcionarios del Ministerio de Salud Pública—1985.* Typescript, Montevideo, 1985.

PHILIP MORRIS INC. *The Activities of Philip Morris in the Third World.* Richmond, Virginia: Philip Morris, Inc., April 1988.

RUOCCO, G., et al. *Encuesta de prevalencia, realizada por el Departamento de Medicina Preventiva y Social de la Facultad de Medicina.* Typescript, Montevideo, 1989.

SARALEGUI, P.J. *Control del tabaquismo en Uruguay.* Typescript, Montevideo: Ministry of Public Health, 1981.

SHULTZ, J.M., NOVOTNY, T.E., RICE, D.P. Quantifying the disease impact of cigarette smoking with SAMMEC II software. *Public Health Reports* 106:326–332, 1991.

SILVA SOSA, R. Country collaborator's report, Uruguay (unpublished data). Pan American Health Organization, 1990.

U.S. DEPARTMENT OF AGRICULTURE. Tobacco, Cotton, and Seeds Division, Foreign Agricultural Service, U.S. Department of Agriculture (unpublished tabulations). Washington, D.C., April 1990.

U.S. DEPARTMENT OF HEALTH AND HUMAN SERVICES. *Reducing the Health Consequences of Smoking: 25 Years of Progress.* A Report of the Surgeon General. U.S. Department of Health and Human Services, Public Health Service, Centers for Disease Control, Center for Chronic Disease Prevention and Health Promotion, Office on Smoking and Health. DHHS Publication No. (CDC) 89–8411, Rockville, Maryland, January 11, 1989.

U.S. FEDERAL TRADE COMMISSION. Federal Trade Commission Report. *"Tar," nicotine, and carbon monoxide of the smoke of 272 varieties of domestic cigarettes.* Washington, D.C.: U.S. Federal Trade Commission, December 1988.

WORLD BANK. *World Development Report 1989.* New York: Oxford University Press, 1989.

WORLD BANK. *World Development Report 1990—Poverty.* New York: Oxford University Press, 1990.

Venezuela

General Characteristics

Venezuela occupies more than 915,000 km² on the Caribbean coast of South America. By 1988, the Venezuelan population was in transition from one characterized by high birth and fertility rates to one with large numbers of adolescents and young adults. In conjunction with this demographic transition, health indicators reflect lower infant mortality, higher life expectancy, and a higher proportion of mortality due to chronic diseases (Table 1).

In the late 1920s, oil pushed ahead of agricultural products to become the leading export product, and Venezuela began rapid modernization. By the 1970s, Venezuela was the wealthiest country of Latin America. A democracy was established in 1958 after dictator Marcos Pérez Jiménez was overthrown, and subsequent political stability has permitted long-term development. With the nationalization of oil companies and the rapid increase in world crude oil prices, the Venezuelan Government gained enough resources to make substantial investments in areas such as health and education. In 1972 Venezuela was spending 10.3 percent of its total budget on defense, but by 1988, defense expenditures had dropped to only 5.8 percent of the total national budget. However, the fall of world oil prices (to 41 percent below inflation-adjusted prices in the peak years of 1979 and 1980) (Herrera 1990) and the regional recession in the early 1980s seriously affected the personal income and spending power of Venezuelans. From 1980 to 1988, Venezuela's per capita gross national product (GNP) declined 25 percent (World Bank 1990). Even so, in 1989 Venezuela still had the second highest per capita GNP among all Latin American countries.

The Tobacco Industry

Agriculture

In 1983, an international study commissioned by the tobacco industry (Agroeconomic Services Ltd. and Tabacosmos Ltd. 1987) reported that 6,890 ha of arable land were used for growing tobacco in Venezuela. In 1988, Venezuela's Ministry of Agriculture reported that 9,108 ha were devoted to tobacco. According to these two sources, the proportion of arable land planted with tobacco increased from 0.2 percent in 1983 (Office of Statistics and Informatics 1988) to 0.5 percent in 1988 (Reyna-Polanco 1989). Tobacco agriculture may generate as many as 25,000 jobs, according to tobacco industry sources, and represent approximately 3 percent of all agricultural workers in Venezuela (Reyna-Polanco 1989; Office of Statistics and Informatics 1990).

In 1983, *tabaco rubio* was grown by 303 farms, 56 percent of which were between 10 and 20 ha and 30 percent of which were larger than 30 ha. In addition, *tabaco negro* was grown by 275 farms, of which 72 percent were smaller than 1 ha (Agroeconomic Services Ltd. and Tabacosmos Ltd. 1987). These figures indicate that *tabaco rubio*, the variety used in most domestic cigarettes, is planted on large farms and that there are few farm owners. In 1989, leaf tobacco accounted for only 0.9 percent of Venezuela's total agricultural production (Reyna-Polanco 1989). The quantity of raw leaf produced remained relatively stable between 1979 and 1989 (Table 2).

The Venezuelan Government recently eliminated its tobacco export incentives, suspended a subsidy for fertilizers used for tobacco agriculture, and removed tobacco price supports (Hernández 1990). Catana de Philip Morris International, a domestic manufacturing company, provides technical assistance and inputs to growers (Philip Morris International Inc. 1988).

Also, Cigarrera Bigott provides grants and loans to farmers in exchange for the privilege of purchasing tobacco at prearranged prices (Fundación Bigott). This is a classic example of a monopsony, a market characterized by a very limited number of buyers who control a less than competi-

Table 1. Health and economic indicators, Venezuela, 1988

Indicator	Year	Value
Population	1988	18.8 million
% < age 15	1988	38.7
% ≥ 65 years	1988	3.6
% urban	1988	83
Life expectancy at birth	1988	70 years
Crude mortality rate per 1,000 persons	1988	5
Crude birth rate per 1,000 persons	1988	30
Infant mortality rate per 1,000 live births	1988	35
Gross domestic product ($US)	1988	$63,750 million
Per capita gross national product ($US)	1988	$3,250

Source: World Bank, 1990.

Table 2. Production, imports, exports, and total consumption (in millions) and per capita consumption of manufactured cigarettes, Venezuela, 1970 to 1989

Year	Production	Imports	Exports	Total consumption	Per capita consumption (≥ 15 years)
1970	11,213	8 (7)	0	11,221	1,947
1971	12,259	14 (12.7)	0	12,273	2,039
1972	13,700	10 (25)	0	13,710 (13,725)	2,184
1973	13,390	26 (28)	0	13,416	2,044
1974	16,219	25 (57)	0	16,244 (16,276)	2,369
1975	16,486	25 (228)	0	16,511 (16,714)	2,334
1976	18,755	25 (292)	0	18,780 (19,047)	2,549
1977	19,880	25 (96)	0	19,905 (19,976)	2,563
1978	21,073 (35,555)	48 (120)	0	21,121 (35,675)	4,388
1979	22,000 (42,179)	30	0 (50)	22,030 (42,159)	4,970
1980	21,300	30 (388)	0 (481)	21,330 (21,207)	2,396
1981	19,800	30 (91)	0 (1,188)	19,830 (18,703)	2,040
1982	19,487	30 (528)	1 (1,211)	19,516 (18,804)	1,980
1983	20,156	25 (18)	1 (1,013)	20,180 (19,161)	1,949
1984	20,643	0 (11)	850 (1,437)	19,793 (19,217)	1,893
1985	19,760	0 (19)	1,342 (1,408)	18,418 (18,371)	1,753
1986	18,377	0 (24)	1,050 (1,554)	17,327 (16,847)	1,558
1987	18,130	0 (23)	1,688 (1,903)	16,442	1,475
1988	18,824	0 (21)	1,700	17,124	1,489
1989	18,400	0	2,000	16,400	1,382

Sources: USDA, 1990; Numbers in parentheses, Ministerio de Agricultura y Cría de Venezuela, Herrera 1990; CELADE, 1990.

tive market. Since 1986, Bigott also operated an agricultural extension program in tobacco-growing regions. As the name indicates, it is not a crop substitution program, but rather a program to provide assistance in the cultivation of corn, sorghum, sesame, rice, and sunflowers (Fundación Bigott).

Manufacturing

In 1988, 37 companies were active in the tobacco-manufacturing industry, including 3 large-scale, 4 medium-scale, and 30 small-scale companies (Office of Statistics and Informatics 1988). By 1990, only two large tobacco manufacturing companies survived; these companies are the only ones that produce cigarettes: Compañía Anónima Tabacalera Nacional (Catana), a privately owned domestic company operating under license to Philip Morris International, and Cigarrera Bigott, a subsidiary of British-American Tobacco. Linked to two well-known multinational companies, these two companies form an oligopoly. Smaller companies produce insignificant amounts of tobacco, usually hand-rolled cigarettes or cigars (Office of Statistics and Informatics 1990).

Cigarrera Bigott holds 76 percent of the market share. The tobacco industry accounted for 3.7 percent of the country's manufactured product in 1988; of this amount, 99.6 percent was generated by the large- and medium-scale companies. In 1988, this sector employed 3,378 persons, which represented only 0.7 percent of all industrial employees (Reyna-Polanco 1989).

Production and Trade

Two sources of published data are used in the following calculations: data reported by the U.S. Department of Agriculture (USDA 1990) and the Venezuelan Ministry of Agriculture (Herrera 1990) (Table 2). For exports and imports, data are available to 1988.

Cigarette production increased steadily between 1970 and 1979, leveled off between 1980 and 1986, and since has begun to fall slightly (Table 2).

Cigarette imports declined substantially since 1983 and are now negligible; most are from the United States. Import duties are 35 percent ad valorem. Exports, on the other hand, recently have increased significantly. In 1989, 10 percent of production was exported, almost entirely in the form of filtered *tabaco rubio* cigarettes. Exports have become profitable since the currency was devalued by 150 percent in 1989, and the manufacturing industry has been using exports to maintain revenues in the face of declining domestic consumption (Tobacco International 1989b). The main port of destination for tobacco exports is Aruba in the Netherlands Antilles, which serves as a distribution center for a large illegal trade in cigarettes to other Caribbean areas, mainly Colombia (Tobacco International 1989b).

Advertising and Promotion

In 1981, the Government banned by decree direct and indirect tobacco product advertising on television; radio advertisements were banned later that year (Gaceta Oficial). Indirect advertising on television (i.e., the use of known cigarette brands in commercials for nontobacco products or contests) during the months of August, September, and October 1989, resulted in three television stations being penalized for violating the spirit of the legislation. All broadcasting from these stations was completely halted for a 24-hour period in November of 1989 (Herrera 1990). Television advertising apparently was an important marketing medium for the tobacco industry despite the ban. In the month in which indirect advertising airtime was highest, sales increased by 46 million units (33 percent) over the preceding month. The investment in television advertisements during that period was approximately $US10 million. The total amount invested in advertising by the cigarette industry during all of 1989 was estimated at $US21 million (Producto 1989).

Advertisements are commonly displayed on billboards, in movie theaters, and in the press with a content similar to that in other countries in the Americas: images of success, popularity, and youth are projected (Herrera 1990). Tobacco companies also use ''cultural workshops,'' which support Venezuela's traditional culture, to promote their public image (Fundación Bigott).

In 1989, the national economic crisis and its negative impact on consumption in general led to stiffer competition in the cigarette market. One promotional strategy used in that year was to release new brands at prices lower than brands already on the market. The prices of some well-known brands were reduced also (Fuentes 1990). Another promotional strategy used was to sell cigarettes in packs of 10, thus using an apparently lower price to en-

courage the use of cigarettes. This practice may also encourage sales of tobacco to children. Currently, there are no restrictions on the sale of cigarettes to minors, and cigarettes are sold singly by street vendors.

Tobacco Use

Per Capita Consumption

Annual adult (age 15 years or older) per capita cigarette consumption increased 16 percent between 1965 and 1973 (Lee and Wilson 1975) and 43.4 percent between 1973 and 1983 (Taylor 1989). However, using Venezuelan Ministry of Agriculture and USDA data on total consumption and population projections of the Latin American Center for Population Studies (CELADE), adult per capita consumption was estimated to increase 33.4 percent between 1970 and 1977 (Table 2). However, if the apparent sharp increase in consumption reported by the Ministry of Agriculture between 1978 and 1979 is reliable, then per capita consumption increased 155 percent during 1970 and 1979. After 1980, there was a sharp decline in per capita consumption. This decline in consumption may be explained in part by the economic crisis of the 1980s, which reduced individual purchasing power. Price increases by the industry were instituted in an effort to maintain profits while cigarettes were taxed at 50 percent of the retail price of a pack of cigarettes (Tobacco International 1989). The cost of a pack of 20 cigarettes was equivalent to 0.5 percent of a worker's average monthly wage in 1990 (Herrera 1990).

The most common form of tobacco used in Venezuela (99.3 percent) is *tabaco rubio* in filtered cigarettes. The production of *tabaco negro* cigarettes has declined since the 1960s.

In 1972, the last year for which data are available on this product, *tabaco negro* cigarettes represented only 1.4 percent of total cigarette production. No data are available on tar and nicotine levels for cigarettes produced in Venezuela.

It is difficult to determine the effect of the 1981 radio and television advertising bans and the vigorous Government antismoking programs in the 1980s on per capita cigarette consumption. The increased sales associated with indirect advertising on television have been noted. The public is generally opposed to tobacco product advertising, as described below. It is thus likely that several different conditions may have caused the decline in per capita cigarette consumption in the late 1980s in Venezuela.

Surveys: Strengths and Weaknesses

Data on the prevalence of smoking by socio-demographic characteristics have been obtained through three surveys of adults in Venezuela (Table 3). These include the 1971 Encuesta Sobre las Características del Hábito de Fumar en América Latina by Pan American Health Organization [PAHO] (Joly 1977), the 1984 Encuesta Sobre las Características del Hábito de Fumar en Venezuela by the Ministry of Health and Social Welfare (Ministry of Health and Social Welfare 1984), and the 1986 Investigaciones en las Comunidades para Programas de Prevención de Enfermedades Crónicas no Transmisibles (ECNT) (Adrianza 1986). None of these reports indicates the sampling method for the surveys; consequently, it is not possible to establish the validity of the reported estimates. In the 1971 PAHO survey (Joly 1977), most of the results are presented as standardized percentages, which allows comparisons among eight cities surveyed.

Each of the studies defined differently the category of "smoker," thus making comparisons between the surveys difficult. For example, in the 1984 Ministry of Health survey, the calculation of "smoking prevalence" included ex-smokers.

Prevalence of Smoking among Adults

In the 16 years between the 1971 PAHO survey and the 1986 Adrianza survey, both conducted in Caracas, the prevalence of cigarette smoking increased by 40 percent from 26.3 percent to 37 percent among women overall, while there was essentially no change in the prevalence among men. The 1971 PAHO survey does not provide data on occasional smokers. It is noteworthy in both the 1984 Ministry of Health survey and the 1986 Adrianza survey that approximately 12 percent of current smokers are occasional smokers; i.e., they do not smoke every day. This behavior was observed for both sexes, in all age groups, and within the various socioeconomic strata. In the United States, less than 10 percent of current smokers are occasional smokers (USDHHS 1989).

In 1989, a public opinion survey of a sample of 400 persons was carried out in Caracas (Ministry of Health and Social Welfare 1989). The survey detected a 36-percent prevalence of smoking (current daily or occasional smokers). If this is the true current smoking prevalence in Caracas, then there has been a 14-percent decline in smoking prevalence over 3 years since the 1986 Adrianza survey. There was a major decline in per capita cigarette consumption in response to the economic depression of the late 1980s, and therefore at least part of this reported decline in prevalence is real. In 1988, the Gallup survey reported that the prevalence of smoking among adults aged 18 to 64 years in urban areas was 27 percent overall (32 percent among men and 23 percent among women). Because the age groups for the Gallup survey differed from those of the other two surveys, and because no information is provided on the sampling frame for the Gallup survey, the validity of the reported prevalences is uncertain.

The prevalence of smoking overall in Venezuela was reported as 37.8 percent by the Ministry of Health in 1984, lower than the level of 42.2 percent reported by Adrianza in 1986 for Caracas.

Table 3. Surveys on smoking by adults and adult current smoking prevalence (percent) by sex, Venezuela, 1971 to 1986

| Survey | Year | Sample | Definition | Ages | Prevalence | | |
					Men	Women	Both
Joly	1971	Caracas N=1,644	≥ 100 cig/ lifetime Current smoker	15–74	48.6	26.3	36.9
Ministry of Health and Social Welfare	1984	Venezuela (cities > 2,000) N=1,175	Smokers	≥ 16			
			Daily		31.8	22.7	27.3
			Occasional		13.6	11.4	12.5
			Total		45.4	34.1	37.8
Adrianza	1986	Caracas N=1,274	Smoked in last 6 months	≥ 15	48.0	37.0	42.2
			Daily		32.6	26.3	29.9
			Occasional		15.6	9.6	12.6

These data suggest that the prevalence of smoking may be higher in urban populations than in rural populations in Venezuela.

The data from both the 1984 Ministry of Health and 1986 Adrianza surveys were stratified by socioeconomic status based on reported income, profession, level of education, and housing. The 1984 Ministry of Health study showed that the prevalence of current smoking was 42 percent among persons in the highest socioeconomic stratum and 33.5 percent among persons in the lowest stratum. Thus, the prevalence of current smoking is positively related to socioeconomic status. In the 1986 Adrianza survey, it was reported that the prevalence of current smoking status was inversely proportional to the respondents' levels of education. Persons with only primary school education had a smoking prevalence of 45.2 percent, which decreased with higher levels of education: from 41.2 percent among persons with secondary school education to 37 percent among those with post-secondary education. However, only 38.1 percent of illiterate persons were smokers. Caracas residents may not be representative of the rest of the country because of greater access to information about the health consequences of smoking.

According to the 1984 Ministry of Health survey, 42.1 percent of smokers consumed 10 or fewer cigarettes per day. Based on the reported frequencies, the average number of cigarettes consumed per day in 1984 in Venezuela was 12 (median=13, mode=5). In the 1986 Adrianza survey, the estimated average daily consumption by smokers in Caracas was 10; most (61.4 percent) smokers smoked fewer than 10 cigarettes per day. Although Venezuela overall (Ministry of Health 1984) was reported to have a lower prevalence of smoking than Caracas (Adrianza 1986), the reported average number of cigarettes smoked per day and the reported percentage of persons smoking 10 or fewer cigarettes per day on these surveys indicate a lower volume of daily consumption in Caracas. These data thus support the notion that Caraqueños may have tried to decrease their consumption of cigarettes, either for health reasons or for economic reasons.

Prevalence of Smoking among Adolescents

In 1980, the Venezuelan Anticancer Society surveyed 576 students aged 10 to 20 years in the cities of Caracas, Maracaibo, and Porlamar, finding that 21.1 percent of those surveyed had begun to smoke between the ages of 10 and 11 (Ministry of Health and Social Welfare 1984).

The 1984 Ministry of Health study included 225 adolescents aged 12 to 15 years. Of these, 6.7 percent had already smoked at least once in their lives, and there was no sex difference in experimentation rates. Of those who had ever smoked, 20 percent were regular smokers, 20 percent were occasional smokers, and 53.3 percent no longer smoked at the time of the survey. Of those in the lowest socioeconomic stratum, 4.1 percent smoked, while 7.4 percent of those from the highest socioeconomic stratum smoked.

Other Uses of Tobacco

The 1971 PAHO survey (Joly 1977) reported a very low prevalence (less than 2 percent) of pipe and cigar smoking in all eight cities surveyed in Latin America, including Caracas. According to the 1984 Ministry of Health study, 1.9 percent of current daily smokers smoked pipes and 4.7 percent smoked cigars. The prevalence of tobacco chewing at some point in the respondents' lives, a habit more common in rural areas of Venezuela, was 5 percent; of these persons, most (84 percent) chewed tobacco only occasionally. Most tobacco chewers were aged 50 years or older.

Another traditional custom in Venezuela is the ingestion of a mixture of tobacco and caustic soda called "chimó." The 1984 Ministry of Health survey found that 5.2 percent of the population had tried chimó and that 1.3 percent ate chimó on a daily basis. The percentages were similar for men and women.

The 1986 Adrianza survey found that 3.4 percent of the Caracas population had chewed tobacco at some point, with a higher prevalence of occasional chewers in the lower socioeconomic strata (3.4 percent in the lowest stratum compared to 0.5 percent in the higher strata). The lower-income groups in the urban areas probably had migrated recently from the countryside to the city and are the groups in which these traditional customs prevail. The study also found a prevalence of 5.6 percent for chimó use, mainly among persons in the lower socioeconomic stratum.

Attitudes, Knowledge, and Opinions about Smoking

Knowledge of the impact of smoking on health

In the 1984 Ministry of Health survey, smokers were asked if they agreed that smoking was harmful to their health: 86.8 percent strongly agreed, 6.7 percent agreed, 1.2 percent agreed somewhat, and 0.4 percent strongly disagreed. When questioned about the harmful effects of smoking on the smoker, 81.7 percent were very aware of these effects and 2.2 percent were unaware of any such effects.

The 1986 Adrianza survey in Caracas found that 75 percent of smokers and 81.4 percent of non-smokers were "very aware" of the harmful effects on other persons of smoking. Of the current smokers, 55.8 percent thought the harm to others was "considerable," 20.3 percent thought there was "some" harm, 16.4 percent "little" harm, and 3 percent thought there was no harm to others. Of nonsmokers, 70 percent replied that smokers caused "considerable" harm to those around them. These data compare favorably with data from the United States, where the issues surrounding environmental tobacco smoke and its control have been publicized widely for several years (Diario El Nacional 1989).

The 1984 Ministry of Health survey asked about adolescents' (aged 12 to 15 years) knowledge about the health impact of smoking. Of smokers, 73 percent believed that smoking is bad only if you smoke daily; 82 percent of those surveyed (including 67 percent of smokers and 83 percent of non-smokers) believed that smoking is harmful only if continued over a long period of time; and 87 percent of smokers and 86 percent of nonsmokers believed that smokers die younger than nonsmokers. Also, 87 percent of smokers and 81 percent of non-smokers believed that everyone who has lung cancer has smoked regularly. Similarly, 80 percent of smokers and 87 percent of nonsmokers believed that nicotine from cigarettes causes damage to blood vessels. Lastly, 95 percent of those surveyed believed that pregnant women smokers are placing their unborn children at risk.

Regarding the addictive nature of nicotine, young people believe that they have considerable control over their smoking. When smokers were asked if they would still be smoking when they turned 18, 33.4 percent answered "probably or definitely not." No smokers and only 14 percent of nonsmokers agreed with the statement that "once you start smoking, you will always depend on smoking."

In general, Venezuelans report high levels of knowledge about the health consequences of smoking. This understanding was greater in the 1986 Adrianza survey in Caracas, which may have sampled a better informed population. The fact that 53 percent of Caraqueños believed that some cigarettes aren't as harmful as others may reflect a distorted understanding based on the advertising of low-tar and low-nicotine brands of cigarettes. Adolescents in Venezuela, as in other parts of the world, may underestimate the potential for addiction to nicotine in cigarettes.

Attitudes on policies restricting smoking in public places

Of the nonsmokers surveyed in the 1989 opinion poll in Caracas, 88 percent responded that they agreed that smoking should not be allowed in either public or private offices. With regard to restricting smoking in public places, 83.3 percent of the respondents in the 1984 Ministry of Health study and 89 percent of the respondents in the 1986 Adrianza study agreed that smoking should be restricted in public places.

Opinions on other tobacco-related policies

In the 1984 national survey by the Ministry of Health, 72.1 percent of respondents, including 73 percent of smokers and 71 percent of nonsmokers, agreed that all forms of cigarette advertising should be banned. In the 1986 Adrianza survey, the percentage agreeing was somewhat higher (80.4 percent, including 81.8 percent of nonsmokers and 83.1 percent of smokers).

Respondents to both surveys were asked about the use of higher cigarette prices as a means of curbing smoking. Of the respondents in the 1984 Ministry of Health study, 60 percent agreed that price increases should be used to decrease smoking. Among respondents to the 1986 Adrianza survey, 70 percent agreed that increased prices might be effective in decreasing tobacco use.

Special mention should be made of the public reaction concerning the use of indirect advertising of tobacco products on television in 1989 mentioned above. Medical, church, and civic authorities, as well as journalists and members of the general population who were interviewed, were strongly opposed to indirect advertising of cigarettes on radio and television (Herrera 1990). The measures taken by the Government to punish the television stations were not disputed by either the industry or the general public. The 1989 Caracas opinion poll conducted by the Ministry of Health, which was taken during this debate, showed that 60 percent of the population agreed with the ban on radio and television advertising. However, when asked about the impact of this measure on smoking, only 13 percent thought that it would be "very effective" in reducing smoking and 24 percent said it would be "somewhat effective," while 49.8 percent thought it would be "totally ineffective."

The 1984 Ministry of Health survey found that equal percentages of adolescent smokers and non-smokers agreed that all tobacco product advertising should be banned.

Almost one-half (47 percent) of the young smokers agreed that smoking should not be allowed in public places. Forty percent of adolescent smokers and 48 percent of the nonsmokers did not agree with increasing cigarette prices to inhibit smoking among young people.

Smoking and Health

General Mortality

Underreporting of deaths in Venezuela is estimated at only 3 percent. However, the quality of data regarding cause-of-death is reported as unsatisfactory because records for 1984 to 1986 show 30 percent of deaths classified as "ill-defined symptoms" and "morbid states" (PAHO 1990). How-

ever, data reported to PAHO (1990) indicate that the proportion of "ill-defined" (ICD-780-799) deaths was only 13.5 percent in 1987.

The mortality rate declined between 1979 and 1987 for the most important cause-of-death groupings (infectious disease, cardiovascular disease, malignant tumors, injuries, and perinatal diseases) except malignant tumors (Table 4). Although differences in proportionate mortality are not significant, there appears to be a smaller proportion of infectious diseases in 1987 than in 1979, with an increase in the proportion due to cardiovascular mortality and cancer mortality. Even by 1979, the mortality structure for Venezuela was clearly more similar to that of an industrialized country than that of other countries of the Andean region.

In a 12-city study (10 cities in Latin America) of urban mortality among persons aged 15 and older carried out by PAHO in 1962 through 1964 (Puffer 1968), causes of death for Caracas were distributed as follows: cardiovascular diseases (22.9 percent), malignant tumors (22.6 percent), infectious diseases (7.9 percent), accidents (6.7 percent), homicides (6.6 percent), "ill-defined symptoms and morbid states" (1.2 percent), and others (32.1 percent). Even at that time, this mortality pattern

Table 4. Deaths, proportionate mortality (of defined causes), and mortality rates per 100,000 population (adjusted to the 1960 Latin American population) for grouped causes of death, Venezuela, 1979 and 1987

Cause and ICD code	1979			1987		
	Cases	%	Age-adjusted rate	Cases	%	Age-adjusted rate
Infectious diseases 001–139, 480–487	9,891	15.7	70.3	8,936	12.7	52.3
Malignant tumors 140–208	7,037	11.2	54.2	9,431	13.4	54
Cardiovascular disease 401–405, 410–438, 440–459	16,612	26.3	132.4	20,011	28.5	115
Conditions originating in the perinatal period 740–759, 767–779	7,875	12.5	50.7	7,509	10.7	45.6
Violence E810–E999	10,743	17	74.3	10,915	15.5	58.7
All other defined causes	10,912	17.3	80.9	13,484	19.2	76.8
Total defined causes	63,070	100	462.8	70,286	100	402.4
Symptoms and ill-defined conditions	10,615	14.4	—	10,705	13.2	—

Source: PAHO, 1990.

Table 5. Proportionate mortality for grouped causes of death, age ≥ 15 years, Caracas, 1962 to 1964, and Venezuela, 1987

	Caracas 1962–1964		Venezuela 1987	
	ICD code	%	ICD code	%
Circulatory diseases	330–334, 420–468	22.9	401–405, 410–438, 440–459	24
Malignant tumors	140–205	22.6	140–208	11.6
Infectious diseases	001–138, 480–502	7.9	001–139, 480–487	8.8
Accidents	E800–E962	6.7	E800–E949	11
Homicides and violence	E964, E965, E980–E999	6.6	E960–E969, E970–E978, E990–E999	2.2
Symptoms and ill-defined conditions	780–795	1.2	780–799	13.7
Others		32.1		28.7

Sources: Puffer and Griffith, 1968; PAHO, 1990.

reflected a Western lifestyle and its accompanying risk behaviors. The current mortality structure for the entire country in 1987 is now similar to that of Caracas in 1962 through 1964 (Table 5).

Lung Cancer Mortality

In the PAHO study on mortality in Caracas (Puffer 1968), lung cancer mortality rates were at an intermediate level compared with the other cities in the study. Higher lung cancer mortality rates were reported for Bristol (England), La Plata (Argentina), and San Francisco (United States). The other seven cities in Latin America (Cali, Lima, Riberão Preto, Bogotá, Guatemala City, Santiago, and Mexico City) had lower age-standardized lung cancer mortality rates. Although information on the prevalence of smoking in Caracas in the 1950s and 1960s is not available, these rates were probably already relatively high compared with the other countries of Latin America, although not as high as in England, Argentina, and the United States. This study found that the lung cancer mortality ratio for men to women was 4.2:1, suggesting a far greater

exposure to tobacco among men. The age-specific lung cancer mortality rate for men aged 45 to 54 was 23.3/100,000, considerably higher than for men aged 55 to 64 (16/100,000) and men aged 65 to 74 (15/100,000). This suggests that the high rates of lung cancer mortality in Caracas are a relatively recent phenomenon. Cigarette smoking had become more common, evidently, in the 1970s, well after peak exposures in the United States (USDHHS 1989).

Mortality from smoking-related diseases in the population aged 25 years and older for 5-year periods between 1950 and 1984 was reported to PAHO in 1986 (PAHO 1987). Lung cancer mortality rates increased until 1975 to 1979 and then leveled off. These data suggest that lung cancer mortality has shifted to younger age groups, similar to the data reported in the 1968 Puffer and Griffith study of urban mortality in 1962 to 1964.

Venezuela was socioeconomically more advanced than most other Latin American countries in the 1930s and 1940s. Thus, tobacco use, as reflected in later lung cancer mortality trends, might have increased substantially during those years, more so than in other countries of the region. Indeed, lung cancer mortality rates increased in the period from 1950 to 1970.

Other Causes of Death Associated with Smoking

Other causes of death associated with smoking (such as cancers of the larynx, pharynx, oral cavity, and esophagus) increased in the 1950s and 1960s. Mortality rates for these causes either remained constant or decreased in the 1970s, with the exception of cancer of the pancreas, cerebrovascular disease, and myocardial infarction.

Health Costs

In 1972, Venezuela spent 11.7 percent of the national budget on health; this proportion declined to 10 percent in 1987. About 57 percent of health spending is used for medical care. Estimates of smoking-associated hospital costs for 1965, 1970, 1975 and 1980 were reported to PAHO in 1986 (PAHO 1987) (Table 6). The length of hospitalization and the cost for smoking-associated diseases both increased between 1965 and 1980. In 1989, the Food and Agriculture Organization of the United Nations (FAO) reported that the Ministry of Health had estimated the costs of smoking-attributable diseases and lost productivity at $US69 million in 1978 and $US110 million in 1985 (FAO 1989).

Table 6. Smoking-attributable hospital discharges, and percentage of total discharges, Venezuela 1965 to 1980

| | 1965 | | 1970 | | | | 1975 | | 1980 | | | |
| | Both sexes | | Men | | Women | | Both sexes | | Men | | Women | |
	No.	%	No.	%	No.	%	No.	%	No.	%	No.	%
Cancer of the lung, trachea, bronchus			113	2.6	50	1.5	328	2.4	464	6.3	208	3.4
Laryngeal cancer	79	2.2	45	1.0	20	0.6	101	0.8	104	1.4	18	0.3
Oropharyngeal cancer	44	1.2	58	1.3	39	1.2	94	0.7	78	1.1	58	0.9
Stomach cancer	68	1.9	55	1.3	25	0.7	108	0.8	89	1.2	36	0.6
Myocardial infarction	1,402	38.5	1,058	24.6	592	17.6	2,895	21.6	695	9.4	311	5.0
Gastroduodenal ulcer	639	17.5	730	17.0	239	7.1	1,245	9.3	938	12.7	347	5.6
Bronchitis, emphysema, asthma	1,366	37.4	2.239	52.2	2,396	71.3	8,643	64.4	5,009	67.9	5,194	84.2
Total	3,645	100	4,298	100	3,361	100	13,414	100	7,377	100	6,172	100

Source: PAHO, 1987.

Tobacco Use Prevention and Control Activities

Government Structure and Policies

Since the early 1950s, medical associations in Venezuela, particularly of lung specialists, have been vocal on tobacco and health issues. The PAHO workshop on the control of smoking in the Andean area reported that ". . . an awareness of the harm caused by tobacco to Venezuelans today is the product of . . . the government support in the last 30 years of democratic development" (PAHO 1987). The Government of Venezuela has espoused, implicitly if not explicitly, a clear policy on smoking. This is evident through the various actions undertaken by the Government, in particular the suspension of television broadcasting when the private channels violated legislation on cigarette advertising. A National Anti-Smoking Program was established in 1984 under the Division of Chronic Diseases of the Ministry of Health and Social Welfare (Official Gazette 1984). It has three basic components: a medical committee, a national multi-institutional council, and a technical unit (Herrera 1990). In November 1985, a smoking-control plan was developed by Ministry of Health (Ministry of Health and Social Welfare 1985). With this plan, Venezuela became one of the leading Latin American nations in efforts to prevent and control chronic diseases caused by tobacco use.

Legislation

Chronologically, the first legislative act on smoking was a law concerning tax and tobacco manufacturing (Official Gazette 1978). This law mandated the printing of the warning **"Cigarette smoking has been determined to be harmful to your health"** on packs of cigarettes, whether domestically produced or imported. This law also stipulated that separate areas for smokers and nonsmokers would be established on public transportation and in establishments open to the public. These regulations became effective on August 27, 1979.

In 1979, the Law on Sports (Official Gazette 1979) banned cigarette advertising at sports facilities. This provision has not been enforced or observed strictly. In 1981, presidential decrees were issued banning direct and indirect advertising on radio and television.

In May 1990, the Government of the Federal District of Caracas issued Decree No. 7. This broad action mandated that all public places have smoking and nonsmoking sections, prohibited cigarette publicity in public places, banned the sale of cigarettes in hospitals and schools, and banned sales of cigarettes to minors. This decree provoked a debate in the print media that confirmed the need for legislative measures to protect the public health against tobacco use (Herrera 1990).

Education

A series of extracurricular activities that address tobacco use by youth ("Educational Communities") has been part of the Ministry of Education's official program since 1987 (Herrera 1990). These activities provide public information on smoking and health and organize parents, students, and teachers to develop formal prevention programs against tobacco for the schools.

Public Information Campaigns

National Smoke-Free Day is celebrated each year in November, and the World Health Organization's World No-Tobacco Day (May 31) has been celebrated since 1984. On these days, substantial media attention is devoted to tobacco and health issues. In addition, the National Anti-Tobacco Program has developed six different 10-minute Public Service Announcements that now rotate on television. During 1990, approximately 10 informational interviews were broadcast on radio channels by the National Anti-Tobacco Program (Herrera 1990).

Taxes

Taxes account for 50 percent of the retail price of cigarettes. From 1979 to 1988, cigarette tax revenues accounted for 2.47 percent on average of total yearly tax revenues, with the lowest percentage (0.96 percent) in 1978 and the highest percentage (4 percent) in 1983. Consumption taxes account for approximately 20 percent of the total State tax revenue in Venezuela. Cigarette taxes provided a yearly average of 16.2 percent of consumption tax revenue from 1979 to 1988, with the highest percentage (23 percent) again reported for 1983 (Herrera 1990). Thus, declining consumption of cigarettes associated with the economic recession of the 1980s may have been accentuated by a relatively high tax rate.

Nongovernmental Action

Venezuelan voluntary groups and medical associations are very active in smoking prevention and control. The Venezuelan Cancer Society has sponsored public information campaigns since 1954. Since 1952, the Venezuelan Tuberculosis and Pneumonology Society has made visible and effective efforts to disseminate information on the health risks of smoking. As it does elsewhere in the hemisphere, the Seventh Day Adventist Church sponsors 5-day smoking cessation programs. Between 1982 and 1986, it was estimated that 27 courses (attended by 2,584 persons) had been provided by this organization. The program has a 6-month abstinence rate of approximately 40 percent (Herrera 1990).

Both private businesses and Government enterprises have made efforts to increase the nonsmoking norm for workplaces. For example, since 1987 the Venezuelan Petroleum Company has pro-

vided support to smokers who want to quit, defended the rights of nonsmokers by ensuring a smokefree workplace, and provided antismoking education to employees' families. In December 1989, an evaluation of this program suggested that the number of smokers in the 900-strong work force had declined by 33 percent (Herrera 1990). In addition, the steel and iron industry, the second largest industry in Venezuela, actively supports worksite-related antismoking activities (Herrera 1990).

Summary and Conclusions

Based on the information presented in this report, the following conclusions can be drawn.

1. Due to the success of its oil industry in the 1960s and 1970s, Venezuela experienced rapid economic growth in the 1970s. As a result, urbanization, industrialization, and the availability of universal education followed. Venezuelans adopted lifestyles and behaviors associated with industrialized nations before most other countries in the Andean subregion; these behaviors include smoking.

2. The sociodemographic transition in Venezuela helps explain the high prevalence of smoking among men and increasing smoking prevalence among women between 1971 and 1986, at least in Caracas. These rates confirm widespread population exposure to tobacco, as do the high levels of adult per capita cigarette consumption reported by the Government and the U.S. Department of Agriculture since 1959.

3. As a result of high levels of exposure to tobacco, the mortality rates for lung cancer and cardiovascular disease have been remarkable for more than two decades in Venezuela. Venezuela has achieved a demographic transition toward the mortality patterns of industrialized nations as well.

4. Venezuela has also pioneered a coherent national antismoking policy, the National Anti-Tobacco Program. As a result of successful public information campaigns and legislative controls on tobacco product advertising, restrictions on smoking in public places, the involvement of several key industries, and general political support, Venezuelans are aware of and better informed on issues of tobacco and health. Unfortunately, social norms have not yet overcome high historical rates of smoking by men and women.

5. The purchasing power of Venezuelans has been

affected by an economic decline due to falling oil prices in the early 1980s and by the general recession in the region. At the same time, the effects of 10 years of antismoking efforts became apparent. Thus, a favorable declining trend in adult per capita cigarette consumption has been established.

6. Venezuela's tobacco industry is dominated by two large multinational corporations that provide some support for tobacco farmers. However, the net economic effect of this industry is in decline, and now accounts for a small proportion of the gross national product and employment.

References

ADRIANZA, M. *Non-Communicable Chronic Diseases.* Ediciones de la Presidencia de la República, Caracas, 1986.

AGROECONOMIC SERVICES AND TABACOSMOS, LTD. *The Employment Tax, Revenue and Wealth that the Tobacco Industry Creates.* September 1987.

BIGOTT. *Su aporte al desarrollo socio-económico de Venezuela.* Brochure. Editorial Altosca. No date.

CENTRO LATINOAMERICANO DEMOGRAFICO. *Boletín Demográfico,* Año XXIII, No. 45. Santiago, Chile, January 1990.

CHAPMAN, S., WONG, W.L. *Tobacco Control in the Third World—a Resource Atlas.* Penang, Malaysia: International Organization of Consumers Unions, 1990.

DIARIO EL 2001. November 7:9, 1989.

DIARIO EL NACIONAL. November 8, 1989.

DIARIO EL UNIVERSAL DE CARACAS. November 1:21, 1989.

DUQUE, G. *Report of the Coordinator of the Smoking Control Program of Lagoven, S.A.* Typescript, January 17, 1990.

FOOD AND AGRICULTURE ORGANIZATION OF THE UNITED NATIONS. Committee on commodity problems. *The Economic Significance of Tobacco.* Fifty-seventh session. Rome, 12–16 June 1989.

FUENTES, M. Mercadeo y ventas. *Cigarreras en la Canicera, el Humo vuelve a su cauce.* El Nacional 12(III):D8, 1990.

FUNDACION BIGOTT. *Programa de extensión agrícola.* Brochure. Editorial Altosca. Venezuela. No date.

FUNDACION BIGOTT. *Talleres de cultura popular.* Brochure. Editorial Altosca. Venezuela. No date.

GACETA OFICIAL. Decree 849 of January 1, 1981. *Official Gazette* 32116, 1981.

GACETA OFICIAL. Decree 996 of April 1, 1981. *Official Gazette* March 2, 1991.

GACETA OFICIAL. Law on Cigarette Taxes and Tobacco Manufacturing. *Official Gazette.* Special issue. Official Gazette No. 2497, 1978.

GACETA OFICIAL. Law on Sports. Official Gazette No. 2492, Special issue of August 17, 1979.

GACETA OFICIAL. Resolución No. 7, October 23, 1984. *Official Gazette* Year CXII. Month I No. 33098. Tuesday, November 6, 1984.

HERNANDEZ, V. *Agro y Cría: productores de tabaco protestan ataques contra esta industria.* El Universal. Caracas, 11-6-1990.

HERRERA, N. Country Collaborator's Report. Unpublished data. Washington, D.C.: Pan American Health Organization, 1990.

JOLY, J.D. *Encuesta sobre las características del hábito de fumar en América Latina.* Washington, D.C.: Pan American Health Organization. Scientific Publication No. 337, 1977.

LEE, P.N., WILSON, M.J. *Tobacco Consumption in Various Countries.* Research Paper 6, 4th Edition. London: Tobacco Research Council, 1975.

MINISTRY OF HEALTH AND SOCIAL WELFARE. *Basis for a Health Program to Control Smoking in Venezuela.* Caracas: Division of Chronic Diseases, November 1985.

MINISTRY OF HEALTH AND SOCIAL WELFARE. *Opinion poll: Cuñas relacionadas con el cigarrillo.* Unpublished report, Caracas, October 1989.

MINISTRY OF HEALTH AND SOCIAL WELFARE. Survey of Smoking in Venezuela. Unpublished data, 1984.

MINISTRY OF HEALTH AND SOCIAL WELFARE. *Yearbook of Epidemiology and Statistics.*

OFICINA DE ESTADISTICA E INFORMATICA. *Statistical Yearbook for Venezuela.* 1988.

OFICINA DE ESTADISTICAS E INFORMATICA. *Venezuela—Principales indicadores.* Caracas, August 13, 1990.

PAN AMERICAN HEALTH ORGANIZATION. *Control del hábito de fumar—Segundo Taller Subregional.* Area Andina. Washington, D.C.: Pan American Health Organization, Technical Paper No. 9. 1987.

PAN AMERICAN HEALTH ORGANIZATION. *Health Conditions in the Americas—1990 Edition.* Washington, D.C.: Pan American Health Organization. Scientific Publication No. 524, 1990.

PAN AMERICAN HEALTH ORGANIZATION. Unpublished tabulations using the mortality database, 1990.

PHILIP MORRIS INTERNATIONAL, INC. *The Activity of Philip Morris in the Third World.* Richmond, Virginia: Philip Morris International Inc., April 1988.

PRODUCTO. El encendido se hizo humo. *Publicidad/Mercadeo/Comunicación* 7(75):34, December 1989.

PUFFER, R., GRIFFITH, G.W. *Characteristics of Urban Mortality.* Washington, D.C.: Pan American Health Organization. Scientific Publication No. 151, May 1968.

REYNA-POLANCO, E. Director Sectorial de la Oficina de Planeación. Ministerio de Agricultura y Cría de Venezuela. Personal communication to Dr. Natasha de Herrera, 1990.

TAYLOR, S. Tobacco and economic growth in developing nations. *Business in the Contemporary World.* Winter:57, 1989.

TOBACCO INTERNATIONAL. Colombia: cigarette smuggling tolerated. *Tobacco International.* Latin American Issue-June 1, 1989:6, 1989a.

TOBACCO INTERNATIONAL. Venezuelan Bolivar cuts menace to tobacco unity. *Tobacco International.* Latin American Issue-June 1:6, 1989b.

U.S. DEPARTMENT OF AGRICULTURE. *Tariffs and Other Import Duties on Tobacco Leaf and Cigarettes, 1988.* Washington, D.C.: U.S. Department of Agriculture, FAS-5-1989.

U.S. DEPARTMENT OF AGRICULTURE. Tobacco, Cotton, and Seeds Division, Foreign Agricultural Service, unpublished tabulations, 1990.

WORLD BANK. *World Development Report 1990—Poverty.* New York: Oxford University Press, 1990.

Glossary of Terms

Adjustment.[1] A summarizing procedure for a statistical measure in which the effects of differences in composition of the populations being compared have been minimized by statistical methods. Examples are adjustment by regression analysis and by standardization. Adjustment often is performed on rates or relative risks, commonly because of differing age distributions in populations that are being compared. The mathematical procedure commonly used to adjust rates for age differences is direct or indirect standardization.

Age-adjusted rate. The number of diseases or deaths per population (usually 100,000 or 1,000 persons) with adjustments to a standard population's age distribution. This adjustment permits trend analyses and between-population comparisons of disease occurrence.

Age of initiation. The age at which an adult or adolescent began using tobacco fairly regularly.

Age-specific rate.[1] A rate for a specified age group. The numerator and denominator refer to the same age group. Example:

$$\text{Age-specific death} = \frac{\substack{\text{Number of deaths} \\ \text{among residents} \\ \text{age 25--34 in an area} \\ \text{in a year}}}{\substack{\text{Average (or mid-year)} \\ \text{population age 25--34 in} \\ \text{the area in that year}}} \times 100{,}000$$

The multiplier (usually 100,000 or 1,000,000) is chosen to produce a rate that can be expressed as a convenient number.

Age standardization.[1] A procedure for adjusting rates, e.g., death rates, designed to minimize the effects of differences in age composition when comparing rates for different populations.

Aging of population.[1] A demographic term meaning an increase over time in the proportion of older persons in the population. It does not necessarily imply an increase in life expectancy or that "people are living longer than they used to." The principal determinant of aging in the population has been a decline in the birth rate: when fewer children are born than in prior years, the result, in the absence of a rise in the death rate at higher ages, has been an increase in the proportion of older persons in the population. In developed societies, however, mortality change is becoming a factor: little further mortality reduction can occur in the first half of life, so reductions are beginning to occur in the third and fourth quarters of life, leading to a rise in the proportion of older persons from this cause.

Birth rate.[1] A summary rate based on the number of live births in a population over a given period, usually one year.

$$\text{Birth rate} = \frac{\substack{\text{Number of births to residents} \\ \text{in an area in a calendar year}}}{\substack{\text{Average or mid-year population} \\ \text{in the area in that year}}} \times 1{,}000$$

Cigarette consumption. The gross number of cigarettes consumed in a given country for a given year. *Total* domestic cigarette consumption is calculated as the total of the estimated metric tonnage of manufactured tobacco produced in the country plus the metric tonnage imported less the metric tonnage exported. The weight of consumed tobacco is converted to cigarettes based on an estimated one gram of tobacco per cigarette. *Per capita cigarette consumption* is the total number of cigarettes consumed domestically (production plus imports less exports) divided by the estimated population aged 15 years and older in a given country for a given year.

Country collaborator. An individual identified by the Pan American Health Organization to provide information and data on tobacco use, disease impact, and prevention and control measures in a given country or other political entity.

Current smoking prevalence. The proportion, expressed as a percentage, of a given population or population subgroup that represents current smokers. In the United States, a current smoker is an ever smoker who is smoking regularly, if even occasionally, at the time of the survey. The World Health Organization defines a current daily smoker as someone who smokes cigarettes every day. An **occasional** smoker is defined as a person who does

---

[1]Taken from: *A Dictionary of Epidemiology* edited by John M. Last, Oxford University Press, 1988.

not smoke every day. Other surveys include **light smokers** (who smoke a few cigarettes every day) as occasional smokers.

Death rate. See mortality rate.

Epidemiologic transition. A complex of changes that include fertility shifts and shifts in mortality and in the age structure of populations, with a rapid increase in the adult and aging populations. In addition, social and economic factors transform the prevalence of health risk factors in these populations. These include urbanization, entry of women into the work force, and exposure to a market-oriented economy. Lifestyle changes, including excessive alcohol use, smoking, and substance abuse, follow these behaviors and lead to increased burdens of chronic disease.

Ever (or lifetime) smoking prevalence. In the United States, ever smoking prevalence is the proportion of adults (usually aged 18 and older) who have smoked 100 or more cigarettes in their lifetimes. Others define "ever smoking" as having smoked even one cigarette in a lifetime.

Excise tax. Taxes levied on cigarettes at the point of wholesale distribution. Cigarettes sold on the black market would escape this tax.

Ex-smokers. Smokers who admit to smoking regularly at some time in their lifetimes but are not smoking at the time of the survey.

Former smoking prevalence. The proportion of a population or a population subgroup that represents former smokers. Former smokers are ever smokers who are not smoking at the time of the survey (i.e., have smoked at least 100 cigarettes at some time in their lives but have quit).

General fertility rate. The annual number of live births divided by the female mid-year population aged 15–49 years, multiplied by 1,000.

Gross domestic product (GDP). Domestic production regardless of its allocation to foreign or domestic payouts.

Gross national product (GNP). The main measure of economic activity in a country. It is the sum of the final output of goods and services produced by the domestic economy plus net receipts of labor and capital from abroad.

Infant mortality rate (IMR).[1] A measure of the yearly rate of deaths in children less than one year old. The denominator is the number of live births in the same year. Defined as:

$$\text{Infant morality rate} = \frac{\text{Number of deaths in a year of children less than 1 year of age}}{\text{Number of live births in the same year}} \times 1{,}000$$

This is often quoted as a useful indicator of the level of health in a community.

Life expectancy at birth.[1] Average number of years a newborn baby can be expected to live if current mortality trends continue. Corresponds to the total number of years a given birth cohort can be expected to live, divided by the number of children in the cohort. Life expectancy at birth is partly dependent on mortality in the first year of life and is lower in poor than in rich countries because of the higher infant and child mortality rates in the former.

Morbidity.[1] Any departure, subjective or objective, from a state of physiological or psychological well-being. In this sense, *sickness, illness,* and *morbid condition* are similarly defined and synonymous.

The WHO Expert Committee on Health Statistics noted in its Sixth report (1959) that morbidity could be measured in terms of three units: (1) persons who were ill; (2) the illnesses (periods or spells of illness) that these persons experienced; and (3) the duration (days, weeks, etc.) of these illnesses.

Morbidity Rate.[1] A term, preferably avoided, used indiscriminately to refer to incidence or prevalence rates of disease.

Mortality Rate (Death Rate).[1] An estimate of the proportion of a population that dies during a specified period. The numerator is the number of persons dying during the period; the denominator is the size of the population, usually estimated as the mid-year population. The death rate in a population is generally calculated by the formula

$$\frac{\text{Number of deaths during a specified period}}{\text{Number of persons at risk of dying during the period}} \times 10^{n}$$

This rate is an estimate of the person-time death rate, i.e., the death rate per 10^{n} person-years. If the rate is low, it is also a good estimate of the cumulative death rate. This rate is also called the crude death rate.

Nongovernmental organization (NGO). Organized groups that may collaborate with governments or may work independently of them on health issues.

Examples include cancer societies, antidrug use citizens' groups, and religious organizations.

Per capita gross national product. GNP divided by the total population in a given year.

Proportionate mortality rate, ratio (PMR).[1] Number of deaths from a given cause in a specific time period, per 100 or 1,000 total deaths in the same time period. PMR can give rise to misleading conclusions if used to compare the mortality experience of populations with different distributions of causes of death.

Register, Registry.[1] In epidemiology the term ''register'' is applied to the file of data concerning all cases of a particular disease or other health-relevant condition in a defined population such that the cases can be related to a population base. With this information incidence rates can be calculated. If the cases are regularly followed up, information on remission, exacerbation, prevalence, and survival can also be obtained. The *register* is the actual document, and the *registry* is the system of ongoing registration.

Smoking-attributable mortality. The total number of deaths that could be postponed or prevented in the absence of smoking in a given population for a given year.

Tabaco negro. Black tobacco, dark tobacco. This type of tobacco was most commonly used in Latin American countries prior to the dominance of tabaco rubio-containing cigarettes manufactured by transnational tobacco companies.

Tabaco rubio. Light tobacco, blond tobacco, Virginia-blend, American-blend tobacco. This variety of tobacco is favored for the manufacture of most mass-produced cigarettes.

Total fertility rate. The sum of specific single-year fertility rates for women 15–49 years of age (if five-year age groups are used, the sum of the rates is multiplied by five). This indicator estimates the approximate ''completed family size,'' that is, the total number of children a woman will bear in her lifetime, assuming no mortality.

Transnational corporations. Also known as multinational corporations. These are companies whose home office may be in a particular country but whose operations and assets are widely held in many countries.

Vertical integration. A characteristic of a particular industry which has influence on several levels of production and sales of a given product. For example, a company is vertically integrated if it directly supports tobacco agriculture, buys the product, manufactures cigarettes from raw tobacco, and controls the sales outlets. Highly vertically integrated companies may be thought of as monopolistic, especially if there are no or few competitors.

World No-Tobacco Day. An internationally coordinated event held on May 31 each year, to support a nonsmoking or nontobacco-using norm. It is sponsored by the World Health Organization as well as national or local advocacy and health groups.